Magnetic Nanoparticles

Magnetic Nanoparticles

Special Issue Editor
Evgeny Katz

MDPI • Basel • Beijing • Wuhan • Barcelona • Belgrade • Manchester • Tokyo • Cluj • Tianjin

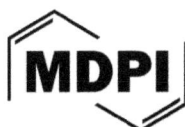

Special Issue Editor
Evgeny Katz
Department of Chemistry and
Biomolecular Science,
Clarkson University
USA

Editorial Office
MDPI
St. Alban-Anlage 66
4052 Basel, Switzerland

This is a reprint of articles from the Special Issue published online in the open access journal *Magnetochemistry* (ISSN 2312-7481) (available at: https://www.mdpi.com/journal/magnetochemistry/special_issues/magnetic_nanoparticles_reviewbook).

For citation purposes, cite each article independently as indicated on the article page online and as indicated below:

LastName, A.A.; LastName, B.B.; LastName, C.C. Article Title. *Journal Name* **Year**, *Article Number*, Page Range.

ISBN 978-3-03928-268-5 (Pbk)
ISBN 978-3-03928-269-2 (PDF)

Cover image courtesy of Wikimedia Foundation

© 2020 by the authors. Articles in this book are Open Access and distributed under the Creative Commons Attribution (CC BY) license, which allows users to download, copy and build upon published articles, as long as the author and publisher are properly credited, which ensures maximum dissemination and a wider impact of our publications.
The book as a whole is distributed by MDPI under the terms and conditions of the Creative Commons license CC BY-NC-ND.

Contents

About the Special Issue Editor vii

Evgeny Katz
Magnetic Nanoparticles
Reprinted from: *Magnetochemistry* 2020, 6, 6, doi:10.3390/magnetochemistry6010006 1

Evgeny Katz
Synthesis, Properties and Applications of Magnetic Nanoparticles and Nanowires—A Brief Introduction
Reprinted from: *Magnetochemistry* 2019, 5, 61, doi:10.3390/magnetochemistry5040061 7

Angelo J. Antone, Zaicheng Sun and Yuping Bao
Preparation and Application of Iron Oxide Nanoclusters
Reprinted from: *Magnetochemistry* 2019, 5, 45, doi:10.3390/magnetochemistry5030045 23

Vlad Socoliuc, Davide Peddis, Viktor I. Petrenko, Mikhail V. Avdeev, Daniela Susan-Resiga, Tamas Szabó, Rodica Turcu, Etelka Tombácz and Ladislau Vékás
Magnetic Nanoparticle Systems for Nanomedicine—A Materials Science Perspective
Reprinted from: *Magnetochemistry* 2020, 6, 2, doi:10.3390/magnetochemistry6010002 39

Kamyar Khoshnevisan, Elahe Poorakbar, Hadi Baharifar and Mohammad Barkhi
Recent Advances of Cellulase Immobilization onto Magnetic Nanoparticles: An Update Review
Reprinted from: *Magnetochemistry* 2019, 5, 36, doi:10.3390/magnetochemistry5020036 75

Maria Hepel
Magnetic Nanoparticles for Nanomedicine
Reprinted from: *Magnetochemistry* 2020, 6, 3, doi:10.3390/magnetochemistry6010003 97

Yolanda Piñeiro, Manuel González Gómez, Lisandra de Castro Alves, Angela Arnosa Prieto, Pelayo García Acevedo, Román Seco Gudiña, Julieta Puig, Carmen Teijeiro, Susana Yáñez Vilar and José Rivas
Hybrid Nanostructured Magnetite Nanoparticles: From Bio-Detection and Theragnostics to Regenerative Medicine
Reprinted from: *Magnetochemistry* 2020, 6, 4, doi:10.3390/magnetochemistry6010004 115

Marcos Luciano Bruschi and Lucas de Alcântara Sica de Toledo
Pharmaceutical Applications of Iron-Oxide Magnetic Nanoparticles
Reprinted from: *Magnetochemistry* 2019, 5, 50, doi:10.3390/magnetochemistry5030050 143

Muhammad Bilal, Shahid Mehmood, Tahir Rasheed and Hafiz M. N. Iqbal
Bio-Catalysis and Biomedical Perspectives of Magnetic Nanoparticles as Versatile Carriers
Reprinted from: *Magnetochemistry* 2019, 5, 42, doi:10.3390/magnetochemistry5030042 163

Ihab M. Obaidat, Venkatesha Narayanaswamy, Sulaiman Alaabed, Sangaraju Sambasivam and Chandu V. V. Muralee Gopi
Principles of Magnetic Hyperthermia: A Focus on Using Multifunctional Hybrid Magnetic Nanoparticles
Reprinted from: *Magnetochemistry* 2019, 5, 67, doi:10.3390/magnetochemistry5040067 183

Oana Hosu, Mihaela Tertis and Cecilia Cristea
Implication of Magnetic Nanoparticles in Cancer Detection, Screening and Treatment
Reprinted from: *Magnetochemistry* 2019, 5, 55, doi:10.3390/magnetochemistry5040055 223

Janja Stergar, Irena Ban and Uroš Maver
The Potential Biomedical Application of NiCu Magnetic Nanoparticles
Reprinted from: *Magnetochemistry* **2019**, 5, 66, doi:10.3390/magnetochemistry5040066 253

Yuko Tada and Phillip C. Yang
Iron Oxide Labeling and Tracking of Extracellular Vesicles
Reprinted from: *Magnetochemistry* **2019**, 5, 60, doi:10.3390/magnetochemistry5040060 279

Sadagopan Krishnan and K. Yugender Goud
Magnetic Particle Bioconjugates: A Versatile Sensor Approach
Reprinted from: *Magnetochemistry* **2019**, 5, 64, doi:10.3390/magnetochemistry5040064 291

Recep Üzek, Esma Sari and Arben Merkoçi
Optical-Based (Bio) Sensing Systems Using Magnetic Nanoparticles
Reprinted from: *Magnetochemistry* **2019**, 5, 59, doi:10.3390/magnetochemistry5040059 313

Reem Khan, Abdur Rehman, Akhtar Hayat and Silvana Andreescu
Magnetic Particles-Based Analytical Platforms for Food Safety Monitoring
Reprinted from: *Magnetochemistry* **2019**, 5, 63, doi:10.3390/magnetochemistry5040063 339

Greta Gaiani, Ciara K. O'Sullivan and Mònica Campàs
Magnetic Beads in Marine Toxin Detection: A Review
Reprinted from: *Magnetochemistry* **2019**, 5, 62, doi:10.3390/magnetochemistry5040062 359

Susana Campuzano, Maria Gamella, Verónica Serafín, María Pedrero, Paloma Yáñez-Sedeño and José Manuel Pingarrón
Magnetic Janus Particles for Static and Dynamic (Bio)Sensing
Reprinted from: *Magnetochemistry* **2019**, 5, 47, doi:10.3390/magnetochemistry5030047 371

About the Special Issue Editor

Evgeny Katz received his Ph.D. in Chemistry from Frumkin Institute of Electrochemistry (Moscow), Russian Academy of Sciences, in 1983. He was Senior Researcher at the Institute of Photosynthesis (Pushchino), Russian Academy of Sciences, during 1983–1991. In 1992–1993 he performed research at München Technische Universität (Germany) as a Humboldt fellow. Later, in 1993–2006, Dr. Katz was Research Associate Professor at the Hebrew University of Jerusalem. He has been serving as Milton Kerker Chaired Professor at the Department of Chemistry and Biomolecular Science, Clarkson University, NY (USA), since his appointment in 2006. He has (co)authored over 470 papers in peer-reviewed journals/books amassing over 35,000 citations (h-index: 88) and holds more than 20 international patents. He has edited five books on different topics, including bioelectronics, molecular and biomolecular computing, implantable bioelectronics, and forensic science. Two books on switchable electrochemical systems and enzyme-based computing, exclusively written by Katz, were published recently. He has also served as Editor-in-Chief for *IEEE Sensors Journal* (2009–2012) and is a member of the editorial boards of numerous other journals. His scientific interests are in the broad areas of bioelectronics, biosensors, biofuel cells, and biomolecular information processing (biocomputing). In 2019, he received the international Katsumi Niki Prize for his contribution to bioelectrochemistry.

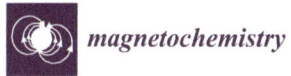

Editorial

Magnetic Nanoparticles

Evgeny Katz

Department of Chemistry and Biomolecular Science, Clarkson University, Potsdam, NY 13699-5810, USA; ekatz@clarkson.edu

Received: 13 January 2020; Accepted: 13 January 2020; Published: 15 January 2020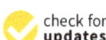

Magnetic nanoparticles are a class of nanoparticle that can be manipulated using magnetic fields. Such particles commonly consist of two components, namely a magnetic material, often iron, nickel, and cobalt, and a chemical component that has functionality, frequently with (bio)catalytic or biorecognition properties. Magnetic nanoparticles, magnetic nanorods, and other magnetic nanospecies have been prepared, and used in many important applications. Particularly, magnetic nanospecies functionalized with biomolecular and catalytic entities have been synthesized and extensively used for many biocatalytic, bioanalytical, and biomedical applications. Different biosensors, including immunosensors and DNA sensors, have been developed using functionalized magnetic nanoparticles for their operation in vitro and in vivo. Their use for magnetic targeting (drugs, genes, radiopharmaceuticals), magnetic resonance imaging, diagnostics, immunoassays, RNA and DNA purification, gene cloning, cell separation, and purification has been developed. Moreover, magnetic nano-objects of complex topology, such as magnetic nanorods and nanotubes, have been produced to serve as parts of various nanodevices, for example, tunable fluidic channels for tiny magnetic particles, data storage devices in nanocircuits, and scanning tips for magnetic force microscopes.

The increasing number of scientific publications focusing on magnetic materials indicates growing interest in the broader scientific community (Figure 1). This Book covers all research areas related to magnetic nanoparticles, magnetic nanorods, and other magnetic nanospecies, as well as their preparation, characterization, and various applications, specifically emphasizing biomedical applications. The chapters written by the leading experts cover different subareas of the science and technology related to various magnetic nanospecies—touching upon the multifaceted area and its applications. The different topics addressed in this Special Issue will be of high interest to the interdisciplinary community active in the fields of nanoscience and nanotechnology. It is hoped that the collection of the different chapters will be important and beneficial for researchers and students working in various areas related to bionanotechnology, materials science, biosensor applications, medicine, and so on. Furthermore, the issue is aimed at attracting young scientists and introducing them to the field, while providing newcomers with an enormous collection of literature references.

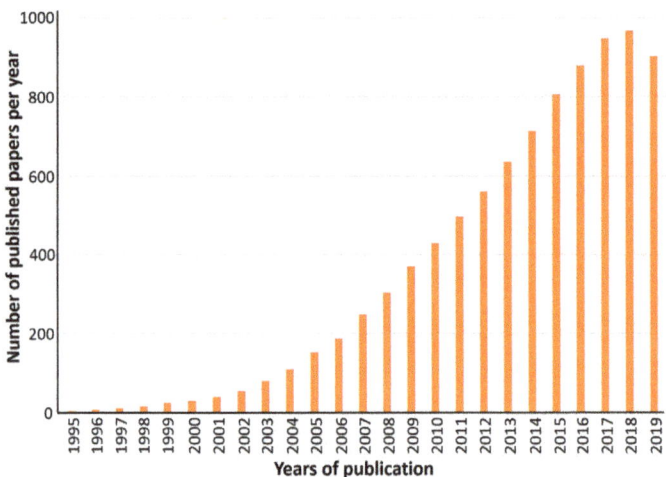

Figure 1. The number of published papers mentioning "magnetic nanoparticles" derived from statistics provided by Web of Science. The search was performed for the key words "magnetic nanoparticles" in the topic. Note the dramatic increase of the publications related to magnetic nanoparticles (the statistics for 2019 was not complete).

The chapters in this book cover the following specific subareas of the research field:

1. General Information—Preparation, Characterization, Modification, and Usage of Various Magnetic Nanoparticles and Nanorods

Advances in nanotechnology led to the development of nanoparticle systems with many advantages due to their unique physicochemical properties. The review article by Katz [1] serves as a brief introduction to the research area and overviews composition and synthetic preparations of various magnetic nanoparticles and nanorods (Figure 2). Another review by Antone et al. [2] focuses specifically on iron oxide nanoclusters and their preparation and use. A review by Socoliuc et al. [3] describes the design and synthesis of single- and multi-core iron oxide nanoparticles and provides an overview on the composition, structural features, surface, and magnetic characterization of the cores. Biomolecular functionalization of magnetic nanoparticles has allowed their numerous applications. Specifically, the modification of magnetic nanoparticles with cellulose enzyme is reviewed in the chapter by Khoshnevisan et al. [4].

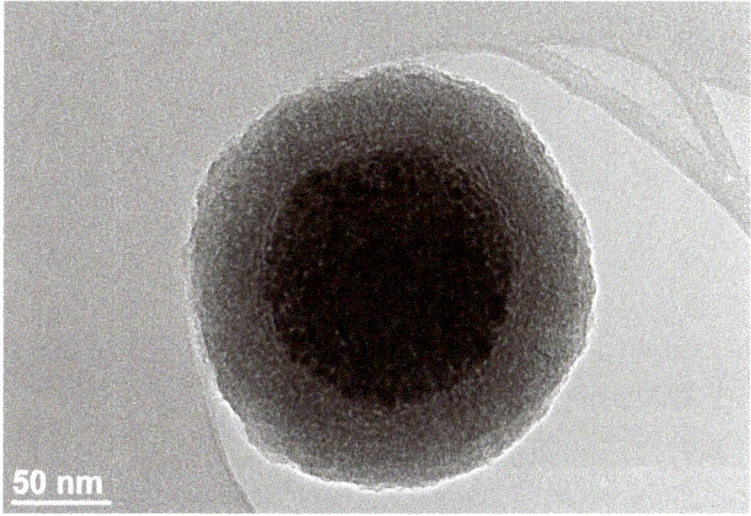

Figure 2. Maghemite silica nanoparticle cluster (scanning electron microscopy (SEM) image): iron oxide (γ-Fe_2O_3) magnetic core and SiO_2 shell—an example of core–shell magnetic nanoparticles. (Adopted from the Wikipedia public domain: https://commons.wikimedia.org/wiki/File:Maghemite_silica_nanoparticle_cluster.jpg).

2. Biomedical Applications of Magnetic Nanoparticles

The comprehensive review by Hepel [5] provides a very broad view on the use of magnetic nanoparticles for various applications in nanomedicine, (Figure 3). Another review by Piñeiro et al. [6] concentrates on the use of magnetic nanoparticles in medical biosensing, theranostics, and tissue engineering. The use of iron oxide magnetic nanoparticles in pharmaceutical areas has increased in the last few decades. The chapter by Luciano Bruschi et al. [7] reviews conceptual information about magnetic nanoparticles, methods of their synthesis, properties useful for pharmaceutical applications, advantages and disadvantages, strategies for nanoparticle assemblies, and use in the production of drug delivery, hyperthermia, theranostics, photodynamic therapy, and as antimicrobial substances. Biocatalysis and biomedical perspectives of magnetic nanoparticles as versatile carriers are highlighted in the review by Bilal et al. [8]. Another chapter article by Obaidat et al. [9] overviews the use of magnetic nanoparticles for hyperthermia, which is a non-invasive method that uses heat for cancer therapy where high temperature has a damaging effect on tumor cells. Magnetic hyperthermia uses magnetic nanoparticles exposed to alternating magnetic fields to generate heat in local regions (tissues or cells). While this therapeutic method is highly important for cancer treatment, the paper is mostly focused on the physical properties of the magnetic nanoparticles, and the intrinsic and extrinsic parameters required for the medical use of magnetic nanoparticles. The implication of magnetic nanoparticles in cancer detection, screening, and treatment is reviewed in the chapter by Hosu et al. [10]. This review summarizes studies about the implications of magnetic nanoparticles in cancer diagnosis, treatment, and drug delivery as well as prospects for future development and challenges of magnetic nanoparticles in the field of oncology. The chapter by Stergar et al. [11] is concentrated on potential biomedical applications of NiCu magnetic nanoparticles. While the most frequently used magnetic nanoparticles are composed of iron oxide (Fe_3O_4), NiCu magnetic nanoparticles, which are not common for biomedical applications, demonstrate some advantages due to their unique features. The chapter by Tada and Yang [12] is a review of iron oxide labeling and tracking of extracellular vesicles. Extracellular vesicles are essential tools for conveying biological information and modulating functions of recipient cells. Therefore, their visualization (imaging), particularly with magnetic nanoparticles, is highly important and the reviewed method is expected to be applicable and useful in clinical analysis.

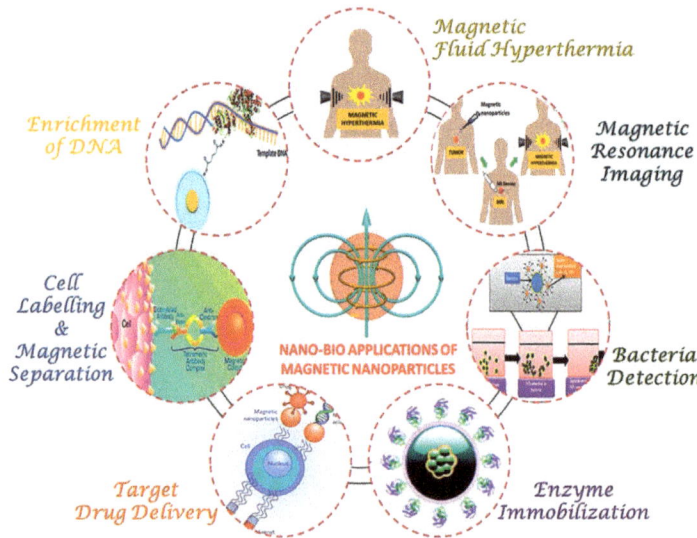

Figure 3. Different biomedical applications of magnetic nanoparticles—schematic presentation. (Adopted from *RSC Adv.* **2016**, *6*, 43989–44012 with permission.)

3. Biosensors Based on Magnetic Nanoparticles

Magnetic nanoparticles conjugated with various biomolecules offer a versatile approach to biosensors, particularly in biomedical applications (Figure 4), as discussed in the chapter by Krishnan and Yugender Goud [13]. Another comprehensive chapter by Üzek et al. [14] focuses on optical biosensing systems based on magnetic nanoparticles. The optical biosensors on the platform of biomolecular-functionalized magnetic nanoparticles are broadly categorized into four types—surface plasmon resonance (SPR), surface-enhanced Raman spectroscopy (SERS), fluorescence spectroscopy (FS), and near-infrared spectroscopy and imaging (NIRS)—that are commonly used in various bioanalytical applications. The use of biosensors based on magnetic nanoparticles specifically for food safety monitoring is highlighted in the chapter by Khan et al. [15]. Due to the expanding occurrence of marine toxins, and their potential impact on human health, there is an increased need for tools for their rapid and efficient detection. The use of magnetic nanoparticles in marine toxin detection is explained in the chapter by Gaiani et al. [16]. Magnetic Janus nanoparticles bring together the ability of Janus particles to perform two different functions at the same time in a single particle with magnetic properties enabling their remote manipulation, which allows headed movement and orientation. The chapter by Campuzano et al. [17] reviews the preparation procedures and applications in the (bio)sensing field of static and self-propelled magnetic Janus nanoparticles. The main progress in the fabrication procedures and the applicability of these nanoparticles are critically discussed, also giving some clues on challenges to be dealt with and future prospects.

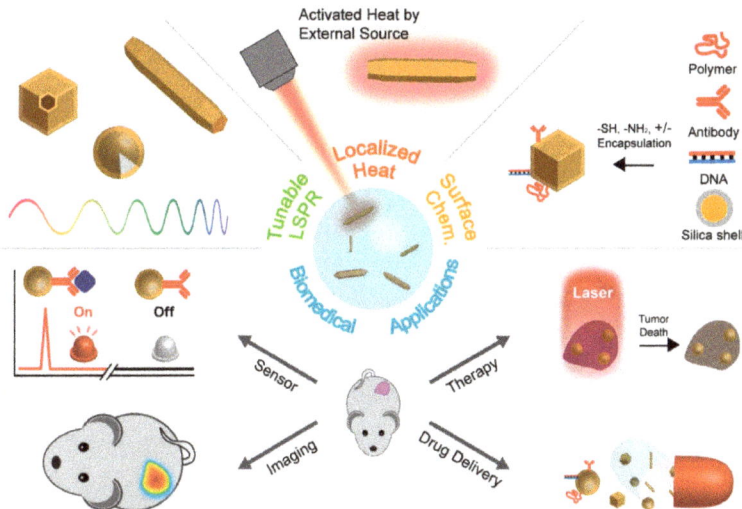

Figure 4. Biomedical applications of magnetic nanoparticles—schematic presentation [18]. (Adopted from *Adv.Sci.* **2019**, *6*, 1900471; open access article under the terms of the Creative Commons Attribution License, which permits use, distribution, and reproduction in any medium.)

References

1. Katz, E. Synthesis, Properties and Applications of Magnetic Nanoparticles and Nanowires—A Brief Introduction. *Magnetochemistry* **2019**, *5*, 61. [CrossRef]
2. Antone, A.J.; Sun, Z.; Bao, Y. Preparation and Application of Iron Oxide Nanoclusters. *Magnetochemistry* **2019**, *5*, 45. [CrossRef]
3. Socoliuc, V.; Peddis, D.; Petrenko, V.I.; Avdeev, M.V.; Susan-Resiga, D.; Turcu, R.; Tombácz, E.; Vékás, L. Magnetoresponsive Nanoparticle Systems in Biorelevant Media. *Magnetochemistry* **2019**, *6*, 2. [CrossRef]
4. Khoshnevisan, K.; Poorakbar, E.; Baharifar, H.; Barkhi, M. Recent Advances of Cellulase Immobilization onto Magnetic Nanoparticles: An Update Review. *Magnetochemistry* **2019**, *5*, 36. [CrossRef]
5. Hepel, M. Magnetic Nanoparticles in Nanomedicine. *Magnetochemistry* **2020**, *6*, 3. [CrossRef]
6. Piñeiro, Y.; González Gómez, M.; de Castro, L.; Arnosa Prieto, A.; García Acevedo, P.; Seco Gudiña, R.; Puig, J.; Teijeiro, C.; Yáñez-Vilar, S.; Rivas, J. Hybrid Nanostructured Magnetite Nanoparticles: From Bio-detection and Theragnostics to Regenerative Medicine. *Magnetochemistry* **2020**, *6*, 4. [CrossRef]
7. Bruschi, M.L.; de Toledo, L.D.A.S. Pharmaceutical Applications of Iron-Oxide Magnetic Nanoparticles. *Magnetochemistry* **2019**, *5*, 50. [CrossRef]
8. Bilal, M.; Mehmood, S.; Rasheed, T.; Iqbal, H.M.N. Bio-Catalysis and Biomedical Perspectives of Magnetic Nanoparticles as Versatile Carriers. *Magnetochemistry* **2019**, *5*, 42. [CrossRef]
9. Obaidat, I.M.; Narayanaswamy, V.; Alaabed, S.; Sambasivam, S.; Muralee Gopi, C.V.V. Principles of Magnetic Hyperthermia: A Focus on Using Multifunctional Hybrid Magnetic Nanoparticles. *Magnetochemistry* **2019**, *5*, 67. [CrossRef]
10. Hosu, O.; Tertis, M.; Cristea, C. Implication of Magnetic Nanoparticles in Cancer Detection, Screening and Treatment. *Magnetochemistry* **2019**, *5*, 55. [CrossRef]
11. Stergar, J.; Ban, I.; Maver, U. The Potential Biomedical Application of NiCu Magnetic Nanoparticles. *Magnetochemistry* **2019**, *5*, 66. [CrossRef]
12. Tada, Y.; Yang, P.C. Iron Oxide Labeling and Tracking of Extracellular Vesicles. *Magnetochemistry* **2019**, *5*, 60. [CrossRef]
13. Krishnan, S.; Goud, K.Y. Magnetic Particle Bioconjugates: A Versatile Sensor Approach. *Magnetochemistry* **2019**, *5*, 64. [CrossRef]

14. Üzek, R.; Sari, E.; Merkoçi, A. Optical-Based (Bio)Sensing Systems Using Magnetic Nanoparticles. *Magnetochemistry* **2019**, *5*, 59. [CrossRef]
15. Khan, R.; Rehman, A.; Hayat, A.; Andreescu, S. Magnetic Particles-Based Analytical Platforms for Food Safety Monitoring. *Magnetochemistry* **2019**, *5*, 63. [CrossRef]
16. Gaiani, G.; O'Sullivan, C.K.; Campàs, M. Magnetic Beads in Marine Toxin Detection: A Review. *Magnetochemistry* **2019**, *5*, 62. [CrossRef]
17. Campuzano, S.; Gamella, M.; Serafín, V.; Pedrero, M.; Yáñez-Sedeño, P.; Pingarrón, J.M. Magnetic Janus Particles for Static and Dynamic (Bio)Sensing. *Magnetochemistry* **2019**, *5*, 47. [CrossRef]
18. Kim, M.; Lee, J.-H.; Nam, J.-M. Plasmonic Photothermal Nanoparticles for Biomedical Applications. *Adv. Sci.* **2019**, *6*, 1900471. [CrossRef] [PubMed]

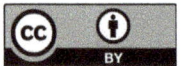

© 2020 by the author. Licensee MDPI, Basel, Switzerland. This article is an open access article distributed under the terms and conditions of the Creative Commons Attribution (CC BY) license (http://creativecommons.org/licenses/by/4.0/).

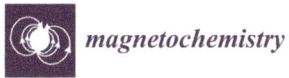

Review

Synthesis, Properties and Applications of Magnetic Nanoparticles and Nanowires—A Brief Introduction

Evgeny Katz

Department of Chemistry and Biomolecular Science, Clarkson University, Potsdam, NY 13699-5810, USA; ekatz@clarkson.edu

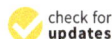

Received: 19 October 2019; Accepted: 7 November 2019; Published: 10 November 2019

Abstract: Magnetic nanoparticles and magnetic nano-species of complex topology (e.g., nanorods, nanowires, nanotubes, etc.) are overviewed briefly in the paper, mostly giving attention to the synthetic details and particle composition (e.g., core-shell structures made of different materials). Some aspects related to applications of magnetic nano-species are briefly discussed. While not being a comprehensive review, the paper offers a large collection of references, particularly useful for newcomers in the research area.

Keywords: magnetic nanoparticles; magnetic nanowires; magnetic nanotubes; core-shell composition; biosensors

1. Magnetic Nanoparticles—Motivations and Applications

Magnetic particles of different size (nano- and micro-) and various composition resulting in different magnetization (superparamagnetic and ferromagnetic) have found numerous applications in biotechnology [1] and medicine [2–5]. Particularly, they are used for magneto-controlled targeting (delivering drugs [6,7], genes [8], radiopharmaceuticals [9]), in magnetic resonance imaging [10], in various diagnostic applications [11], for biosensing [12] (e.g., immunoassays [13]), RNA and DNA purification [14], gene cloning, cell separation and purification [15]. Magnetic nano-species with complex topology (e.g., nanorods, nanowires and nanotubes) [16] have been used in numerous nano-technological devices, including tunable micro-fluidic channels with magnetic control [17], data storage units in nano-circuits [18], and magnetized nano-tips for magnetic force microscopes [19]. Magnetic nano- and micro-particles have been modified with various organic and bioorganic molecules (proteins [20], enzymes [21], antigens, antibodies [22], DNA [23], RNA [24], etc.) as well as with biological cells and cellular components. These species demonstrating magnetic properties and biocatalytic or biorecognition features are usually organized in "core-shell" structures, with the core part made of inorganic magnetic material and the shell composed of biomolecular/biological species chemically bound to the core with organic linkers [25,26]. The chemical (usually covalent) binding of organic linkers to the magnetic core units has been studied and characterized using different analytical methods (e.g., capillary electrophoresis with laser-induced fluorescence detection) [25]. Biomolecular-functionalized magnetic particles have found many applications in various biosensing procedures [27], mostly for immunosensing and DNA analysis, as well as in environmental and homeland security monitoring [28].

2. Core-Shell Structures

The present section is concentrated on the magnetic nanoparticles with a solid magnetic core coated with an organic or bioorganic shell (the shell structures composed of solid materials, e.g., metallic or silicon oxide are overviewed in the next sections). The easiest way of particle modification, particularly with organic polymers, can be based on physical adsorption [29]. However, covalent binding of (bio)organic molecules to the core parts is preferable since it provides more stable immobilization. The core parts of functionalized magnetic particles are frequently made of Fe_3O_4 or γ-Fe_2O_3 [30] having many hydroxyl groups at their surfaces, thus allowing silanization of particles followed by covalent binding of biomolecules to functional groups in the organosilane film [31]. While biomolecules bound to the particles are important for biocatalytic or biorecognition features, the core parts are responsible for magnetic properties. Magnetic nanoparticles with controlled size, specific shape and magnetization have been synthesized according to various methods [32–37] and then successfully used for various biotechnological [35] and biomedical applications [38]. For example, a synthetic procedure was developed for size-controlled preparation of magnetite (Fe_3O_4) nanoparticles in organic solvents [39]. One of the most important characteristics of biocompatible magnetic nanoparticles was their size dispersion characterized by atomic force microscopy and transmission electron microscopy (TEM) [40]. Particular attention was given to the synthesis of monodisperse and uniform nanoparticles [41]. Superparamagnetic iron oxide nanoparticles of controllable size (<20 nm) were prepared in the presence of reduced polysaccharides [42]. Nanoparticles synthesized by this method have an organic shell composed of polysaccharide, which increased the particle stability and offered functional groups for additional modification with various biomolecules and redox species. Biocompatible superparamagnetic Fe_3O_4 nanoparticles were extensively studied and their structural and magnetic features were optimized for their use as labeling units in biomedical applications [43]. Polymer-modified magnetic nanoparticles can be used for isolation and purification of various biomolecules. For example, poly(2-hydroxypropylene imine)-functionalized Fe_3O_4 magnetic nanoparticles were used for high-efficiency DNA isolation, higher than other studied materials at same conditions, and had excellent specificity in presence of some proteins and metal ions [44]. Magnetic nanoparticles modified with a hydrophobic organic shell (e.g., composed of oleic acid) have been tested for magneto-stimulated solvent extraction and demonstrated fast phase disengagement [45].

Highly crystalline iron oxide (Fe_3O_4) nanoparticles with a continuous size-spectrum of 6–13 nm were prepared from monodispersed Fe nanoparticles used as precursors by their oxidation under carefully controlled conditions [46]. Chemical stability of magnetic nanoparticles is an important issue. In order to increase it, the organic shell components can be cross-linked, for example, in iron oxide/polystyrene (core/shell) particles [47]. Cross-linking of polymeric chains in the organic shell resulted in additionally stabilization of the shell structure, also protecting the magnetic core from physical and chemical decomposition. Magnetic properties of nanoparticles can be tuned by varying chemical composition and thickness of the coating materials, as it was reported for the composite FePt-MFe_2O_4 (M = Fe, Co) core-shell nanoparticles [48]. While iron oxide-based magnetic nanoparticles are the most frequently used, some alternative magnetized materials have been suggested for various biomedical and bioanalytical applications [49]. For example, ferromagnetic FeCo nanoparticles demonstrated superior properties that make them promising candidates for magnetically assisted bioseparation methods and analysis, as well as for various electrochemical and bioelectrochemical applications. Magnetic and dielectric properties of magnetic nanoparticles functionalized with organic polymers (a core-shell structure) have been modelled and then the parameters obtained theoretically were compared with the experimental data showing good predictability of the nanoparticle properties using the theoretical model [50].

3. Magnetic Nanoparticles Coated with Noble Metal Shells

Formation of a thin shell-film of noble metals (e.g., Au or Ag) around magnetic cores (e.g., Fe_3O_4 or $CoFe_2O_4$) results in the enhanced chemical stability of the magnetic core [51–56] (Figure 1) also providing high electrical conductivity in particle assemblies, which is an important feature for electrochemical and electronic applications. The enhanced stability of magnetic nanoparticles coated with a Au shell allowed their operation under conditions when non-protected particles degrade rapidly.

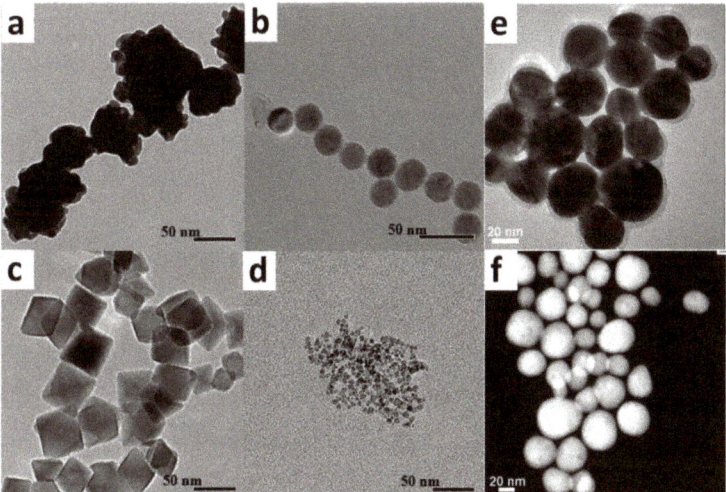

Figure 1. Various magnetic nanoparticles coated with gold shells: (**a–d**) TEM images of Fe_3O_4-core/Au-shell magnetic nanoparticles synthesized according to different experimental procedures: (**a**) [57], (**b**) [58], (**c**) [57,58], (**d**) [59]; see more details in [54]. (**e,f**) TEM and STEM (scanning transmission electron microscopy) images, respectively, of the γ-Fe_2O_3-core/Au-shell magnetic nanoparticles [60] (parts of this figure were adapted from [54] with permission).

For example, Au-coated iron nanoparticles with a specific magnetic moment of 145 emu g^{-1} and a coercivity of 1664 Oe were synthesized for biomedical applications [61]. Also, Au-coated nanoparticles with magnetic Co cores were synthesized for biomedical applications with the controlled size (5–25 nm; ±1 nm) and morphologies (spheres, discs with specific aspect ratio of 5 × 20 nm) tailored for specific applications [62]. Formation of a Au-shell around a magnetic core results in additional options for modification of nanoparticles with (bio)organic molecules. Indeed, Au surfaces are well known for self-assembling of thiolated molecules resulting in a monolayer formation. Au-coated magnetic nanoparticles of different sizes (50 nm, 70 nm and 100 nm) were prepared by the reduction of $AuCl_4^-$ ions with hydroxylamine in the presence of Fe_3O_4 nanoparticles used as seeds [63]. Then, the gold-shell surface was modified with antibodies (rabbit anti-HIVp24 IgG or goat anti-human IgG) through a simple self-assembling of thiolated molecules. The synthesized antibody-functionalized Au-coated magnetic nanoparticles were used in an enzyme-linked immunosorbent assay (ELISA) providing easy separation and purification steps. Importantly for electrochemical and electronic applications, Au-shell-magnetic nanoparticles can be cross-linked with dithiol molecular linkers to yield thin-films with conducting properties [64].

4. Magnetic Nanoparticles Associated with Silicon Oxide Nanoparticles and Nanotubes

Magnetic nanoparticles can be encapsulated in porous silica particles, which were functionalized at their external surfaces with proteins and used for biocatalysis [65,66]. The opposite way of modification resulted in the particles with a magnetic core and a mesoporous silica shell where the pores were filled with biomolecules or drugs [67]. These species allowed magneto-controlled transportation of the molecules included in the porous material of the shells. This approach was successfully used for modifying iron oxide magnetic nanoparticles (γ-Fe_2O_3 20 nm or Fe_3O_4 6–7 nm) with a SiO_2 shell (thickness of 2–5 nm) using wet chemical synthesis [68,69] (Figure 2).

Different approach was used to load magnetic nanoparticles on one-dimensional nano-objects (nanotubes), thus allowing deposition of many particles with a large total magnetization on one nanotube. SiO_2 nanotubes were prepared in an alumina template and then their inner surfaces were modified with Fe_3O_4 magnetic nanoparticles [70]. The resulting magnetic nanotubes were applied for the magnetic-field-assisted bioseparation, biointeraction, and drug delivery, benefiting from a large magnetization originating from the presence of many magnetic nanoparticles and a large external SiO_2 nanotube surface area.

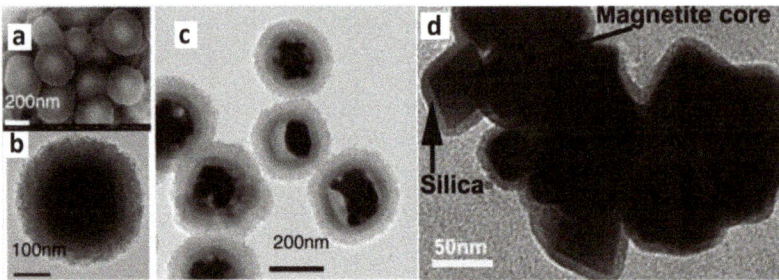

Figure 2. Various magnetic nanoparticles coated with silica shells: Backscattered electrons image (**a**) and TEM image (**b**) of Fe_3O_4-core/SiO_2-mesoporous-shell magnetic nanoparticles [67]. TEM image (**c**) of Fe_3O_4-core/SiO_2-mesoporous-shell magnetic nanoparticles [67]. TEM image (**d**) of Fe_3O_4-core/SiO_2-shell magnetic nanoparticles [71] (parts of this figure were adapted from [67,71] with permission).

5. Magnetic Nanoparticles with Fluorescent Features

Fe_3O_4 magnetic nanoparticles (5–15 nm) with unique optical properties were prepared with an inorganic fluorescent shell composed of ytterbium and erbium co-doped sodium yttrium fluoride ($NaYF_4$/Y/Er), which provided infrared-to-visible up-conversion with the high efficiency [72]. The two-component hybrid core-shell magnetic nanoparticles with fluorescent properties were furthercoated with a second shell made of SiO_2 allowing covalent immobilization of biomolecules (e.g., streptavidin). The produced multi-functional nanoparticles demonstrated efficient magnetization, fluorescence and bioaffinity features, thus allowing magneto-controlled separation of biomolecules, their fluorescent analysis and formation of affinity complexes with complementary biotinylated molecules. Many different approaches have been studied for combining magnetic properties and fluorescent features in one hybrid bi-functional nano-object. For example, magnetic Fe_3O_4 nanoparticles (8.5 nm) were modified with polyelectrolyte films using layer-by-layer deposition of differently charged polyelectrolytes, positively charged polyallylamine and the negatively charged polystyrene sulfonate [73]. The thickness of the polymer-shell around the magnetic core and the charge of the external layer were controlled by the number of deposited layers. The electrical charge of the external layer allowed electrostatic binding of secondary fluorescent nanoparticles. Negatively charged thioglycolic acid-capped CdTe nanoparticles were electrostatically bound to the positively charged polyallylamine exterior layer in the polyelectrolyte shell of the magnetic nanoparticles. The distance between the secondary satellite fluorescent CdTe nanoparticles and the magnetic Fe_3O_4 core was controlled by the number of the deposited polyelectrolyte layers. The developed method allowed further system sophistication by depositing additional layers of polyelectrolytes above the CdTe nanoparticles followed by deposition of another layer of the satellite CdTe nanoparticles. The distance between the primary and secondary fluorescent CdTe nanoparticles was controlled by the number of the polyelectrolyte layers between them, thus allowing tuning of the fluorescent properties of the multi-functional nano-system. Many other magnetic-fluorescent assemblies with different compositions have been reported for different applications. One more example is Co-CdSe core-shell magnetic-fluorescent assembly prepared by deposition of fluorescent CdSe layer on the pre-formed magnetic Co core. The deposition process was performed in a non-aqueous solution using dimethyl cadmium as an organic precursor [74]. Many different magnetic nano-species functionalized with fluorescent labels have been used as versatile labels for biomolecules, demonstrating advantages of both fluorescent reporting part and magnetic separating/transporting part of the assembly. It should be noted that careful optimization of the distance separating the magnetic core and fluorescent species (organic dyes or inorganic quantum dots) should be done to minimize quenching of the photo-excited species by the core part.

6. Magnetic Nanoparticles Combined with Metallic Nano-Species or Quantum Dots

Combining two different nanoparticles (e.g., magnetic and metal or semiconductor) in one nano-assembly where the particles are bound to each other results in unique multi-functional species. In these species two nanoparticles composed of different materials with different properties can be organized as Siamese twins (dumbbell-like bifunctional particles) [75–77]. There are different procedures for binding two nanoparticles in one composite assembly, some of the procedures are based on the controlled growth of the second particle next to the primary particle. For example, magnetic nanoparticles, Fe_3O_4 or FePt, (8 nm) with a protecting/stabilizing organic shell composed of a surfactant were dispersed in an organic solvent (e.g., dichlorobenzene) and added to an aqueous solution of Ag^+ salt [75]. The bi-phase aqueous/organic system was ultrasonicated to yield micelles with the magnetic nanoparticles self-assembled on the liquid/liquid interface. Then, Ag^+ ions penetrated through defects in the surfactant shell being then catalytically reduced by Fe^{2+} sites to yield the seeding of a Ag nanoparticle. Further reduction of Ag^+ ions on the Ag seed resulted in the grows of the seed and formation of a Ag nanoparticle at a side of the magnetic nanoparticle yielding a twin-particles shown in the transmission electron microscopy (TEM) image (Figure 3a). Another Ag nanoparticle was produced at a side of an FePt magnetic nanoparticle in a similar process (Figure 3b). The size of the produced Ag nanoparticle was controlled by the time allowed for the growing process.

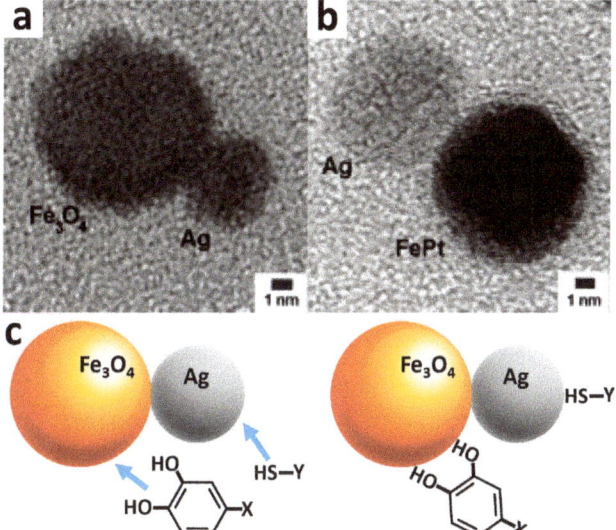

Figure 3. (a,b) TEM images of Fe_3O_4-Ag and FePt-Ag hetero-dimers composed of the magnetic nanoparticle and connected Ag nanoparticle [75]. (c) Directed functionalization of the Fe_3O_4 nanoparticle and Ag nanoparticle with different functional units, such as dopamine-derivatized and thiol-derivatized species, respectively. X and Y might be represented by different molecular and biomolecular species (part of this figure was adapted with permission from [75], American Chemical Society, 2005).

The two parts of the synthesized hetero-dimeric nanoparticles can be conveniently modified with different molecules using the difference of the surface properties of the two parts of the dimer. For example, the Ag nanoparticle in the dimeric hybrid was functionalized with self-assembled thiolated molecules, while the Fe_3O_4 magnetic nanoparticle was modified using dopamine units as anchor groups bound to $Fe^{2+/3+}$ sites of the iron oxide surface (Figure 3c). In a different synthetic approach hetero-dimeric species were produced from FePt two-metal alloy nanoparticles coated by an amorphous CdS shell. The metastable amorphous CdS layer had tendency of changing to a crystalized form upon temperature increase. When the multi-component core-shell nanoparticles were heated, FePt and CdS components were transformed into hetero-dimers due to incompatibility of the FePt and CdS lattices, thus resulting in their separation and formation of individual FePt and CdS nanoparticles (less than 10 nm size) connected to each other [76]. Importantly, the hetero-dimeric species demonstrated superparamagnetism characteristic of the FePt part and fluorescence produced by the CdS quantum dot, providing excellent means for labeling of biomaterials. In a different approach, separately synthesized superparamagnetic γ-Fe_2O_3 nanoparticles (ca. 11.8 nm) and fluorescent CdSe quantum dots (ca. 3.5 nm) were mixed and encapsulated together in a silicon oxide shell yielding a complex multifunctional assembly that demonstrated a unique combination of the magnetic property of γ-Fe_2O_3 and fluorescent features of CdSe [78]. The silicon oxide shell served as a matrix keeping together the functional nano-components, preserving their individual properties, and providing accessibility of the two-component hybrid system for additional chemical modification of both components with different molecules.

7. Modification of Magnetic Nanoparticles with Various Biomolecules

Various organic shells exhibiting different chemical functional groups (e.g., aminosiloxane, dextran or dimercaptosuccinic acid) were prepared around magnetic nanoparticles [71,79,80]. Organic functional groups available at the outer-layer of the organic shell have been used for numerous chemical coupling reactions resulting in covalent immobilization of different (bio)molecules [81,82] to allow various biochemical, bioanalytical and biomedical applications [83]. For example, covalent immobilization of a polyclonal IgG anti-horseradish peroxidase antibody bound to dextran-coated magnetic particles allowed the use of the functionalized particles for the capturing and separation of horseradish peroxidase enzyme from a crude protein extract from *Escherichia coli* [83]. In another example, magnetic core of Fe_3O_4 nanoparticles was silanized and then covalently modified with polyamidoamine (PAMAM) dendrimer [84]. The amino groups added to the nanoparticles upon their modification with PAMAM were used for covalent binding of streptavidin with the load 3.4-fold greater comparing to the direct binding of streptavidin to the silanized magnetite nanoparticles. The increased streptavidin load originated from the increase of the organic shell diameter and the increased number of the amino groups available for the covalent binding of streptavidin. While silanization of metal-oxide magnetic nanoparticles is the most frequently used technique for their primary modification [22], dopamine was also suggested as a robust anchor group to bind biomolecules to magnetic Fe_3O_4 particles [85]. Dopamine ligands bind to iron oxide magnetic nanoparticles through coordination of the dihydroxyphenyl units with Fe^{+2} surface sites of the particles providing amino groups for further covalent attachment of various biomolecules, usually through carbodiimide coupling reactions.

Immobilization of proteins (e.g., bovine serum albumin) [31,86,87] or enzymes (e.g., horseradish peroxidase (HRP) or lipase) [88–91] upon their binding to organic shells of magnetic nanoparticles has been extensively studied and reported for many applications. Immobilization of various enzymes on magnetic nanoparticles preserves the enzyme catalytic activity and, sometimes, results in the enzyme stabilization comparing with the soluble state. For example, alcohol dehydrogenase covalently immobilized on Fe_3O_4 magnetic particles demonstrated excellent biocatalytic activity [92,93]. In many experimentally studied systems magnetic nanoparticles functionalized with redox enzymes demonstrated bioelectrocatalytic activities upon direct contacting with electrode surfaces [91].

While covalent binding or any other permanent immobilization of enzymes on magnetic nanoparticles is beneficial for many applications (e.g., in magneto-controlled biosensors), reversible binding of enzymes might be important for other special applications. Reversible binding of positively charged proteins/enzymes to negatively charged polyacrylic-shell/Fe_3O_4-core magnetic nanoparticles has been reported as an example of electrostatically controlled reversible immobilization [94]. The protein molecules, positively charged at low pH values (pH < pI, isoelectric point), were electrostatically attracted and bound to the negatively charged organic shells, while at higher pH values (pH > pI) the negatively charged protein molecules were electrostatically repulsed and removed from the core-shell magnetic nanoparticles. The demonstrated reversible attraction/repulsion of the proteins controlled by pH values was applied for collecting, purification, and transportation of the proteins with the help of magnetic nanoparticles in the presence of an external magnetic field. Many other applications are feasible, for example, magnetic particles functionalized with carbohydrate oligomers yielding multivalent binding of the magnetic labels to proteins or cells *via* specific carbohydrate-protein interactions have been used in imaging procedures [95].

DNA molecules have been used as templates for formation of magnetic nanoparticles. A mixture of Fe^{2+}/Fe^{3+} ions was deposited electrostatically on the negatively charged single-stranded DNA molecules [96]. Then, the iron ions associated with DNA were used as seeds to produce Fe_3O_4 magnetic particles associated with the DNA molecules. The magneto-labeled single-stranded DNA was hybridized with complementary oligonucleotides yielding the double-stranded DNA complex with the bound magnetic nanoparticles. This allowed magneto-induced separation of the oligonucleotide, which can be later dissociated from the magneto-labeled DNA by the temperature increase.

8. Controlled Aggregation of Magnetic Nanoparticles and Formation of Magnetic Nanowires

The controlled assembling of magnetic nanoparticles using different kinds of cross-linking species or organic matrices has been studied for preparing novel materials with unique properties. Different mechanisms and interactions can be responsible for the nanoparticle assembling. For example, assembling of magnetic nanoparticles in the presence of amino acid-based polymers resulted in the controlled organization of these components due to electrostatic interactions between the block co-polypeptides and nanoparticles [97]. Depending on the kind of the added polypeptide the results of their interaction with magnetic nanoparticles can be different. The addition of polyaspartic acid initiated the aggregation of maghemite (γ-Fe_2O_3) nanoparticles into clusters, without their precipitation. On the other hand, the addition of the block co-polypeptide poly(EG_2-Lys)$_{100}$-b-poly(Asp)$_{30}$ resulted in the assembling of the magnetic nanoparticles in more sophisticated structures composed of micelles with cores consisting of the nanoparticles electrostatically bound to the polyaspartic acid end of the block co-polypeptide. The micelle shell stabilizing the core clusters and controlling their size was composed of the poly(EG_2-Lys) ends of the copolymers. The size and stability of the nanoparticle assembly can be tuned by changing the composition of the block co-polypeptide, thus adjusting the composite structures for their use in different applications.

Magnetic nanowires of different types, sizes and materials have been created for various applications, mostly using alumina membrane template method [98,99]. This method is based on the formation of nanowires inside the pores of the ordered aluminum oxide membrane, usually with electrochemical deposition of the material selected for the nanowires formation, Figure 4. Variation and optimization of the electrochemical deposition parameters allows the control of the nanowires length and structure, while the nanowires diameter depends on the membrane pores. The magnetic properties as well as some other features of the one-dimensional nanowires are unique and allow their use in the fabrication of magnetic nanodevices with high performance and controllability. For example, an ordered hexagonal array of highly aligned strontium ferrite nanowires was produced by dip coating in alumina templates, with magnetic properties dependent on the nanowire diameter and length [100]. The diameter of nanowires, synthesized with high aspect ratios, was changed from 30 to 60 nm while maintaining the same center-to-center distance between the wires. Nickel nanowires (98 nm diameter and 17 μm length) were fabricated by electrodeposition in anodic aluminum oxide membranes [101].

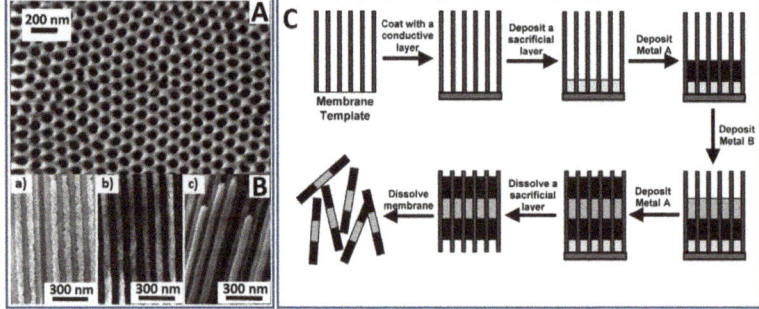

Figure 4. (**A**) Scanning electron micrograph, SEM, (top view) of a typical hexagonally ordered nanoporous alumina template with a pore diameter of 70 nm and an interpore distance of 100 nm. (**B**) SEM cross-sectional view of alumina membranes filled with Fe nanowires deposited from electrolytes containing: (**a**) 0.1 M FeSO$_4$, (**b**) 1 M FeSO$_4$ and (**c**) 0.5 M FeSO$_4$ + 0.4 M H$_3$BO$_3$. (**C**) Schematic description of the membrane-template electrochemical preparation of multifunctional nanowires. (Parts A and B were adapted from [102] with permission; part C was adopted from [103] with permission).

The synthetic method based on the alumina template can be applied to formation of multi-segment nanowires [104], which include magneto-responsive domains (usually represented by metallic Ni or Fe) and domains made of other materials (e.g., Au for deposition of thiolated redox species and biomolecules). The multi-segment nanowires can demonstrate multi-functional behavior with the magnetic properties combined with biocatalytic or biorecognition features depending on the biomolecule species bound to the non-magnetic segments. It is particularly easy to fabricate nanowires made of different metals, each with different properties. For example, Ni-Cu-Co composite magnetic nanowires have been successfully synthesized by electrochemical deposition inside the alumina template [105]. A few examples of magnetic nanowires are shown in Figures 5 and 6.

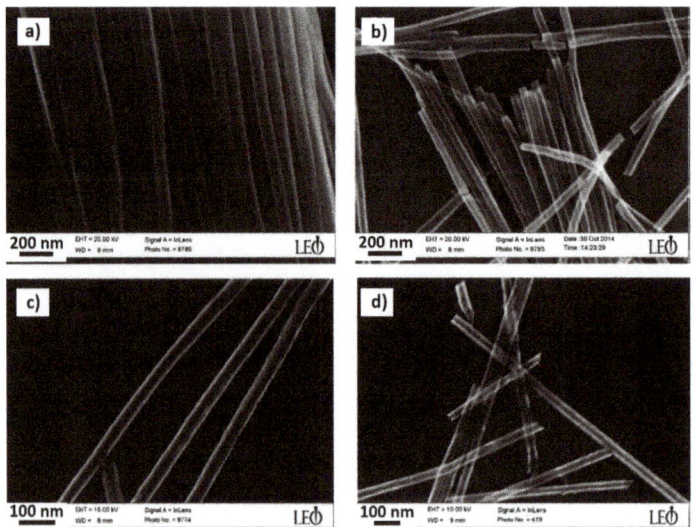

Figure 5. Field emission scanning electron microscope (FESEM) images of released strontium ferrite magnetic nanowires with diameter of (**a**) 60, (**b**) 50, (**c**) 40 and (**d**) 30 nm, after removal of alumina templates (figure adapted from [100] with permission).

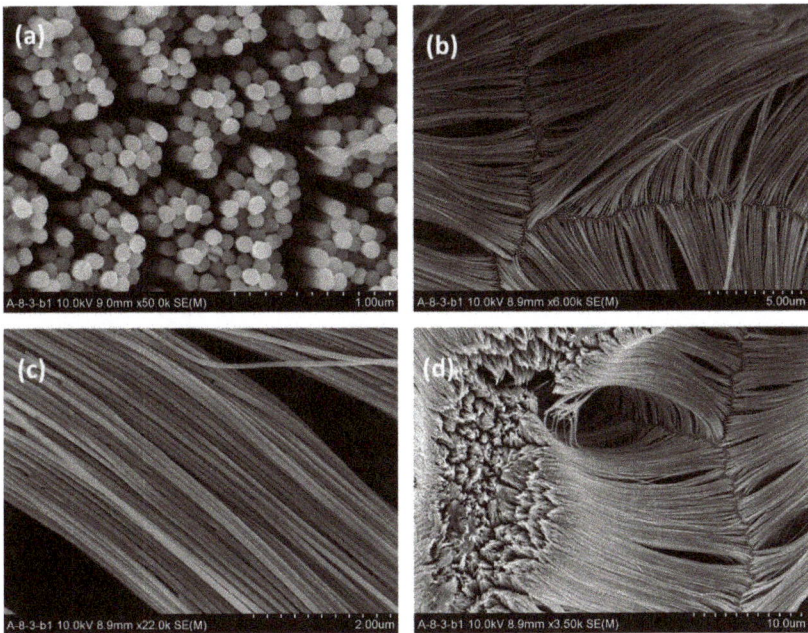

Figure 6. Scanning electron micrographs (SEM) of Ni nanowires with average diameter of 98 nm and length of 17 μm after removal of alumina templates. (The figure was adapted from ref. [101] with permission.). Images (a-d) show various examples of Ni nanowires prepared in alumina templates.

9. Conclusions and Perspectives

The state-of-the-art in the synthesis, functionalization, characterization, and application of (bio)molecule-functionalized magnetic particles and other related micro-/nano-objects, such as nanowires or nanotubes, allows efficient performance of various in vitro and in vivo biosensors and bioelectronic devices. Many of these devices are aimed for biomedical and biotechnological applications. For example, $CoFe_2O_4$-core/Au-shell nanoparticles have been successfully used to design a biosensor for foot-and-mouth viral disease biomarkers [53]. In this example a system with biomimetic oligo peptide-nucleic acid (PNA) was assembled on a gold shell of the magnetic nanoparticles and then hybridized with the complementary DNA sequence which is the disease biomarker. The biosensing was performed upon intercalation of the double-stranded PNA/DNA with a fluorescence probe, Rhodamine 6G. The magnetic features of the nano-species allowed easy separation of the analyzed species from a multi-component biofluid. The present example demonstrates powerful applicability of the biomolecule-functionalized magnetic nanoparticles in biomedical biosensors. Many other applications are feasible using various types of magneto-active nanospecies. Discussion on biological issues related to the biocompatibility, toxicity, etc. are outside the scope of this short review and can be found elsewhere [106–111]. While the present review offers a brief introduction to the topic, interested readers can find comprehensive reviews published recently [112–117].

Funding: This research received no external funding.

Conflicts of Interest: The author declares no conflicts of interest.

References

1. Shen, W.Z.; Cetinel, S.; Montemagno, C. Application of biomolecular recognition via magnetic nanoparticle in nanobiotechnology. *J. Nanoparticle Res.* **2018**, *20*, 130. [CrossRef]
2. Wu, K.; Su, D.Q.; Liu, J.M.; Saha, R.; Wang, J.P. Magnetic nanoparticles in nanomedicine: a review of recent advances. *Nanotechnology* **2019**, *30*, 502003. [CrossRef] [PubMed]
3. Abd Elrahman, A.A.; Mansour, F.R. Targeted magnetic iron oxide nanoparticles: Preparation, functionalization and biomedical application. *J. Drug Deliv. Sci. Technol.* **2019**, *52*, 702–712. [CrossRef]
4. Xu, C.; Akakuru, O.U.; Zheng, J.J.; Wu, A.G. Applications of iron oxide-based magnetic nanoparticles in the diagnosis and treatment of bacterial infections. *Front. Bioeng. Biotechnol.* **2019**, *7*, 141. [CrossRef] [PubMed]
5. Darton, N.J.; Ionescu, A.; Justin Llandro, J. (Eds.) *Magnetic Nanoparticles in Biosensing and Medicine*; Cambridge University Press: Cambridge, UK, 2019.
6. Ziarani, G.M.; Malmir, M.; Lashgari, N.; Badiei, A. The role of hollow magnetic nanoparticles in drug delivery. *RSC Adv.* **2019**, *9*, 25094–25106. [CrossRef]
7. Vangijzegem, T.; Stanicki, D.; Laurent, S. Magnetic iron oxide nanoparticles for drug delivery: Applications and characteristics. *Exp. Opin. Drug Deliv.* **2019**, *16*, 69–78. [CrossRef] [PubMed]
8. Kami, D.; Takeda, S.; Itakura, Y.; Gojo, S.; Watanabe, M.; Toyoda, M. Application of magnetic nanoparticles to gene delivery. *Int. J. Mol. Sci.* **2011**, *12*, 3705–3722. [CrossRef] [PubMed]
9. Jankovic, D.; Radovic, M.; Mirkovic, M.; Vukadinovic, A.; Peric, M.; Petrovic, D.; Antic, B.; Vranjes-Djuric, S. Y-90-labeled of phosphates-coated magnetic nanoparticles as a potential tumor treatment radiopharmaceuticals. *Eur. J. Nuclear Med. Mol. Imaging* **2018**, *45*, S649–S649.
10. Yang, F.; Lei, P.G.; Jiao, J. Recent advances in the use of magnetic nanoparticles in bio-imaging applications. *Nanosci. Nanotechnol. Lett.* **2019**, *11*, 901–922. [CrossRef]
11. Vallabani, N.V.S.; Singh, S.; Karakoti, A.S. Magnetic nanoparticles: Current trends and future aspects in diagnostics and nanomedicine. *Curr. Drug Metab.* **2019**, *20*, 457–472. [CrossRef] [PubMed]
12. Gloag, L.; Mehdipour, M.; Chen, D.F.; Tilley, R.D.; Gooding, J.J. Advances in the application of magnetic nanoparticles for sensing. *Adv. Mater.* **2019**. [CrossRef] [PubMed]
13. Pastucha, M.; Farka, Z.; Lacina, K.; Mikusova, Z.; Skladal, P. Magnetic nanoparticles for smart electrochemical immunoassays: a review on recent developments. *Microchim. Acta* **2019**, *186*, 312. [CrossRef] [PubMed]
14. Percin, I.; Karakoc, V.; Akgol, S.; Aksoz, E.; Denizli, A. Poly(hydroxyethyl methacrylate) based magnetic nanoparticles for plasmid DNA purification from *Escherichia coli* lysate. *Mater. Sci. Eng. C* **2012**, *32*, 1133–1140. [CrossRef]
15. Häfeli, U.; Schütt, W.; Teller, J.; Zborowski, M. (Eds.) *Scientific and Clinical Applications of Magnetic Carriers*; Plenum Press: New York, NY, USA, 2010.
16. Liu, Z.; Zhang, D.; Han, S.; Li, C.; Lei, B.; Lu, W.; Fang, J.; Zhou, C. Single crystalline magnetite nanotubes. *J. Am. Chem. Soc.* **2005**, *127*, 6–7. [CrossRef] [PubMed]
17. Wicke, W.; Ahmadzadeh, A.; Jamali, V.; Unterweger, H.; Alexiou, C.; Schober, R. Magnetic nanoparticle-based molecular communication in microfluidic environments. *IEEE Trans. Nanobiosci.* **2019**, *18*, 156–169. [CrossRef] [PubMed]
18. Sun, X.C.; Huang, Y.H.; Nikles, D.E. FePt and CoPt magnetic nanoparticles film for future high density data storage media. *Int. J. Nanotechnol.* **2004**, *1*, 328–346. [CrossRef]
19. Hendrych, A.; Kubínek, R.; Zhukov, A.V. The magnetic force microscopy and its capability for nanomagnetic studies—The short compendium. In *Modern Research and Educational Topics in Microscopy*; Méndez-Vilas, A., Díaz, J., Eds.; Formatex: Badajoz, Spain, 2007.
20. Talelli, M.; Aires, A.; Marciello, M. Protein-modified magnetic nanoparticles for biomedical applications. *Curr. Org. Chem.* **2016**, *20*, 1252–1261. [CrossRef]
21. Bilal, M.; Zhao, Y.P.; Rasheed, T.; Iqbal, H.M.N. Magnetic nanoparticles as versatile carriers for enzymes immobilization: A review. *Int. J. Biol. Macromol. B* **2018**, *120*, 2530–2544. [CrossRef] [PubMed]
22. Haghighi, A.H.; Faghih, Z.; Khorasani, M.T.; Farjadian, F. Antibody conjugated onto surface modified magnetic nanoparticles for separation of HER2+breast cancer cells. *J. Magn. Magn. Mater.* **2019**, *490*, 165479. [CrossRef]

23. Lee, M.H.; Leu, C.C.; Lin, C.C.; Tseng, Y.F.; Lin, H.Y.; Yang, C.N. Gold-decorated magnetic nanoparticles modified with hairpin-shaped DNA for fluorometric discrimination of single-base mismatch DNA. *Microchim. Acta* **2019**, *186*, 80. [CrossRef] [PubMed]
24. Cruz-Acuna, M.; Halman, J.R.; Afonin, K.A.; Dobson, J.; Rinaldi, C. Magnetic nanoparticles loaded with functional RNA nanoparticles. *Nanoscale* **2018**, *10*, 17761–17770. [CrossRef] [PubMed]
25. Wang, F.-H.; Yoshitake, T.; Kim, D.-K.; Muhammed, M.; Bjelke, B.; Kehr, J. Determination of conjugation efficiency of antibodies and proteins to the superparamagnetic iron oxide nanoparticles by capillary electrophoresis with laser-induced fluorescence detection. *J. Nanoparticle Res.* **2003**, *5*, 137–146. [CrossRef]
26. Bucak, S.; Jones, D.A.; Laibinis, P.E.; Hatton, T.A. Protein separations using colloidal magnetic nanoparticles. *Biotechnol. Prog.* **2003**, *19*, 477–484. [CrossRef] [PubMed]
27. Stanciu, L.; Won, Y.H.; Ganesana, M.; Andreescu, S. Magnetic particle-based hybrid platforms for bioanalytical sensors. *Sensors* **2009**, *9*, 2976–2999. [CrossRef] [PubMed]
28. Andreescu, S.; Njagi, J.; Ispas, C.; Ravalli, M.T. JEM Spotlight: Applications of advanced nanomaterials for environmental monitoring. *J. Environ. Monit.* **2009**, *11*, 27–40. [CrossRef] [PubMed]
29. Yu, S.; Chow, G.M. Carboxyl group (–CO_2H) functionalized ferrimagnetic iron oxide nanoparticles for potential bio-applications. *J. Mater. Chem.* **2004**, *14*, 2781–2786. [CrossRef]
30. Ling, W.H.; Wang, M.Y.; Xiong, C.X.; Xie, D.F.; Chen, Q.Y.; Chu, X.Y.; Qiu, X.Y.; Li, Y.M.; Xiao, X. Synthesis, surface modification, and applications of magnetic iron oxide nanoparticles. *J. Mater. Res.* **2019**, *34*, 1828–1844. [CrossRef]
31. Liu, X.; Xing, J.; Guan, Y.; Shan, G.; Liu, H. Synthesis of amino-silane modified superparamagnetic silica supports and their use for protein immobilization. *Colloids Surf. A Physicochem. Eng. Asp.* **2004**, *238*, 127–131. [CrossRef]
32. Jana, N.R.; Chen, Y.; Peng, X. Size- and shape-controlled magnetic (Cr, Mn, Fe, Co, Ni) oxide nanocrystals via a simple and general approach. *Chem. Mater.* **2004**, *16*, 3931–3935. [CrossRef]
33. Lai, J.; Shafi, K.V.P.M.; Ulman, A.; Loos, K.; Lee, Y.; Vogt, T.; Lee, W.-L.; Ong, N.P. Controlling the size of magnetic nanoparticles using pluronic block copolymer surfactants. *J. Phys. Chem. B* **2005**, *109*, 15–18. [CrossRef] [PubMed]
34. Huber, D.L. Synthesis, properties, and applications of iron nanoparticles. *Small* **2005**, *1*, 482–501. [CrossRef] [PubMed]
35. Tartaj, P.; Morales, M.P.; González-Carreño, T.; Veintemillas-Verdaguer, S.; Serna, C.J. Advances in magnetic nanoparticles for biotechnology applications. *J. Magn. Magn. Mater.* **2005**, *290–291*, 28–34. [CrossRef]
36. Shen, L.; Laibinis, P.E.; Hatton, T.A. Bilayer surfactant stabilized magnetic fluids: Synthesis and interactions at interfaces. *Langmuir* **1999**, *15*, 447–453. [CrossRef]
37. Hyeon, T. Chemical synthesis of magnetic nanoparticles. *Chem. Commun.* **2003**, 927–934. [CrossRef] [PubMed]
38. Gupta, A.K.; Gupta, M. Synthesis and surface engineering of iron oxide nanoparticles for biomedical applications. *Biomaterials* **2005**, *26*, 3995–4021. [CrossRef] [PubMed]
39. Sun, S.; Zeng, H. Size-controlled synthesis of magnetite nanoparticles. *J. Am. Chem. Soc.* **2002**, *124*, 8204–8205. [CrossRef] [PubMed]
40. Silva, L.P.; Lacava, Z.G.M.; Buske, N.; Morais, P.C.; Azevedo, R.B. Atomic force microscopy and transmission electron microscopy of biocompatible magnetic fluids: A comparative analysis. *J. Nanoparticle Res.* **2004**, *6*, 209–213. [CrossRef]
41. Matijević, E. Uniform inorganic colloid dispersions. Achievements and challenges. *Langmuir* **1994**, *10*, 8–16. [CrossRef]
42. Paul, K.G.; Frigo, T.B.; Groman, J.Y.; Groman, E.V. Synthesis of ultrasmall superparamagnetic iron oxides using reduced polysaccharides. *Bioconjugate Chem.* **2004**, *15*, 394–401. [CrossRef] [PubMed]
43. Gamarra, L.F.; Brito, G.E.S.; Pontuschka, W.M.; Amaro, E.; Parma, A.H.C.; Goya, G.F. Biocompatible superparamagnetic iron oxide nanoparticles used for contrast agents: a structural and magnetic study. *J. Magn. Magn. Mater.* **2005**, *289*, 439–441. [CrossRef]
44. Pan, X.H.; Cheng, S.Y.; Su, T.; Zuo, G.C.; Zhang, C.; Wu, L.P.; Jiao, Y.Z.; Dong, W. Poly (2-hydroxypropylene imines) functionalized magnetic polydopamine nanoparticles for high-efficiency DNA isolation. *Appl. Surf. Sci.* **2019**, *498*, 143888. [CrossRef]

45. Lobato, N.C.C.; Ferreira, A.D.; Weidler, P.G.; Franzreb, M.; Mansur, M.B. Improvement of magnetic solvent extraction using functionalized silica coated Fe_3O_4 nanoparticles. *Sep. Purif. Technol.* **2019**, *229*, 115839. [CrossRef]
46. Park, J.; Lee, E.; Hwang, N.-M.; Kang, M.; Kim, S.C.; Hwang, Y.; Park, J.-G.; Noh, H.-J.; Kim, J.-Y.; Park, J.-H.; et al. One-nanometer-scale size-controlled synthesis of monodisperse magnetic iron oxide nanoparticles. *Angew. Chem. Int. Ed.* **2005**, *44*, 2872–2877. [CrossRef] [PubMed]
47. Li, G.; Fan, J.; Jiang, R.; Gao, Y. Cross-linking the linear polymeric chains in the ATRP synthesis of iron oxide/polystyrene core/shell nanoparticles. *Chem. Mater.* **2004**, *16*, 1835–1837. [CrossRef]
48. Zeng, H.; Sun, S.; Li, J.; Wang, Z.L.; Liu, J.P. Tailoring magnetic properties of core/shell nanoparticles. *Appl. Phys. Lett.* **2004**, *85*, 792–794. [CrossRef]
49. Hütten, A.; Sudfeld, D.; Ennen, I.; Reiss, G.; Wojczykowski, K.; Jutzi, P. Ferromagnetic FeCo nanoparticles for biotechnology. *J. Magn. Magn. Mater.* **2005**, *293*, 93–101. [CrossRef]
50. Hu, Z.; Kanagaraj, J.; Hong, H.P.; Yang, K.; Ji, X.H.; Fan, Q.H.; Kharel, P. Characterization of ferrite magnetic nanoparticle modified polymeric composites by modeling. *J. Magn. Magn. Mater.* **2020**, *493*, 165735. [CrossRef]
51. Pita, M.; Tam, T.K.; Minko, S.; Katz, E. Dual magneto-biochemical logic control of electrochemical processes based on local interfacial pH changes. *ACS Appl. Mater. Interfaces* **2009**, *1*, 1166–1168. [CrossRef] [PubMed]
52. Jimenez, J.; Sheparovych, R.; Pita, M.; Narvaez Garcia, A.; Dominguez, E.; Minko, S.; Katz, E. Magneto-induced self-assembling of conductive nanowires for biosensor applications. *J. Phys. Chem. C* **2008**, *112*, 7337–7344. [CrossRef]
53. Pita, M.; Abad, J.M.; Vaz-Dominguez, C.; Briones, C.; Mateo-Martí, E.; Martín-Gago, J.A.; del Puerto Morales, M.; Fernández, V.M. Synthesis of cobalt ferrite core/metallic shell nanoparticles for the development of a specific PNA/DNA biosensor. *J. Colloid Interface Sci.* **2008**, *321*, 484–492. [CrossRef] [PubMed]
54. Silva, S.M.; Tavallaie, R.; Alam, M.T.; Chuah, K.; Gooding, J.J. A comparison of differently synthesized gold-coated magnetic nanoparticles as 'Dispersible Electrodes'. *Electroanalysis* **2016**, *28*, 431–438. [CrossRef]
55. Mandal, M.; Kundu, S.; Ghosh, S.K.; Panigrahi, S.; Sau, T.K.; Yusuf, S.M.; Pal, T. Magnetite nanoparticles with tunable gold or silver shell. *J. Colloid Interface Sci.* **2005**, *286*, 187–194. [CrossRef] [PubMed]
56. Lim, J.K.; Majetich, S.A. Composite magnetic–plasmonic nanoparticles for biomedicine: Manipulation and imaging. *Nano Today* **2013**, *8*, 98–113. [CrossRef]
57. Goon, I.Y.; Lai, L.M.H.; Lim, M.; Munroe, P.; Gooding, J.J.; Amal, R. Fabrication and dispersion of gold-shell-protected magnetite nanoparticles: Systematic control using polyethyleneimine. *Chem. Mater.* **2009**, *21*, 673–681. [CrossRef]
58. Jin, Y.D.; Jia, C.X.; Huang, S.W.; O'Donnell, M.; Gao, X.H. Multifunctional nanoparticles as coupled contrast agents. *Nature Commun.* **2010**, *1*, 41. [CrossRef] [PubMed]
59. Freitas, M.; Viswanathan, S.; Nouws, H.P.A.; Oliveira, M.B.P.P.; Delerue-Matos, C. Iron oxide/gold core/shell nanomagnetic probes and CdS biolabels for amplified electrochemical immunosensing of *Salmonella typhimurium*. *Biosens. Bioelectron.* **2014**, *51*, 195–200. [CrossRef] [PubMed]
60. Riskin, M.; Basnar, B.; Huang, Y.; Willner, I. Magnetoswitchable charge transport and bioelectrocatalysis using maghemite-Au core-shell nanoparticle/polyaniline composites. *Adv. Mater.* **2007**, *19*, 2691–2695. [CrossRef]
61. Chen, M.; Yamamuro, S.; Farrell, D.; Majetich, S.A. Gold-coated iron nanoparticles for biomedical applications. *J. Appl. Phys.* **2003**, *93*, 7551–7553. [CrossRef]
62. Bao, Y.; Krishnan, K.M. Preparation of functionalized and gold-coated cobalt nanocrystals for biomedical applications. *J. Magn. Magn. Mater.* **2005**, *293*, 15–19. [CrossRef]
63. Cui, Y.; Wang, Y.; Hui, W.; Zhang, Z.; Xin, X.; Chen, C. The synthesis of GoldMag nano-particles and their application for antibody immobilization. *Biomed. Microdevices* **2005**, *7*, 153–156. [CrossRef] [PubMed]
64. Wang, L.; Luo, J.; Maye, M.M.; Fan, Q.; Rendeng, Q.; Engelhard, M.H.; Wang, C.; Lin, Y.; Zhong, C.-J. Iron oxide–gold core–shell nanoparticles and thin film assembly. *J. Mater. Chem.* **2005**, *15*, 1821–1832. [CrossRef]
65. Gao, X.; Yu, K.M.K.; Tam, K.Y.; Tsang, S.C. Colloidal stable silica encapsulated nano-magnetic composite as a novel bio-catalyst carrier. *Chem. Commun.* **2003**, 2998–2999. [CrossRef] [PubMed]
66. Yang, H.-H.; Zhang, S.-Q.; Chen, X.-L.; Zhuang, Z.-X.; Xu, J.-G.; Wang, X.-R. Magnetite-containing spherical silica nanoparticles for biocatalysis and bioseparations. *Anal. Chem.* **2004**, *76*, 1316–1321. [CrossRef] [PubMed]

67. Zhao, W.; Gu, J.; Zhang, L.; Chen, H.; Shi, J. Fabrication of uniform magnetic nanocomposite spheres with a magnetic core/mesoporous silica shell structure. *J. Am. Chem. Soc.* **2005**, *127*, 8916–8917. [CrossRef] [PubMed]
68. SYun, S.H.; Lee, C.W.; Lee, J.S.; Seo, C.W.; Lee, E.K. Fabrication of SiO_2-coated magnetic nanoparticles for applications to protein separation and purification. *Mater. Sci. Forum* **2004**, *449*, 1033–1036.
69. He, Y.P.; Wang, S.Q.; Li, C.R.; Miao, Y.M.; Wu, Z.Y.; Zou, B.S. Synthesis and characterization of functionalized silica-coated Fe_3O_4 superparamagnetic nanocrystals for biological applications. *J. Phys. D Appl. Phys.* **2005**, *38*, 1342–1350. [CrossRef]
70. Son, S.J.; Reichel, J.; He, B.; Schuchman, M.; Lee, S.B. Magnetic nanotubes for magnetic-field-assisted bioseparation, biointeraction, and drug delivery. *J. Am. Chem. Soc.* **2005**, *127*, 7316–7317. [CrossRef] [PubMed]
71. del Campo, A.; Sen, T.; Lellouche, J.-P.; Bruce, I.J. Multifunctional magnetite and silica–magnetite nanoparticles: Synthesis, surface activation and applications in life sciences. *J. Magn. Magn. Mater.* **2005**, *293*, 33–40. [CrossRef]
72. Lu, H.; Yi, G.; Zhao, S.; Chen, D.; Guo, L.-H.; Cheng, J. Synthesis and characterization of multi-functional nanoparticles possessing magnetic, up-conversion fluorescence and bio-affinity properties. *J. Mater. Chem.* **2004**, *14*, 1336–1341. [CrossRef]
73. Hong, X.; Li, J.; Wang, M.; Xu, J.; Guo, W.; Li, J.; Bai, Y.; Li, T. Fabrication of magnetic luminescent nanocomposites by a layer-by-layer self-assembly approach. *Chem. Mater.* **2004**, *16*, 4022–4027. [CrossRef]
74. Kim, H.; Achermann, M.; Balet, L.P.; Hollingsworth, J.A.; Klimov, V.I. Synthesis and characterization of Co/CdSe core/shell nanocomposites: Bifunctional magnetic-optical nanocrystals. *J. Am. Chem. Soc.* **2005**, *127*, 544–546. [CrossRef] [PubMed]
75. Gu, H.; Yang, Z.; Gao, J.; Chang, C.K.; Xu, B. Heterodimers of nanoparticles: Formation at a liquid–liquid interface and particle-specific surface modification by functional molecules. *J. Am. Chem. Soc.* **2005**, *127*, 34–35. [CrossRef] [PubMed]
76. Gu, H.; Zheng, R.; Zhang, X.-X.; Xu, B. Facile one-pot synthesis of bifunctional heterodimers of nanoparticles: A conjugate of quantum dot and magnetic nanoparticles. *J. Am. Chem. Soc.* **2004**, *126*, 5664–5665. [CrossRef] [PubMed]
77. Yu, H.; Chen, M.; Rice, P.M.; Wang, S.X.; White, R.L.; Sun, S. Dumbbell-like bifunctional $Au-Fe_3O_4$ nanoparticles. *Nano Lett.* **2005**, *5*, 379–382. [CrossRef] [PubMed]
78. Yi, D.K.; Selvan, S.T.; Lee, S.S.; Papaefthymiou, G.C.; Kundaliya, D.; Ying, J.Y. Silica-coated nanocomposites of magnetic nanoparticles and quantum dots. *J. Am. Chem. Soc.* **2005**, *127*, 4990–4991. [CrossRef] [PubMed]
79. Morais, P.C.; Santos, J.G.; Silveira, L.B.; Gansau, C.; Buske, N.; Nunes, W.C.; Sinnecker, J.P. Susceptibility investigation of the nanoparticle coating-layer effect on the particle interaction in biocompatible magnetic fluids. *J. Magn. Magn. Mater.* **2004**, *272-276*, 2328–2329. [CrossRef]
80. Bruce, I.J.; Sen, T. Surface modification of magnetic nanoparticles with alkoxysilanes and their application in magnetic bioseparations. *Langmuir* **2005**, *21*, 7029–7035. [CrossRef] [PubMed]
81. Tanaka, T.; Matsunaga, T. Fully automated chemiluminescence immunoassay of insulin using antibody–protein A–bacterial magnetic particle complexes. *Anal. Chem.* **2000**, *72*, 3518–3522. [CrossRef] [PubMed]
82. Martin, C.R.; Mitchell, D.T. Peer reviewed: Nanomaterials in analytical chemistry. *Anal. Chem.* **1998**, *70*, 322A–327A. [CrossRef] [PubMed]
83. Fuentes, M.; Mateo, C.; Guisán, J.M.; Fernández-Lafuente, R. Preparation of inert magnetic nano-particles for the directed immobilization of antibodies. *Biosens. Bioelectron.* **2005**, *20*, 1380–1387. [CrossRef] [PubMed]
84. Gao, F.; Pan, B.-F.; Zheng, W.-M.; Ao, L.-M.; Gu, H.-C. Study of streptavidin coated onto PAMAM dendrimer modified magnetite nanoparticles. *J. Magn. Magn. Mater.* **2005**, *293*, 48–54. [CrossRef]
85. Xu, C.; Xu, K.; Gu, H.; Zheng, R.; Liu, H.; Zhang, X.; Guo, Z.; Xu, B. Dopamine as a robust anchor to immobilize functional molecules on the iron oxide shell of magnetic nanoparticles. *J. Am. Chem. Soc.* **2004**, *126*, 9938–9939. [CrossRef] [PubMed]
86. Peng, Z.G.; Hidajat, K.; Uddin, M.S. Adsorption of bovine serum albumin on nanosized magnetic particles. *J. Colloid Interface Sci.* **2004**, *271*, 277–283. [CrossRef] [PubMed]
87. Mikhaylova, M.; Kim, D.K.; Berry, C.C.; Zagorodni, A.; Toprak, M.; Curtis, A.S.G.; Muhammed, M. BSA immobilization on amine-functionalized superparamagnetic iron oxide nanoparticles. *Chem. Mater.* **2004**, *16*, 2344–2354. [CrossRef]

88. Dyal, A.; Loos, K.; Noto, M.; Chang, S.W.; Spagnoli, C.; Shafi, K.V.P.M.; Ulman, A.; Cowman, M.; Gross, R.A. Activity of Candida rugosa lipase immobilized on gamma-Fe_2O_3 magnetic nanoparticles. *J. Am. Chem. Soc.* **2003**, *125*, 1684–1685. [CrossRef] [PubMed]
89. Ma, M.; Zhang, Y.; Yu, W.; Shen, H.; Zhang, H.; Gu, N. Preparation and characterization of magnetite nanoparticles coated by amino silane. *Colloids Surf. A Physicochem. Eng. Asp.* **2003**, *212*, 219–226. [CrossRef]
90. Huang, S.-H.; Liao, M.-H.; Chen, D.-H. Direct binding and characterization of lipase onto magnetic nanoparticles. *Biotechnol. Prog.* **2003**, *19*, 1095–1100. [CrossRef] [PubMed]
91. Cao, D.; He, P.; Hu, N. Electrochemical biosensors utilising electron transfer in heme proteins immobilised on Fe_3O_4 nanoparticles. *Analyst* **2003**, *128*, 1268–1274. [CrossRef] [PubMed]
92. Shinkai, M.; Honda, H.; Kobayashi, T. Preparation of fine magnetic particles and application for enzyme immobilization. *Biocatalysis* **1991**, *5*, 61–69. [CrossRef]
93. Liao, M.-H.; Chen, D.-H. Immobilization of yeast alcohol dehydrogenase on magnetic nanoparticles for improving its stability. *Biotechnol. Lett.* **2001**, *23*, 1723–1727. [CrossRef]
94. Liao, M.-H.; Chen, D.-H. Fast and efficient adsorption/desorption of protein by a novel magnetic nano-adsorbent. *Biotechnol. Lett.* **2002**, *24*, 1913–1917. [CrossRef]
95. Sun, X.-L.; Cui, W.; Haller, C.; Chaikof, E.L. Site-specific multivalent carbohydrate labeling of quantum dots and magnetic beads. *ChemBioChem* **2004**, *5*, 1593–1596. [CrossRef] [PubMed]
96. Mornet, S.; Vekris, A.; Bonnet, J.; Duguet, E.; Grasset, F.; Choy, J.-H.; Portier, J. DNA–magnetite nanocomposite materials. *Mater. Lett.* **2000**, *42*, 183–188. [CrossRef]
97. Euliss, L.E.; Grancharov, S.G.; O'Brien, S.; Deming, T.J.; Stucky, G.D.; Murray, C.B.; Held, G.A. Cooperative assembly of magnetic nanoparticles and block copolypeptides in aqueous media. *Nano Lett.* **2003**, *3*, 1489–1493. [CrossRef]
98. Wang, X.W.; He, Z.C.; Li, J.S.; Yuan, Z.H. Controllable synthesis and magnetic properties of ferromagnetic nanowires and nanotubes. *Curr. Nanoscience* **2012**, *8*, 801–809. [CrossRef]
99. Sousa, C.T.; Leitao, D.C.; Proenca, M.P.; Ventura, J.; Pereira, A.M.; Araujo, J.P. Nanoporous alumina as templates for multifunctional applications. *Appl. Phys. Rev.* **2014**, *1*, 031102. [CrossRef]
100. Ebrahimi, F.; Ashrafizadeh, F.; Bakhshi, S.R. Tuning the magnetic properties of high aligned strontium ferrite nanowires formed in alumina template. *J. Alloys Compd.* **2016**, *656*, 237–244. [CrossRef]
101. Adeela, N.; Maaz, K.; Khan, U.; Karim, S.; Ahmad, M.; Iqbal, M.; Riaz, S.; Han, X.F.; Maqbool, M. Fabrication and temperature dependent magnetic properties of nickel nanowires embedded in alumina templates. *Ceram. Int.* **2015**, *41*, 12081–12086. [CrossRef]
102. Schlörb, H.; Haehnel, V.; Khatri, M.S.; Srivastav, A.; Kumar, A.; Schultz, L.; Fähler, S. Magnetic nanowires by electrodeposition within templates. *Phys. Status Solidi B* **2010**, *247*, 2364–2379. [CrossRef]
103. Wang, J. Adaptive nanowires for on-demand control of electrochemical microsystems. *Electroanalysis* **2008**, *20*, 611–615. [CrossRef]
104. Monzon, L.M.A.; O'Neill, K.; Sheth, Y.; Venkatesan, M.; Coey, J.M.D. Fabrication of multisegmented magnetic wires with micron-length copper spacers. *Electrochem. Commun.* **2013**, *36*, 96–98. [CrossRef]
105. Hussain, M.; Khan, M.; Sun, H.Y.; Nairan, A.; Karim, S.; Nisar, A.; Maqbool, M.; Ahmad, M. Fabrication and temperature dependent magnetic properties of Ni–Cu–Co composite. Nanowires. *Physical B* **2015**, *475*, 99–104. [CrossRef]
106. Jiang, Z.; Shan, K.; Song, J.; Liu, J.; Rajendran, S.; Pugazhendhi, A.; Jacob, J.A.; Chen, B. Toxic effects of magnetic nanoparticles on normal cells and organs. *Life Sci.* **2019**, *220*, 156–161. [CrossRef] [PubMed]
107. Jarockyte, G.; Daugelaite, E.; Stasys, M.; Statkute, U.; Poderys, V.; Tseng, T.-C.; Hsu, S.-H.; Karabanovas, V.; Rotomskis, R. Accumulation and toxicity of superparamagnetic iron oxide nanoparticles in cells and experimental animals. *Int. J. Mol. Sci.* **2016**, *17*, 1193. [CrossRef] [PubMed]
108. Erofeev, A.; Gorelkin, P.; Garanina, A.; Alova, A.; Efremova, M.; Vorobyeva, N.; Edwards, C.; Korchev, Y.; Majouga, A. Novel method for rapid toxicity screening of magnetic nanoparticles. *Sci. Rep.* **2018**, *8*, 7462. [CrossRef] [PubMed]
109. Markides, H.; Rotherham, M.; El Haj, A.J. Biocompatibility and toxicity of magnetic nanoparticles in regenerative medicine. *J. Nanomater.* **2012**, *2012*, 614094. [CrossRef]
110. Patil, R.M.; Thorat, N.D.; Shete, P.B.; Bedge, P.A.; Gavde, S.; Joshi, M.G.; Tofail, S.A.M.; Bohara, R.A. Comprehensive cytotoxicity studies of superparamagnetic iron oxide nanoparticles. *Biochem. Biophys. Rep.* **2018**, *13*, 63–72. [CrossRef] [PubMed]

111. Mahmoudi, M.; Laurent, S.; Shokrgozar, M.A.; Hosseinkhani, M. Toxicity evaluations of superparamagnetic iron oxide nanoparticles: Cell "vision" versus physicochemical properties of nanoparticles. *ACS Nano* **2011**, *5*, 7263–7276. [CrossRef] [PubMed]
112. Zhu, N.; Ji, H.; Yu, P.; Niu, J.; Farooq, M.U.; Akram, M.W.; Udego, I.O.; Li, H.; Niu, X. Surface modification of magnetic iron oxide nanoparticles. *Nanomaterials* **2018**, *8*, 810. [CrossRef] [PubMed]
113. Khan, K.; Rehman, S.; Rahman, H.U.; Khan, Q. Synthesis and application of magnetic nanoparticles. In *Nanomagnetism*; Gonzalez Estevez, J.M., Ed.; One Central Press (OCP): Cheshire, UK, 2014; Chapter 6; pp. 135–159.
114. Boal, A.K. Synthesis and applications of magnetic nanoparticles. In *Nanoparticles: Building Blocks for Nanotechnology*; Rotello, V., Ed.; Springer: Boston, MA, USA, 2004; Chapter 1; pp. 1–27.
115. Fermon, C. Introduction to Magnetic Nanoparticles. In *Nanomagnetism: Applications and Perspectives*; Van de Voorde, M., Fermon, C., Eds.; Wiley: Hoboken, NJ, USA, 2017; Chapter 7; pp. 127–136.
116. Kudr, J.; Haddad, Y.; Richtera, L.; Heger, Z.; Cernak, M.; Adam, V.; Zitka, O. Magnetic nanoparticles: From design and synthesis to real world applications. *Nanomaterials* **2017**, *7*, 243. [CrossRef] [PubMed]
117. Ansari, S.A.M.K.; Ficiarà, E.; Ruffinatti, F.A.; Stura, I.; Argenziano, M.; Abollino, O.; Cavalli, R.; Guiot, C.; D'Agata, F. Magnetic iron oxide nanoparticles: Synthesis, characterization and functionalization for biomedical applications in the central nervous system. *Materials* **2019**, *12*, 465. [CrossRef] [PubMed]

© 2019 by the author. Licensee MDPI, Basel, Switzerland. This article is an open access article distributed under the terms and conditions of the Creative Commons Attribution (CC BY) license (http://creativecommons.org/licenses/by/4.0/).

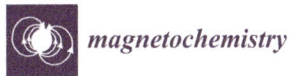

Review

Preparation and Application of Iron Oxide Nanoclusters

Angelo J. Antone [1], Zaicheng Sun [2],* and Yuping Bao [1,2],*

1. Box 870203, Chemical and Biological Engineering, The University of Alabama, Tuscaloosa, AL 35487, USA
2. Beijing Key Lab for Green Catalysis and Separation, Department of Chemistry and Chemical Engineering, School of Environment and Energy Engineering, Beijing University of Technology, 100 Pingleyuan, Chaoyan, Beijing 100124, China
* Correspondence: sunzc@bjut.edu.cn (Z.S.); ybao@eng.ua.edu (Y.B.); Tel.: +001-205-348-9869 (Y.B.)

Received: 10 May 2019; Accepted: 25 July 2019; Published: 1 August 2019

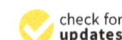

Abstract: Magnetic iron oxide nanoclusters, which refers to a group of individual nanoparticles, have recently attracted much attention because of their distinctive behaviors compared to individual nanoparticles. In this review, we discuss preparation methods for creating iron oxide nanoclusters, focusing on synthetic procedures, formation mechanisms, and the quality of the products. Then, we discuss the emerging applications for iron oxide nanoclusters in various fields, covering traditional and novel applications in magnetic separation, bioimaging, drug delivery, and magnetically responsive photonic crystals.

Keywords: iron oxide nanoclusters; superparticles; magnetically responsive photonic crystals; collective behaviors; magnetic separation; bioimaging

---

1. Introduction

Magnetic iron oxide nanoclusters, which refers to a group of individual nanoparticles, have recently attracted much attention because of their distinctive behaviors compared to individual nanoparticles [1–3]. The magnetic properties of iron oxide nanoparticles are strongly dependent on size, yielding single-domain regimes and a superparamagnetic limit [4]. Because of the superparamagnetic limit, iron oxide nanoparticles with grain sizes above 25 nm (depending on crystal phases (magnetite or maghemite)) are generally ferromagnetic at room temperature. The magnetic interactions between nanoparticles lead to aggregation in solution, which limits their uses in certain applications, such as drug delivery. The superparamagnetic limit also sets a threshold for the maximum moment to be reached. The formation of nanoclusters by assembling individual iron oxide nanoparticles has the potential to overcome this limitation by increasing magnetic moments while at the same time maintaining superparamagnetic behaviors [5].

Magnetic iron oxide nanoclusters combine the properties of individual nanoparticles and exhibit collective behaviors due to interactions between individual nanoparticles [3]. In addition, the collective behaviors of these nanoclusters can be controlled by tuning the size and shape of individual nanoparticles, the interspacing between nanoparticles, and the properties of the capping molecules of individual nanoparticles [2,3,6]. Particularly, magnetic nanoclusters can be manipulated with applied magnetic fields, leading to novel functional materials. Iron oxide nanoclusters have great potential to improve the performance of individual nanoparticles and develop advanced materials with novel functions.

This review will discuss the preparation methods of iron oxide nanoclusters and their applications in various areas. For preparation methods, the discussion will focus on synthetic procedures, formation mechanisms, and the quality of nanoclusters in terms of size distribution, size control, and scalability.

On the other hand, the application discussion will cover the use of improved magnetic properties and novel applications that have been recently developed, such as cell membrane-encapsulated iron oxide nanoclusters for drug screening, drug delivery, and tumor targeting.

2. Preparation of Iron Oxide Nanoclusters

Magnetic iron oxide nanoclusters can be produced either through controlled aggregation of small iron oxide nanoparticles during synthesis (e.g., the polyol method [5]) or the assembly of ligand-capped nanoparticles after synthesis (e.g., solvophobic interactions [7]). Each of these methods has its advantages and disadvantages, which will be discussed in the following section.

2.1. Controlled Aggregation of Nanoparticles during Synthesis

For controlled aggregation methods, small-sized iron oxide nanoparticles (<10 nm) are first formed in a supersaturated solution of iron precursors through nucleation and growth, and then these small-sized nanoparticles spontaneously aggregate into larger nanoclusters (50–300 nm) in a single step. The grain (small nanoparticle) size and final nanocluster size can be controlled by adjusting reaction conditions. Several controlled aggregation methods have been developed to produce iron oxide nanoclusters in a single step, such as the polyol method, solvothermal synthesis, thermal decomposition, and microwave methods.

2.1.1. Polyol Method

The polyol method developed by Yin et al. involves the injection of iron salts (e.g., iron chloride) into a polyol solution (e.g., diethylene glycol) at a high temperature (>200 °C) in the presence of capping molecules (e.g., polyacrylic acid) under basic conditions [5,8]. This method produces highly water-soluble and monodisperse iron oxide nanoclusters (30–200 nm) in a single step [2,5,8,9]. The grain size and nanocluster size are controlled by the amounts of base injected into the reaction [5].

Figure 1a–d shows representative transmission electron microscopy (TEM) images of differently sized iron oxide nanoclusters from the polyol method, where the nanocluster sizes were controlled by the amounts of sodium hydroxide ethylene glycol solution. These nanoclusters consisted of a number of small-sized iron oxide nanoparticles (<10 nm) yielding superparamagnetic behaviors at room temperature but with enhanced saturation magnetization (Figure 1e). In a similar study, control of both the grain size and nanocluster size was achieved by adjusting the concentration and injection speed of the base solution [6]. Because of the polyacrylic acid coatings, iron oxide nanoclusters from this method are highly negatively charged and well dispersed in aqueous solution. These nanoclusters can be directly used for various applications, such as magnetically responsive photonic crystals [6,9].

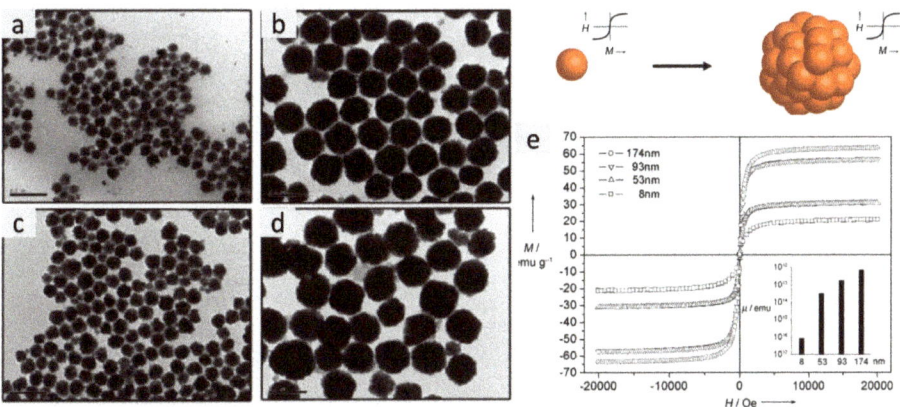

Figure 1. Iron oxide nanoclusters produced with the polyol method: (**a–d**) representative TEM images demonstrating size control, scale bar 200 nm; (**e**) magnetization versus applied field curves, suggesting superparamagnetic behaviors but with increased magnetic moments for larger nanoclusters. (Adapted with permission from Reference [5]).

2.1.2. Solvothermal Synthesis

Solvothermal synthesis involves first mixing reactants (e.g., iron chloride, sodium acetate, capping molecules) in reducing solvents (e.g., ethylene glycol or diethylene glycol) under stirring: Then the mixture reacts in a sealed Teflon-lined stainless steel hydrothermal reactor at a high temperature (>200 °C) to induce iron oxide nanocluster formation [10–14]. This method is highly attractive for several reasons: first, the capping molecules can be selected from a variety of organic acids for different surface chemistries, such as sodium citrate [14], polyacrylic acids [15], and 5-sulfosalicylic acid [13]; and second, the grain and nanocluster size can be controlled easily by adjusting the ratios and concentrations of the reactants [10]. In addition, porous iron oxide nanoclusters can be generated by simply using gas-forming reactants, such as ammonium acetate [16]. Most importantly, the scalable production of the synthetic process (up to 200 g per batch) has been demonstrated without the quality of the iron oxide nanoclusters being affected [14]. Figure 2 shows synthetic procedure, formation mechanism, representative scanning electron microscopy (SEM), and TEM images of iron oxide nanoclusters from gram-scale solvothermal synthesis.

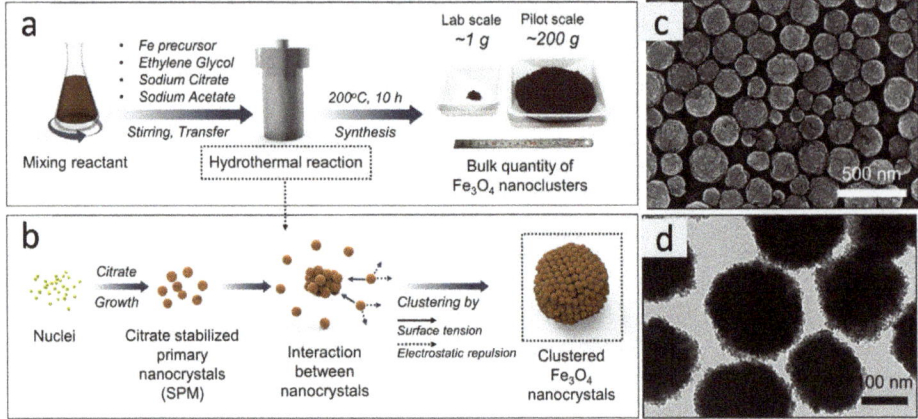

Figure 2. Gram-scale solvothermal synthesis of iron oxide nanoclusters: (**a**) schematic illustration of the procedure; (**b**) proposed mechanism of the nanocluster formation; (**c**,**d**) SEM and TEM images indicating the quality of the nanoclusters (adapted from Reference [14] with permission; copyright American Chemical Society, 2018).

The nanoclusters generated from the solvothermal synthesis are highly soluble in aqueous solution and can be directly used for various applications [14]. Porous iron oxide nanoclusters can also be produced through slight modifications of the process by adding gas forming reagents, and these porous nanoclusters have been explored for magnetically responsive drug delivery with high drug loading capacity [16].

In addition to the polyol method and solvothermal synthesis, other synthetic methods have been explored for the production of iron oxide nanoclusters in a single step, such as thermal decomposition [17] and microwave irritation [18]. However, the quality of the nanoclusters has not been comparable to these two methods. In particular, the size distribution of the nanoclusters from these two methods is much wider.

2.2. Controlled Assembly of Ligand-Capped Nanoparticles

The formation of nanoclusters from the controlled assembly of ligand-capped nanoparticles involves two steps: the synthesis of monodisperse ligand-capped iron oxide nanoparticles (10–20 nm) and the controlled assembly of nanoparticles under specific processing conditions. The processing conditions trigger the assembly process and affect the quality of the final products, such as ligand etching [19] and solvophobic interaction [7,20].

2.2.1. Ligand Etching

Nanoparticles are generally coated with a layer of ligands to prevent them from aggregation. The ligand etching process involves replacing the original capping molecules with weakly bound ligands, which causes the destabilization of nanoparticles and subsequent aggregation and nanocluster formation (Figure 3a). The size and shape of the assembled secondary structures are dependent on the ligands used for the striping process. For example, the addition of diol molecules into the solution of oleic acid-coated iron oxide nanoparticles (~13 nm) led to nanoparticle destabilization and subsequent secondary structure formation [19]. Depending on the types of diol molecules, dimers, oligomers, and nanoclusters were formed during the ligand stripping process. Figure 3b–e shows representative TEM images of the secondary structures with the addition of different diol molecules.

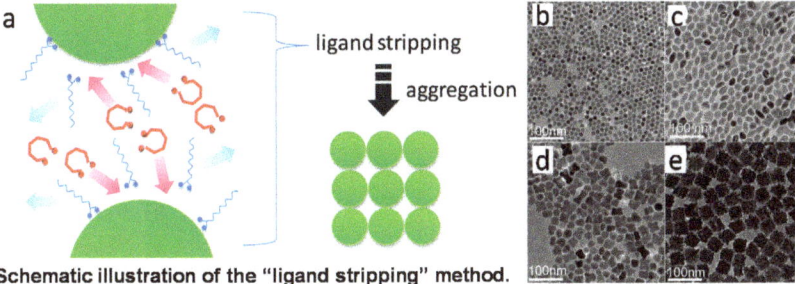

Figure 3. Nanocluster formation via the ligand stripping method: (**a**) illustration of the ligand stripping method process, (**b**) spherical nanoparticles with no diol addition, (**c**) dimer formation induced by the addition of polyethylene glycol 400, (**d**) oligomer induced by the addition of triethylene glycol, and (**e**) nanocluster induced by the addition of diethylene glycol (adapted from Reference [19]; reproduced with permission from the Royal Society of Chemistry).

In a similar study, magnetic iron oxide nanoclusters were prepared using competitive stabilizer desorption, where oleic acid-coated iron oxide nanoparticles were mixed with cyanopropyl-modified silica nanoparticles. The silica particles competed for capping ligands on the iron oxide nanoparticle surfaces, which caused the destabilization of iron oxide nanoparticles and the subsequent formation of magnetic nanoclusters [21]. Compared to the single-step aggregation methods, the nanocluster sizes from ligand stripping are smaller and mainly soluble in organic solvents because of the presence of hydrophobic ligands.

2.2.2. Solvophobic Interactions

The solvophobic interaction method involves mixing hydrophobic ligand-coated (e.g., oleic acid) iron oxide nanoparticles with surfactants (e.g., dodecyltrimethylammonium bromide, DTAB) to form micelle structures. After evaporating away the organic solvent, a group of iron oxide nanoparticles are combined within the micelles. Subsequently, the micelle solution goes through an annealing process in ethylene glycol in the presence of capping molecules at an elevated temperature (e.g., 80 °C), leading to nanocluster formation [7,20]. Figure 4a illustrates the preparation process via solvophobic interactions. The size of the nanoclusters can be controlled by the relative ratios of nanoparticles to surfactants, and the stability of the nanoclusters is affected by the structures of surfactants and capping molecules. Figure 4b,c shows representative TEM and SEM images of iron oxide nanoclusters formed from 6-nm oleic acid–iron oxide nanoparticles using DTAB as a micelle-forming agent and poly(vinylpyrrolidone) as capping molecules. The main advantage of this method is that it is not limited to iron oxide nanoparticles, but can be easily applied to any other type of nanoparticle with a hydrophobic surface coating.

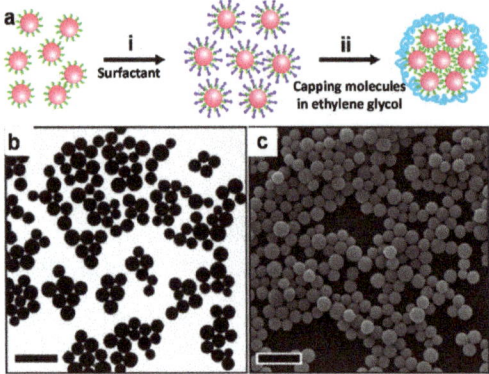

Figure 4. Iron oxide nanoclusters via solvophobic interactions: (**a**) scheme of the formation process, (**b**) TEM image, and (**c**) SEM image, scale bar 500 nm (adapted from Reference [20], with permission; copyright American Chemical Society, 2007).

2.3. Matrix Encapsulation of Nanoparticles

For the matrix encapsulation method, nanocluster formation is assisted by the matrices, where iron oxide nanoparticles are mixed with the selected matrix and the induced matrix crosslinking leads to the formation of nanoclusters. Several types of matrices have been reported to fabricate iron oxide nanoclusters, such as proteins [22], polymers [23–25], silica [26], etc. The control of the aggregation process and the quality of the nanoclusters are highly specific to the choice of matrices. For example, protein encapsulation of iron oxide nanoparticles is normally induced by ethanol addition followed by surface crosslinking with glutaraldehyde [22]. In contrast, polydopamine encapsulation can be easily triggered by changing the pH of the solution [23]. In addition, the salt concentration, amount and addition speed of ethanol, and protein concentration all affect the quality of bovine serum albumin (BSA) encapsulated in ultrasmall iron oxide nanoparticles [22].

Figure 5 shows representative TEM images of iron oxide nanoclusters that were produced with different matrices, where the polymer shells can be clearly seen (Figure 5a), but the silica and protein encapsulation formed matrix–iron oxide composite materials (Figure 5b,c). The matrix-assisted method has several distinctive advantages: first, drug molecules can be simultaneously encapsulated into the nanoclusters during the aggregation process, creating magnetic resonance imaging (MRI)-visible drug delivery vehicles; second, biocompatibility and water solubility can be easily achieved based on the choices of the matrices; and finally, by tuning the nanocluster sizes, other functionality can be achieved, such as ultrasound response [27].

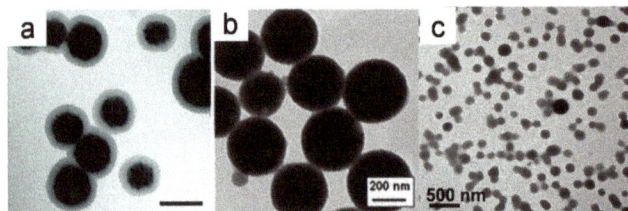

Figure 5. TEM images of matrix-encapsulated iron oxide nanoparticles: (**a**) hydrogel, (**b**) silica, and (**c**) bovine serum albumin protein ((**a**) is adapted from Reference [24] (with permission), copyright American Chemical Society, 2011; (**b**) is adapted from Reference [26] (with permission), copyright American Chemical Society, 2008; (**c**) is adapted from Reference [22], reproduced with permission from the Royal Society of Chemistry).

3. Applications of Iron Oxide Nanoclusters

Iron oxide nanoclusters have been explored for numerous applications [3,28], including rapid magnetic separation [29], MRI contract agents with enhanced sensitivity [30], nanocarriers with high drug loading capacity [16], and magnetically responsive photonic crystals [6,9,31]. The following section will discuss these applications of magnetic nanoclusters in detail to present their potentials as functional materials with improved performance.

3.1. Iron Oxide Nanoclusters for Magnetic Separation

Magnetic separation is the most traditional use for magnetic nanoparticles and utilizes the large surface areas of nanoparticles to enhance adsorption capacity. Subsequently, magnetic fields are applied to extract, enrich, or separate compounds of interest [32–34]. During magnetic separation, the nanoparticles have to overcome the drag forces in solution: therefore, the higher the magnetic moments of nanoparticles, the faster the separation processes. The formation of magnetic nanoclusters increases the magnetic moments, leading to the fast response of separation processes. However, the size increase of nanoclusters causes decreases in the total surface area of nanoclusters per given mass. Therefore, an optimal size range of nanoclusters for magnetic separation needs to be considered for efficient separation and large adsorption capacity. Several nanocluster systems have been designed for the separation, enrichment, and detection of biomolecules [35–37], organisms [38,39], or inorganic ions [40,41].

For example, antibody-functionalized iron oxide nanospheres (~400 nm) (through the assembly of iron oxide nanoparticles onto copolymers) have been used for the quick enrichment of bacteria [38]. The nanospheres showed a fast magnetic response of less than one minute and an over-96% capture efficiency of bacteria at ultralow concentrations (<50 colony-forming unit (CFU)/mL) [38]. Kim et al. have shown the highly selective detection and rapid separation of pathogenic organisms using magnetic iron oxide nanoclusters [39]. In that study, the iron oxide nanoclusters were prepared through solvophobic interactions using polysorbate 80 as a micelle surfactant (Figure 6a). Then, a monoclonal antibody was conjugated on the nanocluster surface for pathogen binding. The magnetic properties of iron oxide nanoclusters were optimized theoretically by calculating size-dependent magnetic forces and Brownian forces of nanoclusters, suggesting that nanoclusters of about 200 nm provided efficient separation and large separation capacity (Figure 6b) [39]. Figure 6c shows the detection principle and the nanoclusters binding to the pathogens via two different binding sites (H and O antigens).

Most recently, we [42] and others [43,44] have developed a new type of magnetic separation method based on cell membrane-encapsulated iron oxide nanoclusters. Compared to traditional magnetic separation techniques using immobilized ligands on nanocluster surfaces to bind the targets, the new technique uses functional transmembrane receptors as binding sites to identify the targets. The complete embedment of iron oxide nanoclusters inside cell membranes overcame the nonspecific binding problems because magnetic nanoclusters were not in direct contact with the analyte solution. Figure 7a illustrates the design of the cell membrane-encapsulated nanoclusters. The choice of the cell membrane depends on the specific targets to be extracted.

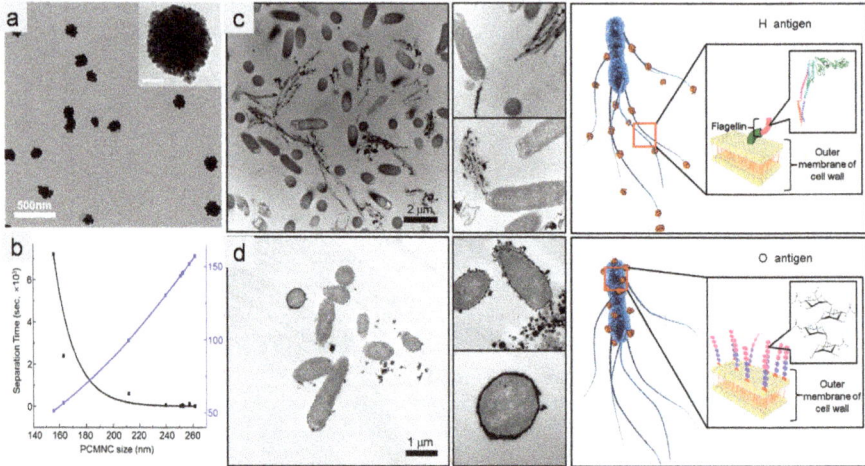

Figure 6. Selective detention of pathogens using iron oxide nanoclusters: (**a**) TEM images of nanoclusters, (**b**) relationship between magnetic separation time (black line) and magnetic force under specific field gradients (blue line), (**c**) H-antigen-specific binding of nanoclusters to flagella, and (**d**) O-antigen-specific binding of the nanoclusters on the surface of the cell body (adapted from Reference [39], with permission; copyright American Chemical Society, 2016).

For example, in order to extract nicotine molecules from tobacco smoke condensates, we created cell membrane-encapsulated nanoclusters using human cell line overexpressing $\alpha_3\beta_4$ receptors, which bind to nicotine molecules specifically. Figure 7b shows representative TEM images of the iron oxide nanoclusters prepared using cell membranes with $\alpha_3\beta_4$ nicotinic receptors. Even though the cell receptors were not visible on the TEM images of the cell membrane-encapsulated iron oxide nanoclusters, the fishing experiments clearly demonstrated binding specificity and efficiency. The nicotine receptors on the surfaces were able to fish out the nicotine molecules from tobacco smoke condensates, and all other compounds without specific binding to the nicotine receptors were washed out, as shown in the washing and elution chromatograms of the high-performance liquid chromatography (HPLC) (Figure 7c). In addition, iron oxide nanoclusters coated with cell membranes without nicotine receptors showed no binding to nicotine in the smoke condensates, suggesting specific binding between nicotine and $\alpha_3\beta_4$ receptors. This new magnetic separation will greatly benefit the discovery of new drug candidate targeting transmembrane receptors. Most importantly, this technique can be easily applied to any other transmembrane receptors.

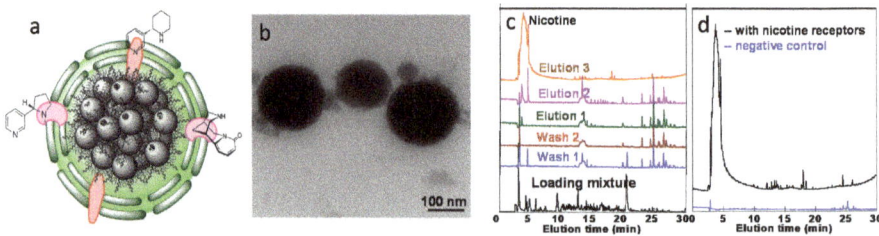

Figure 7. Cell membrane-encapsulated iron oxide nanoclusters: (**a**) design concept, (**b**) TEM image, (**c**) HPLC washing and elution chromatograms of fishing experiments using $\alpha_3\beta_4$ receptors from smoke condensates, (**d**) comparison of elution profiles with and without $\alpha_3\beta_4$ receptors (adapted from Reference [42]; reproduced with permission from the Royal Society of Chemistry).

In a similar study, iron oxide nanoparticles were encapsulated inside red blood cell membranes for virus targeting and isolation [45]. The cell membranes were modified with sialic acid molecules, which formed stable clusters with influenza viruses. The encapsulated superparamagnetic iron oxide nanoparticles enabled the quick enrichment of the influenza virus via magnetic extraction. The enriched viral samples significantly enhanced virus detection through multiple viral quantification methods, such as the immunochromatographic strip test and cell-based tittering assays.

Additionally, iron oxide nanoclusters have been applied to the enhanced removal of molybdate from surface water [40], the reduction of arsenic concentrations below the World Health Organization (WHO) permissible safety limit for drinking water [41], enrichments of chemical molecules for analysis [46], and protein adsorption [37,47].

3.2. Biomedical Applications of Iron Oxide Nanoclusters

The biomedical applications of iron oxide nanoclusters have been focused on magnetically triggered drug release [48–51] and MRI contrast agents with high sensitivity [30,52–54]. For magnetically triggered drug release, either iron oxide nanoparticles (>10 nm) and drugs were colocalized in nanocarriers [55] or porous iron oxide nanoclusters were created to increase drug loading by surface adsorption [16]. Under alternating magnetic fields (AMFs), local heat was generated from iron oxide nanoparticles, which elevated the local temperatures and subsequently caused drug release.

For example, iron oxide nanoparticle-loaded microcapsules were prepared through layer-by-layer deposition of positively and negatively charged polyelectrolytes onto a calcium carbonate template. By replacing the negatively charged electrolyte with negatively charged nanoparticles, the nanoparticles were incorporated inside the shell, as shown in Figure 8a. Figure 8b shows a representative TEM image of a capsule, where the darkness of the shell indicates the successful encapsulation of iron oxide nanoparticles. The drug molecules were loaded inside the capsule after leaking out of the template. Under AMFs, local heat was generated from the nanoparticles inside the shell, which triggered drug release. Compared to samples without applying AMFs, the drug release was significantly enhanced after applying 90 min of AMFs (300 kHz and 24 kAm^{-1}), as shown in Figure 8c. Compared to drug release triggered by photothermal stimulation, magnetic fields have better tissue penetration. In addition, the localization of iron oxide nanoparticles inside the shells decreased the permeability of microcapsules, preventing premature drug release before applying external stimuli [27].

Without matrix assistance, iron oxide nanoclusters are generally made into porous structures for drug delivery applications. The high surface area and cavities of the porous structures increase surface drug adsorption, leading to enhanced drug loading [16,56]. For example, porous iron oxide nanoclusters were prepared using solvothermal synthesis, where sodium acetate was used to create the porous structure because of ammonia gas bubble formation during synthesis [16]. Figure 8d shows an illustration of porous nanoclusters, and Figure 8e shows a representative TEM image of porous iron oxide nanoparticles. These as-prepared porous iron oxide nanoclusters served as great nanocarriers for hydrophobic drugs, with a demonstrated loading capacity as high as 35.0 wt % for paclitaxel (Figure 8f). The antitumor efficacy of paclitaxel-loaded nanoclusters under AFMs was significantly enhanced compared to free drugs.

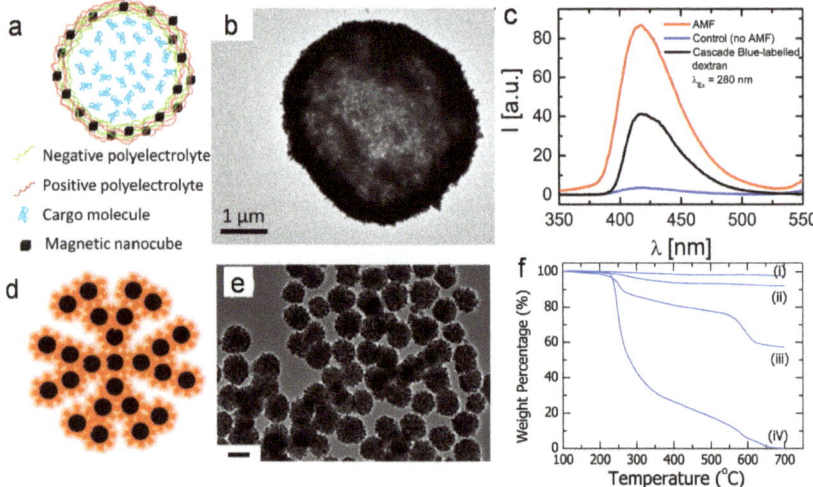

Figure 8. Iron oxide nanoclusters for drug delivery: (**a–c**) design, TEM image, and magnetically triggered drug release profile of iron oxide-decorated microcapsules; and (**d–f**) illustration, TEM image, and thermogravimetric analysis plots representing the drug loading capacity of porous iron oxide nanoclusters (**a–c**) are adapted from Reference [55], reproduced with permission from the Royal Society of Chemistry; (**d–f**) are adapted from Reference [16] (with permission), copyright American Chemical Society, 2011.

Recently, cell membrane-coated iron oxide nanoparticles have been created for tumor targeting and drug delivery [57–60]. For example, macrophage membrane-coated iron oxide nanoparticles have been shown to be effective nanocarriers for tumor targeting and therapy [58]. In that study, the functional transmembrane receptors were able to recognize cancer cells via cell–cell adhesion between macrophage and cancer cell surfaces for effective cell targeting. The encapsulated iron oxide nanoparticles were used as photoabsorbing agents for photothermal therapy. Similar concepts have also been demonstrated for myeloid-derived suppressor cell membrane-coated magnetic nanoparticles, which performed well in immune evasion, active tumor targeting, and photothermal therapy-induced tumor killing [59].

For MRI applications, iron oxide nanoclusters have been explored as both T_1 (positive) and T_2 (negative) contrast agents. The iron oxide-based T_1 contrast agents were mainly either ultrasmall (<4 nm) nanoparticles [22,61,62] or ultrathin (diameter <4 nm) nanowires [63,64]. Nanocluster formation was mainly to overcome the short blood circulation time of these nanostructures due to their small dimensions [22]. For instance, tannic acid-coated ultrasmall iron oxide nanoparticles (3~4 nm) only had about 15 min of blood circulation time and were quickly cleared by the renal system [22]. Encapsulating these ultrasmall iron oxide nanoparticles inside BSA nanoclusters exhibited enhanced T_1 permanence with higher r_1 relaxivity and increased blood circulation times [22]. Figure 9a shows a comparison between phantom MRI images of free nanoparticles and BSA ultrasmall iron oxide nanoclusters, suggesting great T_1 brightening of the nanoclusters. Figure 9b shows MRI images of mice before and 2 h post-injection with BSA ultrasmall iron oxide nanoclusters, where the brain and kidney regions were significantly brightened, suggesting the nanoclusters remained in the blood stream even 2 h after injection. Similarly, ultrasmall iron oxide nanoparticles sandwiched between polymer layers of layer-by-layer assembled microcapsules showed not only increased blood circulation time, but also served as great drug nanocarriers for ultrasound-triggered drug release [27]. Figure 9c shows MRI images of a control mouse and a mouse 48 h post-injection, where the bright region near the heart suggested the long blood circulation time of these nanoparticle-loaded capsules. Because of their larger sizes, these capsules were sensitive to ultrasound, which enhanced drug localization at the tumor site with ultrasound treatment (Figure 9d).

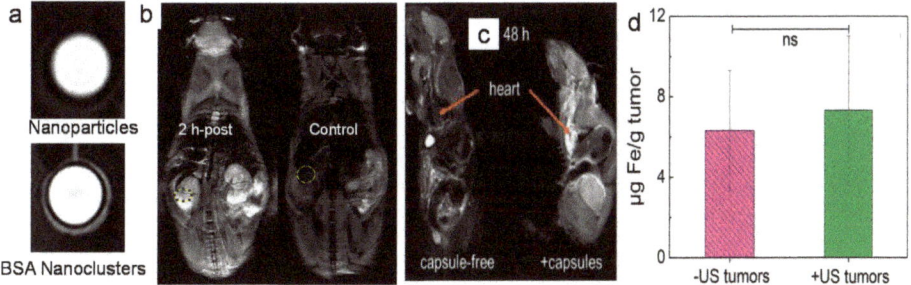

Figure 9. (a) Phantom MRI images of free ultrasmall nanoparticles and bovine serum albumin (BSA) ultrasmall iron oxide nanoclusters, (b) MRI images of mice before and 2 h post-injection with BSA ultrasmall iron oxide nanoclusters, (c) MRI images of a mouse 48 h after injection with ultrasmall iron oxide nanoparticle-loaded capsules (right) and a control (left), and (d) iron quantification showing the increased accumulation of an ultrasound-treated tumor after capsule injection ((a,b) are adapted from Reference [22], reproduced with permission from the Royal Society of Chemistry; (c,d) are adapted from Reference [27]).

T_2 MRI contrast agents are mainly superparamagnetic nanoparticles, and nanocluster formation increases the magnetic signal and subsequently enhances the imaging sensitivity or cell labeling efficiency [24,30,52,53,56,65–67]. For example, differently sized iron oxide nanoclusters via solvothermal synthesis showed higher r_2 relaxivity for nanocluster sizes of around 50–60 nm. The r_2 relaxivity of 63-nm iron oxide nanoclusters was more than three times higher than that of commercial products (Resovist) [30]. In addition, the cellular take efficiency of 63-nm iron oxide nanoclusters by macrophage cells was 10 times higher than that of Resovist [30]. Enhanced MRI sensitivity and increased cellular uptake make iron oxide nanoclusters great candidates for cellular MRI.

3.3. Optical Applications of Iron Oxide Nanoclusters

Iron oxide nanoclusters synthesized by the polyol method are negatively charged and highly water soluble. Under magnetic fields, these nanoclusters assemble into chain-like structures and diffract visible light. Therefore, these nanoclusters are used as building blocks to develop magnetically controlled photonic crystals [6,9,31]. The color of diffracted light can be tuned through adjustments to nanocluster size, interspacing between nanoclusters, and the strength of the applied magnetic fields. Using superparamagnetic polyacrylic acid-coated iron oxide nanoclusters of 120 nm as an example (Figure 10a–c), it was demonstrated that the color of the diffracted lights shifted from blue to red when the applied magnetic fields increased (Figure 10d). The reflection spectra clearly showed the dependence of the refracted light wavelength on the strength of the applied magnetic field, where the field strength was tuned by changing the distance between the magnet and the nanoparticle solution (Figure 10e) [5]. In addition, the optical response of the colloidal photonic crystals to the changes in the external magnetic field was fully reversible.

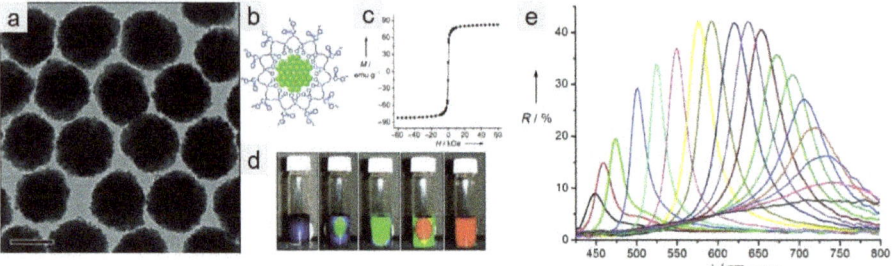

Figure 10. Iron oxide nanoclusters as building blocks for photonic crystals: (**a**) TEM image of iron oxide nanoclusters, scale bar 100 nm; (**b**) schematic illustration of polyacrylate coating on nanocluster surfaces; (**c**) superparamagnetic behavior of nanoclusters at room temperature; (**d**) photographs of photonic crystals formed in response to an external magnetic field; and (**e**) UV-Vis reflectance spectra (adapted with permission from Reference [9]).

In a similar study [6], iron oxide nanoclusters of different cluster and grain sizes were tested for optical response. It was discovered that a critical nanocluster size (~40 nm) existed, below which no changes were observed in light diffraction with applied magnetic fields. In addition, larger nanoclusters (>160 nm) preferably diffracted red light in relatively low magnetic fields, while the smaller nanoclusters (<100 nm) diffracted blue light in stronger magnetic fields.

4. Summary and Outlook

In summary, we have discussed the preparation methods and emerging applications of iron oxide nanoclusters. Compared to individual iron oxide nanoparticles, these nanoclusters are much larger in size (hundreds nm), but remain superparamagnetic. Several synthetic methods have been developed by either directly preparing nanoclusters in a single step (e.g., the polyol method, thermal decomposition, and solvothermal synthesis) or assembling presynthesized ligand-capped nanoparticles under controlled conditions (e.g., solvophobic interaction, ligand etching, and matrix-assisted aggregation). Among the various synthetic methods, solvothermal synthesis is highly attractive, as it produces water-soluble, monodisperse superparamagnetic nanoclusters in a single step. In particular, large-scale production (up to 200 g per batch) has been demonstrated without scarifying the quality of the product. The enhanced magnetic properties and collective behaviors of these nanoclusters have led to a number of emerging applications, such as rapid magnetic separation and magnetically triggered drug delivery. Of all of these discussed applications, cell membrane-encapsulated nanoclusters are particularly attractive because of their enhanced performance. For example, cell membrane-encapsulated nanoclusters for magnetic separation can overcome the nonspecific binding problems associated with current magnetic bead technologies. The functional transmembrane receptors allow for the specific identification and extraction of targets binding to cell receptors. Depending on the choices of cell membranes, cell membrane-encapsulated nanoclusters are also used for drug delivery and tumor targeting. These biomimetic nanocarriers exhibit much better efficiency compared to traditional nanocarriers.

Funding: This work was funded in part by National Science Foundation (NSF) DMR1149931. Z.S. is funded by Beijing Municipal High Level Innovative Team Building Program (IDHT20180504) and the National Natural Science Foundation of China (21805004, 21671011, 21872001 and 51801006).

Acknowledgments: National Science Foundation (NSF) DMR1149931, Beijing Municipal High Level Innovative Team Building Program (IDHT20180504) and the National Natural Science Foundation of China (21805004, 21671011, 21872001 and 51801006).

Conflicts of Interest: The authors declare no conflicts of interest.

References

1. Lee, J.S.; Cha, J.M.; Yoon, H.Y.; Lee, J.K.; Kim, Y.K. Magnetic multi-granule nanoclusters: A model system that exhibits universal size effect of magnetic coercivity. *Sci. Rep.* **2015**, *5*, 12135. [CrossRef]
2. Lu, Z.; Yin, Y. Colloidal nanoparticle clusters: Functional materials by design. *Chem. Soc. Rev.* **2012**, *41*, 6874–6887. [CrossRef] [PubMed]
3. Kostopoulou, A.; Lappas, A. Colloidal magnetic nanocrystal clusters: Variable length-scale interaction mechanisms, synergetic functionalities and technological advantages. *Nanotechnol. Rev.* **2015**, *4*, 595–624. [CrossRef]
4. Krishnan, K.M.; Pakhomov, A.B.; Bao, Y.; Blomqvist, P.; Chun, Y.; Gonzales, M.; Griffin, K.; Ji, X.; Roberts, B.K. Nanomagnetism and spin electronics: Materials, microstructure and novel properties. *J. Mater. Sci.* **2006**, *41*, 793–815. [CrossRef]
5. Ge, J.; Hu, Y.; Biasini, M.; Beyermann, W.P.; Yin, Y. Superparamagnetic magnetite colloidal nanocrystal clusters. *Angew. Chem. Int. Ed.* **2007**, *46*, 4342–4345. [CrossRef]
6. Kostopoulou, A.; Tsiaoussis, I.; Lappas, A. Magnetic iron oxide nanoclusters with tunable optical response. *Photonics Nanostruct. Fundam. Appl.* **2011**, *9*, 201–206. [CrossRef]
7. Zhuang, J.; Wu, H.; Yang, Y.; Cao, Y. Controlling colloidal superparticle growth through solvophobic interactions. *Angew. Chem. Int. Ed.* **2008**, *47*, 2208–2212. [CrossRef]
8. Ge, J.P.; Hu, Y.X.; Biasini, M.; Dong, C.L.; Guo, J.H.; Beyermann, W.P.; Yin, Y.D. One-step synthesis of highly water-soluble magnetite colloidal nanocrystals. *Chem. Eur. J.* **2007**, *13*, 7153–7161. [CrossRef]
9. Ge, J.; Hu, Y.; Yin, Y. Highly tunable superparamagnetic colloidal photonic crystals. *Angew. Chem. Int. Ed.* **2007**, *46*, 7428–7431. [CrossRef]
10. Xuan, S.; Wang, Y.; Yu, J.; Leung, K.C.F. Tuning the grain size and particle size of superparamagnetic Fe_3O_4 microparticles. *Chem. Mater.* **2009**, *21*, 5079–5087. [CrossRef]
11. Gao, J.; Ran, X.; Shi, C.; Cheng, H.; Cheng, T.; Su, Y. One-step solvothermal synthesis of highly water-soluble, negatively charged superparamagnetic Fe_3O_4 colloidal nanocrystal clusters. *Nanoscale* **2013**, *5*, 7026–7033. [CrossRef] [PubMed]
12. Li, S.; Zhang, T.; Tang, R.; Qiu, H.; Wang, C.; Zhou, Z. Solvothermal synthesis and characterization of monodisperse superparamagnetic iron oxide nanoparticles. *J. Magn. Magn. Mater.* **2015**, *379*, 226–231. [CrossRef]
13. Wang, W.; Tang, B.; Wu, S.; Gao, Z.; Ju, B.; Teng, X.; Zhang, S. Controllable 5-sulfosalicylic acid assisted solvothermal synthesis of monodispersed superparamagnetic Fe_3O_4 nanoclusters with tunable size. *J. Magn. Magn. Mater.* **2017**, *423*, 111–117. [CrossRef]
14. Kim, J.; Tran, V.T.; Oh, S.; Kim, C.S.; Hong, J.C.; Kim, S.; Joo, Y.S.; Mun, S.; Kim, M.H.; Jung, J.W.; et al. scalable solvothermal synthesis of superparamagnetic Fe_3O_4 nanoclusters for bioseparation and theragnostic probes. *ACS Appl. Mater. Interfaces* **2018**, *10*, 41935–41946. [CrossRef] [PubMed]
15. Liang, J.; Ma, H.; Luo, W.; Wang, S. Synthesis of magnetite submicrospheres with tunable size and superparamagnetism by a facile polyol process. *Mater. Chem. Phys.* **2013**, *139*, 383–388. [CrossRef]
16. Luo, B.; Xu, S.; Luo, A.; Wang, W.; Wang, S.; Guo, J.; Lin, Y.; Zhao, D.; Wang, C. Mesoporous biocompatible and acid-degradable magnetic colloidal nanocrystal clusters with sustainable stability and high hydrophobic drug loading capacity. *ACS Nano* **2011**, *5*, 1428–1435. [CrossRef] [PubMed]
17. Nikitin, A.A.; Shchetinin, I.V.; Tabachkova, N.Y.; Soldatov, M.A.; Soldatov, A.V.; Sviridenkova, N.V.; Beloglazkina, E.K.; Savchenko, A.G.; Fedorova, N.D.; Abakumov, M.A.; et al. Synthesis of iron oxide nanoclusters by thermal decomposition. *Langmuir* **2018**, *34*, 4640–4650. [CrossRef] [PubMed]
18. Jia, J.; Yu, J.; Zhu, X.; Chan, K.; Wang, Y. Ultra-fast method to synthesize mesoporous magnetite nanoclusters as highly sensitive magnetic resonance probe. *J. Colloid Interface Sci.* **2012**, *379*, 1–7. [CrossRef] [PubMed]
19. Fu, J.; He, L.; Xu, W.; Zhuang, J.; Yang, X.; Zhang, X.; Wu, M.; Yin, Y. Formation of colloidal nanocrystal clusters of iron oxide by controlled ligand stripping. *Chem. Commun.* **2016**, *52*, 128–131. [CrossRef]
20. Zhuang, J.; Wu, H.; Yang, Y.; Cao, Y. Supercrystalline colloidal particles from artificial atoms. *J. Am. Chem. Soc.* **2007**, *129*, 14166–14167. [CrossRef]
21. Ninjbadgar, T.; Brougham, D.F. Epoxy ring opening phase transfer as a general route to water dispersible superparamagnetic Fe_3O_4 nanoparticles and their application as positive MRI contrast agents. *Adv. Funct. Mater.* **2011**, *21*, 4769–4775. [CrossRef]

22. Sherwood, J.; Rich, M.; Lovas, K.; Warram, J.; Bolding, M.S.; Bao, Y. T_1-Enhanced MRI-visible nanoclusters for imaging-guided drug delivery. *Nanoscale* **2017**, *9*, 11785–11792. [CrossRef] [PubMed]
23. Li, X.; Wei, Z.; Lv, H.; Wu, L.; Cui, Y.; Yao, H.; Li, J.; Zhang, H.; Yang, B.; Jiang, J. Iron oxide nanoparticles promote the migration of mesenchymal stem cells to injury sites. *Int. J. Nanomed.* **2019**, *14*, 573–589. [CrossRef]
24. Paquet, C.; de Haan, H.W.; Leek, D.; Lin, H.; Xiang, B.; Tian, G.H.; Kell, A.; Simard, B. Clusters of superparamagnetic iron oxide nanoparticles encapsulated in a hydrogel: A particle architecture generating a synergistic enhancement of the T_2 relaxation. *ACS Nano* **2011**, *5*, 3104–3112. [CrossRef] [PubMed]
25. Xie, X.; Zhang, C. Controllable assembly of sydrophobic superparamagnetic iron oxide nanoparticle with mPEG-PLA copolymer and its effect on MR transverse relaxation rate. *J. Nanomater.* **2011**. [CrossRef]
26. Li, L.; Choo, E.S.G.; Yi, J.; Ding, J.; Tang, X.; Xue, J. Superparamagnetic silica composite nanospheres (SSCNs) with ultrahigh loading of iron oxide nanoparticles via an oil-in-DEG microemulsion route. *Chem. Mater.* **2008**, *20*, 6292–6294. [CrossRef]
27. Alford, A.; Rich, M.; Kozlovskaya, V.; Chen, J.; Sherwood, J.; Bolding, M.; Warram, J.; Bao, Y.; Kharlampieva, E. Ultrasound-triggered delivery of anticancer therapeutics from MRI-visible multilayer microcapsules. *Adv. Therap.* **2018**, 1800051. [CrossRef]
28. Maity, D.; Chandrasekharan, P.; Pradhan, P.; Chuang, K.; Xue, J.; Feng, S.; Ding, J. Novel synthesis of superparamagnetic magnetite nanoclusters for biomedical applications. *J. Mater. Chem.* **2011**, *21*, 14717–14724. [CrossRef]
29. Zhang, H.; Wu, J.; Wang, X.; Li, X.; Wu, M.; Liang, F.; Yang, Y. One-pot solvothermal synthesis of Carboxylatopillar 5 arene-modified Fe_3O_4 magnetic nanoparticles for ultrafast separation of cationic dyes. *Dyes Pigm.* **2019**, *162*, 512–516. [CrossRef]
30. Li, M.; Gu, H.; Zhang, C. Highly sensitive magnetite nano clusters for MR cell imaging. *Nanoscale Res. Lett.* **2012**, *7*, 204. [CrossRef]
31. Yang, P.; Li, H.; Zhang, S.; Chen, L.; Zhou, H.; Tang, R.; Zhou, T.; Bao, F.; Zhang, Q.; He, L.; et al. Gram-scale synthesis of superparamagnetic Fe_3O_4 nanocrystal clusters with long-term charge stability for highly stable magnetically responsive photonic crystals. *Nanoscale* **2016**, *8*, 19036–19042. [CrossRef] [PubMed]
32. Borlido, L.; Azevedo, A.M.; Roque, A.C.A.; Aires-Barros, M.R. Magnetic separations in biotechnology. *Biotechnol. Adv.* **2013**, *31*, 1374–1385. [CrossRef] [PubMed]
33. Ditsch, A.; Lindenmann, S.; Laibinis, P.E.; Wang, D.I.C.; Hatton, T.A. High-gradient magnetic separation of magnetic nanoclusters. *Ind. Eng. Chem. Res.* **2005**, *44*, 6824–6836. [CrossRef]
34. Ezzaier, H.; Marins, J.A.; Claudet, C.; Hemery, G.; Sandre, O.; Kuzhir, P. Kinetics of aggregation and magnetic separation of multicore iron oxide nanoparticles: Effect of the grafted layer thickness. *Nanomaterials* **2018**, *8*, 623. [CrossRef] [PubMed]
35. Zhang, J.; Zhu, M.; Yang, Y.; Cao, J.; Shi, F. Extraction of genomic DNA via superparamagnetic Fe_3O_4 magnetic colloidal nanocrystal clusters. *J. Nanosci. Nanotechnol.* **2018**, *18*, 8105–8110. [CrossRef] [PubMed]
36. Meerod, S.; Deepuppha, N.; Rutnakornpituk, B.; Rutnakornpituk, M. Reusable magnetic nanocluster coated with poly (acrylic acid) and its adsorption with an antibody and an antigen. *J. Appl. Polym. Sci.* **2018**, *135*, 46160. [CrossRef]
37. Long, X.; Li, J.; Sheng, D.; Lian, H. Low-cost iron oxide magnetic nanoclusters affinity probe for the enrichment of endogenous phosphopeptides in human saliva. *RSC Adv.* **2016**, *6*, 96210–96222. [CrossRef]
38. Wen, C.; Jiang, Y.; Li, X.; Tang, M.; Wu, L.; Hu, J.; Pang, D.; Zeng, J. Efficient enrichment and analyses of bacteria at ultralow concentration with quick-response magnetic nanospheres. *ACS Appl. Mater. Interfaces* **2017**, *9*, 9416–9425. [CrossRef]
39. Kim, Y.T.; Kim, K.H.; Kang, E.S.; Jo, G.; Ahn, S.Y.; Park, S.H.; Kim, S.I.; Mun, S.; Baek, K.; Kim, B.; et al. Synergistic effect of detection and separation for pathogen using magnetic clusters. *Bioconjug. Chem.* **2016**, *27*, 59–65. [CrossRef]
40. Ma, W.; Sha, X.; Gao, L.; Cheng, Z.; Meng, F.; Cai, J.; Tan, D.; Wang, R. Effect of iron oxide nanocluster on enhanced removal of molybdate from surface water and pilot scale test. *Colloids Surf. A Physicochem. Eng. Asp.* **2015**, *478*, 45–53. [CrossRef]
41. Lee, S.H.; Cha, J.; Sim, K.; Lee, J.K. Efficient removal of arsenic using magnetic multi-granule nanoclusters. *Bull. Korean Chem. Soc.* **2014**, *35*, 605–609. [CrossRef]

42. Sherwood, J.; Sowell, J.; Beyer, N.; Irvin, J.; Stephen, C.; Antone, A.J.; Bao, Y.P.; Ciesla, L.M. Cell-membrane coated iron oxide nanoparticles for isolation and specific identification of drug leads from complex matrices. *Nanoscale* **2019**, *11*, 6352–6359. [CrossRef]
43. Bu, Y.; Hu, Q.; Ke, R.; Sui, Y.; Xie, X.; Wang, S. Cell membrane camouflaged magnetic nanoparticles as a biomimetic drug discovery platform. *Chem. Comm.* **2018**, *54*, 13427–13430. [CrossRef]
44. Hu, Q.; Bu, Y.; Zhen, X.; Xu, K.; Ke, R.; Xie, X.; Wang, S. Magnetic carbon nanotubes camouflaged with cell membrane as a drug discovery platform for selective extraction of bioactive compounds from natural products. *Chem. Eng. J.* **2019**, *364*, 269–279. [CrossRef]
45. Chen, H.; Fang, Z.; Chen, Y.; Chen, Y.; Yao, B.; Cheng, J.; Chien, C.; Chang, Y.; Hu, C. Targeting and enrichment of viral pathogen by cell membrane cloaked magnetic nanoparticles for enhanced detection. *ACS Appl. Mater. Interfaces* **2017**, *9*, 39953–39961. [CrossRef]
46. Zhang, Y.; Li, L.; Ma, W.; Zhang, Y.; Yu, M.; Guo, J.; Lu, H.; Wang, C. Two-in-one strategy for effective enrichment of phosphopeptides using magnetic mesoporous gamma-Fe_2O_3 nanocrystal clusters. *ACS Appl. Mater. Interfaces* **2013**, *5*, 614–621. [CrossRef]
47. Yang, Q.; Lan, F.; Yi, Q.; Wu, Y.; Gu, Z. A colloidal assembly approach to synthesize magnetic porous composite nanoclusters for efficient protein adsorption. *Nanoscale* **2015**, *7*, 17617–17622. [CrossRef]
48. Bueno, P.V.A.; Hilamatu, K.C.P.; Carmona-Ribeiro, A.M.; Petri, D.F.S. Magnetically triggered release of amoxicillin from xanthan/Fe3O4/albumin patches. *Int. J. Biol. Macromol.* **2018**, *115*, 792–800. [CrossRef]
49. Kuo, C.; Liu, T.; Wang, K.; Hardiansyah, A.; Lin, Y.; Chen, H.; Chiu, W.Y. Magnetic and thermal-sensitive poly(N-isopropylacrylamide)-based microgels for magnetically triggered Controlled release. *J. Vis. Exp.* **2017**. [CrossRef]
50. Benyettou, F.; Flores, J.A.O.; Ravaux, F.; Rezgui, R.; Jouiad, M.; Nehme, S.I.; Parsapur, R.K.; Olsen, J.C.; Selvam, P.; Trabolsi, A. Mesoporous gamma-iron oxide nanoparticles for magnetically triggered release of doxorubicin and hyperthermia treatment. *Chem. Eur. J.* **2016**, *22*, 17018–17026. [CrossRef]
51. Hua, X.; Yang, Q.; Dong, Z.; Zhang, J.; Zhang, W.; Wang, Q.; Tan, S.; Smyth, H.D.C. Magnetically triggered drug release from nanoparticles and its applications in anti-tumor treatment. *Drug Deliv.* **2017**, *24*, 511–518. [CrossRef]
52. Xu, F.; Cheng, C.; Chen, D.; Gu, H. Magnetite nanocrystal clusters with ultra-high sensitivity in magnetic resonance imaging. *ChemPhysChem* **2012**, *13*, 336–341. [CrossRef]
53. Smith, C.E.; Ernenwein, D.; Shkumatov, A.; Clay, N.E.; Lee, J.Y.; Melhem, M.; Misra, S.; Zimmerman, S.C.; Kong, H. Hydrophilic packaging of iron oxide nanoclusters for highly sensitive imaging. *Biomaterials* **2015**, *69*, 184–190. [CrossRef]
54. Wu, M.; Zhang, D.; Liu, X. Nanoclusters of superparamagnetic iron oxide nanoparticles coated with poly(dopamine) for magnetic field-directed, ultrasensitive MRI-guided photothermal cancer therapy. *J. Control. Release* **2015**, *213*, 78. [CrossRef]
55. Carregal-Romero, S.; Guardia, P.; Yu, X.; Hartmann, R.; Pellegrino, T.; Parak, W.J. Magnetically triggered release of molecular cargo from iron oxide nanoparticle loaded microcapsules. *Nanoscale* **2015**, *7*, 570–576. [CrossRef]
56. Dong, F.; Guo, W.; Bae, J.; Kim, S.H.; Ha, C. Highly porous, water-soluble, superparamagnetic, and biocompatible magnetite nanocrystal clusters for targeted drug delivery. *Chem. Eur. J.* **2011**, *17*, 12802–12808. [CrossRef]
57. Lai, P.; Huang, R.; Lin, S.; Lin, Y.; Chang, C. Biomimetic stem cell membrane-camouflaged iron oxide nanoparticles for theranostic applications. *RSC Adv.* **2015**, *5*, 98222–98230. [CrossRef]
58. Meng, Q.; Rao, L.; Zan, M.; Chen, M.; Yu, G.; Wei, X.; Wu, Z.; Sun, Y.; Guo, S.; Zhao, X.; et al. Macrophage membrane-coated iron oxide nanoparticles for enhanced photothermal tumor therapy. *Nanotechnology* **2018**, *29*. [CrossRef]
59. Yu, G.; Rao, L.; Wu, H.; Yang, L.; Bu, L.; Deng, W.; Wu, L.; Nan, X.; Zhang, W.; Zhao, X.; et al. Myeloid-derived suppressor cell membrane-coated magnetic nanoparticles for cancer theranostics by Inducing macrophage polarization and synergizing immunogenic cell death. *Adv. Funct. Mater.* **2018**, *28*, 1801389. [CrossRef]
60. Bu, L.; Rao, L.; Yu, G.; Chen, L.; Deng, W.; Liu, J.; Wu, H.; Meng, Q.; Guo, S.; Zhao, X.; et al. Cancer stem cell-platelet hybrid membrane-coated magnetic nanoparticles for enhanced photothermal therapy of head and neck squamous cell carcinoma. *Adv. Funct. Mater.* **2019**, *29*. [CrossRef]

61. Bao, Y.; Sherwood, J.A.; Sun, Z. Magnetic iron oxide nanoparticles as T_1 contrast agents for magnetic resonance imaging. *J. Mater. Chem. C* **2018**, *6*, 1280–1290. [CrossRef]
62. Lu, Y.; Xu, Y.; Zhang, G.; Ling, D.; Wang, M.; Zhou, Y.; Wu, Y.; Wu, T.; Hackett, M.J.; Hyo Kim, B.; et al. Iron oxide nanoclusters for T1 magnetic resonance imaging of non-human primates. *Nat. Biomed. Eng.* **2017**, *1*, 637–643. [CrossRef]
63. Macher, T.; Totenhagen, J.; Sherwood, J.; Qin, Y.; Gurler, D.; Bolding, M.S.; Bao, Y. Ultrathin iron oxide nanowhiskers as positive contrast agents for magnetic resonance imaging. *Adv. Funct. Mater.* **2015**, *25*, 490–494. [CrossRef]
64. Sherwood, J.; Lovas, K.; Rich, M.; Yin, Q.; Lackey, K.; Bolding, M.S.; Bao, Y. Shape-dependent cellular behaviors and relaxivity of iron oxide-based T-1 MRI contrast agents. *Nanoscale* **2016**, *8*, 17506–17515. [CrossRef]
65. Kostopoulou, A.; Brintakis, K.; Fragogeorgi, E.; Anthousi, A.; Manna, L.; Begin-Colin, S.; Billotey, C.; Ranella, A.; Loudos, G.; Athanassakis, I.; et al. Iron oxide colloidal nanoclusters as theranostic vehicles and their interactions at the cellular level. *Nanomaterials* **2018**, *8*, 315. [CrossRef]
66. Lartigue, L.; Hugounenq, P.; Alloyeau, D.; Clarke, S.P.; Levy, M.; Bacri, J.C.; Bazzi, R.; Brougham, D.F.; Wilhelm, C.; Gazeau, F. Cooperative organization in iron oxide multi-core nanoparticles potentiates their efficiency as heating mediators and MRI contrast agents. *ACS Nano* **2012**, *6*, 10935–10949. [CrossRef]
67. Tang, Y.; Liu, Y.; Li, W.; Xie, Y.; Li, Y.; Wu, J.; Wang, S.; Tian, Y.; Tian, W.; Teng, Z.; et al. Synthesis of sub-100 nm biocompatible superparamagnetic Fe_3O_4 colloidal nanocrystal clusters as contrast agents for magnetic resonance imaging. *RSC Adv.* **2016**, *6*, 62550–62555. [CrossRef]

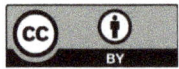

© 2019 by the authors. Licensee MDPI, Basel, Switzerland. This article is an open access article distributed under the terms and conditions of the Creative Commons Attribution (CC BY) license (http://creativecommons.org/licenses/by/4.0/).

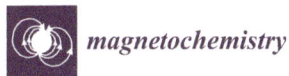

Review

Magnetic Nanoparticle Systems for Nanomedicine—A Materials Science Perspective

Vlad Socoliuc [1], Davide Peddis [2,3], Viktor I. Petrenko [4,5,6], Mikhail V. Avdeev [4], Daniela Susan-Resiga [1,7], Tamas Szabó [8], Rodica Turcu [9], Etelka Tombácz [10,*] and Ladislau Vékás [1,*]

1. Romanian Academy–Timisoara Branch, Center for Fundamental and Advanced Technical Research, Laboratory of Magnetic Fluids, Mihai Viteazu Ave. 24, 300223 Timisoara, Romania; vsocoliuc@gmail.com (V.S.); daniela.resiga@gmail.com (D.S.-R.)
2. Dipartimento di Chimica e Chimica Industriale, Università degli Studi di Genova, Via Dodecaneso 31, 16146 Genova, Italy; davide.peddis@gmail.com
3. Istituto di Struttura della Materia-CNR, 00015 Monterotondo Scalo (RM), Italy
4. Frank Laboratory of Neutron Physics, Joint Institute for Nuclear Research, Joliot-Curie Str. 6, 141980 Dubna, Russia; vip@nf.jinr.ru (V.I.P.); avd@nf.jinr.ru (M.V.A.)
5. BCMaterials, Basque Centre for Materials, Applications and Nanostructures, UPV/EHU Science Park, 48940 Leioa, Spain
6. IKERBASQUE, Basque Foundation for Science, 48013 Bilbao, Spain
7. Faculty of Physics, West University of Timisoara, V. Parvan Ave. 4, 300223 Timisoara, Romania
8. Department of Physical Chemistry and Material Science, University of Szeged, 6720 Szeged, Hungary; sztamas@chem.u-szeged.hu
9. National Institute for Research and Development of Isotopic and Molecular Technologies (INCDTIM), Donat Str. 67-103, 400293 Cluj-Napoca, Romania; rodica.turcu14@gmail.com or rodica.turcu@itim-cj.ro
10. Department of Food Engineering, Faculty of Engineering, University of Szeged, Moszkvai krt. 5-7, H-6725 Szeged, Hungary
* Correspondence: tombacz@chem.u-szeged.hu (E.T.); vekas.ladislau@gmail.com or vekas@acad-tim.tm.edu.ro (L.V.)

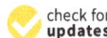

Received: 10 November 2019; Accepted: 19 December 2019; Published: 2 January 2020

Abstract: Iron oxide nanoparticles are the basic components of the most promising magneto-responsive systems for nanomedicine, ranging from drug delivery and imaging to hyperthermia cancer treatment, as well as to rapid point-of-care diagnostic systems with magnetic nanoparticles. Advanced synthesis procedures of single- and multi-core iron-oxide nanoparticles with high magnetic moment and well-defined size and shape, being designed to simultaneously fulfill multiple biomedical functionalities, have been thoroughly evaluated. The review summarizes recent results in manufacturing novel magnetic nanoparticle systems, as well as the use of proper characterization methods that are relevant to the magneto-responsive nature, size range, surface chemistry, structuring behavior, and exploitation conditions of magnetic nanosystems. These refer to particle size, size distribution and aggregation characteristics, zeta potential/surface charge, surface coating, functionalization and catalytic activity, morphology (shape, surface area, surface topology, crystallinity), solubility and stability (e.g., solubility in biological fluids, stability on storage), as well as to DC and AC magnetic properties, particle agglomerates formation, and flow behavior under applied magnetic field (magnetorheology).

Keywords: magnetic nanoparticle systems; bio-ferrofluids; nanomedicine; single core; multi-core; synthesis; functional coating; physical-chemical properties; structural characterization; magnetorheology

1. Magnetism at Nanoscale and Bio-Ferrofluids—A Brief Introduction

Magnetic nanoparticle systems that are relevant for nanomedicine applications [1,2], such as biomedical imaging, magnetically targeted drug delivery, magneto-mechanical actuation of cell surface receptors, magnetic hyperthermia, triggered drug release, and biomarker/cell separation, have some particular features concerning composition, size, morphology, structure, and magnetic behavior, which highly motivated the synthesis, characterization, and post-synthesis application-specific modification of magnetic iron oxide and substituted ferrite nanoparticles [3–10]. These multi-functional magnetoresponsive particles are highly promising in imaging and treating a lesion, simultaneously providing a theranostic approach [11–13]. Microscopic phenomena that are associated with the surface coordination environment, such as canted surface spins, intra- and interparticle interactions (dipolar or exchange, involving surface spins among different particles), and even increased surface anisotropy, which are relevant in improving magnetic field controlled driving and heating, as well as magnetic resonance imaging (MRI) detection, may affect the magnetic behavior of magnetic nanoparticle systems [14,15]. In the case ferrofluids designed for biomedical applications, the magnetic particles dispersed in aqueous carrier involve both single-core and multi-core iron oxide (mainly magnetite and maghemite) nanoparticles (IONPs), consequently *bio-ferrofluids* [16] widely extend the conventional domain of ferrofluids referring only to single core high colloidal stability magnetic nanofluids [17,18].

The interaction of a magnetic nanoparticle (MNP) with an external magnetic field [10] is governed by minimization of the dipole-field interaction energy achieved by the orientation of the particle's magnetic moment parallel to the applied magnetic field [3] and, in case of a non-uniform field, the interaction involves the translation of the particle in the direction of the field gradient, i.e., magnetophoresis [19]. The rotation of the magnetic moment of a particle that is suspended in a liquid carrier can occur either free with respect to the particle (Néel rotation) or together with the particle (Brown rotation) [4,20,21]. The orientation of MNP's magnetic moment in alternating current (AC) magnetic fields shows hysteresis, except for particular situations. The phenomenon of AC magnetic hysteresis is the basis of magnetic particle hyperthermia [21,22] and susceptometric granulometry of single and multicore MNPs [23]. In direct current (DC) magnetic fields, the magnetization of diluted single core particle dispersions follows the Langevin equation, which gives the theoretical framework for the magnetogranulometry of single core particles, due to the permanent magnetic moment of subdomain MNPs [24]. Depending on size, magnetic nanoparticles are subject of various contributions to their anisotropy energy [25–27], influencing the overall magnetic behaviour of the MNP system. The main forms of anisotropy specific to magnetic nanoparticles are summarized in what follows: *(a) Magnetocrystalline Anisotropy:* this property is related to the crystal symmetry and the arrangement of atoms in the crystal lattice. Magneto-crystalline anisotropy can show various symmetries, but uniaxial and cubic forms cover the majority of cases [28,29]. *(b) Magnetostatic anisotropy (shape anisotropy):* this contribution is due to the presence of free magnetic poles on the surface creating a magnetic field inside the system (i.e., demagnetizing field) which is responsible for the magnetostatic energy. Subsequently, for a particle with finite magnetization and non-spherical shape, the magnetostatic energy will be larger for some orientations of the magnetic moments than for others. Thus, the shape determines the magnitude of magnetostatic energy and this type of anisotropy is often called as shape anisotropy [28,30,31]. *(c) Surface anisotropy:* Surface anisotropy, which increases with the increase in surface-to-volume ratio (i.e., a decrease in particle size), gives rise to the lower symmetry of surface atoms with respect to the atoms located within the particle [26,31]. Surface anisotropy is also strictly related to the chemical and/or physical interactions between surface atoms and other chemical species. The coating and functionalization of the nanoparticle surface can induce important modifications in its magnetic properties, referring to the so-called "magnetic dead layer" due to spin-canting [32–34].

Multicore particles have no permanent magnetic moment, provided that the constituent particles are small enough, such that the magnetic dipole-dipole interactions are negligible. The induced (resultant) magnetic moment of multicore particles is parallel to the external magnetic field and it follows the Langevin equation. The multicore particles show magnetic coercivity and remanence due to dipole-dipole interactions if the constituent particles are large, i.e., the anisotropy energy overcomes the thermal energy. The induced magnetic moment of multicore particles at saturation is the sum of the constituent particles' magnetic moments [35]. Many applications of magnetic nanoparticles and nanocomposites in medicine rely on their ability to be manipulated while using magnetic fields. This ability depends on the effectiveness of the magnetophoretic force, being determined by the particle magnetic moment and the field gradient, to fix or to move the particles [19,36,37]. The magnetophoretic force exerted upon single core superparamagnetic nanoparticles is less effective due to their small diameter and magnetic moment implicitly, but, in the case of multicore composites, the resultant field induced magnetic moment is high enough in order to allow magnetic targeting already for moderate values of field intensity and gradient. Multi-core particles with relatively large overall sizes manifest strong magnetic response and, also, preserve the superparamagnetic behavior. Indeed, these multicore composites of sizes well above 20 nm show superparamagnetic properties at room temperature (300 K), while at very low temperature (~2 K) clusters of similar sizes would exhibit typical ferromagnetic hysteresis loops [38]. The particles' magnetic moment is more relevant than mass magnetization in order to assess the magnetic targeting/fixing applicability of magnetic particles [19,39,40].

In this review, we aim to focus on the latest trends in magnetic nanosystem research for nanomedicine applications, involving synthesis, structural, colloidal, magnetic and magnetorheological characterization, as well as demonstrating efficient progress and still existing weaknesses.

2. Designed Synthesis of the Magnetic Core

The preparation of superparamagnetic iron oxide nanoparticles (SPION) dispersions can be approached from two directions [41]: (i) from heterogeneous phases via dispersion (grinding and dispersing solid phase) of iron or iron oxides into aqueous solution and (ii) from homogeneous phases via condensation of precursors from either liquid or gaseous phase [42]. These have recently been called as the top down (mechanical attrition) and bottom up (chemical synthesis) methods of nanoparticle fabrication [43].

The bottom-up synthesis procedures [43–46], for example the coprecipitation of Fe(II) and Fe(III) salts, sol-gel processes, polyol methods, sonolysis [45], thermal decomposition, solvothermal reaction [47], hydrolytic and non-hydrolytic wet chemistry methods [3], liquid phase, polyols, thermal decomposition, microemulsion, and laser evaporation syntheses, biomineralization, [22], are considered to be the most effective ways of fabricating SPIONs. In a recent review [9], referring to the synthesis of shape-controlled magnetic iron oxide nanoparticles, it was emphasized that the nucleation and growth/agglomeration are the main stages in any colloidal or wet chemistry synthesis route. If monodisperse nanoparticles are aimed to be synthesized, the stages should be pulled apart in temperature and time, otherwise the polydisperse system and diverse particle morphology are obtained. For anisometric nanoparticles, like cubes, rods, disks, flowers, and many others, such as hollow spheres, worms, stars, or tetrapods, the growth is the crucial step and the specifically adsorbing ligands are responsible for the final morphology of nanoparticles. Uniform-sized nanoparticles from 3–4 up to 20 nm have been obtained through a seeded growth mechanism. The decomposition of iron stearate at high temperature in the presence of different surfactants allows to synthetize mixed crystals of magnetite and maghemite with sizes between 4 and 28 nm [48]. The synthesis parameters (precursors, additives, and their ratio) and experimental conditions (reaction time, temperature) were changed, and monodisperse, single core (this term was not used in the paper) crystals with different classes of size (e.g., 7–8, 10–11 nm) were made.

The thermal decomposition of organic precursors takes place in the presence of surfactant stabilizers. Nucleation events for the formation of the nanocrystals are controlled and, thus, the size and the use of surfactants allow for monodispersity. In this process, surfactant stabilized hydrophobic particles form that needs further treatments to transfer them into aqueous media. The latter can be achieved by using surfactants (e.g., Na-oleate), forming an oppositely oriented second layer due to hydrophobic interaction with the alkyl chains of first layer chemisorbed on the surface of IONPs [49]. The long-term stability of aqueous magnetic colloids under the effect of magnetic field in biorelevant media has not been evidenced yet [17]. If oleic acid is used in the synthesis, the double bonds of chemisorbed oleate can be oxidized by strong oxidant (e.g., KMnO4 under acidic or alkaline conditions). Azelaic acid forms in an oxidization reaction on the IONPs' surface, and the carboxylated product has good dispersibility in aqueous media [50]. The surfactants with hydrophobic alkyl chains can be replaced by hydrophilic molecules having functional groups (e.g., carboxylic acid, phosphonic acid, aromatic molecules with OH groups in ortho position) that have a higher affinity to ≡Fe-OH sites on IONPs' surface in a ligand-exchange process often used lately [51].

While keeping the superparamagnetic behavior, the synthesis of *multicore* particles proved to be a promising solution for magnetics based imaging, therapeutics, and sensing to improve the manifold magnetic response of particles [40,52–56]. Magnetic nanoparticle clusters embedded in a polymer shell, to sum the magnetic moments of each nanoparticle, were made applying in situ coprecipitation by using gels as microreactors [57,58], and also by strongly polar solvent induced destabilization of a ferrofluid [59]. The miniemulsion technique is also well-established to control clusterization of magnetic nanoparticles [60]. The densely packed magnetic clusters are encapsulated in a polymer shell [61,62]. High magnetization spherical particles in thermoresponsive polymer shell were produced in a ferrofluid miniemulsion procedure [63,64]. Hydrophobic oleic acid coated SPIONs of a light organic carrier (hexane, toluene, tetrahydrofurane) based ferrofluid may also be incorporated into chitosan amphiphile nanoparticles by the ultrasonic emulsification procedure and evaporation of the volatile carrier [65]. The magnetic behavior of nanoparticle assemblies is strongly dependent on interparticle interactions, in particular on dipole-dipole interactions and exchange coupling between surface atoms, with the size and molecular coating of magnetic nanoparticles controlling the resulting arrangements [66].

Various magnetoresponsive nanocomposite particles with adjustable properties (e.g., size, magnetic moment, surface charge, morphology, shell thickness) were synthesized during the last period of time. Figure 1 collects some of these multi-core particles to illustrate the results in the design and manufacture of these magnetic carriers that have to respond to requirements of colloidal stability in aqueous dispersion media, as well as of achievable values of magnetic field strength and gradient. It is essential to ensure high values of the magnetic moment, which is one of the most important requirements, for successful applications in biomedicine of functionalized nanocomposite carriers, in particular in magnetic targeting [19,67,68]. In this respect there are different approaches to distribute a certain amount of magnetic nanoparticles, such as onto the surface of a non-magnetic core [69], or on layered silicate (e.g., montmorillonite) support with high surface area [70], enclosed in a thin vesicle bilayer [71], or close packed to form a magnetic core, the magnetic core-organic shell nanocomposites being favored by their high magnetic response [72]. MNP clusters that are prepared from aqueous [73] and organic [74] ferrofluids can be used to obtain magnetoliposomes [75] with high magnetic response and MRI contrast for in vivo drug and gene delivery into cancer cells. IONPs and anticancer drugs were enclosed into nanocapsules that were designed to be responsive to remote radio frequency (RF) field for ON–OFF switchable drug release [76]. Ferrofluids, as primary materials, provide hydrophobic IONPs to be encapsulated together with camptothecin anticancer drug into PPO (polypropylene oxide) block of Pluronic vesicles. The developed continuous manufacturing procedure is scalable and it provides multi-core theranostic drug delivery vehicles [77].

The usually spherical morphology resulting in oil (ferrofluid)-in-water miniemulsion procedure is modified when the hydrophobic oleic acid coating of MNPs is incomplete and the hydrophobic character of particles significantly reduces. As a consequence, the MNPs accumulate at the ferrofluid drop-water interface, resulting in *strongly non-spherical shape* nanocomposite particles [39]. Magnetic field guided evaporation of ferrofluid droplets [78,79], making use of specific Rosensweig instabilities and tuning the concentration of ferrofluid, allows for preparing various shaped nanocomposites (so-called "supraparticles") and also preserving superparamagnetic behavior. The high evaporation rate organic ferrofluids having oleic acid monolayer coated magnetite NPs were used to fabricate magnetoactive *fibrous nanocomposites* and multi-responsive co-networks [80,81], which exhibit promising characteristics for magnetothermally or pH triggered drug delivery.

More recently *nanoflower type composites* came into the play [82], whose formation is due to exchange interactions between the cores favoring cooperative behavior and a crystal continuity at the core interfaces. The magnetic nanoflowers manifest enhanced susceptibility while maintaining superparamagnetic behavior; their structure (e.g., the contact between cores within a particle, having a strong impact on the collective magnetic properties [83]) critically depends on the synthesis process. Two routes of the latter can be differentiated: the polyol method and thermal decomposition. For example, the 1:2 mixture of Fe(II) and Fe(III) salts was hydrolyzed in organic solvent mixture (diethylene glycol and N-methyldiethanolamine) at high temperature; the clustering and coalescence of seeds took place during the longer period [84]. In this single step process, a big mixture of coalesced flower-like maghemite nanoparticles formed, which was fractionated by increasing salt content of aqueous system at low pH, taking advantage of electrostatic colloidal stability. Figure 2 shows the nanoflowers formed in the one pot synthesis and two fractions selected as examples to distinguish the single and multicore IONPs. Different routes based on the partial oxidation of Fe(OH)$_2$, polyol-mediated synthesis, or the reduction of iron acetylacetonate were used to obtain multicore iron oxide nanoflowers in the size range 25–100 nm [82]. The nanoparticles were either stabilized with well-known agents, such as dextran and citric acid, or, as an alternative, IONPs were embedded in polystyrene to ensure long-term colloidal stability. The first steps toward the standardization of the synthesis and characterization of nanoflowers have been attempted. By now, better quality of magnetite nanoflowers can be also synthesized by thermal decomposition in organic media [25].

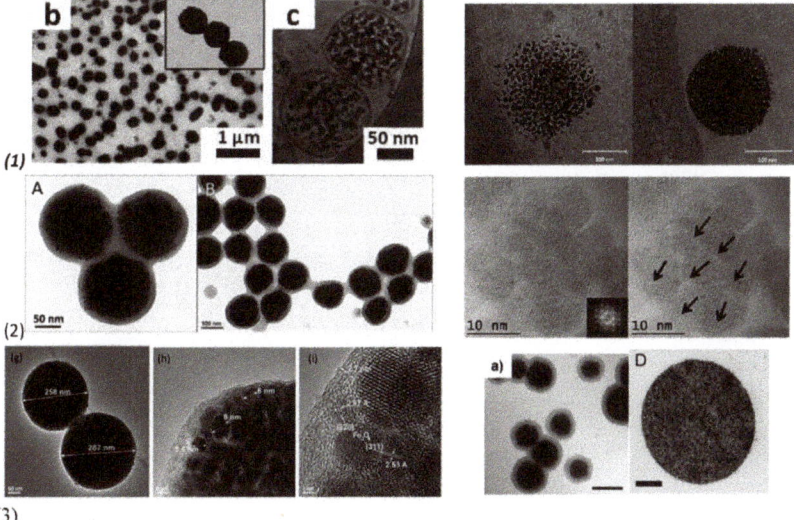

Figure 1. Magnetic multi-core particles obtained by different synthesis procedures: (**1**) *encapsulation of magnetic nanoparticles (MNPs) into liposomes, polymersome*: *left*—TEM (**b**) and cryo-TEM (**c**) micrographs of Ultra Magnetic Liposomes (UMLs) prepared by reverse phase evaporation process (REV) process. MNPs are trapped inside unilamellar vesicles (**c**) and dipole–dipole interaction can occur as exemplified by magnification (**b**) ([73]); *right*—Cryo-TEM image showing iron oxide nanoparticles incorporated in the polymersome membrane with 4.1% iron oxide (left), and 17.4% iron oxide (right) ([77]). (**2**) *thermal decomposition*: *left*—TEM images of polymer encapsulated colloidal ordered assemblies (polymer-COA) at higher (**A**) and lower (**B**) resolution. The dark pattern (**A**) results from the ordering of the closed packed assemblies within the nanobeads, while the brighter gray ring is caused by the polymer shell (lower electron density) of around 20 nm thickness ([59]); *right*—High Resolution TEM of multi-core MNP showing the continuity of the crystal lattice at the grain interfaces. The Fourier transform of this

high resolution image (see inset) shows the monocrystalline fcc structure of the multi-core nanoparticles, oriented along the [001] zone axis ([84]). (3) *miniemulsion*: *left*—TEM images of magnetic microgel with magnetite nanoparticles cluster as a core coated with two layers of cross linked polymer shells poly-N-isopropylacrylamide-polyacrylic acid ([63]); *center*—TEM image of magnetic clusters encapsulated in a copolymer hydrogel poly(N-isopropylacrylamide-acrylic acid). Scale bar: 100 nm ([62]); *right*—TEM image of cross section of superparamagnetic microparticles produced with ferrofluid nanoparticle concentrations of 1 g/L using oil-in water emulsion-templated assembly ([39]). Reprinted with permission from Reference [41].

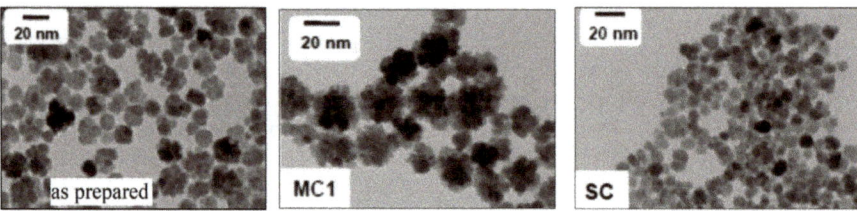

Figure 2. TEM images of the polydisperse mixture of iron oxide nanoparticles (IONPs) (as prepared left side) and its fractions containing multicore (MC1 middle) and single core (SC right side) nanoparticles. Reprinted with permission from Reference [84].

3. Magnetic Nanoparticles in Aqueous Carrier

3.1. Ferrofluids vs. Bioferrofluids

The main distinctive feature of ferrofluids among the larger class of magnetic colloids is their long-term colloidal stability, even in strong and non-uniform magnetic fields specific to most of applications. In the carrier liquid, the overall particle interaction potential should be repulsive, i.e., the attractive van der Waals and magnetic forces have to be balanced by Coulombic, steric or other interactions, in order to keep particles apart from each other [17]. The stabilization of magnetic fluids impeding aggregate formation is more challenging for aqueous than for organic carriers. The necessary increase of magnetic particle concentration also involves an increase of the hydrodynamic volume fraction of surface coated particles determined by the stabilization procedure, electrostatic or electro-steric, which differentiate water-based ferrofluids, to attain high values of saturation magnetization. The steric stabilizing layer (usually a chemisorbed primary and a physisorbed secondary layer of surfactant molecules) has a much greater thickness than the electrostatic one, therefore the hydrodynamic volume fraction at the same magnetic volume fraction is much higher (approx. 7–8 times) for electro-steric (e.g., oleic acid double layer) than for electrostatic stabilized aqueous ferrofluids [85]. The significantly reduced interparticle distance produces colloidal stability issues that involve nanoparticle size and magnetic moment, dipolar interactions, excess surfactant, and agglomerate formation. Ferrofluids designed for biomedical applications—bio-ferrofluids [16]—involve beside single-core particles, a large fraction of multi-core magnetic nanoparticles coated with single or multiple biocompatible surface layers [41], to be discussed in what follows.

3.2. Surface Coating of Magnetic Cores

The surface coating of magnetic iron oxide nanoparticles (IONPs) is inevitable to protect iron leaching, to optimize long term and in-use colloidal stability, to ensure biocompatibility, and to provide specific sites to graft biological functions as well. Therefore, the coating of magnetic nanoparticles should be carefully designed.

The different synthesis methods commonly produce IONP particles that are coated with a protective shell. The preparation of naked IONPs is relatively rare in the literature, probably for the reason that the surface properties of naked IONPs definitely depend on pH and nanoparticles strongly aggregate at neutral pHs, as discussed above [86,87]. The colloidal stability of IONPs under biorelevant conditions, e.g., in blood, at pH~7.4 in physiological salts and protein concentration is the minimum requirement for biomedical applications [71,88]. Therefore, the aggregation of IONPs has to be prevented by protective coating, which can be created either during or after their synthesis. In the literature, in situ coating, post-synthesis adsorption, or post-synthesis grafting are distinguished [68]. In the latter, the functional groups of brush-like polymer chains are anchored to the IONP's surface. Covalently bound molecules can more improve colloidal stability than adsorbed ones, as demonstrated, for example, in the work of Rinaldi and co-authors [89,90]. However, a great disadvantage of the former is the expensive purification process to remove impurities from organic synthesis to reduce the chemical hazard of the formulation. The multipoint adsorption of polyelectrolytes, especially natural polysaccharides, such as chondroitin-sulfate-A (CSA) bound chemically to ≡Fe-OH surface sites of IONPs, is suitable for fabricating biocompatible magnetic fluid (MF) and magnetoresponsive nanocomposites [91–94]. Biopolymer coated magnetite nanoparticles fulfill all assumption of biomedical application, as shown in Figure 3.

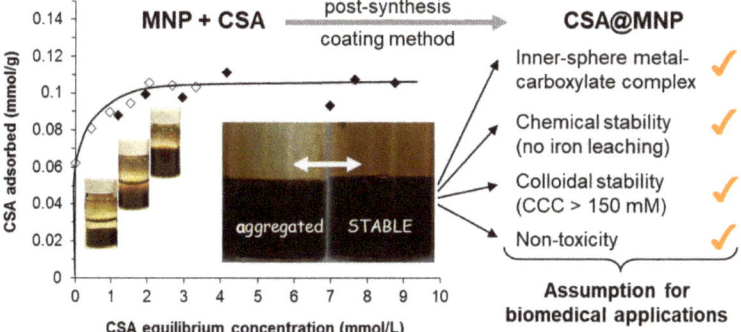

Figure 3. Adsorption isotherm of chondroitin-sulfate-A (CSA) on magnetite nanoparticles (MNP) at pH ~6.3 in aqueous NaCl solution (left side). With increasing CSA concentration, the colloidal state of samples changes characteristically from aggregated to stable, as seen in the vials. The inserted larger photos clearly show the difference between the well stabilized and aggregated magnetic fluids (the amount of CSA is expressed through the number of repeating units in mmol.) Some assumptions of biomedical application are listed in the right side of figure. Reprinted from Reference [94] under the terms of CC by 4.0.

In the literature, the biomedical use of citric acid stabilized IONPs is favored (e.g., the famous VSOP-C184 product) in [45,95,96] or of the multi-core samples in [97]). However, the citrated IONPs coagulate, even at low salt concentration and, moreover, their iron leaching is very high because citric acid has a reducing effect, and it forms complexes with the surface Fe ions [98]; the dissolved iron ions may cause oxidative stress besides the danger of particle aggregation in vivo. Amstad and coworkers [71] reported a similar iron dissolution effect of catechol derivatives (e.g., mimosine) grafted to Fe_3O_4 surfaces, causing the gradual dissolution of Fe_3O_4 nanoparticles through complexation. The other key point is the formation of protein corona of MNPs in biological fluids [99]. Up to now, the coating IONPs with hydrophilic agents is the most widely accepted method for overcoming this problem. Polyethylene oxides or glycols (PEG) and carbohydrates like dextran [3,71] or carbohydrate derivatives (such as mannose, ribose, and rhamnose) [84,100] are the most common of many coating agents, which are chemically bound to the ≡Fe-OH surface sites or by multiple H-bonds, and make IONPs super hydrophilic, inhibiting the adsorption of proteins. However, the formation of protein corona on MNPs covered with dextran and its derivatives has been perceived [101]. Other types of PEG coating on IONPs (grafting with poly(ethylene glycol)-silane [90] or in situ forming in the poly(ethylene glycol) and poly(ethylene imine) mixture [102]), i.e., the PEGylation can generally improve the drug delivery, enhance the drug accumulation, and might improve the blood-brain barrier transport of

IONPs [68]. A new design of PEGylated coating (P(PEGMA-co-AA)@MNPs) provides a non-fouling outer surface that helps the nanoparticles to remain "invisible" for the phagocytic mechanisms, while its free carboxylate moieties can be exploited for grafting specific biologically active molecules or proteins for theranostic applications [103].

Using the synthesis procedure of carboxylic (lauric, myristic or oleic) acid stabilized aqueous ferrofluids [49,104], bovine serum albumin (BSA) coating was applied to rise the colloidal stability of lauric acid-coated IONPs in biological media [105]. The coating greatly reduced the toxicity of nanoparticles and enhanced therapeutic potential of mitoxantrone drug-loaded system. Further cross-linking of BSA coating was performed in order to improve colloidal stability [106], and monoclonal antibodies were covalently bound to BSA coated IONPs promising MRI contrast agents for glioma visualization in brain.

Nanoparticles interact with biological entities in a biological environment, and nano-bio interfaces form [107]. Only the particle surface can be modified to improve in vivo biocompatibility of nanoparticles. Seeing this issue, the size, the sign, and magnitude of surface charge (as manifested in the measurable zeta potential) and dispersibility in aqueous media (hydrophilic/hydrophobic feature) are the main options for change. Experiments have already shown that positively charged particles are probably more toxic than the larger hydrophobic ones clearing rapidly in the reticuloendothelial (RES) system. In biological systems, medium-sized particles with a neutral or weakly negatively charged surface generally tend to promote enhanced permeation and retention (EPR) [107].

A new generation of coating agents P(PEGMA-co-AA), which combine charged functional groups (i.e., carboxyl groups that are capable of anchoring both nanoparticles and bioactive molecules) and superhydrophilic uncharged segments (i.e., PEG chains in comb-like arrangement) has been reported last year [103]. In a post-coating process, these multifunctional molecules are able to spontaneously bind to MNPs' surface sites ≡Fe-OH; stabilize the particles electrostatically via the carboxylate moieties and sterically via the PEG moieties; provide high protein repellency via the structured PEG layer; and, anchor bioactive molecules via chemical bond formation with the free carboxylate groups. The electrosteric (i.e., combined electrostatic and steric) stabilization is efficient down to pH 4 and it tolerates saline media.

In biomedical applications, an optimized coating on SPION surface is required, via which IONPs can interact with different biological entities (proteins, cell membranes, etc.). Only the coating on the engineered NPs can be freely varied at the nanobio interface. The core of nanoparticles has almost all of the desired properties, such as chemical composition, shape and curvature, porosity and surface crystallinity, heterogeneity, and roughness, as listed by Nel and coworkers [107]. The coating layer of core-shell nanosystems provides optimal hydrophobicity/hydrophilicity in a given medium and active sites for anchoring biofunctions. In the same article, the other quantifiable properties of NPs' interactions (dissolution, hydration, zeta potential, aggregation/dispersion, etc.), which are crucially influenced by the ionic strength, pH, temperature, and the presence of large organic molecules (e.g., proteins), or specifically adsorbing molecules or ions (e.g., detergents generally or phosphate ions) of the suspending media, are separately discussed. The composition and structure of interfacial layer on coated NPs, as well as its changes on the nanoscale, definitely affect the microscale and more the macroscale behavior of engineered nanoparticles. The quality of coating interrelates with colloidal stability under biorelevant conditions, as described in [108]. Sedimentation, freezing, and hemocompatibility tests (smears) are recommended for the qualification of good and bad SPION manufacturing for intravenous administration. Besides the colloidal stability of nanosystems, coatings also largely affect the functionality and biological fate of IONPs. Several different functions of NPs' coating can be identified, namely: (i) colloidal stabilization under physiological conditions (protecting against aggregation at biological pHs and salty medium), (ii) inhibiting the corrosion and oxidation of magnetic core (passivation reducing the iron leakage), (iii) hindering non-specific protein adsorption in biological milieu, (iv) providing reactive groups for anchoring drugs and targeting molecules, and (v) controlling nano-bio interfacial interactions (bio/hemocompatibility, reticuloendothelial system

(RES) uptake, blood circulation time, IONP's internalization efficiency, toxicity, targeting efficiency, in vivo fate, etc., as discussed in detail [3,41,68,71,107]). These functions of coating largely overlap with the general concerns of EMA (European Medicines Agency) [109] that should be considered in the development of nanomedicine products.

3.3. Stabilization Mechanisms

The dispersed nanoparticles move freely (thermal motion) in the carrier medium. The colloidal stability of dispersion is the question, whether nanoparticles can retain their separateness during collisions; i.e., whether the particle-particle interactions that are controlled by the frequency and efficiency of collision result in aggregate or not. The latter depends on the extent of attractive and repulsive contributions to the total interaction. The classical DLVO theory of colloidal stability describes the attractive (van der Waals) and repulsive (electrostatic) forces. In addition to these, the hydration, the hydrophobic interactions, and the steric hindrance should be also assessed [110,111]. In the case of magnetic particles, besides the short range exchange interaction especially relevant to formation of multi-core particles, such as nanoflowers [83], the magnetic dipole attraction having a fundamental effect on the collective magnetic properties must also be taken into account [112] to obtain reasonable theoretical stability predictions [90]. In these papers particle aggregation is used as a generic term for coagulation and flocculation independently of the inner structure of aggregates and the reversibility of their formation. Another term, agglomeration, has appeared in the relevant literature, with the same or different meanings as aggregation. Gutiérrez and coworkers [83] reviewed the aggregation of magnetic iron oxide colloids and definitely stated that "nanoparticles tend to form assemblies, either aggregates, if the union is permanent, or agglomerates, if it is reversible", recalling a bit industrial terminology or that used in nanotechnology nowadays. However, there are certain inconsistencies with the classical colloid nomenclature (e.g., in refs. [110,111]), where aggregation involves coagulation and flocculation giving rise to compact and loose structures, respectively. Their reversibility depends on the magnitude of mechanical force against they should exist. For example, coagulum, the aggregate that forms in the coagulation process, is irreversible against thermal motion; however, it disintegrates when subjected to stronger shaking, stirring, or even mild ultrasonication, and, after this, coagulation restarts at rest, so its formation is reversible [111].

In [113], it was emphasized that nanomaterials should be characterized in the relevant medium, and not simply in water, especially in what concerns aggregation (agglomeration) processes. Referring to coagulation kinetics, IONPs' colloidal stability should be acceptable under biorelevant conditions, i.e., at biological pH values, in the presence of salt and proteins, and also in cell culture media. In classical colloid science, coagulation kinetics can correctly characterize colloidal stability, also allowing for predicting the stability of SPIONs' products both on storage and in use. However, the measurements require advanced instrumentation and a lot of time, thus a simpler method would be needed to test SPION preparations [108]. Particle aggregation tests (size evolution, filtration, sedimentation, etc.) under arbitrary conditions are often used [71]. Coagulation kinetics is useful for testing the salt tolerance of IONPs and predicting their resistance against aggregation under physiological condition [87]. A straightforward route of physicochemical (iron dissolution) and colloidal (pH-dependent charging and particle size, salt tolerance from coagulation kinetics) measurements was suggested for assessing the eligibility of IONPs for in vitro and in vivo tests [98].

4. Physical-Chemical Characterization

4.1. Chemical Composition of Magnetic Nanoparticles

X-ray Photoelectron Spectroscopy (XPS) is a very sensitive surface analysis method for the materials chemical composition. The method allows for the determination of the atomic concentrations, the chemical state of the emitting atoms (oxidation degree, valence states, chemical ligands, etc.). This information results from the areas delimited by the photoelectron peaks and from the chemical shifts of the peaks with respect to the elemental state, as induced by the chemical surrounding of the atoms. The electrostatic interaction between the nucleus and the electrons determine the core binding energies of the electrons. The electrostatic shielding of the nuclear charge from all other electrons in the atom reduces this interaction. The removal or addition of electronic charge will alter the shielding: withdrawal of valence electron charge (oxidation) increase in binding energy; addition of valence electron charge decrease in binding energy. Chemical changes can be identified in the photoelectron spectra.

In the case of magnetic nanoparticles, surface properties strongly influence their magnetic performance and their behavior in biological media. The core-shell type magnetic nanoparticle systems consist of the magnetic core and a shell around the core, usually a biocompatible polymer and additionally molecules fulfilling the roles of anchors, spacers, and various functionalities. XPS provides information regarding the chemical composition of the coating layers and, on the other hand, allow for determining the oxidation state of the metal in the magnetic core [63,114–117]. XPS allows for determining the oxidation states of iron and to quantify Fe^{2+} and Fe^{3+} ions in iron oxide nanoparticles. These oxidation states of iron can be determined by Fe2p spectrum employing chemical shift and multiplet splitting and the characteristic satellites [85,118–122].

The organic coating layers of magnetic nanoparticles have major importance for biomedical applications of these nanomaterials. Coating layers ensures the chemical and colloidal stability of magnetic nanoparticles and allow for further functionalization [122–124]. Surface functionalization of magnetic nanoparticles for biomedical applications remains a major challenge. XPS is one of the most appropriate methods for the analysis of the functionalized organic coating of magnetic nanoparticles. The optimization of the required properties for applications requires understanding the nature of the interface between the magnetic core and the shell and the influence of the surface complex formation on the nanoparticle's magnetic properties.

Mazur and coworkers reported a good strategy for surface functionalization of magnetic nanoparticles allowing for the simultaneous attachment of dopamine anchors bearing azide, maleimide, and alkyne terminal groups [125] (Figure 4). This functionalization strategy of nanoparticles by using dopamine derivatives shells has the advantage that, besides the protection of the iron oxide core offering the possibility to integrate in a one-step reaction several reactive sites onto the nanoparticles, making these functionalized nanoparticles very promising for biomedical applications.

XPS allows for a detailed analysis of surface chemical composition of iron oxide nanoparticles before and after functionalization with dopamine derivatives (Figures 5 and 6).

The ratio Fe/O = 0.73 was calculated from XPS spectra, which is in-between that of Fe_3O_4 (0.75) and Fe_2O_3 (0.66). This fact and the peak position and satellite peaks in Fe2p spectrum indicate that the magnetic core contains Fe_3O_4 and Fe_2O_3. The presence of dopamine derivatives shells on the magnetic core was evidenced in the high resolution spectra of N1s and C1s core level spectra. The deconvoluted N1s spectra of Fe_3O_4 that were coated with dopamine derivatives (Figure 6) evidence the characteristic groups of the organic shells. The calculated atomic ratio C/N is a good estimation for the success of the organic coating on magnetic nanoparticles. The XPS spectra and the calculated atomic concentrations for the elements C, O, N, and Fe evidence the coating of the magnetic nanoparticles with dopamine derivatives.

The coating layers largely influence the colloidal stability of magnetic nanoparticles under physiological conditions [3,68,71,107]. The protein corona's effect differs significantly, depending on the surface chemistry of the nanoparticles. The surface chemistry strongly influences the formation of protein corona and the cellular uptake of the nanoparticles. Differences in protein corona formation have been observed for magnetic nanoparticles coated by different organic layers [126,127]. Szekeres et al. undertook a comparative study of the effect of protein corona formation on the colloidal stability of magnetic nanoparticles coated by polyelectrolyte shells, citrate (CA@MNP), and poly(acrylic-co-maleic acid) (PAM@MNP) [128]. PAM coating of MNP ensures a better stability at higher human plasma concentrations as compared with CA coated MNP. XPS determined the chemical composition (atomic concentrations), as well as the chemical state of the atoms at the surface magnetic nanoparticles CA@MNP and PAM@MNP. The relevant differences between the nanoparticles CA@MNP and PAM@MNP can be observed in the XPS spectra for C1s core levels (Figure 7). Both spectra of C1s contain the carboxylic groups and in the case of CA@MNP the C-OH group appears according to the characteristic coating shells.

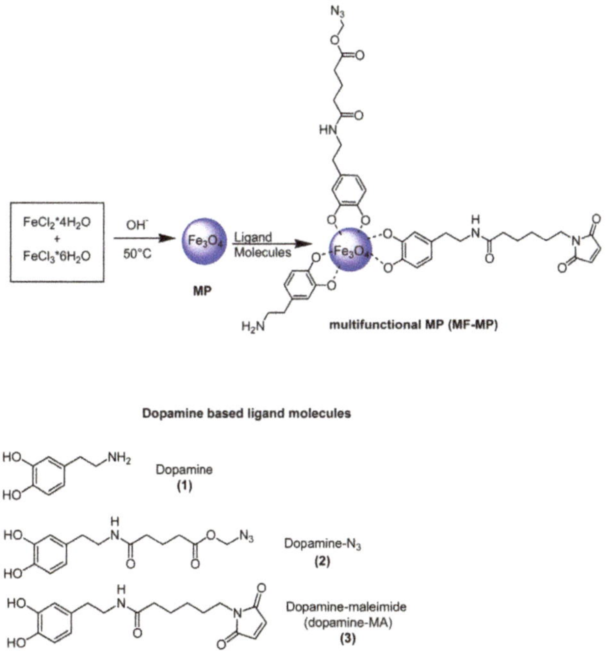

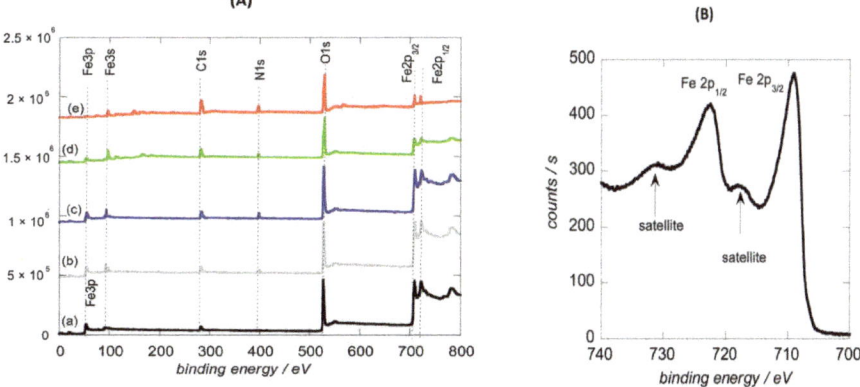

Figure 4. Schematic illustration of the formation of magnetic fluid-multifunctional magnetic nanoparticles (MF-MPs) based on the use of differently functionalized dopamine derivatives. Reprinted with permission from Reference [125].

Figure 5. (A) X-ray Photoelectron Spectroscopy (XPS) survey spectra of as prepared magnetic particles before (a, black) and after modification with dopamine (b, grey), dopamine-N3 (c, blue), dopamine-MA (d, green), and of MF-MP (e, red). (B) High resolution Fe2p spectrum of as-synthesized magnetic particles. Reprinted with permission from Reference [125].

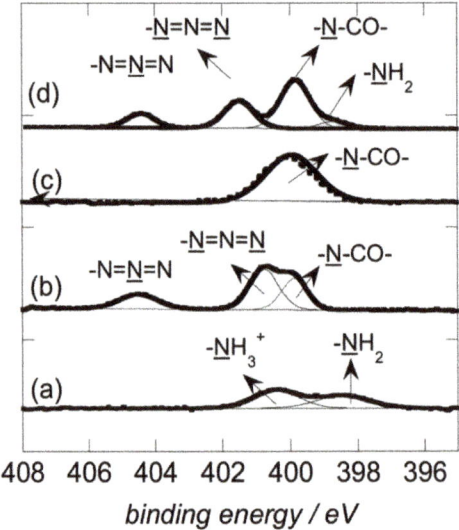

Figure 6. XPS N1s high resolution spectrum of magnetic particles modified with dopamine (**a**), dopamine-N3 (**b**), dopamine-MA (**c**), and MF-MPs (**d**). Reprinted with permission from Reference [125].

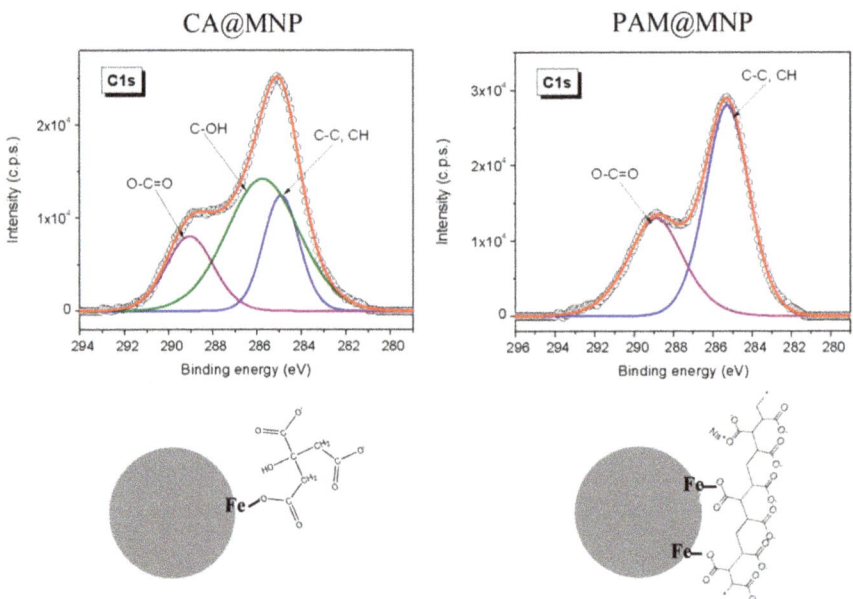

Figure 7. C1s spectra of the core-shell MNPs and the schemes of Fe–O–C(O)–R binding between MNP iron sites and organic carboxylates. Peak positions for CA and PAM coated MNPs: C-C, CH 284.91 and 285.27 eV; O–C=O 289.05 and 288.9 eV, respectively, and C-OH 285.75 eV for CA@MNP. Reprinted with permission from Reference [128].

4.2. Colloidal Stability. Zeta Potential and Hydrodynamic Size

The electrosteric (electrostatic+steric) stabilization has been shown to be quite effective; for example, polyelectrolyte (polyacrylic or polylactic acid, polyethylenimine, etc.) coating on IONPs provides excellent stability [108]. However, outstanding salt tolerance can be achieved through hydrophilic polymer coating, such as dextran, a polysaccharide, which is used commonly in aqueous magnetic fluids [68,95,129]. Silica materials [130], organic molecules (e.g., carboxylates, phosphates, phosphonate, sulfates, amines, alcohols, thiols, etc. [68,88,95]) are often applied as coating agents to ensure colloidal stability. The functional groups of organic agents are mostly chemically bound to the reactive (both charged and uncharged) sites on IONPs' surface. For example, citrate through its OH and COOH groups are chemically linked to ≡Fe-OH sites in the citrated-electrostatic stabilized-magnetic fluids [98] or dopamine by two phenolic OH groups in the favored core-shell products [71,95]). The effect of surface coverage is hardly studied. IONP dispersions coagulate at a pH below PZC (point of zero charge), if polyacids, such as polyacrylic acid, are present in trace amounts, while their higher loading covers completely IONPs' surface and improves the stability and salt tolerance of colloidal iron oxide dispersions [68,131]. Macromolecules adsorb at multiple sites of surface, the so-called multi-site bonding makes the coating layer resistant against dilution and the purification of equilibrium medium easy [110,132].

To illustrate the significance of the stabilization mechanism applied-electrostatic or electrosteric-the zeta potentials and hydrodynamic sizes were measured for citrate and oleate stabilized aqueous ferrofluid samples and are given in Figure 8 to show the characteristic pH-dependence due to the different dissociation behaviors of the acidic groups on the coating molecules [85].

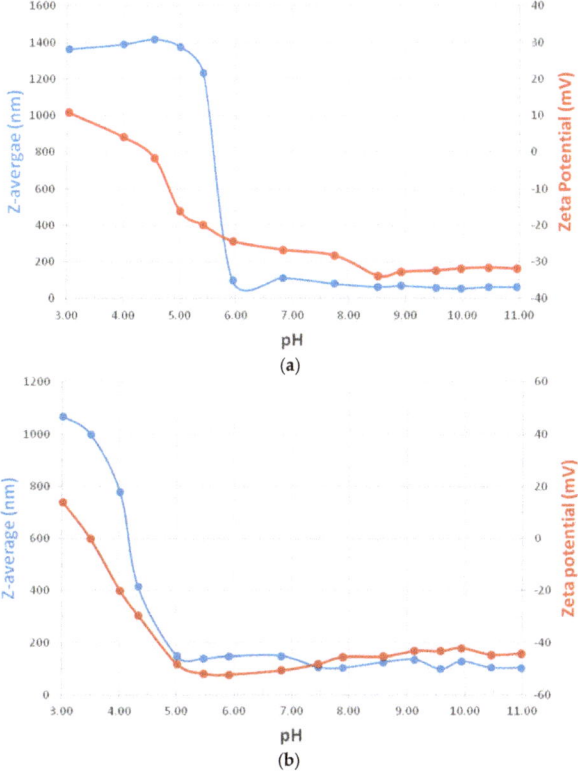

Figure 8. (a) pH dependence of the Z-average particle diameter (blue) and the zeta potential (red) for the citrated (MF/CA) sample. (b) pH dependence of the Z-average particle diameter (blue) and the zeta potential (red) for the oleic acid double layer stabilized (MF/OA) sample. Reprinted with permission from Reference [85].

The MF/CA sample loses colloidal stability below pH6 (Figure 8a) due to the difference in the charged state of citrated and oleic acid double layer coated MNPs, while the MF/OA ferrofluid below pH5 (Figure 8). This behavior is explained by the different dissociability values for citric acid (pKa1 = 3.13, pKa2 = 4.76, and pKa3 = 6.40) and oleic acid (pKa = 5.02). Additionally, from Figure 8a,b, it follows that over a broad range of pH values, where both type of samples are stable, the citrate covered particles have a smaller Z-average diameter than the oleic acid covered nanoparticles.

4.3. Magnetic Properties

The magnetic field dependence of the magnetization, i.e., the magnetization curve, provides information regarding the magnetic properties of single and multicore magnetic nanoparticle systems. The magnetization of single and multicore magnetic nanoparticle systems is conditioned by the magnetic relaxation processes that are specific to the composition, dimension, morphology, etc., as well as external conditions, like temperature.

The direct current (DC) magnetometry is the most frequently used magnetic characterization method. The DC magnetization can be measured by means of vibrating sample magnetometry (VSM), alternative gradient magnetometry (AGM), and superconducting quantum interference device (SQUID). Important characteristics of the sample can be directly obtained from the magnetization curve: initial susceptibility (χ_i), saturation magnetization (M_s), coercive field (H_c), and remanent magnetization (M_r). In the case of superparamagnetic systems, the DC first magnetization curve can be used to determine the statistic of the nanoparticles' magnetic diameter by means of magnetogranulometry [133]. Figure 9 presents the DC magnetization curve and the theoretical fit [24] for a sample of dried magnetic microgels with magnetite nanoparticles [35]. The inset of Figure 9 shows the nanoparticle size distributions that were obtained from magnetogranulometry and TEM.

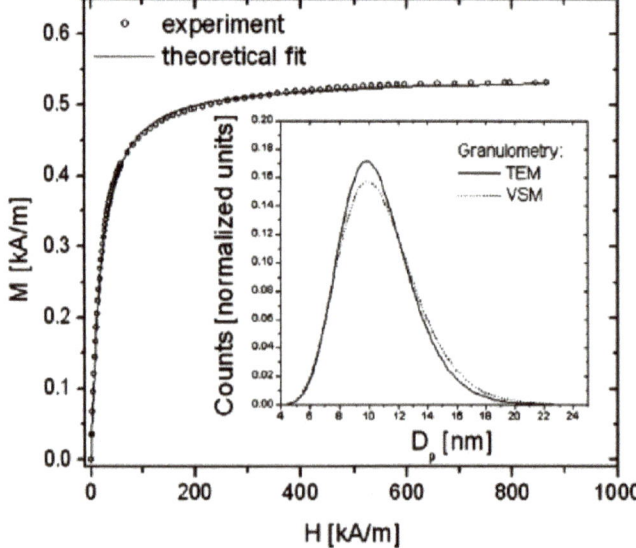

Figure 9. Direct current (DC) magnetization curve and the theoretical fit for a sample of dried magnetic microgels with magnetite nanoparticles. Reprinted with permission from Reference [35].

Several groups recently developed AC magnetometry [134,135] with the aim of determining the hysteresis loss in magnetic nanoparticles used in magnetic hyperthermia applications. The method is generally useful for characterizing the magnetic dynamic response of single and multicore magnetic nanoparticle systems at low and high frequencies in the range 1 kHz–1 MHz. Figure 10 presents the frequency dependent dynamic response for 9 nm (Sample I—Figure 10a) and 21 nm (Sample II—Figure 10b) iron oxide nanoparticles, respectively [134]. The hysteretic loss is significantly larger in the bigger diameter nanoparticle sample.

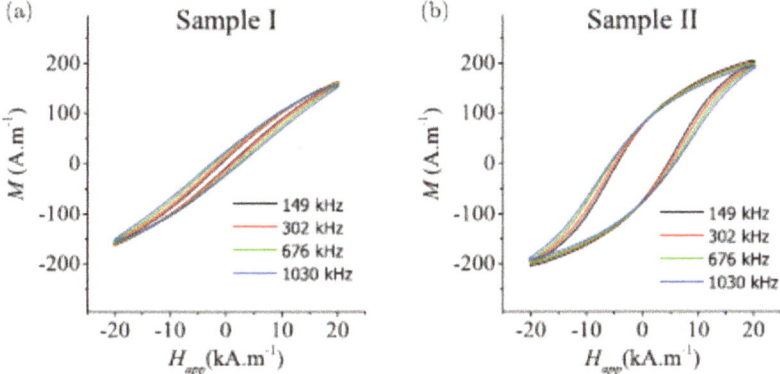

Figure 10. Dynamic hysteresis at different magnetic field frequencies for two iron oxide nanoparticle diameters: (**a**) Sample I 9 nm and (**b**) Sample II 21 nm. Reprinted with permission from Reference [134].

AC susceptometry measures the frequency dependence of the real and imaginary part of the magnetic susceptibility [133]. AC susceptometry is sensitive to the colloidal state of the magnetic nanoparticle dispersion, apart from being useful for the characterization of the relaxation mechanisms of the magnetic moment at the nanoscale. Figure 11a presents the frequency dependence of the normalized components of the complex susceptibility of a ferrofluid sample at different moments of the phase separation process [136]. Figure 11b shows the phase separation in a 10 mT DC field. Thus, it is shown the nontrivial influence of the magnetically induced phase separation on the complex susceptibility spectrum of ferrofluids.

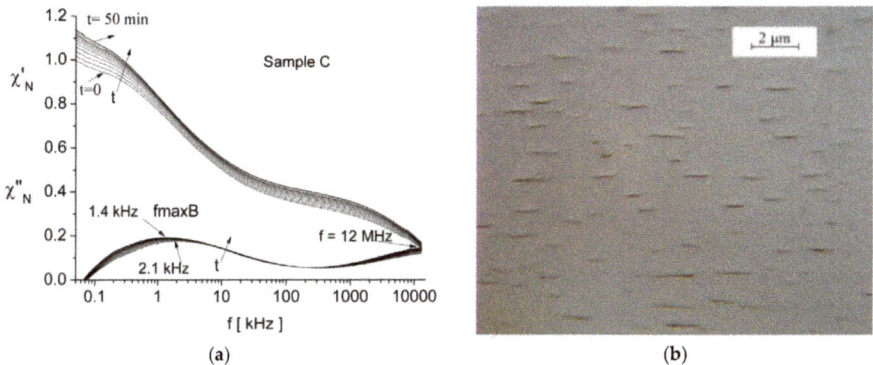

Figure 11. (**a**) Frequency dependence of the normalized components of the complex susceptibility of a ferrofluid sample and (**b**) optical microscopy image of magnetically induced phase separation. Reprinted with permission from Reference [136].

ZFC-FC measurements can characterize the superparamagnetic state of magnetic nanoparticles either isolated or in multi core environments [133]. The sample is cooled down from the superparamagnetic state to the lowest achievable temperature and the magnetization is measured while heating up the sample in an ~100 Oe applied field (ZFC) and afterwards the magnetization is measured while cooling the sample down again under the same applied field (FC).

4.4. Structural Characterization of Magnetic Colloids by Scattering Techniques

4.4.1. Neutron and X-ray Scattering

Scattering methods (neutron or X-rays) are powerful techniques for structural characterization at the nanoscale and contribute much to the development of nanomaterials. It is well known that the properties of the systems containing nanoparticles, such as liquid dispersions, are strongly related to the shape and size of the nanoparticle. Thus, systematic studies of these structural and morphological characteristics are required. Nowadays, small-angle scattering (SAS) and reflectometry are widely applied for nanostructure characterization in bulk and at interfaces, respectively. The main difference between neutron and X-ray scattering is the sensitivity to various chemical elements and their spatial distributions. The sensitivity to magnetic structures in the objects under study is an additional possibility for neutron scattering.

In the course of the SAS experiment, the widening of the neutron or X-ray beam that passed through the sample is analyzed in terms of the differential scattering cross-section per sample volume as a function of scattering vector module. Such dependence is quite sensitive to structural features of the studied systems at the scale interval of 1–300 nm [137], which makes SAS an ideal tool for the structural characterization of ferrofluids [138–140], since the size of particles in them are mostly in this dimensional range. Specific techniques, such as contrast variation and scattering of polarized neutrons, are used in small-angle neutron scattering investigations. From small-angle neutron (SANS) and X-ray (SAXS) scattering, it is possible to derive information regarding particle structure (size, polydispersity, stabilizing shell thickness, composition of particle's core and shell, solvent rate penetration in surfactant layer, structure of possible micelles in solutions), magnetic structure (magnetic size and composition), particle interaction (interparticle potential, magnetic moment correlation, phase separation), and cluster formation (developed aggregation and chain formation). The main task of the SAS experiment is to find out the distribution of scattering length density (SLD), which is defined as a specific sum of the coherent scattering lengths of atoms in a sufficiently small volume and it is usually represented in units of 10^{10} cm^{-2}.

Studying the reflectivity of the radiation (neutrons or X-rays) from planar surfaces is the basic idea of the reflectometry method [141]. The classical analysis of specular reflectivity allows one to determine an SLD profile (thickness, density, and roughness of each layer at interfaces) for the studied object in a direction perpendicular to the interface for a thickness up to hundreds nm with a resolution of 1 nm. The analysis of off-specular (diffuse) neutron scattering makes it possible to characterize lateral correlations on the surface and interlayer boundaries. It should be noted that the active use of the reflectometry method for investigations of ferrofluid structures at interfaces was started about a decade ago (e.g., [142]).

The structural features of several kinds of aqueous magnetic fluids [143–146], as well as surfactant/polymer solutions [147–149], which are used for magnetic nanoparticle stabilization in water, were investigated in detail by SANS (Figures 12 and 13). Additionally, magnetic nanoparticles with bio-macromolecules were successfully studied by SANS and SAXS [150,151] (Figure 14). Thus, investigations of magnetic fluid stability at various amounts of surfactants and aggregation of MNPs were undertaken by SAS for ferrofluids based on non-polar and polar (aqueous) carriers. For water-based ferrofluids with sterical/charge stabilization (double-layer coating of magnetite nanoparticles by sodium oleate (SO) or dodecylbenzene sulfonic acid (DBSA)), the fraction of micelles of formed by non-adsorbed surfactant molecules was found by SANS (Figure 12). It was shown that the different rate of surfactant adsorption on the particle surface depends on the surfactant type. The aggregate reorganization and growth in ferrofluids after 'PEGylation' [145] were observed (Figure 13). The SANS study was performed on mixed SO/polyethylene glycol (PEG) aqueous solutions in order to check the influence of a polymer additive on the surfactants behavior. SANS results revealed drastic morphological and interacting changes of micelles, due to the addition of PEG.

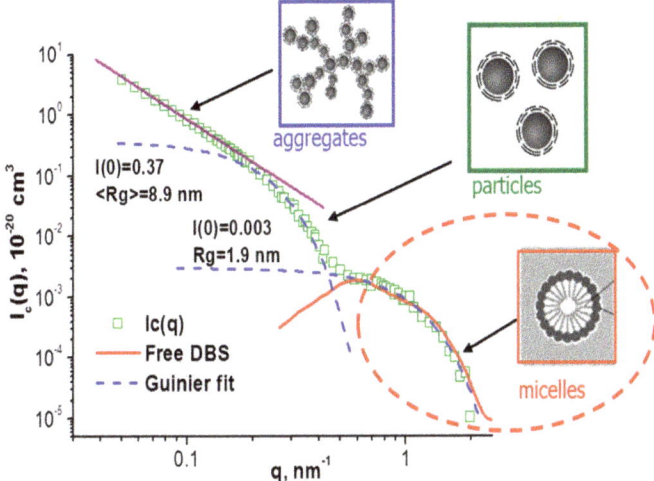

Figure 12. Complex structure of water-based ferrofluids with surfactant excess in its. Reprinted with permission from Reference [152].

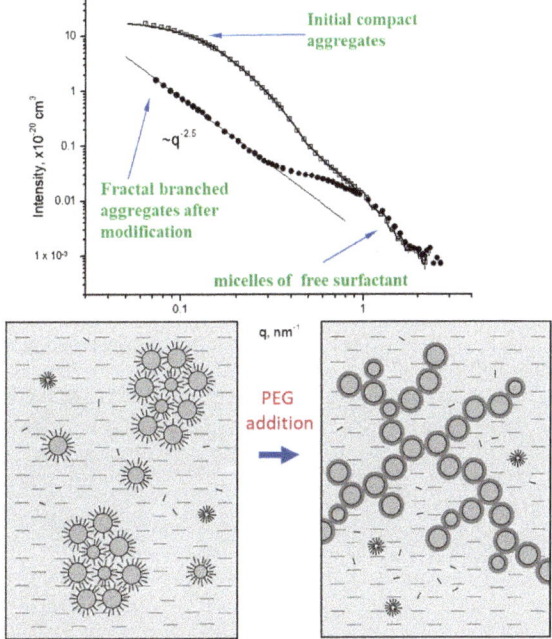

Figure 13. Ferrofluids with surfactant-polymer substitution: Change in aggregate structure according to small-angle neutron (SANS) analysis. SANS signals from different components in the solution were marked by arrows. Reprinted with permission from Reference [145] (https://journals.iucr.org/).

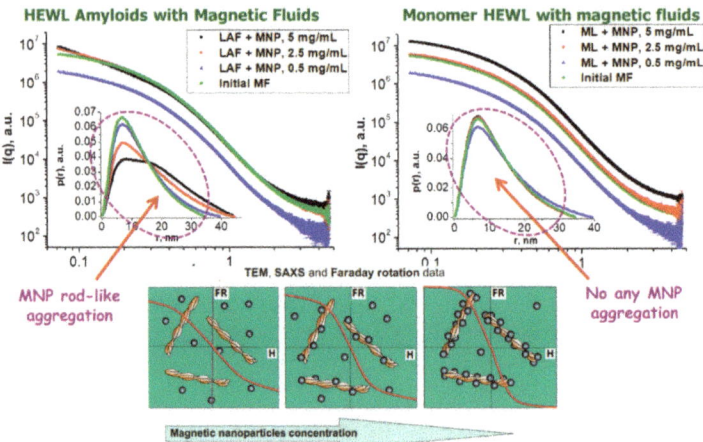

Figure 14. Behavior of magnetic nanoparticles in complex solutions of MNPs with amyloids (left) and with native (not aggregated) protein (right) according to small-angle X-ray scattering (SAXS) data. It's also shown formation of some rod-like aggregates in solutions of MNPs with amyloids and there is no any change in MNPs solutions with native protein at various MNPs concentrations. Sketch of the found adsorption of MNPs on amyloids surface with increase of MNPs concentration according to TEM, SAXS and optical (Faraday rotation) results (bottom). Reprinted with permission from Reference [151].

Neutron reflectometry used to obtain the SLD depth profiles investigated the assembly of magnetite nanoparticles in aqueous magnetic fluids close to a solid (silicon) surface under different external conditions (shear, magnetic field, etc.) [153–156]. The adsorption of surfactant coated magnetic nanoparticles from highly stable magnetic fluids on crystalline functionalized silicon was revealed from the specular reflectivity curves (Figure 15). The detailed analysis of the polarized neutron reflectometry data, together with SANS data, made it possible to obtain the magnetization depth profile and dependence of the resultant magnetic structure on the applied fields, including the distribution of NPs within the adsorption layer. Additionally, the impact of the solvent polarity, as well as bulk structure of ferrofluids, including particle concentration and particle geometry on the structural characteristics of the adsorption layer from magnetic fluids, was considered (Figure 15). The width of the adsorption layer is consistent with the size of single particles, thus showing the preferable adsorption of non-aggregated particles, in spite of the existing aggregate fraction in aqueous magnetic fluids. In the case of PEG-modified ferrofluids, the reorganization of MNP aggregates was observed, which correlates with the changes in the neutron reflectivity. It follows that the single adsorption layer of individual nanoparticles on the oxidized silicon surface for the initial magnetic fluids disappears after PEG modification. Consequently, in case of PEG modified magnetic fluid, all of the particles are in aggregates that are not adsorbed by silicon (Figure 15).

A comprehensive comparative study by small-angle neutron and X-ray scattering (SAXS and SANS) of water-based magnetic fluids with two different stabilization mechanisms—electrostatic (with citric acid (CA) Figure 16) and electro-steric (with oleic acid (OA) double layer; Figure 17)–over a large concentration range up to 30% hydrodynamic volume fraction, identified important differences on the microscopic level for these colloidal systems, as evidenced by the scattering curves in Figures 16 and 17. The electrostatic stabilization ensured high colloidal stability up to the highest magnetization 78.20 kA/m, while the electro-steric stabilized samples already show relatively large agglomerates at reduced volume fraction values [85].

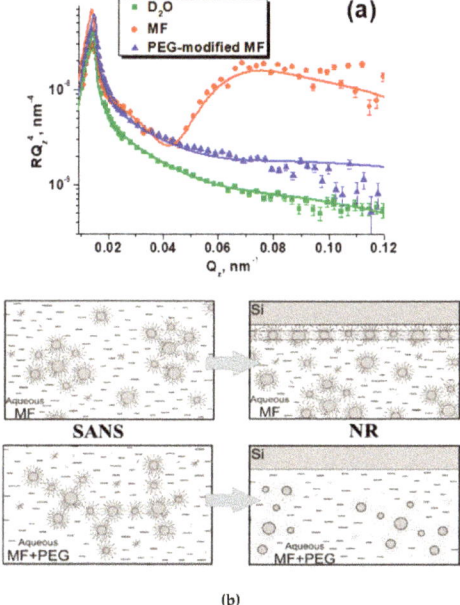

Figure 15. (a) Neutron reflectometry data for initial aqueous ferrofluids, PEG-modified ferrofluids and just buffer (D2O) at interface with solid (Si). It could be seen that reflectivity curves for PEG-modified ferrofluids and just carrier (D2O) are very similar and indicates on the absence of any nanoscale layer at interface. (b) Correlation between bulk structure of ferrofluids according to SANS and at interface ferrofluids/solid according to neutron reflectometry investigations. It is shown that there is no any adsorption of MNPs on solid in case of fractal branched aggregates in ferrofluids bulk. Reprinted with permission from Reference [153].

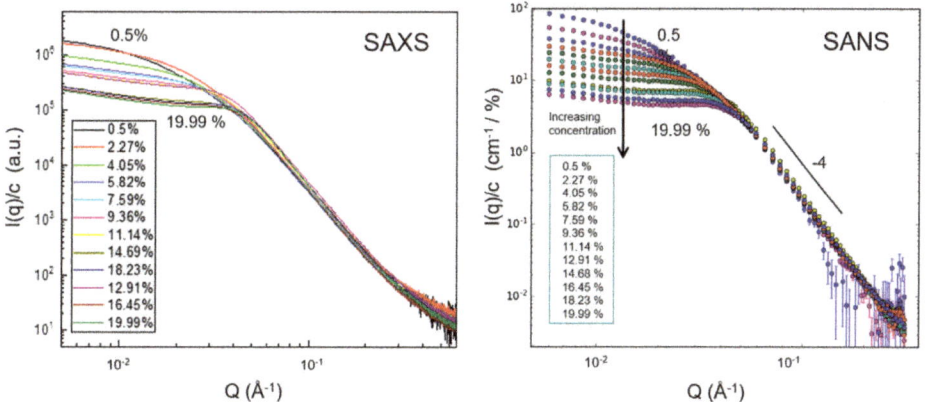

Figure 16. SAXS and SANS intensities normalized to the concentration of MNPs(Fe_3O_4/CA) with varying concentration. The SANS data have been background-subtracted for the H_2O contribution. Reproduced from Reference [85] with permission from The Royal Society of Chemistry.

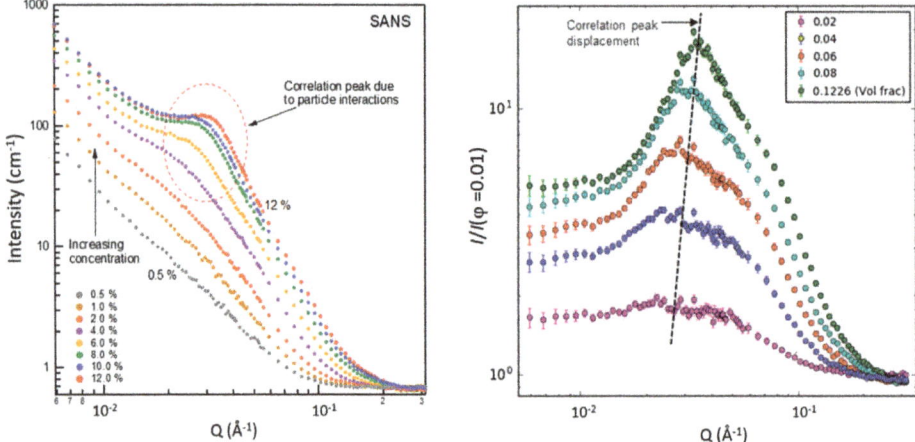

Figure 17. SANS data for the Fe$_3$O$_4$/OA aqueous MF at different concentrations (left). Plot of the "apparent" structure factor (right). The SANS data have been divided by the data for a low-concentration sample (1%), without any further scaling. Reproduced from Reference [85] with permission from The Royal Society of Chemistry.

4.4.2. Light Scattering

Light scattering based structural characterization of magnetic colloids are an affordable laboratory table top alternative to SANS and SAXS. Therefore, a wide spectrum of equipment is already available on the market to help researchers with the fast and accurate characterization of magnetic colloids at nano and mesoscale, both spontaneous and magnetically induced.

Dynamic Light Scattering (DLS) uses the photon correlation spectroscopy to determine the colloidal particle hydrodynamic diameter from the time fluctuations of the light scattered by the colloid sample [157]. Static Light Scattering (SLS) uses the angle dependence of the scattered light intensity to determine the colloidal particle diameter via the Lorentz–Mie light scattering theory [158]. The spontaneous aggregation state of the nanoparticles in the colloid can be assessed while using DLS and SLS together with TEM and/or magnetogranulometry data.

Light scattering is also useful for the characterization of magnetically induced aggregation in magnetic colloids (Figure 18a). An ensemble of parallel prolate objects will scatter light in the plane perpendicular to their shape anisotropy axis, i.e., the scattering plane [158]. The polar angular dependence of the scattered light, i.e., the scattering pattern, can be measured on a projection plane perpendicular to the light propagation direction. 5 s interval scattering patterns from the application of 20 kA/m and 40 kA/m magnetic field, respectively, to a aqueous magnetic nanogel colloid are presented in Figure 17a top and Figure 18a bottom [35]. The scattering patterns themselves and their time evolution show the formation and growth of magnetically induced spindle-like (Figure 18b) aggregates in the colloid. The stronger the magnetic field, the more intense the scattering pattern, and, thus, the more voluminous the aggregated phase. Magnetically induced aggregation in magnetic colloids is of primary concern for practical application due to the potential catastrophic loss of specific surface and/or blood vessels clogging during in vivo experiments. Mesoscale aggregation in magnetic colloids leads to the formation of magnetic field oriented spindle like clusters (Figure 18b), with thickness in the order of microns and lengths in the order of tens to hundreds microns [35,63]. Recently, it was discovered that large scale structuring could be induced by high frequency magnetic fields with amplitude as low as 40 Oe, in suspensions of magnetic multicore-shell nanoparticles (MMCS) [159].

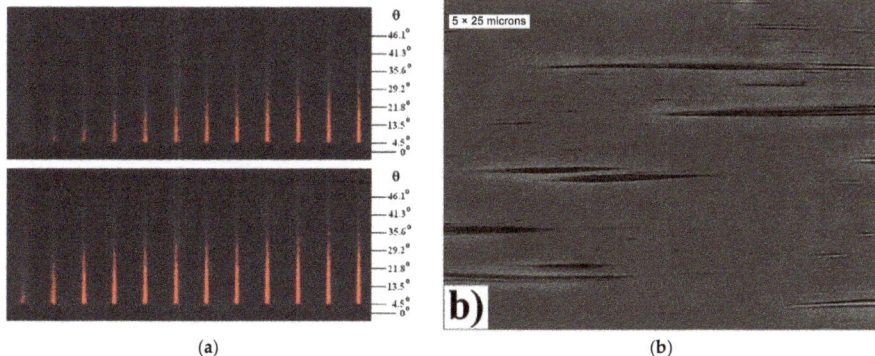

Figure 18. (**a**) Light scattering patterns at 5 s intervals after field onset for 20 kA/m (top) and 40 kA/m (bottom) and (**b**) Optical microscopy image of magnetically induced spindle like aggregates (the scale bar is 25 microns). Reprinted with permission from Reference [35].

Although this large scale structuring can be observed with optical microscopy, light scattering offers the advantage of determining the magnetic supersaturation of the colloid, i.e., the magnetic field dependence of the weight of nanoparticles contained in the aggregates [35].

Figure 19 presents the magnetic field dependence of the supersaturation in three types of MMCS dispersions. The 40 kA/m DC field supersaturation for aqueous dispersions of 60 nm MMCS hardly reaches 0.1% (Figure 19a), while, for 100 nm, MMCSs reach almost 50% (Figure 19b). A 10 kA/m amplitude 100 kHz AC field induces almost 80% supersaturation in 250 nm MMCS dispersion (Figure 19c). Thus, the shear magnitude of the aggregation phenomena should be a priority concern for any practical applications, depending on the composite size and magnetic field intensity.

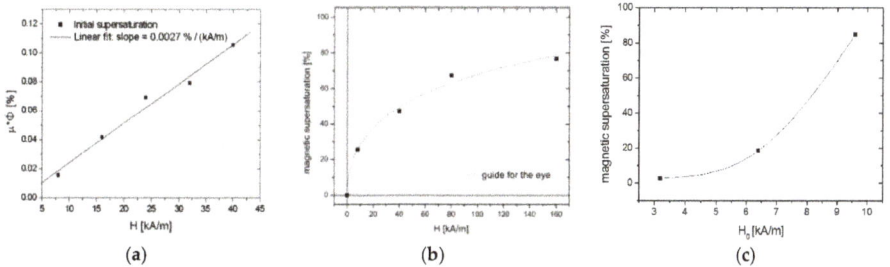

Figure 19. Magnetic field dependence of supersaturation for: (**a**) 60 nm magnetic multicore-shell nanoparticles (MMCS) in DC field. Reprinted with permission from Reference [35], (**b**) 100 nm MMCS in DC field. Reprinted with permission from Reference [63], and (**c**) 250 nm MMCS in AC field [159].

4.5. Rheology and Magnetorheology of Aqueous Ferrofluids

In the case of aqueous bio-ferrofluids usually the multi-core particles in the 50–100 nm size range are predominant. Additionally, while bio-ferrofluids are highly diluted, vector magnetometry and SANS data indicate field dependent "colloidal" anisotropies that arise from the competition between steric repulsion and magnetostatic attraction between particles, having a significant influence on the magnetorheology of these colloids [160].

In the case of concentrated ferrofluids, achieving a high saturation magnetization value requires the increase of physical volume fraction and, thus, a corresponding increase of the hydrodynamic volume fraction, however to different extents, depending on the stabilization mechanism, electrostatic or electro-steric [161]. The electrostatically stabilized ferrofluids have the advantage of reducing the total suspended material at constant magnetic volume fraction when compared with a surfactant stabilized fluid [162], due to the much greater thickness of the steric stabilizing layer.

Vasilescu and colab. made an in-depth analysis on two basic types of water based magnetic fluids (MFs), containing magnetite nanoparticles with electrostatic and with electro-steric stabilization, both being obtained by chemical coprecipitation synthesis under atmospheric conditions [85]. The two sets of magnetic fluid samples, one with citric acid (MF/CA) and the other with oleic acid (MF/OA) coated magnetic nanoparticles, respectively, achieved saturation magnetization values M_S = 78.20 kA/m for the electrostatically and M_S = 48.73 kA/m for the electro-sterically stabilized aqueous ferrofluids, which are among the highest reported to date. These fluids show both similarities and important differences in their microscopic and macroscopic properties.

The two types of ferrofluids manifest different structuring behavior, as evidenced by small angle scattering investigations (Figures 16 and 17); therefore, significant differences are expected in their magnetorheology, in particular concerning the magnitude of the magnetoviscous effect (expressed as the relative field-induced change of viscosity in the presence of a magnetic field, $(\eta_H - \eta_{H=0})/\eta_{H=0}$).

The most concentrated electro-steric stabilized (oleic acid) magnetic fluid sample (MF/OA9) shows shear-thinning (pseudoplastic), both in zero and non-zero magnetic fields—Figure 20, due to particle agglomerates that are progressively destroyed at increasing shear rate values. The applied field induces the formation of new agglomerates, besides those already existing in zero field, as evidenced by the observed magnetoviscous effect (MVE). After demagnetization, the viscosity values remain slightly increased with respect to the initial values, which shows that the agglomerates that formed in the applied field do not fall apart when the field is switched off (are irreversible at the characteristic timescale of measurements).

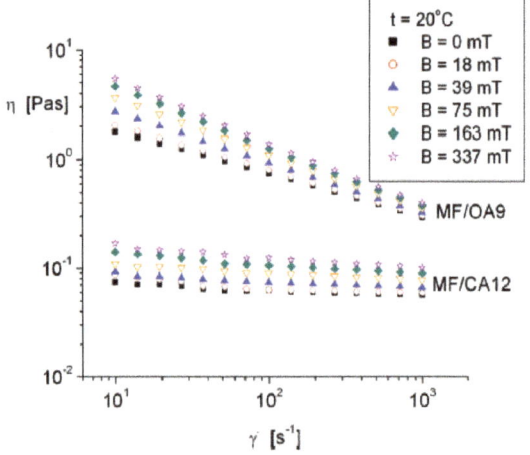

Figure 20. Viscosity curves at different magnetic flux densities for the highest concentration samples: MF/CA12 (physical vol fraction 20%) and MF/OA9 (physical vol fraction 14%). Reproduced from Reference [85] with permission from The Royal Society of Chemistry.

The electrostatic stabilized (citric acid) highest concentration magnetic fluid sample (MF/CA12) has an approximately Newtonian behavior in zero and non-zero magnetic field—Figure 20. From viscosity curves, the MVE is relatively reduced and almost independent of the shear rate. Furthermore, the magnetic field induced agglomeration of particles is partly irreversible; after demagnetization, the viscosities are somewhat higher than the initial values. Moreover, at B = 337 mT, the sample becomes slightly pseudoplastic.

Representing MVE vs. shear rate and vs. magnetic field induction (Figure 21a,b), it was observed that, for small shear rates, the magnetoviscous effect is considerably higher for the MF/OA9 sample.

At shear rates $\gamma > 10^2 \cdot s^{-1}$, the situation changes and the MVE is somewhat greater for the MF/CA12 sample, which indicates the existence of loosely bound agglomerates in the OA stabilized sample, which are disrupted by increasing the shear rate. Abrupt and irreversible changes of the effective viscosity in magnetic fields, which would reflect magnetic field induced phase separation, were not observed. The MVE of the citric acid stabilized magnetic fluid sample is mainly determined by the physical particle volume fraction, which is approx. two times higher than that of the oleic acid stabilized sample.

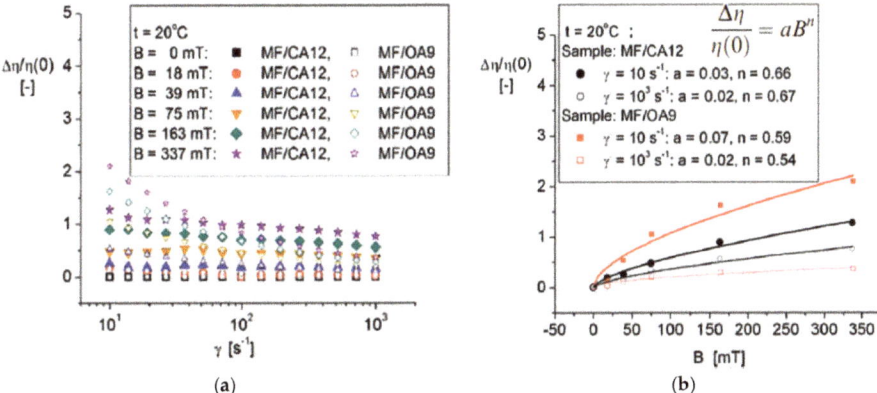

Figure 21. (a) Magnetoviscous effect (MVE) dependence on the shear rate at different magnetic flux densities; (b) MVE dependence on the magnetic flux density at two shear rate values. Reproduced from Reference [85] with permission from The Royal Society of Chemistry.

In good correlation with the results of small-angle scattering, the MVE values at low shear rates were found to be more pronounced for the MF/OA9 sample than for the MF/CA12 sample, which denotes the presence of agglomerates (the existence of correlations) already at small volume fraction values in the case of MF/OA magnetic fluids. However, the observed viscosity increase is moderate when compared to the more than an order of magnitude increase of the effective viscosity in the case of bio-ferrofluids [16].

Bio-ferrofluids having multi-core particles [40,52,53,163–166] demonstrated an increasing interest for the biomedical area during the last years. The higher particle diameter, still guaranteeing a stable suspension, but without magnetized clumps of particles that are caused by remanence, allows for a more effective collection of the particles by the liver. Ferrofluids with multicore particles manifest a rather strong magnetorheological effect, despite the comparatively low concentration of magnetic nanoparticles specific to nanomedicine applications [167,168]. As the concentration of MNPs in blood flow is rather low, for the simulation of the rheological behavior the investigation of dilute ferrofluids is a first step [164,168], including MVE measurements. Nowak and Odenbach developed a capillary viscometer [167], providing a flow situation comparable to the flow in a blood vessel, and having the range of the shear rates adapted to what is expected in the human organism due to the very low zero field viscosity and for a realistic evaluation of MVE. The special capillary viscometer proved to be suitable for measuring the magnetoviscous effect in bio-ferrofluids and the results show good correlation with data measured by rotational rheometry—Figure 22.

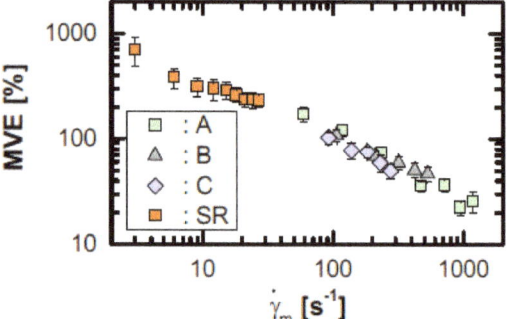

Figure 22. Comparison of MVE data obtained with the capillary viscometer (for three capillaries A, B, C) and with cone-plate setup by rotational rheometry (SR) at the magnetic field strength H = 30 kA/m. Reprinted with permission from Reference [167].

The data from Figure 22 refer to a stable bio-ferrofluid fluidMAG-D-100 nm manufactured by Chemicell GmbH (Berlin, Germany) composed of magnetite as a core material, with starch as surfactant (hydrodynamic diameter was 100 nm, mean single particle diameter was 15.9 nm), and have a concentration in suspension of 25 mg mL^{-1}, a sample also previously investigated in [16].

There are several parameters of the suspended nanoparticles that influence the MVE: the core diameter of the particles, the thickness of the surfactant layer, and the spontaneous magnetization M_0. Regarding the influence of these parameters, in [167] the MVE was compared for three biocompatible ferrofluids with identical composition, except in relation to their hydrodynamic diameter and core composition: the fluidMAG-D-50 nm contains single core particles (hydrodynamic diameter 50 nm), while the other two feature multicore particles: fluidMAG-D-100 nm and fluidMAG-D-200 nm (hydrodynamic diameter 100 nm and 200 nm).

No manifestation of any MV effect was observed for the fluid with single core particles, fluidMAG-D-50 nm. Indeed, the interaction parameter for this ferrofluid

$$\lambda^* = \frac{\mu_0 M_0^2 d^3 \pi}{144 k_B T} \left(\frac{d}{d+2s}\right)^3 \tag{1}$$

was very small: $\lambda^* = 0.09$, and a particle interaction (and implicitly for MVE) is only expected for values of the interaction parameter $\lambda^* > 1$. Here, M_0 is the spontaneous magnetization, μ_0—the vacuum permeability, k_B—the Boltzmann constant, T—the temperature, d—the core diameter, and s—the surfactant thickness.

For the other two ferrofluids that consist of multicore particles, the interaction parameter was calculated with [169]:

$$\lambda_{MC} = \frac{\mu_0 \mu_F \beta^2 (d/2)^3 H_0^2 \pi}{2 k_B T} \left(\frac{d}{d+2s}\right)^3, \quad \text{where } \beta = \frac{\mu_P - \mu_F}{\mu_P + 2\mu_F} \tag{2}$$

in which μ_F represents the relative permeability of the fluid, μ_P—the particles' relative permeability, β—the magnetic contrast factor, and H_0—the magnetic field strength. The interaction parameter at H = 10 kA/m has the values: $\lambda_{MC} = 1.08$ for fluidMAG-D-100 nm and $\lambda_{MC} = 20.1$ for fluidMAG-D-200 nm, which ensures a great MVE—Figure 23.

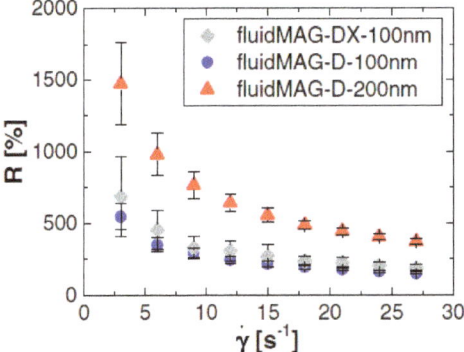

Figure 23. The shear rate dependence of the MVE of three ferrofluid samples at H = 30 kA/m. The commercial fluidMAG-DX-100 nm, investigated in previous studies [167,168], has multicore particles with hydrodynamic diameter 100 nm and stabilized with dextran. Reprinted with permission from Reference [164].

It can be observed from Figure 23 that MVE strongly increases with increasing hydrodynamic diameter, which proves the strong influence of the microscopic makeup of the fluid on this effect. The difference of approx. 20% for MVE for samples fluidMAG-DX-100 nm and fluidMAG-D-100 nm is most likely due to different surfactants (dextran, respective starch) and to different thicknesses of surfactant layers. In addition, MVE increases with intensifying of the magnetic field, due to increasing magnetic interactions between the particles, according to the previously mentioned interaction parameter λ_{MC}, favoring particle agglomeration—Figure 24—and the MVE decreases with increasing shear rate—Figures 23 and 24—due to the rupturing of chain-like structures induced by the magnetic field.

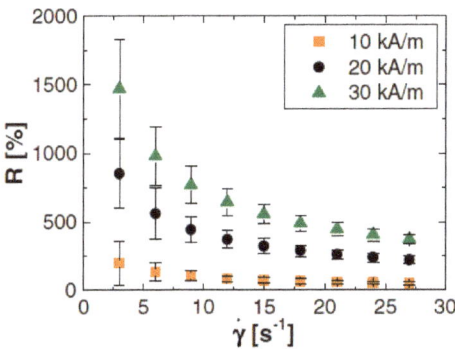

Figure 24. The MVE of the ferrofluid fluidMAG-D-200 nm for three magnetic field strengths depending on the shear rate. Reprinted with permission from Reference [164].

Nowak et al. [167] have comparatively investigated a dilution series starting from two bio-ferrofluids to determine direct connections between the microscopic make-up and the actual rheological behavior as well to establish a condition comparable with the concentration of the fluids in blood flow during the biomedical application: fluidMAG-DX-100 nm (GmbH, Berlin, Germany) and FF054L (provided by the research group of Prof. Alexiou, Erlangen, Germany). Both ferrofluids are based on multi-core magnetite/maghemite particles with 100 nm mean particle diameter. Both ferrofluids have Newtonian behavior in the absence of a magnetic field—Figure 25.

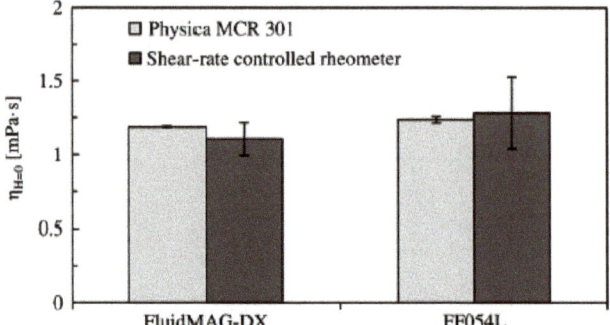

Figure 25. Newtonian viscosity of fluidMAG-DX-100 nm and FF054L samples without the influence of a magnetic field. Reprinted with permission from Reference [16].

The measurements revealed that the magnetorheology of these samples is quite similar; their behavior becomes shear-thinning and MVE is great and strongly dependent on magnetic field intensity—Figure 26.

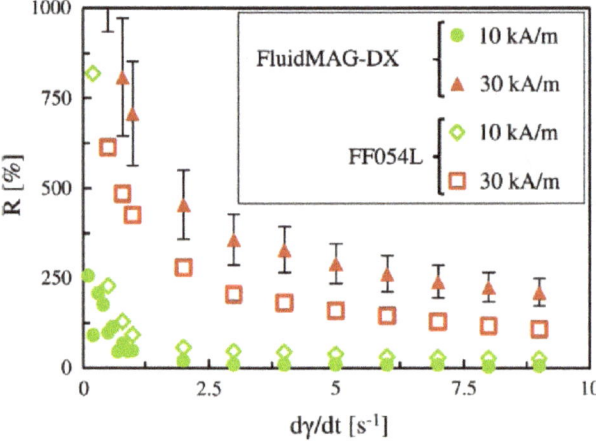

Figure 26. The MVE in the fluidMAG-DX-100 nm in comparison with the FF054L for two values of intensity of magnetic field. Reprinted with permission from Reference [16].

At H = 10 kA/m It is observed from Figure 26 that the MVE is higher for FF054L, despite its lower concentration of suspended magnetic material (0.12% vs. 0.28% in fluidMAG-DX-100 nm). For H > 10 kA/m, the effect is higher for the commercial fluid MAG-DX, as shown in Figure 26 for H = 30 kA/m. This change in the strength of the MVE for the two fluids can be understood while referring to the particle size distribution (a slightly higher fraction of larger particles in the FF054L fluid) as well as to the parameters of the investigated ferrofluids (saturation magnetization: M_S = 1275.5 A/m for fluidMAG-DX-100 nm and M_S = 520.77 A/m for FF054L, volume fraction of magnetic material: Φ = 0.28% for fluidMAG-DX-100 nm and Φ = 0.12% for FF054L), and to the size dependence of the interparticle interaction. The stronger MVE of the FF054L at low field strength is related to the slightly wider particle size distribution involving comparatively larger particles that can contribute to the formation of chains at a H = 10 kA/m. On the contrary, at H > 10 kA/m, the higher volume fraction of magnetic material in fluidMAG-DX-100 nm leads to a stronger MVE in this fluid.

For most biomedical applications, the ferrofluids are supposed to a dilution after injection into the blood flow; therefore, both samples investigated in [16] were diluted with distilled water. Measurements for the dilution series revealed that there is still a strong MVE for a dilution factor $K < 5$ $\left(K = \left(V_{FF} + V_{diluting\,agent}\right)/V_{FF}\right)$—when magnetoviscous effect exceeds about 300%, but, if $K > 10$, the MVE is hardly detectable. For diluted ferrofluids, the shear dependency of the MVE is still manifestly present.

5. Concluding Remarks and Theranostic Prospects

The development of various nanoparticle systems for nanomedicine is a challenging task of present day's material science. In this context, iron oxide nanoparticle systems are among of the most promising nanomaterials in clinical diagnostic and therapeutic applications (theranostics); therefore, the review was focused on efficient manufacturing procedures and manifold characterization methods of these magneto-responsive systems. The recent progress in designed synthesis and multiple functional coating of single- and multicore magnetic nanocomposite particles for imaging, drug delivery, hyperthermia, or point-of-care diagnostics was thoroughly evaluated in correlation with the results of advanced physical-chemical characterization methods, among them X-ray photoelectron spectroscopy, AC susceptometry, small-angle neutron and X-ray scattering, neutron reflectometry, and magnetorheology, beside the more frequently used techniques, such as high resolution transmission electron microscopy, dynamic and static light scattering, or zeta potential measurements. The reviewed manifold physical, chemical, and colloidal characterization is undoubtedly required in order to ensure the desired outcome in the near future of standardized manufacturing of magnetic nanoparticle systems for nanomedicine applications before the translation of novel laboratory creation into the viable clinical product including safety, regulatory, and ethical requirements.

Author Contributions: Writing—original draft, Writing—review & editing, V.S.; Conceptualization, Writing—original draft, D.P., M.V.A. and R.T.; Writing—original draft, V.I.P., D.S.-R. and T.S.; Conceptualization, Writing—original draft, Writing—review & editing, E.T.; Conceptualization, Writing—original draft, Writing—review & editing, Supervision, L.V. All authors have read and agree to the published version of the manuscript.

Funding: The work of D.S.-R., L.V. and V.S. was mainly supported by the RA-TB/CFATR/LMF multiannual research program 2016–2020 and by a grant of the Romanian Ministry of Research and Innovation, CCCDI-UEFISCDI, project number PN-III-PI-1,2-PCCDI-2017-0871, contract c47PCCDI/2018. D.P., L.V. and V.S. are indebted for the partial support from the bilateral agreement between Romanian Academy and Italian National research Council project *Ferro-Tera*. R.T. acknowledges the support from the grant of the Romanian Ministry of Research and Innovation, CCCDI-UEFISCDI, project number PN-III-P1-1.2-PCCDI-2017-0769, contract no. 64, within PNCDI III and from the JINR-RO project 04-4-1121-2015/2020. The work of E.T. and T.S. was supported by the Hungarian National Research, Development and Innovation Office via the Grants FK-124851.

Conflicts of Interest: The authors declare no conflict of interest.

References

1. Pelaz, B.; Alexiou, C.; Alvarez-Puebla, R.A.; Alves, F.; Andrews, A.M.; Ashraf, S.; Bosi, S.; Carril, M.; Chen, C.; Cheng, Z.; et al. Diverse Applications of Nanomedicine. *ACS Nano* **2017**, *11*, 2313–2381. [CrossRef] [PubMed]
2. Thanh, N.T.K. (Ed.) *Clinical Applications of Magnetic Nanoparticles Design to Diagnosis Manufacturing to Medicine*; CRC Press Taylor & Francis Group: Boca Raton, FL, USA, 2018.
3. Colombo, M.; Carregal-Romero, S.; Casula, M.F.; Gutiérrez, L.; Morales, M.P.; Böhm, I.B.; Heverhagen, J.T.; Prosperi, D.; Parak, W.J. Biological applications of magnetic nanoparticles. *Chem. Soc. Rev.* **2012**, *41*, 4306–4334. [CrossRef] [PubMed]
4. Kuncser, V.; Palade, P.; Kuncser, A.; Greculeasa, S.; Schinteie, G. Engineering Magnetic Properties of Nanostructures via Size Effects and Interphase Interactions. In *Size Effects in Nanostructures*; Kuncser, V., Miu, L., Eds.; Springer: Berlin, Germany, 2014; pp. 169–237.
5. Wells, J.; Kazakova, O.; Posth, O.; Steinhoff, U.; Petronis, S.; Bogart, L.K.; Southern, P.; Pankhurst, Q.; Johansson, C. Standardisation of magnetic nanoparticles in liquid suspension. *J. Phys. D Appl. Phys.* **2017**, *50*, 383003-28. [CrossRef]

6. Bogren, S.; Fornara, A.; Ludwig, F.; Morales, M.P.; Steinhoff, U.; Hansen, M.F.; Kazakova, O.; Johansson, C. Classification of Magnetic nanoparticle systems-synthesis, standardization and analysis methods in the NanoMag project. *Int. J. Mol. Sci.* **2015**, *16*, 20308–20325. [CrossRef]
7. Nedyalkova, M.; Donkova, B.; Romanova, J.; Tzvetkov, G.; Madurga, S.; Simeonov, V. Iron oxide nanoparticles—In vivo/in vitro biomedical applications and in silico studies. *Adv. Colloid Interface Sci.* **2017**, *249*, 192–212. [CrossRef]
8. Song, C.; Sun, W.; Xiao, Y.; Shi, X. Ultrasmall iron oxide nanoparticles: Synthesis, surface modification, assembly, and biomedical applications. *Drug Discov. Today* **2019**, *24*, 835–844. [CrossRef]
9. Roca, A.G.; Gutiérrez, L.; Gavilán, H.; Brollo, M.E.F.; Veintemillas-Verdaguer, S.; Morales, M.P. Design strategies for shape-controlled magnetic iron oxide nanoparticles. *Adv. Drug Deliv. Rev.* **2019**, *138*, 68–104. [CrossRef]
10. Savliwala, S.; Chiu-Lam, A.; Unni, M.; Rivera-Rodriguez, A.; Fuller, E.; Sen, K.; Threadcraft, M.; Rinaldi, C. Magnetic nanoparticles. In *Nanoparticles for Biomedical Applications: Fundamental Concepts, Biological Interactions and Clinical Applications*; A Volume in Micro and Nano Technologies; Chapter 13; Chung, E.J., Leon, L., Rinaldi, C., Eds.; Elsevier: Amsterdam, The Netherlands, 2019; pp. 195–221.
11. Sun, Z.; Worden, M.; Thliveris, J.A.; Hombach-Klonisch, S.; Klonisch, T.; van Lierop, J.; Hegmann, T.; Miller, D.W. Biodistribution of negatively charged iron oxide nanoparticles (IONPs) in mice and enhanced brain delivery using lysophosphatidicacid(LPA). *Nanomed. Nanotechnol. Biol. Med.* **2016**, *12*, 1775–1784. [CrossRef]
12. Khandhar, A.P.; Keselman, P.; Kemp, S.J.; Ferguson, R.M.; Goodwill, P.W.; Conolly, S.M.; Krishnan, K.M. Evaluation of PEG-coated iron oxide nanoparticles as blood pool tracers for preclinical Magnetic Particle Imaging. *Nanoscale* **2017**, *9*, 1299–1306. [CrossRef]
13. Gul, S.; Khan, S.B.; Rehman, I.U.; Khan, M.A.; Khan, M.I. A Comprehensive Review of Magnetic Nanomaterials Modern Day Theranostics. *Front. Mater.* **2019**, *6*, 179. [CrossRef]
14. Kostopoulou, A.; Lappas, A. Colloidal magnetic nanocrystal clusters: Variable length-scale interaction mechanisms, synergetic functionalities and technological advantages. *Nanotechnol. Rev.* **2015**, *4*, 595–624. [CrossRef]
15. Muscas, G.; Yaacoub, N.; Concas, G.; Sayed, F.; Sayed Hassan, R.; Greneche, J.M.; Cannas, C.; Musinu, A.; Foglietti, V.; Casciardi, S.; et al. Evolution of the magnetic structure with chemical composition in spinel iron oxide nanoparticles. *Nanoscale* **2015**, *7*, 13576–13585. [CrossRef] [PubMed]
16. Nowak, J.; Wolf, D.; Odenbach, S. A rheological and microscopical characterization of biocompatible ferrofluids. *J. Magn. Magn. Mater.* **2014**, *354*, 98–104. [CrossRef]
17. Vékás, L.; Avdeev, M.V.; Bica, D. Magnetic nanofluids: Synthesis and structure. In *Nanoscience in Biomedicine*; Shi, D., Ed.; Springer: Berlin, Germany, 2009; pp. 650–720.
18. Susan-Resiga, D.; Socoliuc, V.; Boros, T.; Borbáth, T.; Marinica, O.; Han, A.; Vékás, L. The influence of particle clustering on the rheological properties of highly concentrated magnetic nanofluids. *J. Colloid Interface Sci.* **2012**, *373*, 110–115. [CrossRef]
19. Silva, A.K.A.; Di Corato, R.; Gazeau, F.; Pellegrino, T.; Wilhelm, C. Magnetophoresis at the nanoscale: Tracking the magnetic targeting efficiency of nanovectors. *Nanomedicine* **2012**, *7*, 1–15.
20. Shliomis, M.I. Magnetic fluids. *Sov. Phys. Usp.* **1974**, *17*, 153. [CrossRef]
21. Krishnan, K.M. Biomedical Nanomagnetics: A Spin through Possibilities in Imaging, Diagnostics, and Therapy. *IEEE Trans. Magn.* **2010**, *46*, 2523–2558. [CrossRef]
22. Dutz, S.; Hergt, R. Magnetic particle hyperthermia—A promising tumour therapy? *Nanotechnology* **2014**, *25*, 452001–452028. [CrossRef]
23. Wiekhorst, F.; Steinhoff, U.; Eberbeck, D.; Trahms, L. Magnetorelaxometry assisting biomedical applications of magnetic nanoparticles. *Pharm. Res.* **2012**, *29*, 1189–1202. [CrossRef]
24. Ivanov, A.O.; Kantorovich, S.S.; Reznikov, E.N.; Holm, C.; Pshenichnikov, A.F.; Lebedev, A.V.; Chremos, A.; Camp, P.J. Magnetic properties of polydisperse ferrofluids: A critical comparison between experiment, theory, and computer simulation. *Phys. Rev. E* **2007**, *75*, 061405. [CrossRef]
25. Suber, L.; Peddis, D. Approaches to synthesis and characterization of spherical and anisometric metal oxide magnetic nanomaterials. In *Magnetic Nanomaterials*; Kumar, C., Ed.; WILEY-VCH Verlag GmbH & Co. KgaA: Weinheim, Germany, 2010; Volume 4, Chapter 12; pp. 431–487.

26. Peddis, D. Magnetic Properties of Spinel Ferrite Nanoparticles: Influence of the Magnetic Structure. In *Magnetic Nanoparticle Assemblies*; Trohidou, K.N., Ed.; Pan Stanford Publishing: Singapore, 2014; Volume 7, pp. 978–981.
27. Dormann, J.L.; Fiorani, D. (Eds.) *Magnetic Properties of Fine Particles*, 1st ed.; North-Holland Delta Series; Elsevier Science Publishers B.V.: Amsterdam, The Netherlands, 1992.
28. Crangle, J. *Solid State Magnetism*; Great Britain Edward Arnold: London, UK, 1991.
29. Coey, J.M.D. *Magnetism and Magnetic Materials*; Cambrige University Press: New York, NY, USA, 2010.
30. Bodker, F.; Morup, S.; Linderoth, S. Surface Effects in Metallic Iron Nanoparticles. *Phys. Rev. Lett.* **1994**, *72*, 282. [CrossRef] [PubMed]
31. Muscas, G.; Yaacoub, N.; Peddis, D. Chapter 4—Magnetic Disorder in Nanostructured Materials. In *Novel Magnetic Nanostructures Rentschler*; Domracheva, N., Caporali, M., Eva, B.T., Eds.; Elsevier: Amsterdam, The Netherlands, 2018; pp. 127–163.
32. Daou, T.J.; Greneche, J.M.; Pourroy, G.; Buathong, S.; Derory, A.; Ulhaq-Bouillet, C.; Donnio, B.; Guillon, D.; Begin-Colin, S. Coupling Agent Effect on Magnetic Properties of Functionalized Magnetite-Based Nanoparticles. *Chem. Mater.* **2008**, *20*, 5869–5875. [CrossRef]
33. Peddis, D.; Orrù, F.; Ardu, A.; Cannas, C.; Musinu, A.; Piccaluga, G. Interparticle Interactions and Magnetic Anisotropy in Cobalt Ferrite Nanoparticles: Influence of Molecular Coating. *Chem. Mater.* **2012**, *24*, 1062–1071. [CrossRef]
34. Vasilakaki, M.; Ntallis, N.; Yaacoub, N.; Muscas, G.; Peddis, D.; Trohidou, K.N. Optimising the Magnetic Performance of Co Ferrite Nanoparticles via Organic Ligand Capping. *Nanoscale* **2018**, *10*, 21244–21253. [CrossRef] [PubMed]
35. Socoliuc, V.; Vékás, L.; Turcu, R. Magnetically induced phase condensation in an aqueous dispersion of magnetic nanogels. *Soft Matter* **2013**, *9*, 3098–3105. [CrossRef]
36. Bernad, S.I.; Susan-Resiga, D.; Vekas, L.; Bernad, E.S. Drug targeting investigation in the critical region of the arterial bypass graft. *J. Magn. Magn. Mater.* **2019**, *475*, 14–23. [CrossRef]
37. Bernad, S.I.; Susan-Resiga, D.; Bernad, E.S. Hemodynamic Effects on Particle Targeting in the Arterial Bifurcation for Different Magnet Positions. *Molecules* **2019**, *24*, 2509. [CrossRef]
38. Ge, J.; Hu, Y.; Biasini, M.; Beyermann, W.P.; Yin, Y. Superparamagnetic magnetite colloidal nanocrystal clusters. *Angew. Chem. Int. Ed.* **2007**, *46*, 4342–4345. [CrossRef]
39. O'Mahony, J.J.; Platt, M.; Kilinc, D.; Lee, G. Synthesis of superparamagnetic particles with tunable morphologies: The role of nanoparticle-nanoparticle interactions. *Langmuir* **2013**, *29*, 2546–2553. [CrossRef]
40. Yoon, K.Y.; Mehrmohammadi, M.; Borwankar, A.; Emelianov, S.Y.; Johnston, K.P. Synthesis of Iron Oxide Nanoclusters with Enhanced Magnetization and Their Applications in Pulsed Magneto-Motive Ultrasound Imaging. *NANO Brief Rep. Rev.* **2015**, *10*, 1550073. [CrossRef]
41. Tombácz, E.; Turcu, R.; Socoliuc, V.; Vékás, L. Magnetic iron oxide nanoparticles: Recent trends in design and synthesis of magnetoresponsive nanosystems. *Biochem. Biophys. Res. Comm.* **2015**, *468*, 442–453. [CrossRef] [PubMed]
42. Charles, S.W. The preparation of magnetic fluids. In *Ferrofluids*; Odenbach, S., Ed.; Springer: Berlin, Germany, 2002; pp. 3–18.
43. Veiseh, O.; Gunn, J.W.; Zhang, M. Design and fabrication of magnetic nanoparticles for targeted drug delivery and imaging. *Adv. Drug Deliv. Rev.* **2010**, *62*, 284–304. [CrossRef] [PubMed]
44. Gupta, A.K.; Gupta, M. Synthesis and surface engineering of iron oxide nanoparticles for biomedical applications. *Biomaterials* **2005**, *26*, 3995–4021. [CrossRef] [PubMed]
45. Laurent, S.; Forge, D.; Port, M.; Roch, A.; Robic, C.; Vander Elst, L.; Muller, R.N. Magnetic Iron Oxide Nanoparticles: Synthesis, Stabilization, Vectorization, Physicochemical Characterizations, and Biological Applications. *Chem. Rev.* **2008**, *108*, 2064–2110. [CrossRef]
46. Tartaj, P.; Morales, M.P.; Veintemillas-Verdaguer, S.; Gonzalez-Carreno, T.; Serna, C.J. Synthesis, Properties and Biomedical Applications of Magnetic Nanoparticles. *Handb. Magn. Mater.* **2006**, *16*, 403–482.
47. Oh, J.K.; Park, J.M. Iron oxide-based superparamagnetic polymeric nanomaterials: Design, preparation, and biomedical application. *Prog. Polym. Sci.* **2011**, *36*, 168–189. [CrossRef]
48. Baaziz, W.; Pichon, B.P.; Fleutot, S.; Liu, Y.; Lefevre, C.; Grenéche, J.-M.; Toumi, M.; Mhiri, T.; Begin-Colin, S. Magnetic iron oxide nanoparticles: Reproducible tuning of the size and nanosized-dependent composition, defects, and spin canting. *J. Phys. Chem. C* **2014**, *118*, 3795–3810. [CrossRef]

49. Bica, D.; Vékás, L.; Avdeev, M.; Marinică, O.; Socoliuc, V.; Bălăsoiu, M.; Garamus, V.M. Sterically stabilized water based magnetic fluids: Synthesis, structure and properties. *J. Magn. Magn. Mater.* **2007**, *311*, 17–21. [CrossRef]
50. Herranz, F.; Morales, M.P.; Roca, A.G.; Desco, M.; Ruiz-Cabello, J. A new method for the rapid synthesis of water stable superparamagnetic nanoparticles. *Chem. A Eur. J.* **2008**, *14*, 9126–9130. [CrossRef]
51. Palma, S.I.C.J.; Marciello, M.; Carvalho, A.; Veintemillas-Verdaguer, S.; Puerto Morales, M.; Roque, A.C.A. Effects of phase transfer ligands on monodisperse iron oxide magnetic nanoparticles. *J. Coll. Interf. Sci.* **2015**, *437*, 147–155. [CrossRef]
52. Yoon, T.-J.; Lee, H.; Shao, H.; Hilderbrand, S.A.; Weissleder, R. Multicore Assemblies Potentiate Magnetic Properties of Biomagnetic Nanoparticles. *Adv. Mater.* **2011**, *23*, 4793–4797. [CrossRef] [PubMed]
53. Dutz, S.; Kettering, M.; Hilger, I.; Müller, R.; Zeisberger, M. Magnetic multicore nanoparticles for hyperthermia—Influence of particle immobilization in tumour tissue on magnetic properties. *Nanotechnology* **2011**, *22*, 265102. [CrossRef] [PubMed]
54. Dennis, C.L.; Krycka, K.L.; Borchers, J.A.; Desautels, R.D.; van Lierop, J.; Huls, N.F.; Jackson, A.J.; Gruettner, C.; Ivkov, R. Internal magnetic structure of nanoparticles dominates time-dependent relaxation processes in a magnetic field. *Adv. Funct. Mater.* **2015**, *25*, 4300–4311. [CrossRef]
55. Lee, H.; Shin, T.-H.; Cheon, J.; Weissleder, R. Recent Developments in Magnetic Diagnostic Systems. *Chem. Rev.* **2015**, *115*, 10690–10724. [CrossRef]
56. Ahrentorp, F.; Blomgren, J.; Jonasson, C.; Sarwe, A.; Sepehri, S.; Eriksson, E.; Kalaboukhov, A.; Jesorka, A.; Winkler, D.; Schneiderman, J.; et al. Sensitive magnetic biodetection using magnetic multi-core nanoparticles and RCA coils. *J. Magn. Magn. Mater.* **2017**, *427*, 14–18. [CrossRef]
57. Timko, M.; Molcan, M.; Hashim, A.; Skumiel, A.; Muller, M.; Gojzewski, H.; Jozefczak, A.; Kovac, J.; Rajnak, M.; Makowski, M.; et al. Hyperthermic effect in suspension of magnetosomes prepared by various methods. *IEEE Trans. Magn.* **2013**, *49*, 250–254. [CrossRef]
58. Baumgartner, J.; Bertinetti, L.; Widdrat, M.; Hirt, A.M.; Faivre, D. Formation of Magnetite Nanoparticles at Low Temperature: From Superparamagnetic to Stable Single Domain Particles. *PLoS ONE* **2013**, *8*, e57070. [CrossRef]
59. Bigall, N.C.; Wilhelm, C.; Beoutis, M.-L.; García-Hernandez, M.; Khan, A.A.; Giannini, C.; Sánchez-Ferrer, A.; Mezzenga, R.; Materia, M.E.; Garcia, M.A.; et al. Colloidal ordered assemblies in a polymer shell—A novel type of magnetic nanobeads for theranostic applications. *Chem. Mater.* **2013**, *25*, 1055–1062. [CrossRef]
60. Landfester, K. Synthesis of Colloidal Particles in Miniemulsions. *Annu. Rev. Mater. Res.* **2006**, *36*, 231–279. [CrossRef]
61. Qiu, P.; Jensen, C.; Charity, N.; Towner, R.; Mao, C. Oil phase evaporation-induced self-assembly of hydrophobic nanoparticles into spherical clusters with controlled surface chemistry in an oil-in-water dispersion and comparison of behaviors of individual and clustered iron oxide nanoparticles. *J. Am. Chem. Soc.* **2010**, *132*, 17724–17732. [CrossRef]
62. Paquet, C.; de Haan, H.W.; Leek, D.M.; Lin, H.-Y.; Xiang, B.; Tian, G.; Kell, A.; Simard, B. Clusters of superparamagnetic iron oxide nanoparticles encapsulated in a hydrogel: A particle architecture generating a synergistic enhancement of the T2 relaxation. *ACS Nano* **2011**, *5*, 3104–3112. [CrossRef]
63. Turcu, R.; Socoliuc, V.; Craciunescu, I.; Petran, A.; Paulus, A.; Franzreb, M.; Vasile, E.; Vekas, L. Magnetic microgels, a promising candidate for enhanced magnetic adsorbent particles in bioseparation: Synthesis, physicochemical characterization, and separation performance. *Soft Matter* **2015**, *11*, 1008–1018. [CrossRef] [PubMed]
64. Turcu, R.; Craciunescu, I.; Garamus, V.M.; Janko, C.; Lye, S.R.; Tietze, R.; Alexiou, C.; Vékás, L. Magnetic microgels for drug targeting applications: Physical–chemical properties and cytotoxicity evaluation. *J. Magn. Magn. Mater.* **2015**, *380*, 307–314. [CrossRef]
65. Hobson, N.J.; Weng, X.; Siow, B.; Veiga, C.; Ashford, M.; Thanh, N.T.K.; Schatzlein, A.G.; Uchegbu, I.F. Clustering superparamagnetic iron oxide nanoparticles produces organ-targeted high-contrast magnetic resonance images. *Nanomedicine* **2019**, *14*, 1135–1152. [CrossRef] [PubMed]
66. Peddis, D.; Cannas, C.; Musinu, A.; Ardu, A.; Orrù, F.; Fiorani, D.; Laureti, S.; Rinaldi, D.; Muscas, G.; Concas, G.; et al. Beyond the Effect of Particle Size: Influence of $CoFe_2O_4$ Nanoparticle Arrangements on Magnetic Properties. *Chem. Mater.* **2013**, *25*, 2005–2013. [CrossRef]

67. Vangijzegem, T.; Stanicki, D.; Laurent, S. Magnetic iron oxide nanoparticles for drug delivery: Applications and characteristics. *Expert Opin. Drug Deliv.* **2019**, *16*, 69–78. [CrossRef]
68. Laurent, S.; Saei, A.A.; Behzadi, S.; Panahifar, A.; Mahmoudi, M. Superparamagnetic iron oxide nanoparticles for delivery of therapeutic agents: Opportunities and challenges. *Expert Opin. Drug Deliv.* **2014**, *11*, 1–22. [CrossRef]
69. Qu, H.; Tong, S.; Song, K.; Ma, H.; Bao, G.; Pincus, S.; Zhou, W.; O'Connor, C. Controllable in situ synthesis of magnetite coated silica-core water-dispersible hybrid nanomaterials. *Langmuir* **2013**, *29*, 10573–10578. [CrossRef]
70. Szabo, T.; Bakandritsos, A.; Tzitzios, V.; Papp, S.; Korosi, L.; Galbacs, G.; Musabekov, K.; Bolatova, D.; Petridis, D.; Dekany, I. Magnetic iron oxide/clay composites: Effect of the layer silicate support on the microstructure and phase formation of magnetic nanoparticles. *Nanotechnology* **2007**, *18*, 285602. [CrossRef]
71. Amstad, E.; Textor, M.; Reimhult, E. Stabilization and functionalization of iron oxide nanoparticles for biomedical applications. *Nanoscale* **2011**, *3*, 2819–2843. [CrossRef]
72. Laurenti, M.; Guardia, P.; Contreras-Cáceres, R.; Pérez-Juste, J.; Fernandez-Barbero, A.; Lopez-Cabarcos, E.; Rubio-Retama, J. Synthesis of thermosensitive microgels with a tunable magnetic core. *Langmuir* **2011**, *27*, 10484–10491. [CrossRef] [PubMed]
73. Béalle, G.; Di Corato, R.; Kolosnjaj-Tabi, J.; Dupuis, V.; Clément, O.; Gazeau, F.; Wilhelm, C.; Ménager, C. Ultra magnetic liposomes for MR imaging, targeting, and hyperthermia. *Langmuir* **2012**, *28*, 11834–11842. [CrossRef] [PubMed]
74. Namiki, Y.; Namiki, T.; Yoshida, H.; Ishii, Y.; Tsubota, A.; Koido, S.; Nariai, K.; Mitsunaga, M.; Yanagisawa, S.; Kashiwagi, H.; et al. A novel magnetic crystal-lipid nanostructure for magnetically guided in vivo gene delivery. *Nat. Nanotechnol.* **2009**, *4*, 598–606. [CrossRef] [PubMed]
75. Mikhaylov, G.; Mikac, U.; Magaeva, A.A.; Itin, V.I.; Naiden, E.P.; Psakhye, I.; Babes, L.; Reinheckel, T.; Peters, C.; Zeiser, R.; et al. Ferri-liposomes as an MRI-visible drug-delivery system for targeting tumours and their microenvironment. *Nat. Nanotechnol.* **2011**, *6*, 594–602. [CrossRef]
76. Kong, S.D.; Choi, C.; Khamwannah, J.; Jin, S. Magnetically Vectored Delivery of Cancer Drug Using Remotely On–Off Switchable NanoCapsules. *IEEE Trans. Magn.* **2013**, *49*, 349–352. [CrossRef]
77. Bleul, R.; Thiermann, R.; Marten, G.U.; House, M.J.; St Pierre, T.G.; Häfeli, U.O.; Maskos, M. Continuously manufactured magnetic polymersomes—A versatile tool (not only) for targeted cancer therapy. *Nanoscale* **2013**, *5*, 11385–11393. [CrossRef]
78. Bannwarth, M.B.; Utech, S.; Ebert, S.; Weitz, D.A.; Crespy, D.; Landfester, K. Colloidal Polymers with Controlled Sequence and Branching Constructed from Magnetic Field Assembled Nanoparticles. *ACS Nano* **2015**, *9*, 2720–2728. [CrossRef]
79. Hu, M.; Butt, H.-J.; Landfester, K.; Bannwarth, M.B.; Wooh, S.; Thérien-Aubin, H. Shaping the Assembly of Superparamagnetic Nanoparticles. *ACS Nano* **2019**, *13*, 3015–3022. [CrossRef]
80. Savva, I.; Odysseos, A.D.; Evaggelou, L.; Marinica, O.; Vasile, E.; Vekas, L.; Sarigiannis, Y.; Krasia-Christoforou, T. Fabrication, Characterization, and Evaluation in Drug Release Properties of Magnetoactive Poly(ethylene oxide)-Poly(L-lactide) Electrospun Membranes. *Biomacromolecules* **2013**, *14*, 4436–4446. [CrossRef]
81. Papaphilippou, P.; Christodoulou, M.; Marinica, O.; Taculescu, A.; Vekas, L.; Chrissafis, K.; Krasia-Christoforou, T. Multiresponsive Polymer Conetworks Capable of Responding to Changes in pH, Temperature, and Magnetic Field: Synthesis, Characterization, and Evaluation of Their Ability for Controlled Uptake and Release of Solutes. *ACS Appl. Mater. Interfaces* **2012**, *4*, 2139–2147. [CrossRef]
82. Gavilan, H.; Kowalski, A.; Heinke, D.; Sugunan, A.; Sommertune, J.; Varon, M.; Bogart, L.K.; Posth, O.; Zeng, L.; Gonzalez-Alonso, D.; et al. Colloidal Flower-Shaped Iron Oxide Nanoparticles: Synthesis Strategies and Coatings. *Part. Part. Syst. Charact.* **2017**, *34*, 1700094. [CrossRef]
83. Gutiérrez, L.; de la Cueva, L.; Moros, M.; Mazarío, E.; Bernardo, S.; de la Fuente, J.M.; Morales, M.P.; Salas, G. Aggregation effects on the magnetic properties of iron oxide colloids. *Nanotechnology* **2019**, *30*, 112001. [CrossRef] [PubMed]
84. Lartigue, L.; Hugounenq, P.; Alloyeau, D.; Clarke, S.P.; Lévy, M.; Bacri, J.-C.; Bazzi, R.; Brougham, D.F.; Wilhelm, C.; Gazeau, F. Cooperative organization in iron oxide multi-core nanoparticles potentiates their efficiency as heating mediators and MRI contrast agents. *ACS Nano* **2012**, *6*, 10935–10949. [CrossRef] [PubMed]

85. Vasilescu, C.; Latikka, M.; Knudsen, K.D.; Garamus, V.M.; Socoliuc, V.R.; Tombácz, E.; Susan-Resiga, D.; Ras, R.H.A.; Vékás, L. High concentration aqueous magnetic fluids: Structure, colloidal stability, magnetic and flow properties. *Soft Matter* **2018**, *14*, 6648. [CrossRef]
86. Tombácz, E.; Illés, E.; Majzik, A.; Hajdú, A. Ageing in the Inorganic Nanoworld: Example of Magnetite Nanoparticles in Aqueous Medium. *Croat. Chem. Acta* **2007**, *80*, 503–515.
87. Forge, D.; Laurent, S.; Gossuin, Y.; Roch, A.; Van der Elst, L.; Muller, R.N. An original route to stabilize and functionalize magnetite nanoparticles for theranosis applications. *J. Magn. Magn. Mater.* **2011**, *323*, 410–415. [CrossRef]
88. Ramimoghadam, D.; Bagheri, S.; Abd Hamid, S.B. Stable monodisperse nanomagnetic colloidal suspensions: An overview. *Colloids Surf. B Biointerfaces* **2015**, *133*, 388–411. [CrossRef]
89. Creixell, M.; Herrera, A.P.; Latorre-Esteves, M.; Ayala, V.; Torres-Lugo, M.; Rinaldi, C. The effect of grafting method on the colloidal stability and in vitro cytotoxicity of carboxymethyl dextran coated magnetic nanoparticles. *J. Mater. Chem.* **2010**, *20*, 8539–8547. [CrossRef]
90. Barrera, C.; Herrera, A.P.; Bezares, N.; Fachini, E.; Olayo-Valles, R.; Hinestroza, J.P.; Rinaldi, C. Effect of poly(ethylene oxide)-silane graft molecular weight on the colloidal properties of iron oxide nanoparticles for biomedical applications. *J. Colloid Interface Sci.* **2012**, *377*, 40–50. [CrossRef] [PubMed]
91. Mihai, M.; Socoliuc, V.; Doroftei, F.; Ursu, E.-L.; Aflori, M.; Vekas, L.; Simionescu, B.C. Calcium Carbonate–Magnetite–Chondroitin Sulfate Composite Microparticles with Enhanced pH Stability and Superparamagnetic Properties. *Cryst. Growth Des.* **2013**, *13*, 3535–3545. [CrossRef]
92. Bunia, I.; Socoliuc, V.; Vekas, L.; Doroftei, F.; Varganici, C.; Coroaba, A.; Simionescu, B.C.; Mihai, M. Superparamagnetic Composites Based on Ionic Resin Beads/CaCO$_3$/Magnetite. *Chem. A Eur. J.* **2016**, *22*, 18036–18044. [CrossRef] [PubMed]
93. Biliuta, G.; Secarescu, L.; Socoliuc, V.; Iacob, M.; Gheorghe, L.; Negru, D.; Coseri, S. Carboxylated Polysaccharides Decorated with Ultrasmall Magnetic Nanoparticles with Antibacterial and MRI Properties. *Macromol. Chem. Phys.* **2017**, *218*, 1700062. [CrossRef]
94. Tóth, I.Y.; Illés, E.; Szekeres, M.; Zupkó, I.; Turcu, R.; Tombácz, E. Chondroitin-Sulfate-A-Coated Magnetite Nanoparticles: Synthesis, Characterization and Testing to Predict Their Colloidal Behavior in Biological Milieu. *Int. J. Mol. Sci.* **2019**, *20*, 4096. [CrossRef] [PubMed]
95. Boyer, C.; Whittaker, M.R.; Bulmus, V.; Liu, J.; Davis, T.P. The design and utility of polymer-stabilized iron-oxide nanoparticles for nanomedicine applications. *NPG Asia Mater.* **2010**, *2*, 23–30. [CrossRef]
96. Kumar, C. *Magnetic Nanomaterials*; Wiley-VCH: Weinheim, Germany, 2009.
97. Blanco-Andujar, C.; Ortega, D.; Southern, P.; Pankhurst, Q.A.; Thanh, N.T.K. High performance multi-core iron oxide nanoparticles for magnetic hyperthermia: Microwave synthesis, and the role of core-to-core interactions. *Nanoscale* **2015**, *7*, 1768–1775. [CrossRef] [PubMed]
98. Szekeres, M.; Tóth, I.Y.; Illés, E.; Hajdú, A.; Zupkó, I.; Farkas, K.; Oszlánczi, G.; Tiszlavicz, L.; Tombácz, E. Chemical and colloidal stability of carboxylated core-shell magnetite nanoparticles designed for biomedical applications. *Int. J. Mol. Sci.* **2013**, *14*, 14550–14574. [CrossRef]
99. Jedlovszky-Hajdú, A.; Bombelli, F.B.; Monopoli, M.P.; Tombácz, E.; Dawson, K.A. Surface coatings shape the protein corona of SPIONs with relevance to their application in vivo. *Langmuir* **2012**, *28*, 14983–14991. [CrossRef] [PubMed]
100. Lartigue, L.; Innocenti, C.; Kalaivani, T.; Awwad, A.; Mar Sanchez Duque, M.; Guari, Y.; Larionova, J.; Guerin, C.; Montero, J.G.; Barragan-Montero, V.; et al. Water-Dispersible Sugar-Coated Iron Oxide Nanoparticles. An Evaluation of their Relaxometric and Magnetic Hyperthermia Properties. *J. Am. Chem. Soc.* **2011**, *133*, 10459–10472. [CrossRef]
101. Weidner, A.; Gräfe, C.; von der Lühe, M.; Remmer, H.; Clement, J.H.; Eberbeck, D.; Ludwig, F.; Müller, R.; Schacher, F.H.; Dutz, S. Preparation of Core-Shell Hybrid Materials by Producing a Protein Corona Around Magnetic Nanoparticles. *Nanoscale Res. Lett.* **2015**, *10*, 282. [CrossRef]
102. Wang, J.; Zhang, B.; Wang, L.; Wang, M.; Gao, F. One-pot synthesis of water-soluble superparamagnetic iron oxide nanoparticles and their MRI contrast effects in the mouse brains. *Mater. Sci. Eng. C* **2015**, *48*, 416–423. [CrossRef]
103. Illés, E.; Szekeres, M.; Tóth, I.Y.; Szabó, Á.; Iván, B.; Turcu, R.; Vékás, L.; Zupkó, I.; Jaics, G.; Tombácz, E. Multifunctional PEG-carboxylate copolymer coated superparamagnetic iron oxide nanoparticles for biomedical application. *J. Magn. Magn. Mater.* **2018**, *451*, 710–720. [CrossRef]

104. Socoliuc, V.-M.; Vékás, L. Hydrophobic and hydrophilic magnetite nanoparticles: Synthesis by chemical coprecipitation and physico-chemical characterization. In *Upscaling of Bio-Nano-Processes*; Nirschl, H., Keller, K., Eds.; Springer: Berlin, Germany, 2014; pp. 39–55.
105. Zaloga, J.; Janko, C.; Nowak, J.; Matuszak, J.; Knaup, S.; Eberbeck, D.; Tietze, R.; Unterweger, H.; Friedrich, R.P.; Duerr, S.; et al. Development of a lauric acid/albumin hybrid iron oxide nanoparticle system with improved biocompatibility. *Int. J. Nanomed.* **2014**, *9*, 4847–4866. [CrossRef] [PubMed]
106. Abakumov, M.A.; Nukolova, N.V.; Sokolsky-Papkov, M.; Shein, S.A.; Sandalova, T.O.; Vishwasrao, H.M.; Grinenko, N.F.; Gubsky, I.L.; Abakumov, A.M.; Kabanov, A.V.; et al. VEGF-targeted magnetic nanoparticles for MRI visualization of brain tumor. Nanomedicine Nanotechnology. *Biol. Med.* **2015**, *11*, 825–833.
107. Nel, A.E.; Mädler, L.; Velegol, D.; Xia, T.; Hoek, E.M.V.; Somasundaran, P.; Klaessig, F.; Castranova, V.; Thompson, M. Understanding biophysicochemical interactions at the nano-bio interface. *Nat. Mater.* **2009**, *8*, 8543–8557. [CrossRef] [PubMed]
108. Tombacz, E.; Farkas, K.; Foldesi, I.; Szekeres, M.; Illes, E.; Toth, I.Y.; Nesztor, D.; Szabo, T. Polyelectrolyte coating on superparamagnetic iron oxide nanoparticles as interface between magnetic core and biorelevant media. *Interface Focus* **2016**, *6*, 20160068. [CrossRef] [PubMed]
109. EMA. *EMA/325027/2013. Reflection Paper on Surface Coatings: General Issues for Consideration Regarding Parenteral Administration of Coated Nanomedicine Products*; European Medicines Agency: Amsterdam, The Netherlands, 22 May 2013. Available online: https://www.ema.europa.eu/en/documents/scientific-guideline/reflection-paper-surface-coatings-general-issues-consideration-regarding-parenteral-administration_en.pdf (accessed on 19 December 2019).
110. Elimelech, M.; Gregory, J.; Jia, X.; Williams, R. *Particle Deposition and Aggregation, Measurement, Modelling and Simulation*; Butterworth-Heinemann Ltd.: Oxford, UK, 1995.
111. Gregory, J. *Particles in Water, Properties and Processes*; CRC Press Taylor & Francis Group: Boca Raton, FL, USA, 2006.
112. Eberbeck, D.; Wiekhorst, F.; Steinhoff, U.; Trahms, L. Aggregation behaviour of magnetic nanoparticle suspensions investigated by magnetorelaxometry. *J. Phys. Condens. Matter.* **2006**, *18*, 2829–2846. [CrossRef]
113. Nel, A.E.; Brinker, C.J.; Parak, W.J.; Zink, J.I.; Chan, W.C.W.; Pinkerton, K.E.; Xia, T.; Baer, D.R.; Hersam, M.C.; Weiss, P.S. Where Are We Heading in Nanotechnology Environmental Health and Safety and Materials Characterization? *ACS Nano* **2015**, *9*, 5627–5630. [CrossRef]
114. Kolen'ko, Y.V.; Bañobre-López, M.; Rodríguez-Abreu, C.; Carbó-Argibay, E.; Sailsman, A.; Piñeiro-Redondo, Y.; Fátima Cerqueira, M.; Petrovykh, D.Y.; Kovnir, K.; Lebedev, O.I.; et al. Large-Scale Synthesis of Colloidal Fe_3O_4 Nanoparticles Exhibiting High Heating Efficiency in Magnetic Hyperthermia. *J. Phys. Chem. C* **2014**, *118*, 8691–8701. [CrossRef]
115. Di Corato, R.; Aloisi, A.; Rella, S.; Greneche, J.M.; Pugliese, G.; Pellegrino, T.; Malitesta, C.; Rinaldi, R. Maghemite Nanoparticles with Enhanced Magnetic Properties: One-Pot Preparation and Ultrastable Dextran Shell. *ACS Appl. Mater. Interfaces* **2018**, *10*, 20271–20280. [CrossRef]
116. Tóth, Y.I.; Szekeres, M.; Turcu, R.; Sáringer, S.; Illes, E.; Nesztor, D.; Tombácz, E. Mechanism of in Situ Surface Polymerization of Gallic Acid in an Environmental-Inspired Preparation of Carboxylated Core-Shell Magnetite Nanoparticles. *Langmuir* **2014**, *30*, 15451–15461. [CrossRef]
117. Nan, A.; Radu, T.; Turcu, R. Poly(glycidyl methacrylate)-functionalized magnetic nanoparticles as platforms for linking functionalities, bioentities and organocatalysts. *RSC Adv.* **2016**, *6*, 43330–43338. [CrossRef]
118. Willis, A.L.; Turro, N.J.; O'Brien, S. Spectroscopic Characterization of the Surface of Iron Oxide Nanocrystals. *Chem. Mater.* **2005**, *17*, 5970–5975. [CrossRef]
119. Daou, T.J.; Pourroy, G.; Begin-Colin, S.; Greneche, J.M.; Ulhaq-Bouillet, C.; Legare, P.; Bernhardt, P.; Leuvrey, C.; Rogez, G. Hydrothermal synthesis of monodisperse magnetite nanoparticles. *Chem. Mater.* **2006**, *18*, 4399–4404. [CrossRef]
120. Wilson, D.; Langell, M.A. XPS analysis of oleylamine/oleic acid capped Fe_3O_4 nanoparticles as a function of temperature. *Appl. Surf. Sci.* **2014**, *303*, 6–13. [CrossRef]
121. Roth, H.-C.; Schwaminger, S.P.; Schindler, M.; Wagner, F.E.; Berensmeier, S. Influencing factors in the CO-precipitation process of superparamagnetic iron oxide nano particles: A model based study. *J. Magn. Magn. Mater.* **2015**, *377*, 81–89. [CrossRef]

122. Daou, T.J.; Begin-Colin, S.; Greneche, J.M.; Thomas, F.; Derory, A.; Bernhardt, P.; Legare, P.; Pourroy, G. Phosphate Adsorption Properties of Magnetite-Based Nanoparticles. *Chem. Mater.* **2007**, *19*, 4494–4505. [CrossRef]
123. Walter, A.; Garofalo, A.; Parat, A.; Martinez, H.; Felder-Flesch, D.; Begin-Colin, S. Functionalization strategies and dendronization of iron oxide nanoparticles. *Nanotechnol. Rev.* **2015**, *4*, 581–593. [CrossRef]
124. Palanisamy, S.; Wang, Y.-M. Superparamagnetic Iron oxide Nanoparticulate System: Synthesis, Targeting, Drug Delivery and Therapy in Cancer. *Dalton Trans.* **2019**, *48*, 9490–9515. [CrossRef]
125. Mazur, M.; Barras, A.; Kuncser, V.; Galatanu, A.; Zaitzev, V.; Turcheniuk, K.V.; Woisel, P.; Lyskawa, J.; Laure, W.; Siriwardena, A.; et al. Iron oxide magnetic nanoparticles with versatile surface functions based on dopamine anchors. *Nanoscale* **2013**, *5*, 2692–2702. [CrossRef]
126. Safi, M.; Courtois, J.; Seigneuret, M.; Conjeaud, H.; Berret, J.-F. The effects of aggregation and protein corona on the cellular internalization of iron oxide nanoparticles. *Biomaterials* **2011**, *32*, 9353–9363. [CrossRef]
127. Calatayud, M.P.; Sanz, B.; Raffa, V.; Riggio, C.; Ibarra, M.R.; Goya, G.F. The effect of surface charge of functionalized Fe_3O_4 nanoparticles on protein adsorption and cell uptake. *Biomaterials* **2014**, *35*, 6389–6399. [CrossRef] [PubMed]
128. Szekeres, M.; Tóth, I.Y.; Turcu, R.; Tombácz, E. The effect of polycarboxylate shell of magnetite nanoparticles on protein corona formation in blood plasma. *J. Magn. Magn. Mater.* **2017**, *427*, 95–99. [CrossRef]
129. Dürr, S.; Janko, C.; Lyer, S.; Tripal, P.; Schwarz, M.; Jan, Z.; Tietze, R.; Alexiou, C. Magnetic Nanoparticles for Cancer Therapy. *Nanotechnol. Rev.* **2013**, *2*, 395–409. [CrossRef]
130. Pinho, S.L.C.; Pereira, G.A.; Voisin, P.; Kassem, J.; Bouchaud, V.; Etienne, L.; Peters, J.A.; Carlos, L.; Mornet, S.; Geraldes, C.F.G.C.; et al. Fine Tuning of the Relaxometry of gamma-Fe_2O_3@SiO_2 Nanoparticles by Tweaking the Silica Coating Thickness. *ACS Nano* **2010**, *4*, 5339–5349. [CrossRef] [PubMed]
131. Tombácz, E.; Szekeres, M.; Hajdú, A.; Tóth, I.Y.; Bauer, R.A.; Nesztor, D.; Illés, E.; Zupkó, I.; Vékás, L. Colloidal stability of carboxylated iron oxide nanomagnets for biomedical use. *Period. Polytech. Chem. Eng.* **2014**, *58*, 3–10. [CrossRef]
132. Toth, I.Y.; Illes, E.; Bauer, R.A.; Nesztor, D.; Szekeres, M.; Zupko, I.; Tombacz, E. Designed polyelectrolyte shell on magnetite nanocore for dilution-resistant biocompatible magnetic fluids. *Langmuir* **2012**, *28*, 16638–16646. [CrossRef]
133. Socoliuc, V.; Turcu, R.; Kuncser, V.; Vekas, L. Magnetic Characterization. In *Contrast Agents for MRI-Experimental Methods*; Pierre, V.C., Allen, M.J., Eds.; Royal Society of Chemistry: Brighton, UK, 2018; pp. 391–426.
134. Garaio, E.; Collantes, J.M.; Plazaola, F.; Garcia, J.A.; Castellanos-Rubio, I. A multifrequency eletromagnetic applicator with an integrated AC magnetometer for magnetic hyperthermia experiments. *Meas. Sci. Technol.* **2014**, *25*, 115702. [CrossRef]
135. Lenox, P.; Plummer, L.K.; Paul, P.; Hutchison, J.E.; Jander, A.; Dhagat, P. High-Frequency and High-Field Hysteresis Loop Tracer for Magnetic Nanoparticle Characterization. *IEEE Magn. Lett.* **2018**, *9*, 6500405. [CrossRef]
136. Fannin, P.; Marin, C.N.; Malaescu, I.; Raj, K.; Popoiu, C. Local arrangement of particles in magnetic fluids due to the measurement alternating field. *J. Magn. Magn. Mater.* **2017**, *438*, 116–120. [CrossRef]
137. Pedersen, J.S. Analysis of small-angle scattering data from colloids and polymer solutions: Modeling and least-squares fitting. *Adv. Colloid Interface Sci.* **1997**, *70*, 171–210. [CrossRef]
138. Mühlbauer, S.; Honecker, D.; Périgo, É.A.; Bergner, F.; Disch, S.; Heinemann, A.; Erokhin, S.; Berkov, D.; Leighton, C.; Ring Eskildsen, M.; et al. Magnetic small-angle neutron scattering. *Rev. Mod. Phys.* **2019**, *91*, 015004. [CrossRef]
139. Avdeev, M.V.; Aksenov, V.L. Small-angle neutron scattering in structure research of magnetic fluids. *Phys. Usp.* **2010**, *53*, 971–993. [CrossRef]
140. Avdeev, M.V.; Petrenko, V.I.; Gapon, I.V.; Bulavin, L.A.; Vorobiev, A.A.; Soltwedel, O.; Balasoiu, M.; Vekas, L.; Zavisova, V.; Kopcansky, P. Comparative structure analysis of magnetic fluids at interface with silicon by neutron reflectometry. *Appl. Surf. Sci.* **2015**, *352*, 49–53. [CrossRef]
141. Daillant, J.; Gibaud, A. (Eds.) *X-Ray and Neutron Reflectivity: Principles and Applications*; Springer: Berlin/Heidelberg, Germany, 2009.
142. Vorobiev, A.; Major, J.; Dosch, H.; Gordeev, G.; Orlova, D. Magnetic field dependent ordering in ferrofluids at SiO_2 interfaces. *Phys. Rev. Lett.* **2004**, *93*, 267203. [CrossRef] [PubMed]

143. Nagornyi, A.V.; Petrenko, V.I.; Avdeev, M.V.; Yelenich, O.V.; Solopan, S.O.; Belous, A.G.; Gruzinov, A.Y.; Ivankov, O.I.; Bulavin, L.A. Structural aspects of magnetic fluid stabilization in aqueous agarose solutions. *J. Magn. Magn. Mater.* **2017**, *431*, 16–19. [CrossRef]
144. Petrenko, V.I.; Aksenov, V.L.; Avdeev, M.V.; Bulavin, L.A.; Rosta, L.; Vekas, L.; Garamus, V.M.; Willumeit, R. Analysis of the structure of aqueous ferrofluids by the small-angle neutron scattering method. *Phys. Solid State* **2010**, *52*, 974–978. [CrossRef]
145. Avdeev, M.V.; Feoktystov, A.V.; Kopcansky, P.; Lancz, G.; Garamus, V.M.; Willumeit, R.; Jurikova, A.J.; Timiko, M.; Zavisova, V.; Csach, K.; et al. Structure of water-based ferrofluids with sodium oleate and polyethylene glycol stabilization by small-angle neutron scattering: contrast-variation experiments. *J. Appl. Cryst.* **2010**, *43*, 959–969. [CrossRef]
146. Petrenko, V.I.; Artykulnyi, O.P.; Bulavin, L.A.; Almásy, L.; Garamus, V.M.; Ivankov, O.I.; Grigoryeva, N.A.; Vekas, L.; Kopcansky, P.; Avdeev, M.V. On the impact of surfactant type on the structure of aqueous ferrofluids. *Colloids Surf. A* **2018**, *541*, 222–226. [CrossRef]
147. Petrenko, V.I.; Avdeev, M.V.; Garamus, V.M.; Bulavin, L.A.; Kopcansky, P. Impact of polyethylene glycol on aqueous micellar solutions of sodium oleate studied by small-angle neutron scattering. *Colloids Surf. A* **2015**, *480*, 191–196. [CrossRef]
148. Lancz, G.; Avdeev, M.V.; Petrenko, V.I.; Garamus, V.M.; Koneracká, M.; Kopčanský, P. SANS study of poly(ethylene glycol) solutions in D2O. *Acta Phys. Polonica A* **2010**, *118*, 980–982. [CrossRef]
149. Artykulnyi, O.P.; Petrenko, V.I.; Bulavin, L.A.; Ivankov, O.I.; Avdeev, M.V. Impact of poly (ethylene glycol) on the structure and interaction parameters of aqueous micellar solutions of anionic surfactants. *J. Mol. Liq.* **2019**, *276*, 806–811. [CrossRef]
150. Melníková, L.; Petrenko, V.I.; Avdeev, M.V.; Garamus, V.M.; Almásy, L.; Ivankov, O.I.; Bulavin, L.A.; Mitróová, Z.; Kopcansky, P. Effect of iron oxide loading on magnetoferritin structure in solution as revealed by SAXS and SANS. *Colloids Surf. B* **2014**, *123*, 82–88.
151. Majorosova, J.; Petrenko, V.I.; Siposova, K.; Timko, M.; Tomasovicova, N.; Garamus, V.M.; Koralewski, M.; Avdeev, M.V.; Leszczynski, B.; Jurga, S.; et al. On the adsorption of magnetite nanoparticles on lysozyme amyloid fibrils. *Colloids Surf. B* **2016**, *146*, 794–800. [CrossRef] [PubMed]
152. Petrenko, V.I.; Nagornyi, A.V.; Gapon, I.V.; Vekas, L.; Garamus, V.M.; Almasy, L.; Feoktystov, A.V.; Avdeev, M.V. Magnetic Fluids: Structural Aspects by Scattering Techniques. In *Modern Problems of Molecular Physics*; Bulavin, L., Chalyi, A., Eds.; Springer: Cham, Switzerland, 2018; Volume 197, pp. 205–226.
153. Kubovcikova, M.; Gapon, I.V.; Zavisova, V.; Koneracka, M.; Petrenko, V.I.; Soltwedel, O.; Almasy, L.; Avdeev, M.V.; Kopcansky, P. On the adsorption properties of magnetic fluids: Impact of bulk structure. *J. Magn. Magn. Mater.* **2017**, *427*, 67–70. [CrossRef]
154. Avdeev, M.V.; Petrenko, V.I.; Feoktystov, A.V.; Gapon, I.V.; Aksenov, V.L.; Vekás, L.; Kopčanský, P. Neutron investigations of ferrofluids. *Ukr. J. Phys.* **2015**, *60*, 728–736. [CrossRef]
155. Theis-Bröhl, K.; Gutfreund, P.; Vorobiev, A.; Wolff, M.; Toperverg, B.P.; Dura, J.A.; Borchers, J.A. Self assembly of magnetic nanoparticles at silicon surfaces. *Soft Matter* **2015**, *11*, 4695–4704. [CrossRef] [PubMed]
156. Theis-Bröhl, K.; Vreeland, E.C.; Gomez, A.; Huber, D.L.; Saini, A.; Wolff, M.; Maranville, B.B.; Brok, E.; Krycka, K.L.; Dura, J.A.; et al. Self-assembled layering of magnetic nanoparticles in a ferrofluid on silicon surfaces. *ACS Appl. Mater. Interfaces* **2018**, *10*, 5050–5060.
157. Berne, B.J.; Pecora, R. *Dynamic Light Scattering*; John Wiley: New York, NY, USA, 1976.
158. Bohren, C.F.; Huffmann, D.R. *Absorption and Scattering of Light by Small Particles*; Wiley-Interscience: New York, NY, USA, 2010.
159. Socoliuc, V.; Turcu, R. Large scale aggregation in magnetic colloids induced by high frequency magnetic fields. *J. Magn. Magn. Mater.* **2019**, accepted. [CrossRef]
160. Dennis, C.L.; Jackson, A.J.; Borchers, J.A.; Gruettner, C.; Ivkov, R. Correlation between physical structure and magnetic anisotropy of a magnetic nanoparticle colloid. *Nanotechnology* **2018**, *29*, 215705. [CrossRef]
161. Massart, R. *Magnetic Fluids and Applications Handbook*; Berkovski, B.M., Bashtovoy, V.G., Eds.; Begell House: Washington, DC, USA, 1996; pp. 24–27.
162. Odenbach, S. Ferrofluids. In *Handbook of Magnetic Materials*; Buschow, K.H.J., Ed.; Elsevier Science: Amsterdam, The Netherlands, 2006; Volume 16, pp. 127–208.

163. Roger, S.; Sang, Y.Y.C.; Bee, A.; Perzynski, R.; Di Meglio, J.M.; Ponton, A. Structural and multi-scale rheophysical investigation of diphasic magneto-sensitive materials based on biopolymers. *Eur. Phys. J. E Soft Matter Biol. Phys.* **2015**, *38*, 88. [CrossRef]
164. Nowak, J.; Wiekhorst, F.; Trahms, L.; Odenbach, S. The influence of hydrodynamic diameter and core composition on the magnetoviscous effect of biocompatible ferrofluids. *J. Phys. Condens. Matter* **2014**, *26*, 176004. [CrossRef]
165. Dutz, S.; Clement, J.H.; Eberbeck, D.; Gelbrich, T.; Hergt, R.; Müller, R.; Wotschadlo, J.; Zeisberger, M. Ferrofluids of magnetic multicore nanoparticles for biomedical applications. *J. Magn. Magn. Mater.* **2009**, *321*, 1501–1504. [CrossRef]
166. Bender, P.; Bogart, L.K.; Posth, O.; Szczerba, W.; Rogers, S.E.; Castro, A.; Nilsson, L.; Zeng, L.J.; Sugunan, A.; Sommertune, J.; et al. Structural and magnetic properties of multi-core nanoparticles analysed using a generalized numerical inversion method. *Sci. Rep.* **2017**, *7*, 45990. [CrossRef]
167. Nowak, J.; Odenbach, S. A capillary viscometer designed for the characterization of biocompatible ferrofluids. *J. Magn. Magn. Mater.* **2016**, *411*, 49–54. [CrossRef]
168. Nowak, J.; Odenbach, S. Magnetoviscous effect in a biocompatible ferrofluid. *IEEE Trans. Magn.* **2013**, *49*, 208–212. [CrossRef]
169. Bossis, G.; Volkova, O.; Lacis, S.; Meunier, A. Magnetorheology: Fluids, structures and rheology. In *Ferrofluids*; Springer: Berlin/Heidelberg, Germany, 2002; Volume 594, pp. 202–230.

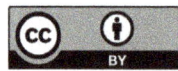

© 2020 by the authors. Licensee MDPI, Basel, Switzerland. This article is an open access article distributed under the terms and conditions of the Creative Commons Attribution (CC BY) license (http://creativecommons.org/licenses/by/4.0/).

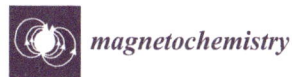

Review

Recent Advances of Cellulase Immobilization onto Magnetic Nanoparticles: An Update Review

Kamyar Khoshnevisan [1,*], Elahe Poorakbar [2], Hadi Baharifar [3] and Mohammad Barkhi [4]

1. Biosensor Research Center, Endocrinology and Metabolism Molecular-Cellular Sciences Institute, Tehran University of Medical Sciences, Tehran 1411713137, Iran
2. Department of Biology, Faculty of Sciences, University of Payame Noor, Tehran 19395-3697, Iran; epoor2000@yahoo.com
3. Department of Medical Nanotechnology, Applied Biophotonics Research Center, Science and Research Branch, Islamic Azad University, Tehran 1477893855, Iran; baharifar.h@gmail.com
4. Zar Center, University of Applied Science and Technology (UAST), Karaj 1599665111, Iran; mbarkhi@gmail.com
* Correspondence: k-khoshnevisan@razi.tums.ac.ir or kamyar.khoshnevisan@gmail.com; Tel.: +964-9888220068; Fax: +964-9888220052

Received: 25 April 2019; Accepted: 4 June 2019; Published: 10 June 2019

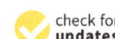

Abstract: Cellulosic enzymes, including cellulase, play an important role in biotechnological processes in the fields of food, cosmetics, detergents, pulp, paper, and related industries. Low thermal and storage stability of cellulase, presence of impurities, enzyme leakage, and reusability pose great challenges in all these processes. These challenges can be overcome via enzyme immobilization methods. In recent years, cellulase immobilization onto nanomaterials became the focus of research attention owing to the surface features of these materials. However, the application of these nanomaterials is limited due to the efficacy of their recovery process. The application of magnetic nanoparticles (MNPs) was suggested as a solution to this problem since they can be easily removed from the reaction mixture by applying an external magnet. Recently, MNPs were extensively employed for enzyme immobilization owing to their low toxicity and various practical advantages. In the present review, recent advances in cellulase immobilization onto functionalized MNPs is summarized. Finally, we discuss enhanced enzyme reusability, activity, and stability, as well as improved enzyme recovery. Enzyme immobilization techniques offer promising potential for industrial applications.

Keywords: cellulase immobilization; magnetic nanoparticles; stability; functionalized nanoparticles

1. Introduction

The environmental pollution produced by fossil fuels, the increasing growth of population, and the expensive costs of traditional energy sources compel researchers to develop novel approaches toward ecofriendly and biodegradable energy sources. Biomass, specifically cellulose, nature's most abundant biopolymer, is a low-cost energy source which can be degraded as biomaterials to yield chemical products applicable in many industrial applications [1,2].

Cellulosic enzymes such as cellulases are catalysts which convert cellulose to glucose, and are widely used in different industries, including food, pulp and paper, laundry, beverages, textile, agriculture, pharmaceutics, medicine, and especially in biofuel production [3]. Glucose is the main product of cellulose conversion, which is applied as a precursor for the production of various valuable products. Cellulase, which is synthesized by microorganisms including bacteria and fungi [4,5], is the most powerful hydrolyzing enzyme and can be easily employed [6].

Chemical, physical, and biological methods were employed for cellulosic hydrolysis, from which the enzymatic conversion gained much attention because of its mild reaction conditions. Therefore, these methods provide high yield with no inhibitory by-products and are considered environmentally friendly. Cellulases are highly selective catalysts and the degradation process is naturally carried out in pH 4.5–5.5 at 40–50 °C [7–9].

Cellulases are responsible for biochemical conversion processes and convert the lignocellulosic biomass (hemicellulose and cellulose) into an intermediate sugar, which further acts as the substrate for ethanol production [10–14]. Biocatalysts have limitations such as limited availability, substrate scope, and operational stability [15]. Recent findings can help scientists overcome these limitations. The main challenge in the application of biocatalysts is their high cost; therefore, reusability and recovery of the enzymes are two significant factors that should be considered for industrial applications [16,17]. In industrial processes, enzymatic reactions are generally performed in high-temperature conditions which can lead to changes in the natural structure of cellulase [18,19]. For this reason, enzyme properties must be greatly improved. Immobilization is a powerful tool to increase the stability and reusability of enzymes.

Enzyme immobilization on support materials is a well-established approach for enhancement of enzyme features such as activity, stability, reusability, purification, reduction of inhibition, and selectivity. Enzyme immobilization on a solid support provides good distribution of the catalysts with less aggregation. On the other hand, covalent binding between the support and the enzyme results in increased enzymatic stability, which in turn leads to enhanced enzymatic activity [1,20,21].

Different methods for enzyme immobilization exist, including covalent binding, adsorption, ionic bonding, entrapment, and encapsulation [22–27]. There are also numerous approaches to facilitate enzyme immobilization on nanomaterials, including enzymatic modifications, enzymatic immobilization and biosensor development [28,29], enzymatic degradation, enzyme nanoparticles, and enzyme mimics of nanomaterials [30–33]. Among several available nanoparticles, magnetic nanoparticles (MNPs) received more attention owing to their advantageous features including low toxicity and high surface area, which allows a large number of enzyme molecules to be loaded to their surface [30,34,35].

In recent decades, most research studies on cellulase immobilization illustrated that the enzyme structure was improved, and bound cellulase maintains high activity for a long time. Furthermore, the immobilized cellulase is more resistant to structural alterations induced by increased temperature [36–39]. The activity of bounded cellulase was shown to be higher at most pH values than the free form due to enhanced stability [40–42].

Fe_3O_4 MNPs obtained great attention due to their low toxicity, simple preparation, unique size, strong magnetic properties, and proper physical properties, as well as simple recovery from the media with an external magnetic field [43,44]. Although, magnetite nanoparticles tend to agglomerate and be easily oxidized upon air exposure, it is very important to functionalize its surface in order to avoid oxidization.

The enzymes can bind to the surface of MNPs through van der Waals and electrostatic forces, hydrophobic, or π–π stacking connections by means of non-covalent binding. However, the main challenge of non-covalent immobilization is protein leakage from the surface of the MNPs. Thus, the covalent binding using cross-linkers is widely applied to resolve this problem. Among the cross-linkers, glutaraldehyde is commonly employed as the coupling agent for covalent cellulase immobilization to the support since it is soluble in aqueous solvents and provides firm inter- and intra-covalent bonds [45–49].

A summary of different methods used for MNP functionalization for cellulase immobilization is presented in Figure 1. These functionalization methods are further described and their advantageous features are thoroughly discussed. The current review is focused on recent findings on immobilized cellulases on MNP supports with various functionalized groups and their advantages.

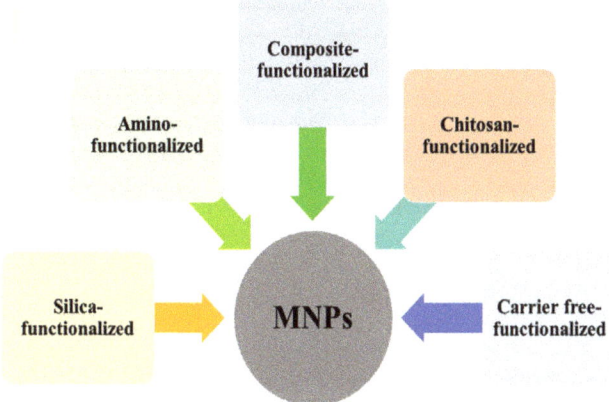

Figure 1. An overview of magnetic nanoparticles (MNPs) functionalized by different methods.

2. Cellulase Immobilization on Silica-Functionalized MNPs

Silica functionalized MNPs provide suitable supports with low aggregation in solutions. Silica functionalization enhances biocompatibility, as well as thermal and chemical stability, of the MNP surface [34,50]. Co-immobilization of tri-enzymes consisting of cellulase, pectinase, and xylanase was investigated for industrial applications. The results revealed that kinetic parameters (i.e., V_{max} and K_m) of the tri-enzyme were not affected by the immobilization process. It can be concluded that the immobilization process significantly enhances thermal and chemical stability [18].

Zhang et al. reported an enzymatic catalysis with chemocatalysis in an iPrOH/water solvent mixture by employing a novel approach for green conversion of ionic liquid (IL) while pretreating cellulose with 5-hydroxymethylfurfural (HMF). This pretreatment of media converted cellulose to glucose and glucose to HMF, while HMF and glucose yields were 43.6% and 86.2%, respectively (Scheme 1). The results obtained from enzymatic cascades and reaction systems prove that this method can be applied as an operative route for biomass energy maintenance [51].

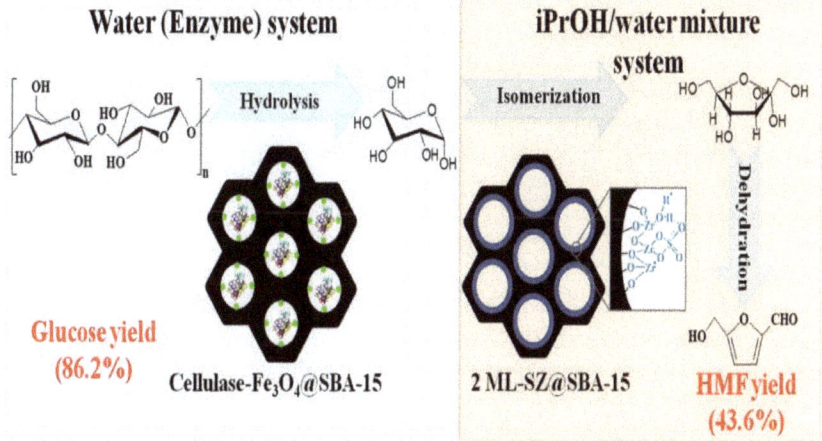

Scheme 1. Schematic representation of the cascaded enzymatic and chemical steps for ionic liquid (IL) pretreated cellulose into 5-hydroxymethylfurfural (HMF) in water (enzyme) and iPrOH/water solvent mixtures with enzyme and SBA-15 grafted sulfated zirconium dioxide (SZ) conformed monolayers, respectively. Reproduced with permission from Reference [51].

In another study, *Trichoderma reesei* cellulase was immobilized on two different nanomatrices (MNPs and silica nanoparticles (SNPs)) to improve enzymatic efficiency. Then, 1-ethyl-3-methylimidazoliumacetate [EMIM][Ac] was applied as an IL for cellulase immobilization and was used for pretreatment of sugarcane bagasse and wheat straw. The results obtained from this study revealed a great hydrolysis yield (89%). This process, due to IL reusability and the enhanced stability of the immobilized enzyme, can be potentially used for biorefineries [52].

The immobilization and characterization of holocellulase from *Aspergillus niger* on five different nanoparticles (NPs) via available methods was reported by Kuma et al. Enzyme molecules were covalently immobilized on magnetic enzyme–nanoparticle complexes (MENC), and the results obtained from this study revealed that the immobilization of indigenous enzymes and their consumption can be used for saccharification of paddy straw [53].

Jia et al. established and applied novel MNP cross-linked cellulase aggregates (Figure 2) in order to improve enzyme reusability and stability for biomass bioconversion. The immobilized cellulase further represented suitable activity and stability following reusability in biomass applications [54].

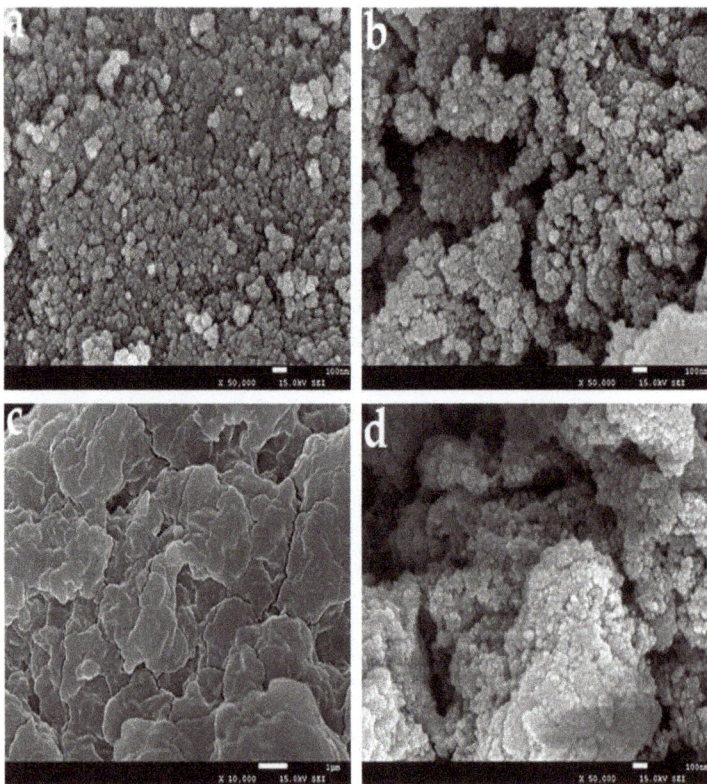

Figure 2. Scanning electron microscopy (SEM) images of (**a**) Fe_3O_4; (**b**) 3-aminopropyl triethoxysilane (APTES)-Fe_3O_4; (**c**) cellulase cross-linked enzyme aggregates (CLEAs); (**d**) magnetic cellulase CLEAs. Reproduced from Reference [54].

The key parameters of enzyme immobilization such as pH, temperature, efficiency, reusability, and coupling agents, as well as supports and substrates, are presented in Table 1. As mentioned before, glutaraldehyde is the most commonly used cross-linker for enzyme immobilization. Our findings suggest that biocompatible, biodegradable, and nontoxic polymers such as polyethylene glycol (PEG) can also be used as an alternative cross-linker for this process.

Table 1. Cellulase immobilization on silica-functionalized magnetic nanoparticles (MNPs).

Enzyme	Substrate	Support	Coupling Agent	Amount *	pH	Temperature	Reusability Cycle	Reusability Efficiency	Ref.
Pectinase Xylanase Cellulase	Polygalacturonic acid Xylan CMC	(Fe$_3$O$_4$) on APTES	Glutaraldehyde	12, 5, 31 mg/mL	4.8	70 °C	5	87%, 69%, and 58%	[18]
Cellulase	Cellulose	Fe$_3$O$_4$ encapsulated with SBA-15	PEG-1000	1.6 mg	4.8	25–85 °C	5	87.5%	[51]
Cellulase	Wheat straw and sugarcane	[EMIM][Ac] functionalized-MNPs and SNP	Glutaraldehyde	10 and, 7.5 mg/mL	3.5–9.5	20–80 °C	10	85% and 76%	[52]
Holocellulase	FP, CMC, and xylan	APTES-Fe$_3$O$_4$	Glutaraldehyde	2 mg/mL	3–7	40–80 °C	2	60–80%	[53]
Cellulase	CMC	APTES-Fe$_3$O$_4$	Glutaraldehyde	176 mg/g	3–8	30–80 °C	6	88%	[54]

Abbreviations: 1-ethyl-3-methylimidazoliumacetate [EMIM][Ac]; silica nanoparticles (SNPs); filter paper (FP); polyethylene glycol (PEG); carboxyl methyl cellulose (CMC); 3-aminopropyltriethoxysilane (APTES); * amount of immobilized enzyme.

3. Carrier Free Cellulase Immobilization Strategy

In recent years, MNPs were commonly applied as a solid support for recovery systems [55]. Carrier-free immobilization approaches like co-immobilization by cross-linked enzyme crystals (CLECs) and cross-linking enzyme aggregates (CLEAs) are conceivable methods to boost the enzyme stability [56–59]. Tri-enzyme was co-immobilized on MNPs to improve reusability by cross-linking with glutaraldehyde. In this study, co-immobilized MNPs remained stable for more than a month at 5 °C and also retained activity for up to four cycles. It was suggested that this platform can be effectively applied for the extraction of different plants [19]. In another similar study, enzymes including xylenes, cellulases, and amylases were derived from bacteria and applied for cellulase immobilization on MNPs to enhance stability and facilitate reusability (Figure 3). The results obtained demonstrated that the enzyme-coupled MNPs exhibited excellent stability and recovery. Tri-enzyme immobilized MNPs can be potentially applied in plant biomass production [60].

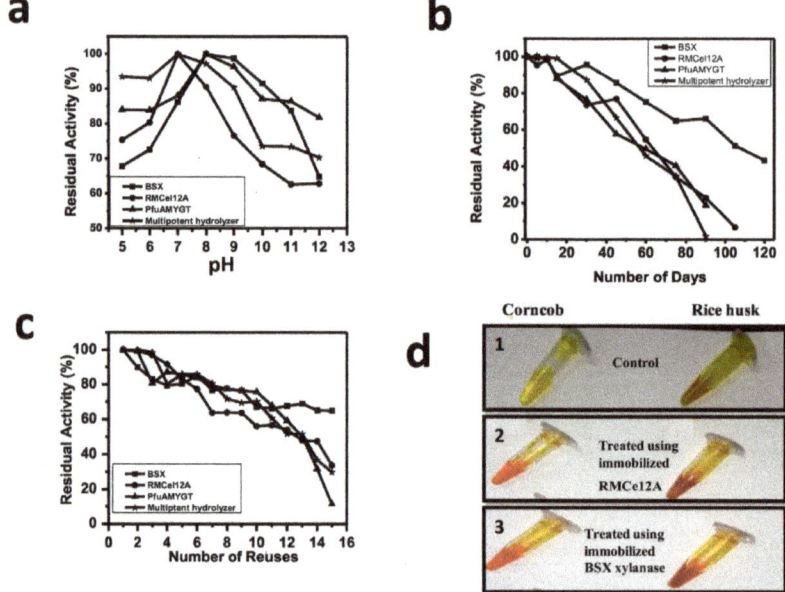

Figure 3. Functional characterization of immobilized enzyme-carrying magnetic nanoparticles (MNPs) and untreated (control) nanoparticles where fitting. The text insets describe individual plots or photographs relating to nanoparticles carrying BSX, RMCel12A, or PfuAmyGT, or all the tri-enzymes (multipotent). (**a**) Effect of pH; (**b**) variations in stability upon storage; (**c**) reusability of immobilized enzyme preparations; (**d**) visual evidence for degradation of biomass (corn cob or rice husk) by RMCel12A or BSX. Reproduced with permission from Reference [60].

Different MNPs were prepared and characterized, while the significance of MNP characterization was exclusively discussed by Schwaminger and his colleagues (Scheme 2). Moreover, electrostatic and hydrophobic interactions between the enzyme molecules and MNPs were also investigated. Results from infrared (IR) spectroscopy revealed a high affinity for β-sheet formation in the tertiary structure content of enzyme molecules. In this study, cellulase loading on different MNPs was studied, and the results showed that higher loading efficiencies would be achieved by using a higher α-helical section [61].

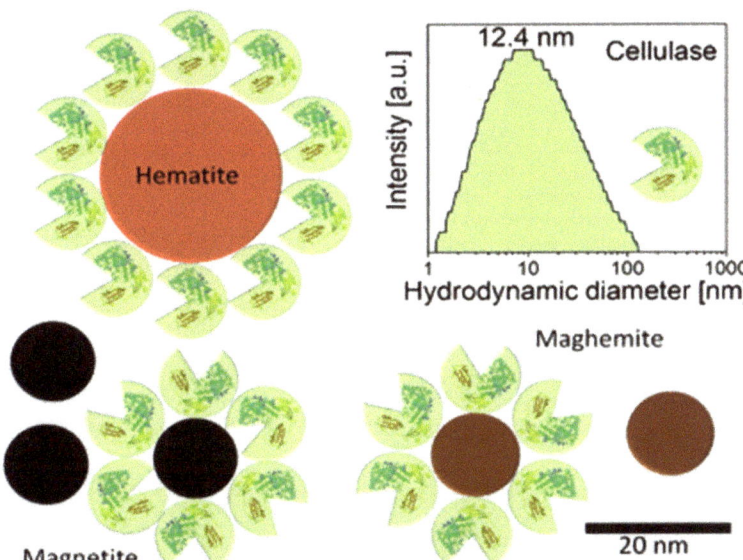

Scheme 2. Schematic representation of cellulase immobilization onto three types of MNPs. Reproduced with permission from Reference [61].

In another study, fungus cell filtrate was applied to synthesize MNPs, which was further characterized. The results obtained from this study revealed that the free enzyme was more efficient than the immobilized form and that cellulase molecules retained high activity following immobilization. The authors suggested that cellulase immobilization on MNPs provides good reusability, making the process more efficient for sustainable bioethanol production [62]. As summarized in Table 2, the significant parameters of cellulase immobilization such as pH, temperature, reusability, and coupling agents, as well as supports and substrates, are presented for carrier-free immobilization approach.

Table 2. Carrier-free MNP systems for cellulase immobilization.

Enzyme	Substrate	Support	Coupling Agent	Amount	pH	Temperature	Reusability Cycle	Efficiency	Ref.
Cellulase, pectinase, and xylanase	CMC, pectin, and xylan	Fe_3O_4	Glutaraldehyde	5.06 ± 0.46 mg/mL 3.39 ± 0.12 mg/mL 2.95 ± 0.14 mg/mL	5.5	55–75 °C	4	80.25 ± 1.03% 84.76 ± 1.71% 75.62 ± 0.76%	[19]
Xylanase, cellulase, amylase	Xylan, CMC, starch	MNPs	Glutaraldehyde	3 mg/mL	2–12	Thermostable up to 70 °C	13	69, 48, and 50%	[60]
Cellulase	N/A *	magnetite, maghemite, and hematite MNPs	N/A	0.6 g·g^{-1}	N/A	NA	N/A	N/A	[61]
Cellulase	Microcrystalline	Fe_3O_4	Glutaraldehyde	250 mg	N/A	27 °C, 40 °C, 50 °C and 60 °C	3	52%	[62]

* Not available.

4. Cellulase Immobilization on Amino-Functionalized MNPs

Functionalization of MNPs is a commonly used strategy for tri-enzyme immobilization via covalent bonding. Amines are among the most common functionalized groups that can be linked to proteins via cross-linking agents. Cellulase (from *Trichoderma reesei*) and pectinase (from *Aspergillus aculeatus*) were simultaneously immobilized on amino-functionalized MNPs (AMNPs) for antioxidant extraction from waste fruit peels. This immobilization method led to increased thermal stability, half-life, and V_{max} for both enzymes; however, it caused a slight decrease in their activity. Immobilized enzymes on MNPs show increased reusability of the biocatalyst. Results showed that glutaraldehyde's concertation is an important factor affecting the activity of immobilized enzyme [63]. In a similar study, pectinase and cellulase were immobilized on AMNPs and utilized in the extraction of tomato peel lycopene. The immobilization process decreased enzyme activity while increasing its stability. Ultrasonic irradiation is used to highly activate immobilized cellulase, as well as increase the efficiency of biocatalyst. Results also showed that the biocatalyst decreased extraction time in comparison to free enzyme forms [64]. Hyperactivity of immobilized cellulase on AMNPs was investigated in another study. Application of ultrasound irradiation enhanced cellulase activity up to 3.6-fold. Sonication also increased V_{max} and decreased K_m of cellulase. The results obtained from this study showed that MNP/enzyme ratio, concentration of cross-linking agent, and cross-linking time affected the enzyme activity [65].

Co-immobilization of cellulase and lysozyme on AMNPs was performed for extraction of lipids from microalgae (Scheme 3). Their findings showed that enzyme stability and catalytic efficiency were increased; however, the activity and kinetic parameters of both enzymes decreased following immobilization [66].

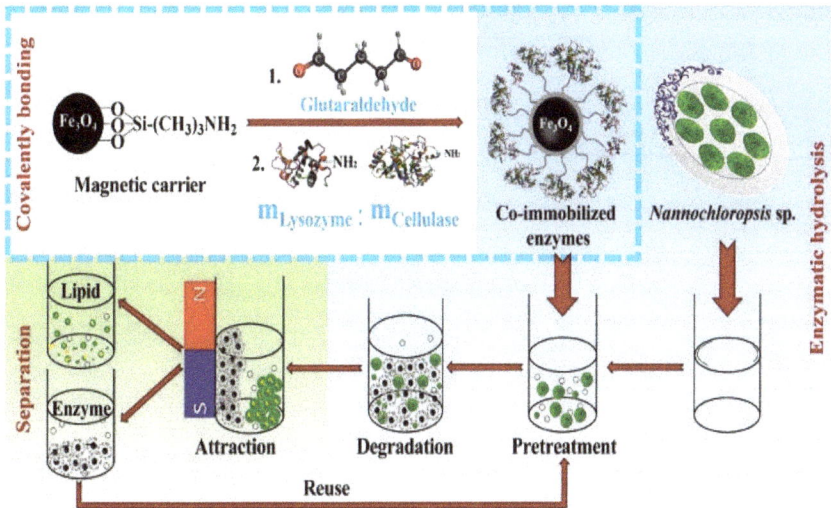

Scheme 3. Co-immobilization of cellulase and lysozyme on amino-functionalized MNPs (AMNPs) for extraction of lipid. Reproduced with permission from Reference [66].

It is believed that co-immobilization of cellulose is greatly influenced by the enzyme concentration on the MNP surface. In addition, the immobilization process increases the efficiency of biocatalyst via multiple enzymes; however, applicable enzyme concentration is limited and enzyme activity is reduced due to low availability of surface area. As summarized in Table 3, enzyme immobilization on AMNPs via covalent bonding can increase thermal and chemical stability while generally reducing enzyme activity. MNPs provide biocatalyst reusability, while sonication hyperactivates immobilized cellulase which can compensate for the enzyme activity. It can be concluded that enzyme immobilization on AMNPs can be used for industrial applications.

Table 3. Cellulase immobilization on amino-functionalized MNPs (AMNPs).

Enzyme	Substrate	Support	Coupling Agent	Amount	pH	Temperature	Reusability		Ref.
							Cycle	Efficiency	
Pectinase, cellulase	Carboxymethyl cellulose (CMC)	AMNPs	Glutaraldehyde	9 and 3 mg/mL	6.5	50–70 °C	8	87% and 82%	[63]
Pectinase, cellulase	pectin, cellulose	AMNPs	Glutaraldehyde	50 mg	5	25–35 °C	8	85% and 80%	[64]
Cellulase	cellulose	AMNPs	Glutaraldehyde	N/A	3–8	30–80 °C	7	58%	[65]
Cellulase, lysozyme	cell walls	AMNPs	Glutaraldehyde	0.5 mg	3–7	60–80 °C	6	78.1% and 69.6%	[66]
Cellulase	CMC	Cu/AMNPs	APTES	N/A	2–7	20–80 °C	5	73%	[67]

Amino-functionalized MNPs (AMNPs); 3-aminopropyl-triethoxysilane (APTES).

In a recent study, AMNPs in combination with copper (Cu) (as an affinity ligand) were employed for immobilization of *A. niger*-derived cellulase. Metal affinity ligands are commonly used due to their high chemical stability, low cost, and modifying capability. Loading concentration and cellulase activity were investigated by full factorial design, considering pH, and Cu/MNP and enzyme/MNP ratios as independent variables. Obtained data revealed that Cu improved the immobilized enzyme's activity, storage stability, and loading capacity (i.e., 164 mg/g MNPs). The biocatalyst remained stable under a wide range of pHs and temperatures [67].

5. Cellulase Immobilization on Composite-Functionalized MNPs

MNPs used as enzyme immobilization supports can be coated with various nanomaterials. MNP coating prevents nanoparticles oxidation, improves enzyme immobilization efficacy, and may decrease toxicity of the support materials. The coating process should not alter the magnetic properties of nanoparticles, which are essential for the biocatalyst's reusability through a magnetic field. Different composite coatings were prepared for cellulase immobilization, and the effects of coating on enzyme activity and stability were studied.

In recent years, metallic, metallic oxide, and carbon-related materials were widely applied and blended with different polymers to prepare novel nanocomposites for enzyme immobilization. Specifically, gold, MgO, and graphene oxide (GO) were blended with different polymers such as PEG, glutamic acid, and poly(methyl methacrylate) for enhancing the enzyme stability.

Immobilized cellulase on MNPs coated with layered double hydroxide (LDH) nanosheets were used to reduce the magneto-induced effect on the enzyme. Results showed that utilizing nanocomposite materials could increase specific enzyme activity and loading efficiency, but could reduce enzyme reusability. Immobilized cellulase also demonstrated higher stability in a wide range of temperatures and pH values [68]. MgO-coated MNPs were used as a support for covalent immobilization of cellulase from *Chlorella* sp. CYB2. MgO played a significant role for improvement of immobilization yield, activity recovery, and hydrolysis of the substrate [69].

In another study, poly(methyl methacrylate)-coated MNPs were used for cellulase immobilization as shown in Scheme 4. Enzyme stability and activity were affected by the immobilization process as detailed in Table 4. The results obtained revealed that poly(methyl methacrylate) as a coating polymer did not have any significant effect on the particles' magnetic properties (Figure 4) [70].

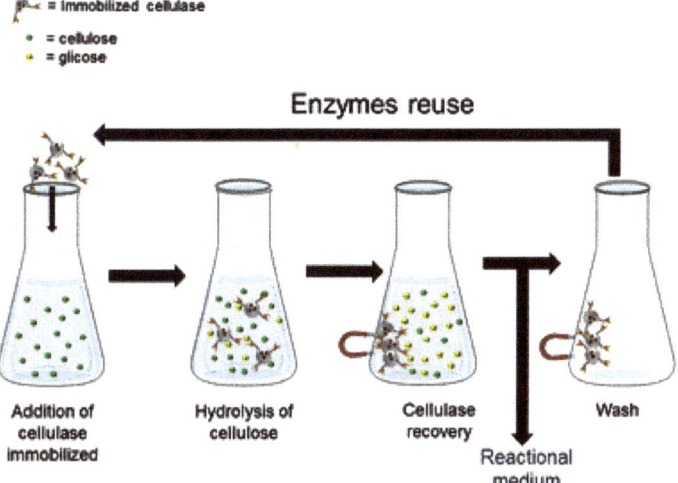

Scheme 4. Overview of hydrolysis of cellulose by poly(methyl methacrylate)-coated MNPs applied for enzyme immobilization and enzyme reusability. Reproduced with permission from Reference [70].

Table 4. Cellulase immobilization on composite functionalized MNPs.

Enzyme	Substrate	Support	Coupling Agent	Amount	pH	Temperature	Reusability Cycle	Efficiency	Ref.
Cellulase	CMC	(Fe_3O_4) layered double hydroxides (LDHs)	Glutaraldehyde	1.2 g/L	5.5	50 °C	6	31.8%	[68]
Cellulase	cellulose	MgO-Fe_3O_4	Xylan aldehyde	150 mg/g	4.5–6.5	50–70 °C	7	84.5%	[69]
Cellulase	CMC	Poly(methyl methacrylate) MNPs	N/A	5% (w/v)	3–8	35–75 °C	8	69%	[70]
Cellulase	Microcrystalline cellulose or filter paper	Fe_3O_4-NH_2@4-arm-PEG-NH_2	Glutaraldehyde	132 mg/g	3–7	30–80 °C	6	76%.	[45]
Cellulase	Microcrystalline cellulose or filter paper	GO@Fe_3O_4@4arm PEG NH_2	Glutaraldehyde	2–8 mg	3.5–5.5	30–80 °C	7	65% and 70%	[71]
Cellulase	Microcrystalline or filter paper	Glu@PEGylated mAu@PSN	Glutamic acid	25 mg	3–8	35–75 °C	5	76%	[72]

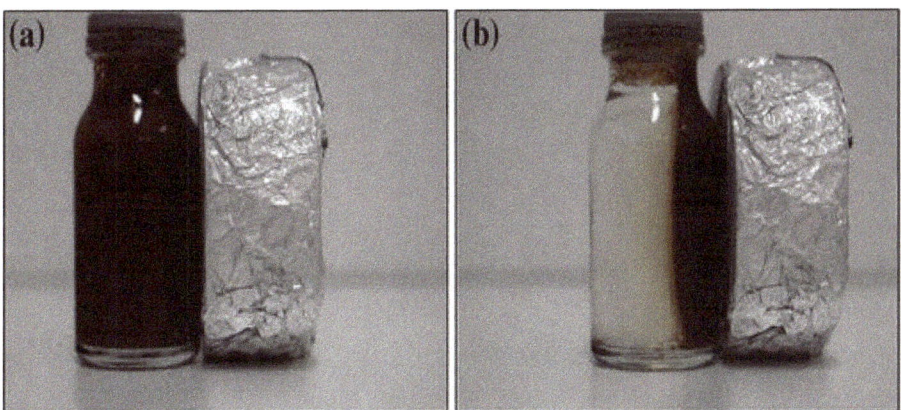

Figure 4. Magnetic behavior of poly(methyl methacrylate)-coated MNPs before (**a**) and after (**b**) separation. Reproduced with permission from Reference [70].

Four-arm dendritic polymers composed of PEG-NH$_2$ (Scheme 5) were used as coating materials for immobilization of cellulase derived from *Trichoderma viride* onto MNPs. The enzyme was covalently bonded to the dendrimer via coupling agents. The dendrimer improved the thermal stability and activity of cellulase [45]. GO-decorated four-arm PEG-NH$_2$ was applied as a coating composite of MNPs in another study (Scheme 6). The obtained results showed that polymers with higher molecular weights can increase loading capacity, enzymatic activity, and storage stability of cellulase [71].

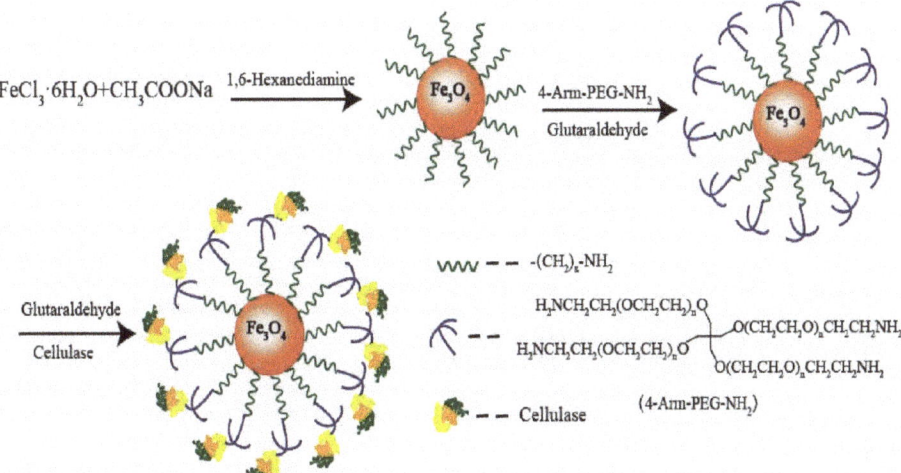

Scheme 5. Preparation process of four-arm dendritic polymers comprising polyethylene glycol (PEG)-NH$_2$. Reproduced with permission from Reference [45].

Core–shell magnetic gold mesoporous silica was exploited as a support for cellulase immobilization (Scheme 7). Thermal and chemical stabilities were considerably augmented in a wide range of pH values and temperatures. Vibrating-sample magnetometer (VSM) study results showed that the magnetic behavior of MNPs was not altered following the coating process [72].

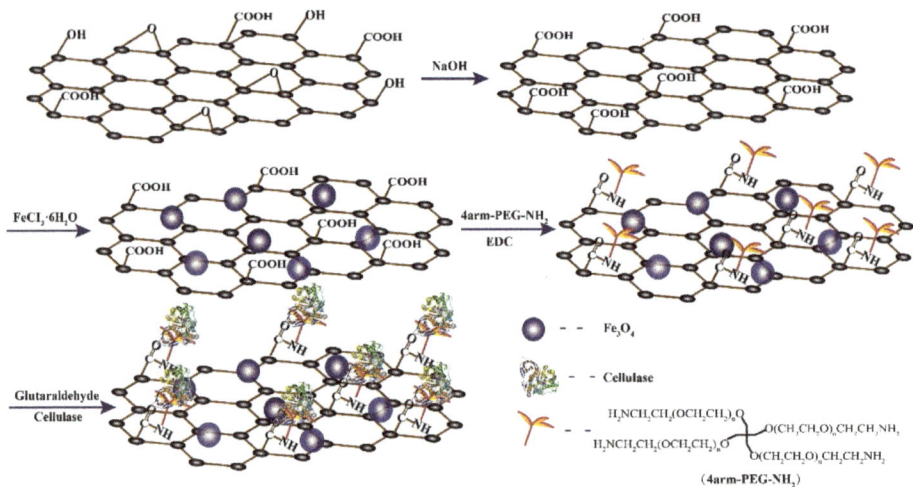

Scheme 6. Graphene oxide (GO)-decorated four-arm PEG-NH$_2$ coating composite of MNPs. Reproduced with permission from Reference [71].

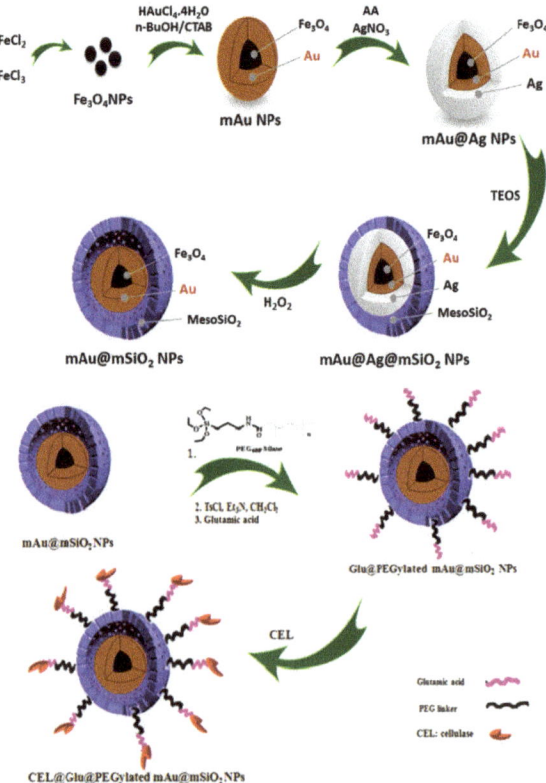

Scheme 7. Cellulase immobilization on core–shell magnetic gold mesoporous silica support. Reproduced with permission from Reference [72].

As presented in Table 4, cellulase was immobilized on MNP surfaces via different coating materials. Polymers are extensively applied as preferred coating materials for cellulase immobilization. The immobilization of cellulase on MNPs via covalent binding improves biocatalyst activity and stability, regardless of coating type.

6. Cellulase Immobilization on Chitosan-Functionalized MNPs

Chitosan, a biocompatible and biodegradable polymer, is exclusively used as a coating agent in enzyme immobilization processes. Chitosan can provide a positively charged coating, while acting as a toxicity reducing agent or adhesive enhancer for simple immobilization processes or in vivo applications.

Cellulase enzyme was covalently immobilized on chitosan-coated MNPs (Ch-MNPs) using coupling agents. The immobilization of cellulase decreased enzyme activity compared to free enzyme, while thermal stability and reusability of the enzyme was improved. The immobilization process significantly increased the K_m value and the biocatalyst efficiently hydrolyzed lignocellulosic materials from *Agave atrovirens* leaves with acceptable yield [37]. In a similar study, cellulase was immobilized on MNPs using a cross-linking agent (Scheme 8), and the optimal enzyme loading efficiency and standard recovery ratio were studied [46].

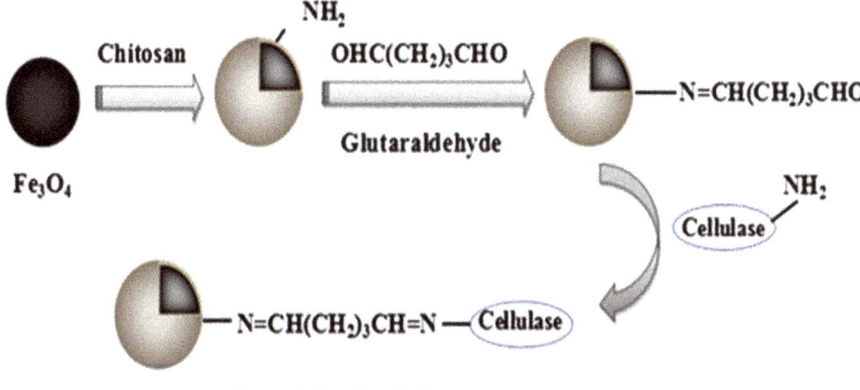

Scheme 8. Immobilization of cellulase on chitosan-coated (Ch)-MNPs using glutaraldehyde as a cross-linking agent. Reproduced with permission from Reference [46].

Maximizing the rate of cellulase and xylanase immobilization onto Ch-MNP was studied, and the obtained data showed that 12 mg of protein was cross-linked per gram of MNPs. The results also showed that size distribution, shape, and surface chemistry of MNPs affected the coating process and immobilization efficiency [73]. In the case of enzymatic saccharification, laccase from *Trametes versicolor* was immobilized onto Ch-MNPs (Scheme 9). It was concluded that the catalytic activity, thermal and chemical stability, and the K_m value were improved significantly following enzyme immobilization [74].

Chitosan as a coating material for MNPs was utilized for enzyme cross-linking in order to enhance the stability parameters (Table 5). Chitosan-coated MNPs are prepared in a one-step process which can be a simple and cost-effective method for enzyme immobilization.

Table 5. Cellulase immobilization on chitosan-functionalized MNPs.

Enzyme	Substrate	Support	Coupling Agent	Amount	pH	Temperature	Reusability		Ref.
							Cycle	Efficiency	
Cellulase	CMC	Chitosan-coated MNPs (Ch-MNPs)	Glutaraldehyde	26.06 mg	2.5–8.5	20–70 °C	15	80%	[37]
Cellulase	CMC	Magnetic $Fe_3O_4^-$ chitosan	Glutaraldehyde	32.29 mg	3–7	30–70 °C	5	80%	[46]
Xylanase and cellulase 1:0.5	N/A	Chitosan-coated magnetite particles	Glutaraldehyde	N/A	N/A	N/A	N/A	N/A	[73]
Laccase	Lignin	Chitosan (C)-MNP	Glutaraldehyde	25 mg	2–7	25–75 °C	5	50%	[74]

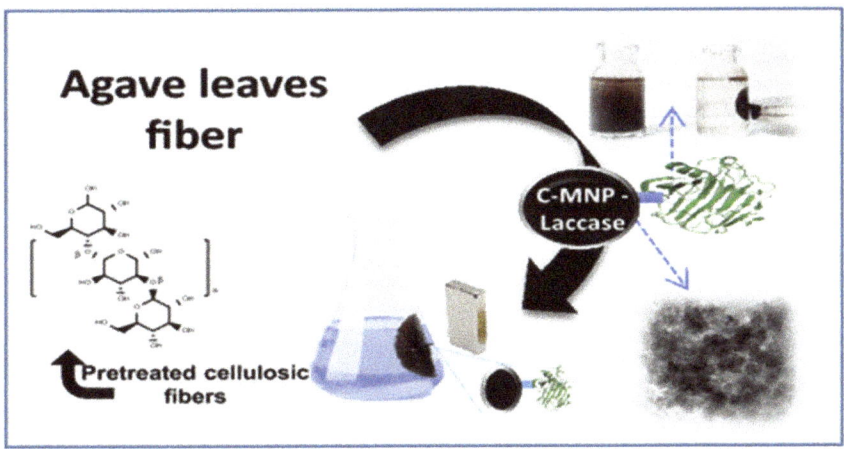

Scheme 9. Enzymatic saccharification and reusability of immobilized laccase onto Ch-MNPs. Reproduced with permission from Reference [74].

7. An Overview of Principal Factors Affecting Cellulase Immobilization onto MNPs

Among the different methods available for cellulase immobilization on functionalized MNPs, covalent binding by applying glutaraldehyde as the coupling agent is the most efficient process. Different types of functionalized MNPs were studied for cellulase immobilization [39,75–77]. Gold magnetic silica nanoparticles were used as a promising platform for cellulase immobilization. Graphene oxide is another candidate which retains high enzymatic activity. In addition to functionalized groups, chitosan- and silica-coated MNPs could be used as efficient solid supports for biomaterials hydrolysis. The application of ultrasound is another approach for improving the properties of immobilized enzyme. Different functionalization methods of MNPs for the cellulase immobilization approach and the attributes of each approach are outlined in Table 6.

Table 6. Recent advances in immobilizing cellulase onto MNPs.

Different Functionalized MNPs Applied in Cellulase Immobilization Approaches		
Immobilization Approach	Attributes	Ref.
Silica-based surface functionalization	Enhanced chemical stability while avoiding the aggregation of nanoparticles	[51–54]
Composite-based surface functionalization	Providing unique physical and electronic properties and also providing a large surface area for biomolecules to anchor	[69–72]
Amino-based surface functionalization	Novel strategies to enhance the enzyme's thermal and chemical stability	[63–67]
Chitosan-based surface functionalization	Providing an appropriate surface for biomolecules to anchor	[46,74]
Carrier-free immobilization	Novel strategies to improve enzyme activity	[60–62]

8. Summary and Outlook

Biotechnology opened new horizons for human beings, especially in the field of industry. Due to increased environmental pollution, and of the increase in human population, biotechnology employs nano-biomaterials in order to enhance product yield. Cellulase is one of the most widely used biocatalysts that converts cellulosic materials into monosaccharides such as glucose, which are further used for biofuel production. However, biomass conversion to glucose needs to be efficient and cost-effective; as a result, researchers are focusing on the development of novel approaches with enhanced enzyme reusability and lower cost, along with easy enzyme recovery from the reaction mixture. During the last two years, studies showed that immobilized cellulases on nanocarrier supports provide promising potential as novel nano-biocatalysts which can be further exploited for achieving higher enzyme activity and storage stability in the immobilization processes. Meanwhile, MNPs are suitable nano-carriers to separate enzymes from the reaction mixture by using an external magnet while being efficient by reducing recycling costs. Various MNPs with different functional groups as solid supports exist, including inorganic metals, graphene, chitosan, and organic compounds. Despite recent advances, novel approaches are still required for achieving more efficient nano-biocatalysts. The increasing demand for low-cost immobilized cellulase and the ever-increasing applications in different industries are the main reasons for research attention in this field.

Author Contributions: Conceptualization, methodology, writing, original draft preparation, table preparation, review, and editing, K.K.; writing, original draft preparation, table preparation, and review E.P.; writing, original draft preparation, and table preparation, H.B.; original draft preparation, schemes and figures preparation, M.B.

Funding: Private funds were applied to carry out this study.

Acknowledgments: The authors would like to express special thanks to F. Vakhshiteh, A.K. Bordbar, and H. Stamatis for their practical and valuable collaboration in our previous study.

Conflicts of Interest: The authors declare no conflicts of interest.

References

1. Khoshnevisan, K.; Vakhshiteh, F.; Barkhi, M.; Baharifar, H.; Poor-Akbar, E.; Zari, N.; Stamatis, H.; Bordbar, A.-K. Immobilization of cellulase enzyme onto magnetic nanoparticles: Applications and recent advances. *Mol. Catal.* **2017**, *442*, 66–73. [CrossRef]
2. Coseri, S. Cellulose: To depolymerize . . . or not to? *Biotechnol. Adv.* **2017**, *35*, 251–266. [CrossRef] [PubMed]
3. Phitsuwan, P.; Laohakunjit, N.; Kerdchoechuen, O.; Kyu, K.L.; Ratanakhanokchai, K. Present and potential applications of cellulases in agriculture, biotechnology, and bioenergy. *Folia Microbiol.* **2013**, *58*, 163–176. [CrossRef] [PubMed]
4. Kuhad, R.C.; Gupta, R.; Singh, A. Microbial Cellulases and Their Industrial Applications. *Enzym. Res.* **2011**, *2011*, 280696. [CrossRef]
5. Aftab, M.N.; Zafar, A.; Awan, A.R. Expression of thermostable β-xylosidase in Escherichia coli for use in saccharification of plant biomass. *Bioengineered* **2017**, *8*, 665–669. [CrossRef] [PubMed]
6. Meenu, K.; Singh, G.; Vishwakarma, R.A. *Chapter 22—Molecular Mechanism of Cellulase Production Systems in Trichoderma*; Gupta, V.K.; Schmoll, M., Herrera-Estrella, A., Upadhyay, R.S., Druzhinina, I., Tuohy, M., Eds.; Elsevier: Amsterdam, The Netherlands, 2014; pp. 319–324, ISBN 978-0-444-59576-8.
7. Pan, X.; Arato, C.; Gilkes, N.; Gregg, D.; Mabee, W.; Pye, K.; Xiao, Z.; Zhang, X.; Saddler, J. Biorefining of softwoods using ethanol organosolv pulping: Preliminary evaluation of process streams for manufacture of fuel-grade ethanol and co-products. *Biotechnol. Bioeng.* **2005**, *90*, 473–481. [CrossRef]
8. Klein-Marcuschamer, D.; Simmons, B.A.; Blanch, H.W. Techno-economic analysis of a lignocellulosic ethanol biorefinery with ionic liquid pre-treatment. *Biofuels Bioprod. Biorefin.* **2011**, *5*, 562–569. [CrossRef]
9. Zhang, Y.-H.P.; Ding, S.-Y.; Mielenz, J.R.; Cui, J.-B.; Elander, R.T.; Laser, M.; Himmel, M.E.; McMillan, J.R.; Lynd, L.R. Fractionating recalcitrant lignocellulose at modest reaction conditions. *Biotechnol. Bioeng.* **2007**, *97*, 214–223. [CrossRef]
10. Gupta, V.K.; Kubicek, C.P.; Berrin, J.-G.; Wilson, D.W.; Couturier, M.; Berlin, A.; Filho, E.X.F.; Ezeji, T. Fungal Enzymes for Bio-Products from Sustainable and Waste Biomass. *Trends Biochem. Sci.* **2016**, *41*, 633–645. [CrossRef]
11. Kossatz, H.L.; Rose, S.H.; Viljoen-Bloom, M.; van Zyl, W.H. Production of ethanol from steam exploded triticale straw in a simultaneous saccharification and fermentation process. *Process Biochem.* **2017**, *53*, 10–16. [CrossRef]
12. Binod, P.; Gnansounou, E.; Sindhu, R.; Pandey, A. Enzymes for second generation biofuels: Recent developments and future perspectives. *Bioresour. Technol. Rep.* **2019**, *5*, 317–325. [CrossRef]

13. Poudel, S.; Giannone, R.J.; Rodriguez, M.; Raman, B.; Martin, M.Z.; Engle, N.L.; Mielenz, J.R.; Nookaew, I.; Brown, S.D.; Tschaplinski, T.J.; et al. Integrated omics analyses reveal the details of metabolic adaptation of Clostridium thermocellum to lignocellulose-derived growth inhibitors released during the deconstruction of switchgrass. *Biotechnol. Biofuels* **2017**, *10*, 14. [CrossRef] [PubMed]
14. Avanthi, A.; Kumar, S.; Sherpa, K.C.; Banerjee, R. Bioconversion of hemicelluloses of lignocellulosic biomass to ethanol: An attempt to utilize pentose sugars. *Biofuels* **2017**, *8*, 431–444. [CrossRef]
15. Sheldon, R.A.; Brady, D. The limits to biocatalysis: Pushing the envelope. *Chem. Commun.* **2018**, *54*, 6088–6104. [CrossRef] [PubMed]
16. Ye, L.; Yang, C.; Yu, H. From molecular engineering to process engineering: Development of high-throughput screening methods in enzyme directed evolution. *Appl. Microbiol. Biotechnol.* **2018**, *102*, 559–567. [CrossRef]
17. Naeem, M.; Rehman, A.U.; Shen, B.; Ye, L.; Yu, H. Semi-rational engineering of carbonyl reductase YueD for efficient biosynthesis of halogenated alcohols with in situ cofactor regeneration. *Biochem. Eng. J.* **2018**, *137*, 62–70. [CrossRef]
18. Perwez, M.; Ahmad, R.; Sardar, M. A reusable multipurpose magnetic nanobiocatalyst for industrial applications. *Int. J. Biol. Macromol.* **2017**, *103*, 16–24. [CrossRef]
19. Muley, A.B.; Thorat, A.S.; Singhal, R.S.; Harinath Babu, K. A tri-enzyme co-immobilized magnetic complex: Process details, kinetics, thermodynamics and applications. *Int. J. Biol. Macromol.* **2018**, *118*, 1781–1795. [CrossRef]
20. Waifalkar, P.P.; Parit, S.B.; Chougale, A.D.; Sahoo, S.C.; Patil, P.S.; Patil, P.B. Immobilization of invertase on chitosan coated γ-Fe_2O_3 magnetic nanoparticles to facilitate magnetic separation. *J. Colloid Interface Sci.* **2016**, *482*, 159–164. [CrossRef]
21. Dosadina, E.E.; Savelyeva, E.E.; Belov, A.A. The effect of immobilization, drying and storage on the activity of proteinases immobilized on modified cellulose and chitosan. *Process Biochem.* **2018**, *64*, 213–220. [CrossRef]
22. Bilal, M.; Rasheed, T.; Zhao, Y.; Iqbal, H.M.N.; Cui, J. "Smart" chemistry and its application in peroxidase immobilization using different support materials. *Int. J. Biol. Macromol.* **2018**, *119*, 278–290. [CrossRef] [PubMed]
23. Liu, D.-M.; Chen, J.; Shi, Y.-P. Advances on methods and easy separated support materials for enzymes immobilization. *TrAC Trends Anal. Chem.* **2018**, *102*, 332–342. [CrossRef]
24. Lonappan, L.; Liu, Y.; Rouissi, T.; Pourcel, F.; Brar, S.K.; Verma, M.; Surampalli, R.Y. Covalent immobilization of laccase on citric acid functionalized micro-biochars derived from different feedstock and removal of diclofenac. *Chem. Eng. J.* **2018**, *351*, 985–994. [CrossRef]
25. Zaak, H.; Sassi, M.; Fernandez-Lafuente, R. A new heterofunctional amino-vinyl sulfone support to immobilize enzymes: Application to the stabilization of β-galactosidase from Aspergillus oryzae. *Process Biochem.* **2018**, *64*, 200–205. [CrossRef]
26. Vaghari, H.; Jafarizadeh-Malmiri, H.; Mohammadlou, M.; Berenjian, A.; Anarjan, N.; Jafari, N.; Nasiri, S. Application of magnetic nanoparticles in smart enzyme immobilization. *Biotechnol. Lett.* **2016**, *38*, 223–233. [CrossRef]
27. Royvaran, M.; Taheri-Kafrani, A.; Landarani Isfahani, A.; Mohammadi, S. Functionalized superparamagnetic graphene oxide nanosheet in enzyme engineering: A highly dispersive, stable and robust biocatalyst. *Chem. Eng. J.* **2016**, *288*, 414–422. [CrossRef]
28. Baharifar, H.; Honarvarfard, E.; Haji Malek-kheili, M.; Maleki, H.; Barkhi, M.; Ghasemzadeh, A.; Khoshnevisan, K. The Potentials and Applications of Cellulose Acetate in biosensor technology. *Nanomed. Res. J.* **2017**, *2*, 216–223.
29. Khoshnevisan, K.; Maleki, H.; Honarvarfard, E.; Baharifar, H.; Gholami, M.; Faridbod, F.; Larijani, B.; Faridi Majidi, R.; Khorramizadeh, M.R. Nanomaterial based electrochemical sensing of the biomarker serotonin: A comprehensive review. *Microchim. Acta* **2019**, *186*, 49. [CrossRef]
30. Chen, M.; Zeng, G.; Xu, P.; Lai, C.; Tang, L. How Do Enzymes 'Meet' Nanoparticles and Nanomaterials? *Trends Biochem. Sci.* **2017**, *42*, 914–930. [CrossRef]
31. Nasir, M.; Nawaz, M.H.; Latif, U.; Yaqub, M.; Hayat, A.; Rahim, A. An overview on enzyme-mimicking nanomaterials for use in electrochemical and optical assays. *Microchim. Acta* **2017**, *184*, 323–342. [CrossRef]
32. Wu, J.; Wang, X.; Wang, Q.; Lou, Z.; Li, S.; Zhu, Y.; Qin, L.; Wei, H. Nanomaterials with enzyme-like characteristics (nanozymes): Next-generation artificial enzymes (II). *Chem. Soc. Rev.* **2019**, *48*, 1004–1076. [CrossRef] [PubMed]

33. Hemmati, M.; Barkhi, M.; Baharifar, H.; Khoshnevisan, K. Removal of Malachite Green by Using Immobilized Glucose Oxidase Onto Silica Nanostructure-Coated Silver Metal-Foam. *J. Nanoanal.* **2017**, *4*, 196–204.
34. Bilal, M.; Iqbal, H.M.N. Chemical, physical, and biological coordination: An interplay between materials and enzymes as potential platforms for immobilization. *Coord. Chem. Rev.* **2019**, *388*, 1–23. [CrossRef]
35. Pandiyaraj, K.N.; Ramkumar, M.C.; Arun Kumar, A.; Padmanabhan, P.V.A.; Pichumani, M.; Bendavid, A.; Cools, P.; De Geyter, N.; Morent, R.; Kumar, V.; et al. Evaluation of surface properties of low density polyethylene (LDPE) films tailored by atmospheric pressure non-thermal plasma (APNTP) assisted co-polymerization and immobilization of chitosan for improvement of antifouling properties. *Mater. Sci. Eng. C* **2019**, *94*, 150–160. [CrossRef] [PubMed]
36. Tedersoo, L.; Sánchez-Ramírez, S.; Kõljalg, U.; Bahram, M.; Döring, M.; Schigel, D.; May, T.; Ryberg, M.; Abarenkov, K. High-level classification of the Fungi and a tool for evolutionary ecological analyses. *Fungal Divers.* **2018**, *90*, 135–159. [CrossRef]
37. Sánchez-Ramírez, J.; Martínez-Hernández, J.L.; Segura-Ceniceros, P.; López, G.; Saade, H.; Medina-Morales, M.A.; Ramos-González, R.; Aguilar, C.N.; Ilyina, A. Cellulases immobilization on chitosan-coated magnetic nanoparticles: Application for Agave Atrovirens lignocellulosic biomass hydrolysis. *Bioprocess Biosyst. Eng.* **2017**, *40*, 9–22. [CrossRef] [PubMed]
38. Xu, J.; Xiong, P.; He, B. Advances in improving the performance of cellulase in ionic liquids for lignocellulose biorefinery. *Bioresour. Technol.* **2016**, *200*, 961–970. [CrossRef]
39. Cipolatti, E.P.; Valério, A.; Henriques, R.O.; Moritz, D.E.; Ninow, J.L.; Freire, D.M.G.; Manoel, E.A.; Fernandez-Lafuente, R.; de Oliveira, D. Nanomaterials for biocatalyst immobilization—State of the art and future trends. *RSC Adv.* **2016**, *6*, 104675–104692. [CrossRef]
40. Malgas, S.; Thoresen, M.; van Dyk, J.S.; Pletschke, B.I. Time dependence of enzyme synergism during the degradation of model and natural lignocellulosic substrates. *Enzym. Microb. Technol.* **2017**, *103*, 1–11. [CrossRef]
41. Molina, G.; de Lima, E.A.; Borin, G.P.; de Barcelos, M.C.S.; Pastore, G.M. *Chapter 7—Beta-Glucosidase From Penicillium*; Gupta, V.K., Rodriguez-Couto, S.B.T.-N., Eds.; Elsevier: Amsterdam, The Netherlands, 2018; pp. 137–151, ISBN 978-0-444-63501-3.
42. Khoshnevisan, K.; Bordbar, A.-K.; Zare, D.; Davoodi, D.; Noruzi, M.; Barkhi, M.; Tabatabaei, M. Immobilization of cellulase enzyme on superparamagnetic nanoparticles and determination of its activity and stability. *Chem. Eng. J.* **2011**, *171*, 669–673. [CrossRef]
43. Khoshnevisan, K.; Barkhi, M.; Zare, D.; Davoodi, D.; Tabatabaei, M. Preparation and Characterization of CTAB-Coated Fe$_3$O$_4$ Nanoparticles. *Synth. React. Inorg. Met. Org. Nano-Met. Chem.* **2012**, *42*, 644–648. [CrossRef]
44. Khoshnevisan, K.; Barkhi, M.; Ghasemzadeh, A.; Tahami, H.V.; Pourmand, S. Fabrication of Coated/Uncoated Magnetic Nanoparticles to Determine Their Surface Properties. *Mater. Manuf. Process.* **2016**, *31*, 1206–1215. [CrossRef]
45. Han, J.; Wang, L.; Wang, Y.; Dong, J.; Tang, X.; Ni, L.; Wang, L. Preparation and characterization of Fe$_3$O$_4$-NH$_2$@4-arm-PEG-NH$_2$, a novel magnetic four-arm polymer-nanoparticle composite for cellulase immobilization. *Biochem. Eng. J.* **2018**, *130*, 90–98. [CrossRef]
46. Lin, Y.; Liu, X.; Xing, Z.; Geng, Y.; Wilson, J.; Wu, D.; Kong, H. Preparation and characterization of magnetic Fe3O4–chitosan nanoparticles for cellulase immobilization. *Cellulose* **2017**, *24*, 5541–5550. [CrossRef]
47. Yang, C.; Mo, H.; Zang, L.; Chen, J.; Wang, Z.; Qiu, J. Surface functionalized natural inorganic nanorod for highly efficient cellulase immobilization. *RSC Adv.* **2016**, *6*, 76855–76860. [CrossRef]
48. Zang, L.; Qiao, X.; Hu, L.; Yang, C.; Liu, Q.; Wei, C.; Qiu, J.; Mo, H.; Song, G.; Yang, J.; et al. Preparation and Evaluation of Coal Fly Ash/Chitosan Composites as Magnetic Supports for Highly Efficient Cellulase Immobilization and Cellulose Bioconversion. *Polymers* **2018**, *10*, 523. [CrossRef] [PubMed]
49. Carli, S.; de Campos Carneiro, L.A.B.; Ward, R.J.; Meleiro, L.P. Immobilization of a β-glucosidase and an endoglucanase in ferromagnetic nanoparticles: A study of synergistic effects. *Protein Expr. Purif.* **2019**, *160*, 28–35. [CrossRef]
50. Cacicedo, M.L.; Manzo, R.M.; Municoy, S.; Bonazza, H.L.; Islan, G.A.; Desimone, M.; Bellino, M.; Mammarella, E.J.; Castro, G.R. Chapter 7—Immobilized Enzymes and Their Applications. In *Biomass, Biofuels, Biochemicals*; Singh, R.S., Singhania, R.R., Pandey, A., Larroche, C.B.T.-A., Eds.; Elsevier: Amsterdam, The Netherlands, 2019; pp. 169–200, ISBN 978-0-444-64114-4.

51. Zhang, Y.; Jin, P.; Liu, M.; Pan, J.; Yan, Y.; Chen, Y.; Xiong, Q. A novel route for green conversion of cellulose to HMF by cascading enzymatic and chemical reactions. *AIChE J.* **2017**, *63*, 4920–4932. [CrossRef]
52. Grewal, J.; Ahmad, R.; Khare, S.K. Development of cellulase-nanoconjugates with enhanced ionic liquid and thermal stability for in situ lignocellulose saccharification. *Bioresour. Technol.* **2017**, *242*, 236–243. [CrossRef]
53. Kumar, A.; Singh, S.; Tiwari, R.; Goel, R.; Nain, L. Immobilization of indigenous holocellulase on iron oxide (Fe_2O_3) nanoparticles enhanced hydrolysis of alkali pretreated paddy straw. *Int. J. Biol. Macromol.* **2017**, *96*, 538–549. [CrossRef]
54. Jia, J.; Zhang, W.; Yang, Z.; Yang, X.; Wang, N.; Yu, X. Novel Magnetic Cross-Linked Cellulase Aggregates with a Potential Application in Lignocellulosic Biomass Bioconversion. *Molecules* **2017**, *22*, 269. [CrossRef] [PubMed]
55. Gaikwad, S.; Ingle, A.P.; da Silva, S.S.; Rai, M. Immobilized Nanoparticles-Mediated Enzymatic Hydrolysis of Cellulose for Clean Sugar Production: A Novel Approach. *Curr. Nanosci.* **2019**, *15*, 296–303. [CrossRef]
56. Cui, J.D.; Jia, S.R. Optimization protocols and improved strategies of cross-linked enzyme aggregates technology: Current development and future challenges. *Crit. Rev. Biotechnol.* **2015**, *35*, 15–28. [CrossRef] [PubMed]
57. Xu, M.-Q.; Wang, S.-S.; Li, L.-N.; Gao, J.; Zhang, Y.-W. Combined Cross-Linked Enzyme Aggregates as Biocatalysts. *Catalysts* **2018**, *8*, 460. [CrossRef]
58. Bilal, M.; Asgher, M.; Parra-Saldivar, R.; Hu, H.; Wang, W.; Zhang, X.; Iqbal, H.M.N. Immobilized ligninolytic enzymes: An innovative and environmental responsive technology to tackle dye-based industrial pollutants—A review. *Sci. Total Environ.* **2017**, *576*, 646–659. [CrossRef] [PubMed]
59. Jafari Khorshidi, K.; Lenjannezhadian, H.; Jamalan, M.; Zeinali, M. Preparation and characterization of nanomagnetic cross-linked cellulase aggregates for cellulose bioconversion. *J. Chem. Technol. Biotechnol.* **2016**, *91*, 539–546. [CrossRef]
60. Kumari, A.; Kaila, P.; Tiwari, P.; Singh, V.; Kaul, S.; Singhal, N.; Guptasarma, P. Multiple thermostable enzyme hydrolases on magnetic nanoparticles: An immobilized enzyme-mediated approach to saccharification through simultaneous xylanase, cellulase and amylolytic glucanotransferase action. *Int. J. Biol. Macromol.* **2018**, *120*, 1650–1658. [CrossRef] [PubMed]
61. Schwaminger, S.P.; Fraga-García, P.; Selbach, F.; Hein, F.G.; Fuß, E.C.; Surya, R.; Roth, H.-C.; Blank-Shim, S.A.; Wagner, F.E.; Heissler, S.; et al. Bio-nano interactions: Cellulase on iron oxide nanoparticle surfaces. *Adsorption* **2017**, *23*, 281–292. [CrossRef]
62. Ingle, A.P.; Rathod, J.; Pandit, R.; da Silva, S.S.; Rai, M. Comparative evaluation of free and immobilized cellulase for enzymatic hydrolysis of lignocellulosic biomass for sustainable bioethanol production. *Cellulose* **2017**, *24*, 5529–5540. [CrossRef]
63. Nadar, S.S.; Rathod, V.K. A co-immobilization of pectinase and cellulase onto magnetic nanoparticles for antioxidant extraction from waste fruit peels. *Biocatal. Agric. Biotechnol.* **2019**, *17*, 470–479. [CrossRef]
64. Ladole, M.R.; Nair, R.R.; Bhutada, Y.D.; Amritkar, V.D.; Pandit, A.B. Synergistic effect of ultrasonication and co-immobilized enzymes on tomato peels for lycopene extraction. *Ultrason. Sonochem.* **2018**, *48*, 453–462. [CrossRef] [PubMed]
65. Ladole, M.R.; Mevada, J.S.; Pandit, A.B. Ultrasonic hyperactivation of cellulase immobilized on magnetic nanoparticles. *Bioresour. Technol.* **2017**, *239*, 117–126. [CrossRef] [PubMed]
66. Chen, Q.; Liu, D.; Wu, C.; Yao, K.; Li, Z.; Shi, N.; Wen, F.; Gates, I.D. Co-immobilization of cellulase and lysozyme on amino-functionalized magnetic nanoparticles: An activity-tunable biocatalyst for extraction of lipids from microalgae. *Bioresour. Technol.* **2018**, *263*, 317–324. [CrossRef]
67. Abbaszadeh, M.; Hejazi, P. Metal affinity immobilization of cellulase on Fe_3O_4 nanoparticles with copper as ligand for biocatalytic applications. *Food Chem.* **2019**, *290*, 47–55. [CrossRef] [PubMed]
68. Pei, J.; Huang, Y.; Yang, Y.; Yuan, H.; Liu, X.; Ni, C. A Novel Layered Anchoring Structure Immobilized Cellulase via Covalent Binding of Cellulase on MNPs Anchored by LDHs. *J. Inorg. Organomet. Polym. Mater.* **2018**, *28*, 1624–1635. [CrossRef]
69. Velmurugan, R.; Incharoensakdi, A. MgO-Fe_3O_4 linked cellulase enzyme complex improves the hydrolysis of cellulose from *Chlorella* sp. CYB2. *Biochem. Eng. J.* **2017**, *122*, 22–30. [CrossRef]
70. Lima, J.S.; Araújo, P.H.H.; Sayer, C.; Souza, A.A.U.; Viegas, A.C.; de Oliveira, D. Cellulase immobilization on magnetic nanoparticles encapsulated in polymer nanospheres. *Bioprocess Biosyst. Eng.* **2017**, *40*, 511–518. [CrossRef]

71. Han, J.; Luo, P.; Wang, Y.; Wang, L.; Li, C.; Zhang, W.; Dong, J.; Ni, L. The development of nanobiocatalysis via the immobilization of cellulase on composite magnetic nanomaterial for enhanced loading capacity and catalytic activity. *Int. J. Biol. Macromol.* **2018**, *119*, 692–700. [CrossRef]
72. Poorakbar, E.; Shafiee, A.; Saboury, A.A.; Rad, B.L.; Khoshnevisan, K.; Ma'mani, L.; Derakhshankhah, H.; Ganjali, M.R.; Hosseini, M. Synthesis of magnetic gold mesoporous silica nanoparticles core shell for cellulase enzyme immobilization: Improvement of enzymatic activity and thermal stability. *Process Biochem.* **2018**, *71*, 92–100. [CrossRef]
73. Díaz-Hernández, A.; Gracida, J.; García-Almendárez, B.E.; Regalado, C.; Núñez, R.; Amaro-Reyes, A. Characterization of Magnetic Nanoparticles Coated with Chitosan: A Potential Approach for Enzyme Immobilization. *J. Nanomater.* **2018**, *2018*, 9468574. [CrossRef]
74. Sánchez-Ramírez, J.; Martínez-Hernández, J.L.; López-Campos, R.G.; Segura-Ceniceros, E.P.; Saade, H.; Ramos-González, R.; Neira-Velázquez, M.G.; Medina-Morales, M.A.; Aguilar, C.N.; Ilyina, A. Laccase Validation as Pretreatment of Agave Waste Prior to Saccharification: Free and Immobilized in Superparamagnetic Nanoparticles Enzyme Preparations. *Waste Biomass Valorization* **2018**, *9*, 223–234. [CrossRef]
75. Zhou, M.; Ju, X.; Li, L.; Yan, L.; Xu, X.; Chen, J. Immobilization of cellulase in the non-natural ionic liquid environments to enhance cellulase activity and functional stability. *Appl. Microbiol. Biotechnol.* **2019**, *103*, 2483–2492. [CrossRef] [PubMed]
76. Saha, K.; Verma, P.; Sikder, J.; Chakraborty, S.; Curcio, S. Synthesis of chitosan-cellulase nanohybrid and immobilization on alginate beads for hydrolysis of ionic liquid pretreated sugarcane bagasse. *Renew. Energy* **2019**, *133*, 66–76. [CrossRef]
77. Bohara, R.A.; Thorat, N.D.; Pawar, S.H. Immobilization of cellulase on functionalized cobalt ferrite nanoparticles. *Korean J. Chem. Eng.* **2016**, *33*, 216–222. [CrossRef]

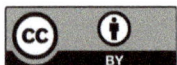

© 2019 by the authors. Licensee MDPI, Basel, Switzerland. This article is an open access article distributed under the terms and conditions of the Creative Commons Attribution (CC BY) license (http://creativecommons.org/licenses/by/4.0/).

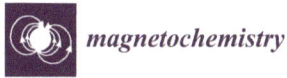

Review

Magnetic Nanoparticles for Nanomedicine

Maria Hepel

Department of Chemistry, State University of New York, Potsdam, NY 13676, USA; hepelmr@potsdam.edu;
Tel.: +1-315-267-2267

Received: 8 December 2019; Accepted: 7 January 2020; Published: 9 January 2020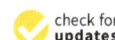

Abstract: The field of nanomedicine has recently emerged as a product of the expansion of a range of nanotechnologies into biomedical science, pharmacology and clinical practice. Due to the unique properties of nanoparticles and the related nanostructures, their applications to medical diagnostics, imaging, controlled drug and gene delivery, monitoring of therapeutic outcomes, and aiding in medical interventions, provide a new perspective for challenging problems in such demanding issues as those involved in the treatment of cancer or debilitating neurological diseases. In this review, we evaluate the role and contributions that the applications of magnetic nanoparticles (MNPs) have made to various aspects of nanomedicine, including the newest magnetic particle imaging (MPI) technology allowing for outstanding spatial and temporal resolution that enables targeted contrast enhancement and real-time assistance during medical interventions. We also evaluate the applications of MNPs to the development of targeted drug delivery systems with magnetic field guidance/focusing and controlled drug release that mitigate chemotherapeutic drugs' side effects and damage to healthy cells. These systems enable tackling of multiple drug resistance which develops in cancer cells during chemotherapeutic treatment. Furthermore, the progress in development of ROS- and heat-generating magnetic nanocarriers and magneto-mechanical cancer cell destruction, induced by an external magnetic field, is also discussed. The crucial roles of MNPs in the development of biosensors and microfluidic paper array devices (µPADs) for the detection of cancer biomarkers and circulating tumor cells (CTCs) are also assessed. Future challenges concerning the role and contributions of MNPs to the progress in nanomedicine have been outlined.

Keywords: magnetic nanoparticles; nanocarriers; controlled drug delivery; high-resolution medical imaging; cancer biomarkers; circulating cancer cells; fluorescent probes

1. Introduction

Considerable research effort has recently been extended into developing novel nanotechnologies aimed at biomedical advancements [1–11]. This effort has greatly benefited human health and enabled improvements in disease control [12]. In the meantime, nanomedicine created in the process has become a powerhouse of innovative technologies [12,13] for diagnosing, monitoring, and treating the most challenging human diseases, such as neoplasia, neurological disorders, and others. In this comprehensive review, novel applications of magnetic nanoparticles in nanomedicine are evaluated, including those in the area of controlled drug delivery, gene neutralizing or replacement therapy, medical imaging, drug distribution, extenuating drug side effects, mitigating multiple drug resistance, and assisting during invasive medical interventions.

Among the many applications of magnetic nanoparticles (MNPs) in nanomedicine, some of the most interesting are those involving MNPs as probes analyzing the status of the disease and providing drugs to mitigate the problem. MNPs have been successfully utilized in biosensor preparation, fluorescent-magnetic bioimaging probe design, as well as in the synthesis of drug delivery nanocarriers. Specially modified magnetic nanoparticles have also been applied for the detection of cancer and circulating tumor cells (CTCs) in addition to the recognition and binding to the cell membrane receptors. Therefore, MNPs have been developed as fluorescent–magnetic probes for cellular/subcellular targeting, imaging and therapy.

Various kinds of magnetic materials can be utilized for MNP development [14,15]. The key challenge is to obtain NPs that are stable in biological environments, are non-toxic, and show the desired magnetic properties. The strong magnets of rare earth elements are not chemically stable in biological media and are cytotoxic [16]. Pure metallic magnets are prone to corrosion. One of the simplest solutions is to utilize iron oxide NPs (magnetite Fe_3O_4 [14,17] or hematite Fe_2O_3 [18]) which are non-toxic and highly biocompatible, although their saturation magnetization is not as high as for lanthanide magnetic materials. Small size NPs of this kind are referred to as superparamagnetic iron oxide nanoparticles (SPION). Recently, the Krishnan group reported obtaining monodispersed magnetite nanoparticles with near-ideal saturation magnetization [19]. On the other hand, intermetallic compounds in the transition metal group exhibit quite strong magnetic properties and are relatively stable in biological media. For instance, Fe_xNi_y alloys have been synthesized in form of superparamagnetic nanoparticles [20]. They offer higher magnetization strength than magnetite but are more difficult to synthesize. Very important is the particle size dependence of magnetic properties of MNPs. Larger particles with several magnetic domains often show permanent ferromagnetic properties resulting in MNP aggregation. Smaller particles may form only a single magnetic domain and their superparamagnetic properties are most suitable for the application as MNPs for nanomedicine. It has been shown that particle sizes of approximately 20–30 nm are critical [14,21,22]. Although the large particles show stronger magnetic properties, they cannot be applied as MNP probes for nanomedicine, due to permanent magnetization leading to MNPs aggregation.

Generally, all MNPs, even the most stable ones, require some kind of a protection against the biological environment [15]. Thus, coatings of MNPs may include silica shells [23], gold film [24], polymer coats [16], or a dense self-assembled monolayer of impenetrable ligands [25].

The MNPs designed for controlled drug delivery and those for targeted activity require immobilization of drugs and targeting ligands on their surface. Hence, these active molecules must be attached to the nanocarrier shell or a surface-protecting film. Various chemistries have been developed to effectively bind these molecules to the nanocarriers [3,8,9,15,26–28]. Other ligands, such as those preventing nonspecific binding of proteins and enhancing biocompatibility must also be incorporated in the surface film of nanocarriers.

2. Magnetic Nanoparticles (MNP)-Enhanced Sensors for Disease Biomarkers

In the rapidly growing field of biosensors, the utilization of nanomaterials opens new opportunities for enhancing sensitivity and selectivity of biosensing platforms. Here, magnetic nanoparticles serve two main purposes: (i) to provide convenient means for transferring nanoparticles between different media in sensor fabrication processes, thus facilitating the MNP surface functionalization; and (ii) to serve as a part of the sensory material of biosensors by providing their own functionalized surface for biorecognition of analytes. The optical biosensors based on MNPs have recently been evaluated in an excellent review by Merkoci and coworkers [11]. Different molecular recognition probes and analytes, including disease biomarkers, that can be determined with functionalized MNP-based biosensors have also been reviewed by Krishnan and colleagues [29].

Among the novel biosensors utilizing unique properties of nanomaterials are sensors based on nanophotonic arrays, plasmonic enhancements, and multi-tier amplification schemes. Examples range from optical enhancement by AgNP films [30,31] and plasmon-controlled fluorescence [32–35], to modulation of fluorescence resonance energy transfer (FRET) by protein films on plasmonic NPs [36,37] and a variety of biorecognition processes followed by FRET [38] and intramolecular fluorescence resonance energy transfer (iFRET) [39], resonance elastic light scattering (RELS) [28,40,41], Raman scattering [6,7], or enzymatic detection [42]. The presence of MNPs in sensory films facilitates the amplification of biorecognition processes, as evidenced in seminal works on magnetic field-activated sensing of mRNA in vivo [4,5,43].

The enhanced Raman plasmonic grid biosensors based on an Au-coated superparamagnetic Fe$_2$Ni nanoparticle core (Fe$_2$Ni@Au) have been successfully designed and characterized [20]. These plasmonic-magnetic core-shell NPs have subsequently been employed in SERS studies of DNA damage caused by the chemotherapeutic drug doxorubicin (DOX) [6] (Figure 1) and in designing of a microfluidic platform with a "hot-spot"-enriched and magnetically held SERS nanogrid sensor for the detection of cancer biomarkers [7] (Figure 2). Experimental findings obtained for the carcinoembryonic antigen (CEA) antibody–antigen sandwich structure using NiFe@Au and Au NPs were corroborated by theoretically simulated plasmonic coupling resulting in E-field enhancement based on a core–shell type model with an Au core and protein shell. An excellent CEA detection limit, LOD = 0.1 pM, has been obtained.

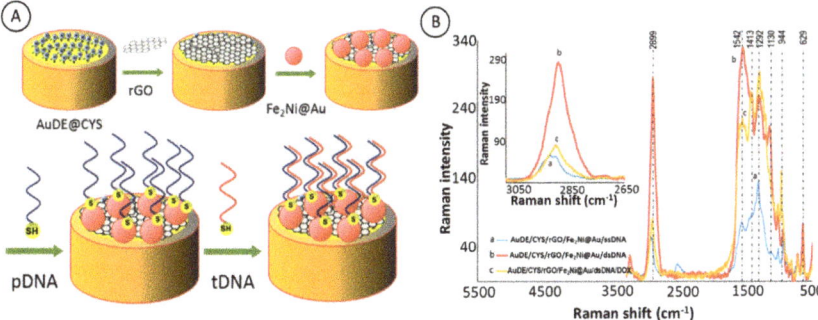

Figure 1. SERS biosensors for testing of doxorubicin (DOX) interactions with DNA. (**A**) Scheme of the modification of gold disc coated with cysteine (AuDE), reduced graphene oxide (rGO), Fe$_2$Ni@Au nanoparticles and probe ssDNA (pDNA) followed by interaction with complementary DNA (tDNA); (**B**) SERS spectra for (a) nanobiosensor, (b) after hybridization with tDNA, (c) after incubation of dsDNA with doxorubicin (DOX). Inset: details of high frequency peak. Reprinted with permission [6].

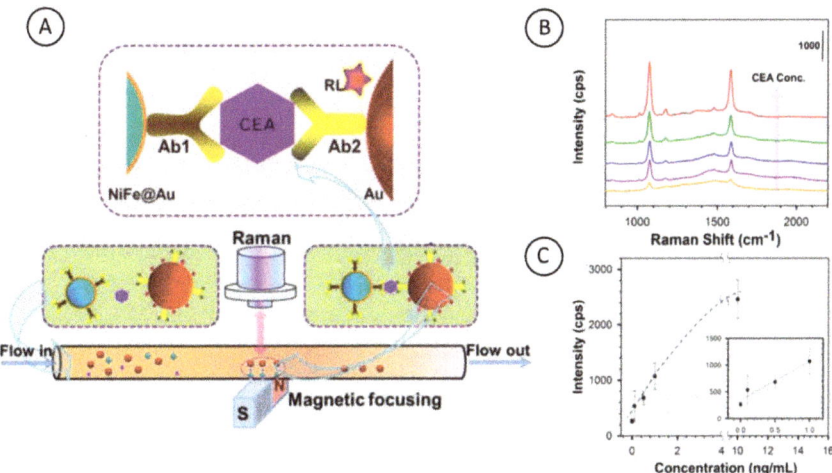

Figure 2. (**A**) Scheme of experimental setup; (**B**) SERS spectra of sandwich conjugates of NiFe@Au and AuNPs with antibodies, in response to the different concentrations of CEA (0.0, 0.1, 0.5, 1.0, 10.0 ng/mL); (**C**) plot of peak intensity at 1076 cm^{-1} vs. CEA concentration. Insert: a magnified view of the low-concentration range data. Reprinted with permission [7].

Experimental and theoretical assessments of the high field spots formed in the interparticle area in a particle dimer bound via DNA duplex linkages have recently been performed for Au- or Ag-coated magnetite SPIONs [24].

Magnetic nanoparticles have also been employed in high-sensitivity hyphenated analytical methods. A combination of: (i) cell labeling with multiple magnetic metal beads; (ii) hybridization chain reaction amplification; and (iii) detection using inductively coupled plasma–mass spectrometry (ICP–MS), has been proposed by He et al. [44] for distinguishing and simultaneous counting of multiple cancer cells. The labelling of cells with MNPs was described by Kolosnjaj-Tabi et al. [45]. This technique was applied for simultaneous counting of human hepatocellular carcinoma cells (SMMC-7721) and human lung carcinoma cells (A549) with high sensitivity and specificity. Simultaneous detection of CTCs and cancer biomarkers in an immunomagnetic flow system was first described by Huang et al. [46].

3. MNP-Core Nanocarriers for Controlled Drug and Gene Delivery

Various types of nanocarriers have been investigated for possible application in theranostics, including plasmonic metal NPs, liposomes, micelles, protein nanostructures, graphene oxide nanosheets, biopolymers, synthetic polymers, and others [8–10,26,27,47,48]. These nanocarriers must combine a high capacity for carrying drugs or genes, biocompatibility-enhancing agents, and targeting ligands able to recognize the sites for a drug release (e.g., receptors in a cancer cell membrane). The same requirement concerns nanocarriers for gene delivery where an oligonucleotide strand is immobilized on a nanocarrier in place of drug molecules [10,28,47,49]. The nanocarriers must also be able to release the drugs under specific local conditions (acidity, GSH level) [50–52] or under external stimuli, such as a light pulse, an X-ray signal, or a heat wave. The novel nanocarriers now include also functionalized magnetic core-based NPs [3,6,7,53–55], where the magnetic core is protected against degradation in biological environments by coating with a silica shell [23], gold film [24], a tight polymeric coat (e.g., PEG, poly-L-lysine, carboxydextran) [16], or a dense self-assembled monolayer of impenetrable ligands [25]. The protective shell provides also an easy means for the attachment of drugs, adjuvants, targeting ligands, and agents ensuring the nanocarrier biocompatibility [53,54,56]. The magnetic properties of such carriers enable magnetic field-based guidance of nanocarriers to the target tissue. Recently, the magnetic actuation of a drug release at the target sites has been proposed [5,43].

The effects of particle surface corona on cancer cell targeting were investigated in simulated physiological fluids by Zhao et al. [57]. Studies of advanced cancer cell targeting have been carried out by many research groups [15,58] and an interesting range of suitable chemistries, including "click chemistry", has been devised.

Further issues in controlled drug delivery are related to the nanocarriers internalization, i.e., entering into a target cell, either by endocytosis, receptor-mediated entry (e.g., via binding to folate receptors), or by penetrating the cell membrane (for hydrophobic nanocarriers, e.g., graphene or graphene oxide nanocarriers that partially dissolve in the membrane disrupting its tightness). The same mechanisms as observed for other types of solid nanocarriers, are expected for MNP-based nanocarriers.

The drug and gene release from MNP-based nanocarriers is also expected to be similar to other solid nanocarriers because binding of these ligands to both types of nanocarriers are of the same type.

4. Magnetic Particle Imaging (MPI) for Cancer Diagnostics, Staging, and Medical Intervention

Magnetic Particle Imaging (MPI) is a novel non-invasive and radiation-free tomographic technique where in contrast to X-ray computed tomography (CT) and magnetic resonance imaging (MRI), the imaging is performed by tracking the superparamagnetic iron oxide nanoparticle (SPION) tracers with simultaneous generation of 3D images with extraordinary spatial and temporal resolution [59]. The direct 3D volume rendering (DVR) enables real-time 3D guidance in vascular interventions, such as in the real-time percutaneous transluminal angioplasty [60,61] with the insertion of a stent or balloon in a blocked artery. It can also be utilized for the direct visualization of thromboembolic material within the lumen of the middle cerebral artery (MCA), carotid arteries, or a hepatic artery [62].

The first commercial preclinical MPI scanners, with small chambers able to accommodate a mouse or rabbit, have recently been developed and are under testing. A new scanner with large field of view (up to 45 mm) with a resolution to 500 µm, based on a traveling wave MPI and an array of electromagnets enabling magnetic field gradients up to 10 T/m, has recently been announced by the Vogel group [2,63]. A human-sized MPI research system for brain applications has been designed by Graeser and colleagues [1]. First MPI angiography in human-sized organs (pig kidney perfusion system) has been obtained by Molwitz and coworkers [64]. The principles and applications of MPI in biomedical research have been evaluated in a review by Talebloo and coworkers [65].

The effect of the magnetic nanoparticle core size on the MPI sensitivity has been investigated by Shasha et al. [66]. They have demonstrated that the magnetic core diameter of SPION nanoparticle tracers of 28 nm is optimal for use in MPI. For larger NPs, the relaxation effects and interparticle interactions begin to dominate, reducing the colloid stability. The optimized SPION probes were applied in studies of their intracellular dynamics for MPI applications [67]. The monodispersed single-phase magnetite NPs have been well characterized and size-optimized for MPI [21,22]. The utilization of MPI for in-vivo cancer imaging with systemic tracer administration was reported by Collony's group [68] (Figure 3). A whole-body biodistribution of the tracer NPs was monitored with a large field of view (FOV). Another scanner, with decoupled harmonics generation and field-free point handling, was recently reported by Bagheri and coworkers [69]. Harmonics are generated due to the non-linear magnetization characteristics of tracer MNPs. This new approach provides more flexibility for exploring and optimizing tracer particle responses to obtain the best spatial resolution of images in the sub-millimeter range.

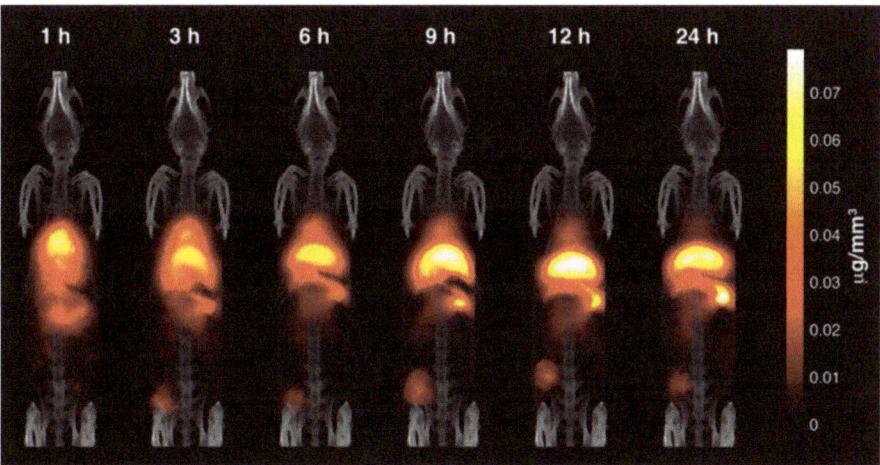

Figure 3. Maximum intensity projection of 3D magnetic particle imaging (MPI) volumes co-registered with a CT skeletal reference. The whole-body tracer dynamics along with the tumor are clearly visualized. Reprinted with permission [68].

The non-targeted MPI can be utilized for cancer detection and therapy due to the enhanced permeability and retention (EPR) effect caused by leaky blood vessels, poor drainage of lymphatic system, and misalignment of endothelial cells.

So far, the outstanding performance of the MPI scanning technique has been demonstrated in the following applications [70]:

- vasculature visualization and monitoring of blood flow;
- detection of neoplasia and monitoring of outcomes of therapeutic intervention;
- detection of arterial aneurisms;

- guidance for catheterization in percutaneous angioplasty, including procedures performed during cardiac infarction;
- cancer thermotherapy.

Research studies on the utilization of MPI techniques in other fields of nanomedicine are under way.

In summary, the novel MPI technique based on magnetically tracking SPION probes offers very high spatial and temporal resolutions, is radiation-free, depth-independent, and causes virtually no side-effects. Therefore, it can successfully compete with the well-established imaging techniques, such as MRI, CT, and PET. Also, MPI does not require allergenic and highly nephrotoxic iodine-based contrast agents [71]. Note that Schlorf and coworkers [72] have used the SPION nanoparticles as the contrast agents and as the labels for cell tagging for MRI imaging. They have found that the retention of the magnetic nanoparticles in cells lasts for about two weeks.

The utilization of superparamagnetic iron oxide nanoparticles in conjunction with the new MPI technique has the potential to detect and diagnose cancer at an earlier stage than current imaging methods [3].

5. Hyperthermic Treatment of Malignant Cells with MNPs

Hyperthermia has been applied as a method of anticancer therapy, in which nanoparticles highly absorbing electromagnetic radiation are administered to the cancer tissue and then excited with a precision laser beam to destroy cancer cells by the rising temperature of the nanoparticles. For nanocarriers with a magnetic core, the temperature rise can also be achieved by vibrating or rotating the nanocarriers via stimulation by alternating magnetic field [73–78]. It has been successfully applied for treatment of malignant glioma [79]. The advantage of using MNP carriers is clear in the deep penetration of magnetic field modulation stimulating the nanocarriers, whereas light stimulation is applicable only to a near-surface tissue.

Wu et al. [80] have successfully synthesized porous carbon-coated magnetite nanoparticles (PCCMNs) by a one-pot solvothermal method. A hyaluronic acid-modified PCCMN with fluorescent carbon quantum dots has been applied for efficient photothermal cancer therapy (PTT) in vivo with MRI monitoring and fluorescent imaging. The nanocarriers served both as the contrast agent for MRI and the heat generator upon absorbing a NIR laser beam at 808 nm wavelength and 1.5 W/cm^2 energy. The proposed nanocarriers can also carry chemotherapeutic drugs.

A new drug delivery system based on magnetic hollow porous carbon nanoparticle nanocarriers (MHPCNs) was also developed by the same group [81]. To cap the pores in the nanocarrier shell, a poly(γ-glutamic acid) was used. The photothermal conversion of carbon and magnetite (Fe_3O_4) shells enabled photothermal therapy to be performed with no anticancer drug leakage during the systemic distribution. The proposed drug delivery in sealed nanocages and controlled photothermal release enabled the multidrug resistance induced by chemotherapeutic treatment to be overcome [82,83]. The MPI was not used in these experiments. Therefore, monitoring of the therapeutic outcomes was limited to the resolution of the magnetic resonance imaging. These experiments have demonstrated the effective tumor growth inhibition through the hyperthermia/chemotherapy synergistic action.

The conditions for efficient heat generation have been discussed by many researchers and high-performance frequency tuners for resonant inverters suitable for magnetic hyperthermia have been designed [84].

6. Magneto-Mechanical Destruction of Cytoskeletal Scaffolds and Permeabilization of Lysosome Membranes by Alternating Magnetic Field-Driven MNP Vibrations for Cancer Treatment

Alternating magnetic field-driven vibration and rotation of MNPs accumulated in cancer cells may result in relaxation with heat generation resulting in local temperature increase, as discussed in the case of hyperthermia. However, for small MNPs, generally less than 20 nm in diameter, magnetic field stimulation would not result in enough heat generation to cause sufficient temperature increase to kill cancer cells [74]. Yet, in experiments performed by several groups, the magnetic field-driven MNP vibrations clearly resulted in cancer cell death [18,85–92]. Recently, Kabanov's group [93] provided a completely new mechanism of cancer cell death under such conditions. Their experiments, conducted with 7–8 nm MNPs and a low-frequency magnetic field of 50 Hz, confirmed no temperature rise of the medium. They demonstrated that the cancer cell killing ability of this low energy magnetic stimulation is due to the disruption of the cytoskeletal framework of cancer cells by magneto-mechanical movement and inelastic impact of MNPs leading to apoptosis. Klyachko et al. [91] and Hoffmann et al. [94] have found that magnetic field-driven MNPs can be used to control enzymatic processes. Further studies of the discovered phenomenon will help to uncover biochemical pathways driving the cells to self-destruction.

7. Magnetically Guided MNPs for ROS Generation and Cancer Treatment

Reactive oxygen species (ROS) are highly potent radicals able to damage DNA, lipids and other biomolecules. They are generated in the mitochondrial respiration system and used by the organism to protect against invasion of microbes. The generation of ROS may also be utilized in the fight with cancer. Hence, this concept has recently gained new attention [95–101] which concentrates on enhancing the ROS generation in mitochondria with various drugs and in Fenton-like cascade processes based on decomposition of H_2O_2 to HO* radicals, catalyzed by Fe^{2+} or Cu^{2+} and catechol moiety [102]. Cell death caused by ROS generation by Fenton-like cascades has been dubbed oxytosis [97] or ferroptosis [95]. Unlike a typical apoptosis, it is not driven by the caspase 3 pathway and does not lead to chromatin condensation [97].

A new kind of interesting magnetic nanoparticles, consisting of a magnetic iron carbide Fe_5C_2 (MIC NP), has been developed by Yu and coworkers [103]. These MIC NPs are able to release Fe^{2+} ions upon entering the zone of high acidity in the tumor environment. Since Fe^{2+} ions catalyze the decomposition of H_2O_2 through the Fenton cascade mechanism and since H_2O_2 is overproduced and available in cancer cells, the reactive oxygen species, in particular HO* radicals, are formed and aid in the destruction of cancer cell DNA [102]. To enhance the release of Fe^{2+} ions from MIC NPs, a coating of a magnetite film on Fe_5C_2 core was applied, forming the final MIC NPs with the composition: $Fe_5C_2@Fe_3O_4$. A schematic illustration of the MIC NP endocytosis, followed by Fe^{2+} release and ROS generation is presented in Figure 4, together with T2-weighted MR images of 4T1 tumor-bearing mice. Monitoring of MIC NPs distribution can be carried out using a magnetic resonance imaging (MRI) scanner. Interestingly, it has been found that the magnetism of MIC NPs decreases upon Fe^{2+} release and the T2 signal in MRI decreased. At the same time, the released Fe^{2+} causes the increase in the T1 MRI signal. Therefore, the presence of a tumor tissue with a low pH and the release of Fe^{2+}, leading to the generation of ROS and apoptosis of cancer cells, can be sensitively monitored by MRI.

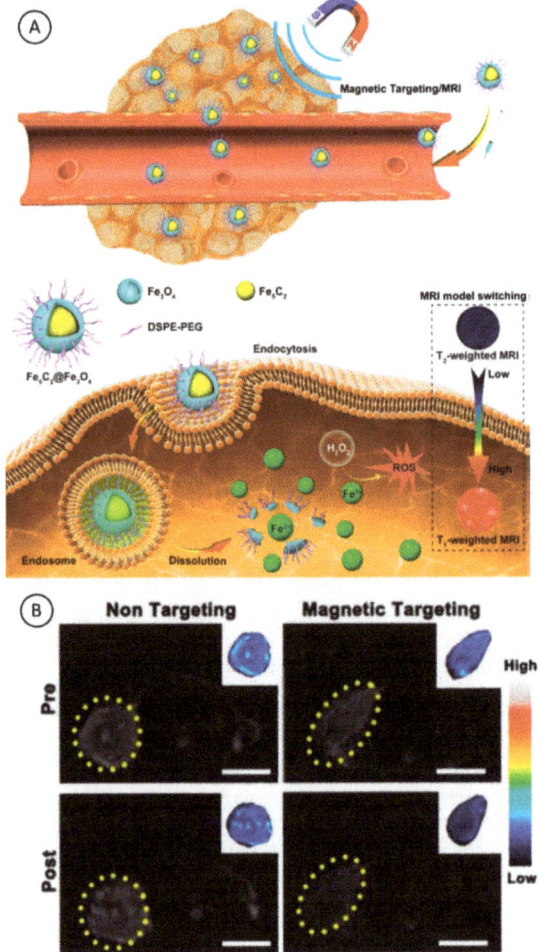

Figure 4. (**A**) A schematic illustration of MNPs for pH-responsive Fe^{2+} releasing, ROS generation and T2/T1 signal conversion; (**B**) representative T2-weighted MR images of 4T1 tumor-bearing mice before (Pre) and one day after (Post) injection of $PEG/Fe_5C_2@Fe_3O_4$ NPs with or without magnetic targeting. The tumor sites are circled by a yellow dashed line. Reprinted with permission [103].

Applications of high-frequency alternating magnetic fields (HF-AMF) with MNPs accumulated in tissues [90] have demonstrated permeabilization of lysosome membranes in cancer cells but not in healthy cells. The appearance of ROS, generated in mitochondria, was detected 30 min after the AMF application. These experiments show that using MNPs stimulated with HF-AMF, it becomes possible to generate ROS in targeted cancer cells, mitigating collateral damage to healthy cells as well as reversing drug resistance established by overexpression of GSH in cancer cells in response to oxidative stress [41,104,105] introduced by chemotherapeutic drugs.

8. Detection of Circulating Cancer Cells

In the critical stage of tumor development, some cancer cells begin to detach from the original neoplasia and enter the blood stream and lymphatic highway system to become circulating tumor cells (CTCs), able to settle on the way and proliferate into new tumor outcrops, marking the onset of metastasis, i.e., the spread of the original tumor into distal sites. The detection of CTCs is therefore an important and challenging task in cancer therapy. The key issue is the low concentration of CTCs. Hence, special efforts have been made to develop highly sensitive techniques for the detection and identification of CTCs. So far, the microfluidic format of CTCs isolation and identification is the only format that can offer successful outcomes and rapid analysis without sample preparation. It integrates all procedures in a small microfluidic chip and requires minimal sample volume, as envisioned by the device inventors [106].

In one such effort, Green et al. [107] have designed a microfluidic device for high-sensitivity profiling of CTCs in patients with metastatic castration-resistant prostate cancer (mCRPC). The circulating cells were first sorted according to protein expression levels. For that purpose, EpCAM antibody-functionalized magnetic nanoparticles were developed. The blood samples analyzed were from patients undergoing treatment with abiraterone or enzalutamide, two drugs used to treat advanced prostate cancer. The samples taken during treatment (9–22 weeks) were compared to the baseline (week 0). It has been shown that the number of low-EpCAM CTCs increased with the treatment time for progressive patients. The proposed microfluidic device with antibody functionalized MNP probes offered higher efficiency compared to the commercially available CellSearch device.

Mandal et al. [108] have developed AIEgen-based fluorescent magnetic nanoparticle probes, with a hydrodynamic size ranging from 25 to 50 nm and rich surface chemistry enabling attachment of ligands able to recognize and bind to cell membrane receptors. The AIEgen molecules exhibit a unique aggregation-induced fluorescence emission (AIE) property. To construct the MNP@AIEgen probes, the hydrophobic γ-Fe_2O_3 nanoparticles were first converted into hydrophilic nanoparticles by a polyacrylate overcoat of N-(3-aminopropyl)-methacrylamide hydrochloride with/without 3-sulfopropyl methacrylate. The obtained primary amine-terminated hydrophilic nanoparticles were then conjugated with tetraphenylethene (TPE), an AIEgen molecule, further derivatized with various functional groups. The study's authors have demonstrated that the AIEgen-based fluorescent MNPs can act as the cellular imaging probes. Furthermore, the labeled cells can be magnetically separated.

An immunomagnetic flow system for simultaneous detection of CTCs and cancer biomarkers in blood was developed by Huang et al. [46]. In his microfluidic device, folate receptors (FR) in membrane of cancer cells were detected using fluorescence microscope while cells marked with anti-FR antibody-coated magnetic beads were captured with a magnetic field on the microfluidic channel wall. Using a microfluidic device with magnetic separation of CTCs and electric impedance cytometry, Han and Han [109] were able to detect colorectal cancer cell line DLD-1 in peripheral blood by enrichment of ca. 500-fold. Recently, Wang and coworkers [110] have developed a rapid and highly efficient method to isolate and identify heterogeneous CTCs (F-MNPs+, Hoechst 33342+, and CD45−) from patient blood samples using fluorescent MNPs (F-MNPs). An F-MNP consisted of a Fe_3O_4 core and a SiO_2 shell decorated with a fluorescent dye 1,1′-dioctadecyl-3,3,3′,3′-tetramethyl-indocarbocyanine perchlorate (DiI). On the surface of F-MNPs, a layer of a zwitterionic polymer, poly(carboxybetaine methacrylate) (pCBMA), able to decrease the nonspecific cell adhesion with anti-EpCAM and anti-N-cadherin antibodies, was formed (Figure 5).

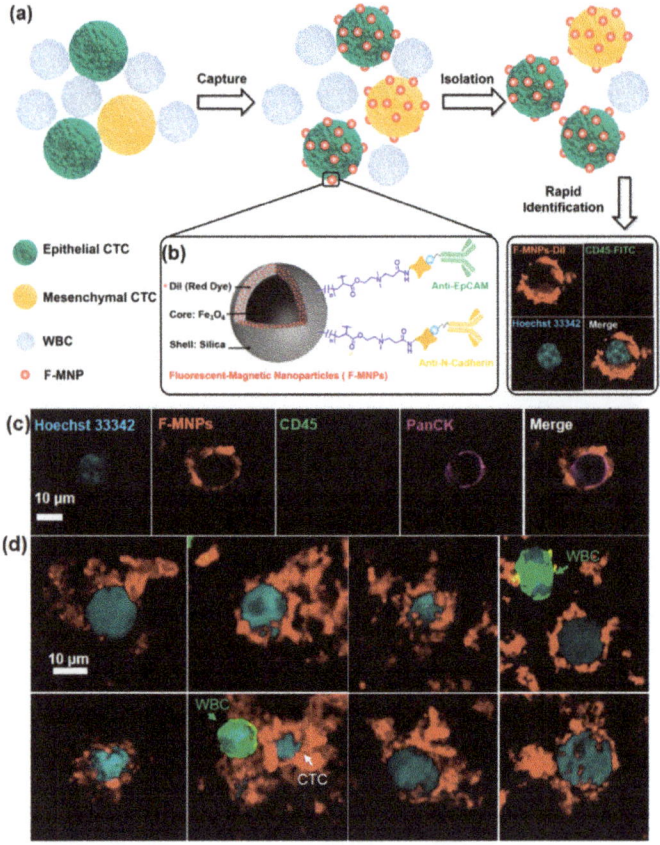

Figure 5. (a) Illustration of the isolation and identification of heterogeneous circulating tumor cells (CTCs) from breast cancer patients' blood samples using fluorescent magnetic nanoparticles (F-MNPs); (b) the construction of F-MNPs; (c) fluorescent images of one CTC identified by immunostaining of anti-PanCK-647 and F-MNPs for breast cancer sample BrC01; (d) fluorescent images of eight CTCs (Hoechst 33342+, F-MNPs+, CD45−) and WBCs (Hoechst 33342+, CD45+) from the BrC05 patient sample identified by F-MNPs with immunostaining of anti-CD45-FITC and Hoechst 33342. Reprinted with permission [110].

9. Protective Coating of MNPs

Magnetic nanoparticles operating in a biological environment generally require a protective coating against adverse effects of dissolved oxygen, ROS, and bioactive compounds. Hence, compact and chemically stable shells are grown on the cores. Biomedical applications require robust MNPs that are properly coated by hydrophilic polymers. Firstly, surface coatings are important to prevent MNPs from agglomeration in a physiological environment. Therefore, the MNP coatings have to show a net non-zero charge and have limited zwitterionic and hydrophobic properties. Secondly, coatings must act as a barrier, effectively shielding the magnetic core against the attack of chemical species in the aqueous solution. A silica shell or gold film can fulfill these requirements, but a tight polymer shell is also suitable for this purpose. Further functionalization of the shell material should be considered to avoid non-specific adsorption of biomolecules. Thirdly, different functional groups can be attached to the coatings (e.g., amine, carboxyl) that can be used for immobilization of functional molecules, such as drugs, adjuvants, targeting ligands, fluorescent molecules, biocompatibility enhancing agents, and molecules preventing non-specific adsorption [8,27,48,111] (Figure 6).

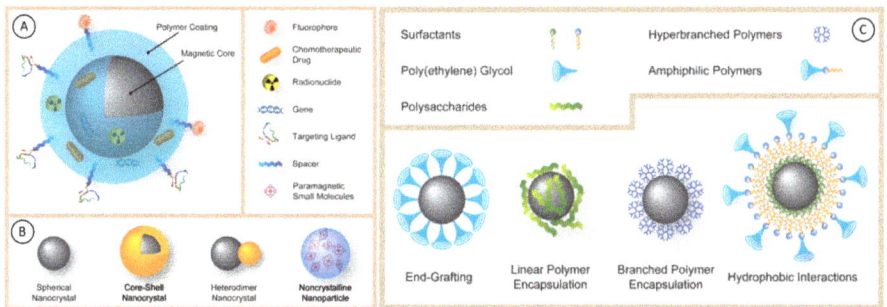

Figure 6. (**A**) Illustration of the structure of a multifunctional/multimodality MNP with a magnetic core, a polymeric coating, and targeting ligands extended from the surface of MNP with the aid of polymeric spacers; (**B**) schematic representation of different types of magnetic cores; (**C**) illustration of different types of coating strategies for hydrophilic MNPs. Reprinted with permission [111].

10. Toxicity of MNPs and Systemic Clearance

The protected core-shell MNPs are generally nontoxic and are well tolerated in vivo, independently of the administration routes. However, the toxicity of newly developed MNPs should always be carefully evaluated. For instance, Feng et al. [112] have performed a detailed investigation of the in vitro cell uptake and cytotoxicity, as well as the in vivo distribution, clearance and toxicity of commercially available and well-characterized iron oxide nanoparticles (IONPs) with different sizes and coatings. It has been found that the polyethyleneimine (PEI)-coated IONPs exhibited significantly higher uptake than PEGylated ones in both macrophages and cancer cells and caused severe cytotoxicity through multiple mechanisms such as ROS production and apoptosis. In that respect, replacing PEI with a biocompatible poly-L-lysine coating also bearing positive charge may solve the problem [28].

11. Conclusions: Advantages, Disadvantages, and Future Challenges

Emerging nanotechnologies provide new perspectives in medicine for solving challenging problems caused by complex human diseases such as neoplasia and debilitating neurodegenerative diseases. In particular, novel applications of magnetic nanoparticles in nanomedicine now involve MNPs in a variety of tasks, such as medical imaging, controlled drug and gene delivery, drug distribution, mitigating the side effects and multiple drug resistance, as well as the aid the MNPs provide in the invasive medical interventions. The advantages of nanotechnologies based on magnetic nanoparticles include the unique electromagnetic and magneto-mechanical properties of MNPs allowing for communication and controlling of their vibration, rotation and translational movement, absorption of electromagnetic energy, and remote heating and actuation. The deep penetration of magnetic fields through living tissues without any effect on healthy cells is a great attribute. The possibility of surface functionalization provides the feasibility to accumulate MNPs at specific locations, e.g., in cancer cells, and enables destruction of the targeted cells by releasing chemotherapeutic drugs, nucleic acids for gene therapy, or a disruption of the cytoskeletal framework of the cell on a remote command. The MNP-based imaging is becoming one of the most versatile imaging techniques with its high spatial and temporal resolution and can serve for cancer diagnosing and grading, and to guide surgical interventions. The MNPs are generally biocompatible and relatively stable, especially when protected by a dense self-assembling monolayer or by coating with a shell of gold, silica, or carbons. A great advantage of MNPs is the feasibility of attaching them to targeted cells that permits cell sorting, e.g., removal of circulating tumor cells or collecting them for analysis. The disadvantages of common

MNPs are mainly related to their weak magnetic properties and the requirement of large size particles, especially when applied in hyperthermia treatment (usually for SPION, particle diameter should be >250 nm [74,93]) and the large size creates then problems with their retrieval from the body. Since the hyperthermia involves larger area of the tissue due to the high thermal conductivity of water and thus encases also healthy cells, this procedure is less likely to be at the forefront of MNP-based technologies. On the other hand, the theranostic, controlled drug release and magneto-mechanical disruption of cytoskeletal framework of cancer cells, as well as the lysosomal membrane permeabilization processes are likely to be among the favorite development strategies.

Future challenges will certainly involve the development of smaller superparamagnetic NPs with stronger magnetic responsivity to maintain the high spatial and temporal sensitivity for the emerging magnetic particle imaging (MPI) technology while enabling an enhanced renal clearance (NP diameter ~2 nm or less). Further development of the new MPI technology and its application for whole-body scanning will enable radiation-free tomographic monitoring of medical interventions, tumorigenesis, and therapeutic outcomes. Extensive research will be needed to develop rapid and convenient microfluidic techniques for the challenging detection of circulating tumor cells, cell sorting, and sensor arrays (µPADs) for testing sets of cancer biomarkers to enable reliable cancer diagnostics and monitoring of cancer therapy at points-of-care with high efficacy. The use of MNPs in development of these analytical devices (µPADs, biosensors, lateral flow sensors, etc.) is crucial as it allows for rapid handling of NPs and separation of MNP-labelled CTCs.

Funding: This research received no external funding.

Conflicts of Interest: The authors declare no conflict of interest.

References

1. Graeser, M.; Thieben, F.; Szwargulski, P.; Werner, F.; Gdaniec, N.; Boberg, M.; Griese, F.; Moddel, M.; Ludewig, P.; van de Ven, D.; et al. Human-sized magnetic particle imaging for brain applications. *Nat. Commun.* **2019**, *10*, 1936. [CrossRef] [PubMed]
2. Vogel, P.; Markert, J.; Ruckert, M.A.; Herz, S.; Kessler, B.; Dremel, K.; Althoff, D.; Weber, M.; Buzug, T.M.; Bley, T.A.; et al. Magnetic particle imaging meets computed tomography: First simultaneous imaging. *Sci. Rep.* **2019**, *9*, 12627. [CrossRef] [PubMed]
3. Gobbo, O.L.; Sjaastad, K.; Radomski, M.W.; Volkov, Y.; Prina-Mello, A. Magnetic nanoparticles in cancer theranostics. *Theranostics* **2015**, *5*, 1249–1263. [CrossRef] [PubMed]
4. Bakshi, S.; Zakharchenko, A.; Mino, S.; Kolpashchikov, D.M.; Katz, E. Towards nanomaterials for cancer theranostics: A system of DNA-modified magnetic nanoparticles for detection and suppression of RNA marker in cancer cells. *Magnetochemistry* **2019**, *5*, 24. [CrossRef]
5. Bakshi, S.F.; Guz, N.; Zakharchenko, A.; Deng, H.; Tumanov, A.V.; Woodworth, C.D.; Minko, S.; Kolpashchikov, D.M.; Katz, E. Magnetic field-activated sensing of mRNA in living cells. *J. Am. Chem. Soc.* **2017**, *139*, 12117–12120. [CrossRef]
6. Ilkhani, H.; Hughes, T.; Li, J.; Zhong, C.J.; Hepel, M. Nanostructured SERS-electrochemical biosensors for testing of anticancer drug interactions with DNA. *Biosens. Bioelectron.* **2016**, *80*, 257–264. [CrossRef]
7. Li, J.; Skeete, Z.; Shan, S.; Yan, S.; Kurzatkowska, K.; Zhao, W.; Ngo, Q.M.; Holubovska, P.; Luo, J.; Hepel, M.; et al. Surface Enhanced Raman Scattering Detection of Cancer Biomarkers with Bifunctional Nanocomposite Probes. *Anal. Chem.* **2015**, *87*, 10698–10702. [CrossRef]
8. Santiago, T.; DeVaux, R.S.; Kurzatkowska, K.; Espinal, R.; Herschkowitz, J.I.; Hepel, M. Surface-enhanced Raman scattering investigation of targeted delivery and controlled release of gemcitabine. *Int. J. Nanomed.* **2017**, *12*, 7763–7776. [CrossRef]
9. Ratajczak, K.; Krazinski, B.E.; Kowalczyk, A.E.; Dworakowska, B.; Jakiela, S.; Stobiecka, M. Hairpin–Hairpin Molecular Beacon Interactions for Detection of Survivin mRNA in Malignant SW480 Cells. *ACS Appl. Mater. Interfaces* **2018**, *10*, 17028–17039. [CrossRef]

10. Stobiecka, M.; Dworakowska, B.; Jakiela, S.; Lukasiak, A.; Chalupa, A.; Zembrzycki, K. Sensing of Survivin mRNA in Malignant Astrocytes Using Graphene Oxide Nanocarrier-Supported Oligonucleotide Molecular Beacons. *Sens. Actuators B* **2016**, *235*, 136–145. [CrossRef]
11. Uzek, R.; Sari, E.; Merkoci, A. Optical-based (bio) sensing systems using magnetic nanoparticles. *Magnetochemietry* **2019**, *5*, 59. [CrossRef]
12. Ferrari, M. Cancer nanotechnology: Opportunities and challenges. *Nat. Rev. Cancer* **2005**, *5*, 161–171. [CrossRef] [PubMed]
13. Allen, T.M. Ligand-targeted therapeutics in anticancer therapy. *Nat. Rev. Drug Discov.* **2002**, *2*, 750–763. [CrossRef] [PubMed]
14. Park, H.Y.; Schadt, M.J.; Wang, L.; Lim, I.I.S.; Njoki, P.N.; Kim, S.H.; Jang, M.Y.; Luo, J.; Zhong, C.J. Fabrication of magnetic core@shell Fe oxide @Au nanoparticles for interfacial bioactivity and bio-separation. *Langmuir* **2007**, *23*, 9050–9056. [CrossRef]
15. Skeete, Z.; Cheng, H.; Crew, E.; Lin, L.; Zhao, W.; Joseph, P.; Shan, S.; Cronk, H.; Luo, J.; Zhang, Q.; et al. Design of functional nanoparticles and assemblies for theranostic applications. *ACS Appl. Mater. Interface* **2014**, *6*, 21752–21768. [CrossRef]
16. Oyewumi, M.O.; Mumper, R.J. Comparison of cell uptake, biodistribution and tumor retention of folate-coated and PEG-coated gadolinium nanoparticles in tumor-bearing mice. *J. Control. Release* **2004**, *95*, 613–626. [CrossRef]
17. Hufschmid, R.; Landers, J.; Shasha, C.; Salamon, S.; Wende, H.; Krishnan, K.M. Nanoscale physical and chemical structure of iron oxide nanoparticles for magnetic particle imaging. *Phys. Status Solidi A* **2018**. [CrossRef]
18. Bergey, E.J.; Levy, L.; Wang, X.; Krebs, L.J.; Lal, M.; Kim, K.S.; Pakatchi, S.; Liebow, C.; Prasad, P.N. DC Magnetic Field Induced Magnetocytolysis of Cancer Cells Targeted by LH-RH Magnetic Nanoparticles in vitro. *Biomed. Microdev.* **2002**, *4*, 293–299. [CrossRef]
19. Kemp, S.J.; Ferguson, R.M.; Khandhar, A.P.; Krishnan, K.M. Monodisperse magnetite nanoparticles wit nearly ideal saturation magnetization. *RSC Adv.* **2016**, *6*, 77452–77464. [CrossRef]
20. Liu, Y.; Chi, Y.; Shan, S.; Yin, J.; Luo, J.; Zhong, C.J. Characterization of magnetic NiFe nanoparticles with controlled bimetallic composition. *J. Alloys Compd.* **2014**, *587*, 260–266. [CrossRef]
21. Ziemian, S.; Lowa, N.; Kosch, O.; Bajj, D.; Wiekhorst, F.; Schutz, G. Optimization of iron oxide tracer synthesis for magnetic particle imaging. *Nanomaterials* **2018**, *8*, 180. [CrossRef] [PubMed]
22. Bao, N.; Shen, L.; Wang, Y.; Padhan, P.; Gupta, A. Fe_3O_4 superparamagnetic size 19.8 nm. *J. Am. Chem. Soc.* **2007**, *129*, 12374. [CrossRef] [PubMed]
23. Yan, F.; Kopelman, R.; Reddy, R. Synthesis and characterization of silica-embedded iron oxide nanoparticles for magnetic resonance imaging. *J. Nanosci. Nanotechnol.* **2004**, *4*, 72–76. [CrossRef]
24. Skeete, Z.; Cheng, H.W.; Li, J.; Salazar, C.; Sun, W.; Ngo, Q.M.; Lin, L.; Luo, J.; Zhong, C.J. Assessing Interparticle Spatial Characteristics of DNA-Linked Core–Shell Nanoparticles with or without Magnetic Cores in Surface Enhanced Raman Scattering. *J. Phys. Chem. C* **2017**, *121*, 15767–15776. [CrossRef]
25. Zhang, Y.; Shang, M. Self-assembled coatings on individual monodisperse magnetite nanoparticles for efficient intracellular uptake. *Biomed. Microdev.* **2004**, *6*, 33–40. [CrossRef]
26. Kydd, J.; Jadia, R.; Velpurisiva, O.; Gad, A.; Pallwal, S.; Rai, P. Targeting strategies for the combination treatment of cancer using drug delivery systems. *Pharmaceutics* **2017**, *9*, 46. [CrossRef]
27. Smith, M.; Hepel, M. Controlled release of targeted anti-leukemia drugs azacitidine and decitabine monitored using surface-enhanced Raman scattering (SERS) spectroscopy. *Mediterr. J. Chem.* **2017**, *6*, 125–132. [CrossRef]
28. Stobiecka, M.; Hepel, M. Double-shell gold nanoparticle-based DNA-carriers with poly-L-lysine binding surface. *Biomaterials* **2011**, *32*, 3312–3321. [CrossRef]
29. Krishnan, S.; Goud, K.Y. Magnetic particle bioconjugates: A versatile sensor approach. *Magnetochemistry* **2019**, *5*, 64. [CrossRef]
30. Lakowicz, J.R.; Ray, K.; Chowdhury, M.; Szmacinski, H.; Fu, Y.; Zhang, J.; Nowaczyk, K. Plasmon-controlled fluorescence: A new paradigm in fluorescence spectroscopy. *Analyst* **2008**, *133*, 1308–1346. [CrossRef]
31. Ray, K.; Chowdhury, M.H.; Zhang, J.; Fu, Y.; Szmacinski, H.; Nowaczyk, K.; Lakowicz, J.R. Plasmon-controlled fluorescence towards high-sensitivity optical sensing. *Adv. Biochem. Engng. Biotechnol.* **2009**, *116*, 29–72.
32. Xie, F.; Pang, J.S.; Centeno, A.; Ryan, M.P.; Riley, D.J.; Alford, N.M. Nanoscale control of Ag nanostructures for plasmonic fluorescence enhancement of near-infrared dyes. *Nano Res.* **2013**, *6*, 496–510. [CrossRef]

33. Zheng, Y.B.; Kiraly, B.; Weiss, P.S.; Huang, T.J. Molecular plasmonics for biology and nanomedicine. *Nanomedicine* **2012**, 751–770. [CrossRef] [PubMed]
34. Aroca, R.F.; Teo, G.Y.; Mohan, H.; Guerrero, A.R.; Albella, P.; Moreno, F. Plasmon-Enhanced Fluorescence and Spectral Modification in SHINEF. *J. Phys. Chem. C* **2011**, *115*, 20419–20424. [CrossRef]
35. Feng, A.L.; You, M.L.; Tian, L.; Singamaneni, S.; Liu, M.; Duan, Z.; Lu, T.J.; Xu, F.; Lin, M. Distance-Dependent Plasmon-Enhanced Fluorescence of Upconversion Nanoparticles using Polyelectrolyte Multilayers as Tunable Spacers. *Sci. Rep.* **2015**, *5*, 7779. [CrossRef] [PubMed]
36. Stobiecka, M. Novel plasmonic field-enhanced nanoassay for trace detection of proteins. *Biosens. Bioelectron.* **2014**, *55*, 379–385. [CrossRef]
37. Stobiecka, M.; Chalupa, A. Modulation of Plasmon-Enhanced Resonance Energy Transfer to Gold Nanoparticles by Protein Survivin Channeled-Shell Gating. *J. Phys. Chem. B* **2015**, *119*, 13227–13235. [CrossRef]
38. Xu, H.; Wallace, R.; Hepel, M. Interactions of antifouling monolayers: Energy transfer from excitedalbumin molecule to phenol red dye. *Chem. Pap.* **2015**, *69*, 227–236. [CrossRef]
39. Ratajczak, K.; Lukasiak, A.; Grel, H.; Dworakowska, B.; Jakiela, S.; Stobiecka, M. Monitoring of dynamic ATP level changes by oligomycin-modulated ATP synthase inhibition in SW480 cancer cells using fluorescent "On-Off" switching DNA aptamer. *Anal. Bioanal. Chem.* **2019**, *411*, 6899–6911. [CrossRef]
40. Stobiecka, M.; Hepel, M. Rapid functionalization of metal nanoparticles by moderator-tunable ligand-exchange process for biosensor designs. *Sens. Actuators B* **2010**, *149*, 373–380. [CrossRef]
41. Hepel, M.; Stobiecka, M. Detection of Oxidative Stress Biomarkers Using Functional Gold Nanoparticles. In *Fine Particles in Medicine and Pharmacy*; Matijević, E., Ed.; Springer: Boston, MA, USA, 2012; pp. 241–281.
42. Hutter, E.; Maysinger, D. Gold-nanoparticle-based biosensors for detection of enzyme activity. *Trends Pharmacol. Sci.* **2013**, *34*, 497–507. [CrossRef] [PubMed]
43. Bakshi, S.F.; Guz, N.; Zakharchenko, A.; Deng, H.; Tumanov, A.V.; Woodworth, C.D.; Minko, S.; Kolpashchikov, D.M.; Katz, E. Nanoreactors Based on DNAzyme-Functionalized Magnetic Nanoparticles Activated by Magnetic Field. *Nanoscale* **2018**, *10*, 1356–1365. [CrossRef] [PubMed]
44. He, Y.; Chen, S.; Huang, L.; Wang, Z.; Wu, Y.; Fu, F. Combination of Magnetic-Beads-Based Multiple Metal Nanoparticles Labeling with Hybridization Chain Reaction Amplification for Simultaneous Detection of Multiple Cancer Cells with Inductively Coupled Plasma Mass Spectrometry. *Anal. Chem.* **2019**, *91*, 1171–1177. [CrossRef] [PubMed]
45. Kolosnjaj-Tabi, J.; Wilhelm, C.; Clement, O.; Gazeau, F. Cell labelling with magnetic nanoparticls: Opportunity for magnetic cell imaging and cell manipulation. *J. Nanobiotechnol.* **2013**, *11*, S7. [CrossRef] [PubMed]
46. Huang, W.; Chang, C.L.; Chan, B.D.; Jalal, S.I.; Matei, D.E.; Low, P.S.; Savran, C.A. Concurrent detection of cellular and molecular cancer markers using an immunomagnetic flow system. *Anal. Chem.* **2015**, *87*, 10205–10212. [CrossRef] [PubMed]
47. Ratajczak, K.; Krazinski, B.E.; Kowalczyk, A.E.; Dworakowska, B.; Jakiela, S.; Stobiecka, M. Optical biosensing system for the detection of survivin mRNA in colorectal cancer cells using a graphene oxide carrier-bound oligonucleotide molecular beacon. *Nanomaterials* **2018**, *8*, 510. [CrossRef]
48. Running, L.; Espinal, R.; Hepel, M. Controlled release of targeted chemotherapeutic drug dabrafenib for melanoma cancers monitored using surface-enhanced Raman scattering (SERS) spectroscopy. *Mediterr. J. Chem.* **2018**, *7*, 18–27. [CrossRef]
49. Hepel, M.; Stobiecka, M. *Interactions of Herbicide Atrazine with DNA*; Nova Science Publishers: New York, NY, USA, 2010; ISBN 978-1-6172-8908-8.
50. Kamaly, N.; Yameen, B.; Wu, J.; Farokhzad, O.C. Degradable controlled release polymers and polymeric nanoparticles: Mechanisms of controlling drug release. *Chem. Rev.* **2016**, *116*, 2602–2663. [CrossRef]
51. Wong, P.T.; Choi, S.K. Mechanisms of drug release in nanotherapeutic delivery systems. *Chem. Rev.* **2015**, *115*, 3388–3432. [CrossRef]
52. Hong, R.; Han, G.; Fernández, J.M.; Kim, B.J.; Forbes, N.S.; Rotello, V.M. Glutathione-mediated delivery and release using monolayer protected nanoparticle carriers. *J. Am. Chem. Soc.* **2006**, *128*, 1078–1079. [CrossRef]
53. Mosayebi, J.; Kiyasatfar, M.; Laurent, S. Synthesis, functionalization, and design of magnetic nanoparticles for theranostic applications. *Adv. Healthc. Mater.* **2017**, *6*, 1700306. [CrossRef]
54. McBain, S.C.; Yiu, H.H.P.; Dobson, J. Magnetic nanoparticles for gene and drug delivery. *Int. J. Nanomed.* **2008**, *3*, 169–180.

55. Gul, S.; Khan, S.B.; Rehman, I.U.; Khan, M.A.; Khan, M.I. A comprehensive review of magnetic nanomaterials modern day theranostics. *Front. Mater.* **2019**, *6*, 179. [CrossRef]
56. Latorre, A.; Couleaud, P.; Aires, A.; Cortajarena, A.L.; Somoza, A. Multifunctionalization of magnetic nanoparticles for controlled drug release: A general approach. *Eur. J. Med. Chem.* **2014**, *82*, 355–362. [CrossRef]
57. Zhao, J.; Wu, S.; Qin, J.; Shi, D.; Wang, Y. Electrical-Charge-Mediated Cancer Cell Targeting via Protein Corona-Decorated Superparamagnetic Nanoparticles in a Simulated Physiological Environment. *ACS Appl. Mater. Interfaces* **2018**, *10*, 41986–41998. [CrossRef]
58. Connell, J.J.; Patrick, P.S.; Yu, Y.; Lythgoe, M.F.; Kalber, T.L. Advanced cell therapies: Targeting, tracking and actuation of cells with magnetic particles. *Regenerat. Med.* **2015**, *10*, 757–772. [CrossRef]
59. Gleich, B.; Weizenecker, J. Tomographic imaging using the nonlinear response of magnetic particles. *Nature* **2005**, *435*, 1214. [CrossRef]
60. Herz, S.; Vogel, P.; Dietrich, P.; Kampf, T.; Ruckert, M.A.; Kickuth, R.; Behr, V.C.; Bley, T.A. Magnetic particle imaging guided real-time percutaneous transluminal angioplasty in a phantom model. *Cardiovasc. Intervent. Radiol.* **2018**. [CrossRef]
61. Herz, S.; Vogel, P.; Kampf, T.; Dietrich, P.; Veldhoen, S.; Ruckert, M.A.; Kickuth, R.; Behr, V.C.; Bley, T.A. Magnetic particle imaging-guided stenting. *J. Endovasc. Ther.* **2019**, *26*, 512–519. [CrossRef]
62. Weller, A.; Salamon, J.M.; Frolich, A.; Moddel, M.; Knopp, T.; Werner, R. Combining direct 3D volume rendering and magnetic particle imaging to advance radiation-free real-time 3D guidance of vascular interventions. *Cardiovasc. Intervent. Radiol.* **2019**. [CrossRef]
63. Vogel, P.; Ruckert, M.A.; Kemp, S.J.; Khandhar, A.P.; Ferguson, R.M.; Herz, S.; Vilter, A.; Klauer, P.; Bley, T.A.; Krishnan, K.M.; et al. Micro-traveling wave magnetic particle imaging-sub-millimeter resolution with optimized tracer LS-008. *IEEE Trans. Magnet.* **2019**. [CrossRef]
64. Molwitz, I.; Ittrich, H.; Knopp, T.; Mummert, T.; Jung, J.S.C.; Adam, G.; Kaul, M.G. First magnetic particle imaging angiography in human sized organs by employing a multimodal ex vivo pig kidney perfusion system. *Physiol. Meas.* **2019**. [CrossRef] [PubMed]
65. Talebloo, N.; Gudi, M.; Robertson, N.; Wang, P. Magnetic particle imaging: Current applications in biomedical research. *J. Magnet. Resonace Imag.* **2019**. [CrossRef] [PubMed]
66. Shasha, C.; Teeman, E.; Krishnan, K.M. Nanoparticle core size optimization for magnetic particle imaging. *Biomed. Phys. Engng. Expr.* **2019**. [CrossRef]
67. Teeman, E.; Shasha, C.; Evans, J.E.; Krishnan, K.M. Intracellular dynamics of superparamagnetic iron oxide nanoparticles for magnetic particle imaging. *Nanoscale* **2019**. [CrossRef] [PubMed]
68. Yu, E.Y.; Bishop, M.; Zheng, B.; Ferguson, R.M.; Khandhar, A.P.; Kemp, S.J.; Krishnan, K.M.; Goodwill, P.W.; Conolly, S.M. Magnetic Particle Imaging: A Novel in Vivo Imaging Platform for Cancer Detection. *Nano Lett.* **2017**, *17*, 1648–1654. [CrossRef]
69. Bagheri, H.; Kierans, C.A.; Nelson, K.J.; Andrade, B.A.; Wong, C.L.; Frederick, A.L.; Hayden, M.E. A mechanically driven magnetic particle imaging scanner. *Appl. Phys. Lett.* **2018**, *113*, 183703. [CrossRef]
70. Bakenecker, A.C.; Ahlborg, M.; Debbeler, C.; Kaethner, C.; Buzug, T.M.; Ludtke-Buzug, K. Magnetic particle imaging in vascular medicine. *Innov. Surg. Sci.* **2018**, *3*, 179–192.
71. Bartorelli, A.L.; Marenzi, G. Contrast-induced nephropathy. *J. Interv. Cardiol.* **2008**, *21*, 74–85. [CrossRef]
72. Schlorf, T.; Meincke, M.; Kossel, E.; Glüer, C.C.; Jansen, O.; Mentlein, R. Biological properties of iron oxide nanoparticles for cellular and molecular magnetic resonance imaging. *Int J. Mol. Sci.* **2010**, *12*, 12–23. [CrossRef]
73. Vallejo-Fernandez, G.; Whear, O.; Roca, A.G.; Hussain, S.; Timmis, J.; Patel, V.; O'Grady, K. Mechanisms of hyperthermia in magnetic nanoparticles. *J. Phys. D Appl. Phys.* **2013**, *46*, 312001. [CrossRef]
74. Carrey, J.; Mehdaoui, B.; Respaud, M. Simple models for dynamic hysteresis loop calculations of magnetic single-domain nanoparticles: Application to magnetic hyperthermia optimization. *J. Appl. Phys.* **2011**, *109*, 083921. [CrossRef]
75. Lachowicz, D.; Kaczyńska, A.; Wirecka, R.; Kmita, A.; Szczerba, W.; Bodzoń-Kułakowska, A.; Sikora, M.; Karewicz, A.; Zapotoczny, S. A hybrid system for magnetic hyperthermia and drug delivery: SPION functionalized by curcumin conjugate. *Materials* **2018**, *11*, 2388. [CrossRef] [PubMed]

76. Drašler, B.; Drobne, D.; Novak, S.; Valant, J.; Boljte, S.; Otrin, L.; Rappolt, M.; Sartori, B.; Iglič, A.; Kralj-Iglič, V.; et al. Effects of magnetic cobalt ferrite nanoparticles on biological and artificial lipid membranes. *Int. J. Nanomed.* **2014**, *9*, 1559–1581. [CrossRef] [PubMed]
77. Verde, E.L.; Landi, G.T.; Gomes, J.A.; Sousa, M.H.; Bakuzis, A.F. Magnetic hyperthermia investigation of cobalt ferrite nanoparticles: Comparison between experiment, linear response theory, and dynamic hysteresis simulations. *J. Appl. Phys.* **2012**, *111*. [CrossRef]
78. Hilger, I. In vivo applications of magnetic nanoparticle hyperthermia. *Int. J. Hyperthermia* **2013**, *29*, 828–834. [CrossRef]
79. Sun, J.; Guo, M.; Pang, H.; Qi, J.; Zhang, J.; Ge, Y. Treatment of malignant glioma using hyperthermia. *Neural Regen. Res.* **2013**, *8*, 2775–2782.
80. Wu, F.; Sun, B.; Chu, X.; Zhang, Q.; She, Z.; Song, S.; Zhou, N.; Zhang, J.; Yi, X.; Wu, D.; et al. Hyaluronic Acid-Modified Porous Carbon-Coated Fe_3O_4 Nanoparticles for Magnetic Resonance Imaging-Guided Photothermal/Chemotherapy of Tumors. *Langmuir* **2019**, *35*, 13135–13144. [CrossRef]
81. Wu, F.; Zhang, M.; Lu, H.; Liang, D.; Huang, Y.; Xia, Y.; Hu, Y.; Hu, S.; Wang, J.; Yi, X.; et al. Triple Stimuli-Responsive Magnetic Hollow Porous Carbon-Based Nanodrug Delivery System for Magnetic Resonance Imaging-Guided Synergistic Photothermal/Chemotherapy of Cancer. *ACS Appl. Mater. Interfaces* **2018**, *10*, 21939–21949. [CrossRef]
82. Lee, S.M.; Kim, H.J.; Kim, S.Y.; Kwon, M.K.; Kim, S.; Cho, A.; Yun, M.; Shin, J.S.; Yoo, K.H. Drug-loaded gold plasmonic nanoparticles for treatment of multidrug resistance in cancer. *Biomaterials* **2014**, *35*, 2272–2282. [CrossRef]
83. Bar-Zeev, M.; Livney, Y.D.; Assaraf, Y.G. Targeted nanomedicine for cancer therapeutics: Towards precision medicine overcoming drug resistance. *Drug Resist. Updates* **2017**, *31*, 15–30. [CrossRef] [PubMed]
84. Mazon, E.E.; Samano, A.H.; Calleja, H.; Quintero, L.H.; Paz, J.A.; Cano, M.E. A frequency tuner for resonant inverters suitable for magnetic hyperthermia applications. *Meas. Sci. Technol.* **2017**, *28*, 095901. [CrossRef]
85. Villanueva, A.; Presa, P.d.l.; Alonso, J.M.; Rueda, T.; Martınez, A.; Crespo, P.; Morales, M.P.; Gonzalez-Fernandez, M.A.; Valdes, J.; Rivero, G. Hyperthermia HeLa cell treatment with silica-coated manganese oxide nanoparticles. *J. Phys. Chem. C* **2010**, *114*, 1976–1981. [CrossRef]
86. Creixell, M.; Bohorquez, A.C.; Torres-Lugo, M.; Rinaldi, C. EGFR-targeted magnetic nanoparticle heaters kill cancer cells without a perceptible temperature rise. *ACS Nano* **2011**, *5*, 7124–7129. [CrossRef]
87. Domenech, M.; Marrero-Berrios, I.; Torres-Lugo, M.; Rinaldi, C. Lysosomal membrane permeabilization by targeted magnetic nanoparticles in alternating magnetic fields. *ACS Nano* **2013**, *7*, 5091–5101. [CrossRef]
88. Sanchez, C.; Diab, D.E.H.; Connord, V.; Clerc, P.; Meunier, E.; Pipy, B.; Fourmy, D. Targeting a G-protein-coupled receptor overexpressed in endocrine tumors by magnetic nanoparticles to induce cell death. *ACS Nano* **2014**, *8*, 1350–1363. [CrossRef]
89. Zhang, E.; Kircher, M.F.; Koch, X.M.; Eliasson, L.; Goldberg, S.N.; Renstrom, E. Dynamic magnetic fields remote-control apoptosis via nanoparticle rotation. *ACS Nano* **2014**, *8*, 3192–3201. [CrossRef]
90. Connord, V.; Clerc, P.; Hallali, N.; Diab, D.E.H.; Fourmy, D.; Gigoux, V.; Carrey, J. Real-time analysis of magnetic hyperthermia experiments on living cells under a confocal microscope. *Small* **2015**, *11*, 2437–2445. [CrossRef]
91. Klyachko, N.L.; Sokolsky-Papkov, M.; Pothayee, N.; Efremova, M.V.; Gulin, D.A.; Pothayee, N.; Kuznetsov, A.A.; Majouga, A.G.; Riffle, J.S.; Golovin, Y.I.; et al. Changing the enzyme reaction rate in magnetic nanosuspensions by a non-heating magnetic field. *Angew. Chem. Int. Ed.* **2012**, *51*, 12016–12019. [CrossRef]
92. Kim, D.H.; Rozhkova, E.A.; Ulasov, I.V.; Bader, S.D.; Rajh, T.; Lesniak, M.S.; Novosad, V. Biofunctionalized magnetic-vortex microdiscs for targeted cancer-cell destruction. *Nat. Mater.* **2010**, *9*, 165–171. [CrossRef]
93. Master, A.M.; Williams, P.N.; Pothayee, N.; Pothayee, N.; Zhang, R.; Vishwasrao, H.M.; Golovin, Y.I.; Riffle, J.S.; Sokolsky, M.; Kabanov, A.V. Remote actuation of magnetic nanoparticles for cancer cell selective treatment through cytoskeletal disruption. *Sci. Rep.* **2016**, *6*, 33560. [CrossRef] [PubMed]
94. Hoffmann, C.; Mazari, E.; Lallet, S.; Borgne, R.L.; Marchi, V.; Gosse, C.; Gueroui, Z. Spatiotemporal control of microtubule nucleation and assembly using magnetic nanoparticles. *Nat. Nanotechnol.* **2013**, *8*, 199–205. [CrossRef] [PubMed]

95. Dixon, S.J.; Lemberg, K.M.; Lamprecht, M.R.; Skouta, R.; Zaitsev, E.M.; Gleason, C.E.; Patel, D.N.; Bauer, A.J.; Cantley, A.M.; Yang, W.S.; et al. Ferroptosis: An iron-dependent form of nonapoptotic cell death. *Cell* **2012**, *149*, 1060–1072. [CrossRef] [PubMed]
96. Dixon, S.J.; Stockwell, B.R. The role of iron and reactive oxygen species in cell death Scott J Dixon1,5* & Brent R Stockwell. *Nat. Chem. Biol.* **2014**, *10*, 9–17. [CrossRef] [PubMed]
97. Tan, S.; Schubert, D.; Maher, P. Oxytosis: A novel form of programmed cell death. *Curr. Top. Med. Chem.* **2001**, *1*, 497–506. [CrossRef]
98. Trachootham, D.; Alexandre, J.; Huang, P. Targeting cancer cells by ROS-mediated mechanisms: A radical therapeutic approach? *Nat. Rev. Drug Discov.* **2009**, *8*, 579–591. [CrossRef]
99. Prasad, S.; Gupta, S.C.; Tyagi, A.K. Reactive oxygen species (ROS) and cancer: Role of antioxidative nutraceuticalas. *Cancer Lett.* **2017**, *387*, 95–105. [CrossRef]
100. Wang, N.; Wu, Y.; Bian, J.; Qian, X.; Lin, H.; Sun, H.; You, Q.; Zhang, X. Current development of ROS-modulating agents as novel antitumor therapy. *Curr. Cancer Drug Targets* **2017**, *17*, 122–136. [CrossRef]
101. Shen, Z.; Song, J.; Yung, B.C.; Zhou, Z.; Wu, A.; Chen, X. Emerging strategies of cancer therapy based on ferroptosis. *Adv. Mater.* **2018**, *30*, 1704007. [CrossRef]
102. Hepel, M.; Stobiecka, M.; Peachey, J.; Miller, J. Intervention of glutathione in pre-mutagenic catechol-mediated DNA damage in the presence of copper(II). *Mutat. Res.* **2012**, *735*, 1–11. [CrossRef]
103. Yu, J.; Zhao, F.; Gao, W.; Yang, X.; Ju, Y.; Zhao, L.; Guo, W.; Xie, J.; Liang, X.; Tao, X.; et al. Magnetic Reactive Oxygen Species Nanoreactor for Switchable Magnetic Resonance Imaging Guided Cancer Therapy Based on pH-Sensitive Fe_5C_2@Fe_3O_4 Nanoparticles. *ACS Nano* **2019**, *13*, 10002–10014. [CrossRef] [PubMed]
104. Hepel, M.; Stobiecka, M. Comparative kinetic model of fluorescence enhancement in selective binding of monochlorobimane to glutathione. *J. Photochem. Photobiol. A Chem.* **2011**, *225*, 72–80. [CrossRef]
105. Hepel, M.; Stobiecka, M. Supramolecular interactions of oxidative stress biomarker glutathione with fluorone black. *Spectrochim. Acta A* **2018**, *192*, 146–152. [CrossRef] [PubMed]
106. Hong, J.W.; Quake, S.R. Integrated nanoliter systems. *Nat. Biotechnol.* **2003**, *21*, 1179–1183. [CrossRef] [PubMed]
107. Green, B.J.; Nguyen, V.; Atenafu, E.; Weeber, P.; Duong, B.T.V.; Thiagalingam, P.; Labib, M.; Mohamadi, R.M.; Hansen, A.R.; Joshua, A.M.; et al. Phenotypic Profiling of Circulating Tumor Cells in Metastatic Prostate Cancer Patients Using Nanoparticle-Mediated Ranking. *Anal. Chem.* **2019**, *91*, 9348–9355. [CrossRef] [PubMed]
108. Mandal, K.; Jana, D.; Ghorai, B.K.; Jana, N.R. AIEgen-Conjugated Magnetic Nanoparticles as Magnetic–Fluorescent Bioimaging Probes. *ACS Appl. Nano Mater.* **2019**, *2*, 3292–3299. [CrossRef]
109. Han, S.I.; Han, K.H. Electrical detection method for circulating tumor cells using graphene nanoplates. *Anal. Chem.* **2015**, *87*, 10585–10592. [CrossRef]
110. Wang, Z.; Sun, N.; Liu, H.; Chen, C.; Ding, P.; Yue, X.; Zou, H.; Xing, C.; Pei, R. High-Efficiency Isolation and Rapid Identification of Heterogeneous Circulating Tumor Cells (CTCs) Using Dual-Antibody-Modified Fluorescent-Magnetic Nanoparticles. *ACS Appl. Mater. Interfaces* **2019**, *11*, 39586–39593. [CrossRef]
111. Fang, C.; Zhang, M. Multifunctional magnetic nanoparticles for medical imaging applications. *J. Mater. Chem.* **2009**, *19*, 6258–6266. [CrossRef]
112. Feng, Q.; Liu, Y.; Huang, J.; Chen, K.; Huang, J.; Xiao, K. Uptake, distribution, clearance, and toxicity of iron oxide nanoparticles with different sizes and coatings. *Sci. Rep.* **2018**, *8*, 2082. [CrossRef]

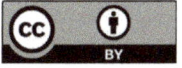

© 2020 by the author. Licensee MDPI, Basel, Switzerland. This article is an open access article distributed under the terms and conditions of the Creative Commons Attribution (CC BY) license (http://creativecommons.org/licenses/by/4.0/).

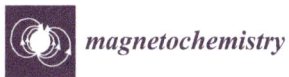

Review

Hybrid Nanostructured Magnetite Nanoparticles: From Bio-Detection and Theragnostics to Regenerative Medicine

Yolanda Piñeiro *, Manuel González Gómez, Lisandra de Castro Alves, Angela Arnosa Prieto, Pelayo García Acevedo, Román Seco Gudiña, Julieta Puig, Carmen Teijeiro, Susana Yáñez Vilar * and José Rivas

Applied Physics Department, Nanomag Laboratory, Universidade de Santiago de Compostela, 15782 Santiago de Compostela, Spain; manuelantonio.gonzalez@usc.es (M.G.G.); lisandracristina.decastro@usc.es (L.d.C.A.); angela.arnosa@usc.es (A.A.P.); pelayo.garcia.acevedo@usc.es (P.G.A.); romanseco@hotmail.es (R.S.G.); julieta.puig@usc.es (J.P.); carmen.teijeiro@usc.es (C.T.); jose.rivas@usc.es (J.R.)
* Correspondence: y.pineiro.redondo@usc.es (Y.P.); susana.yanez@usc.es (S.Y.V.); Tel.: +34-881813062 (Y.P.); +34-881813062 (S.Y.V.)

Received: 5 November 2019; Accepted: 27 December 2019; Published: 10 January 2020

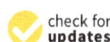

Abstract: Nanotechnology offers the possibility of operating on the same scale length at which biological processes occur, allowing to interfere, manipulate or study cellular events in disease or healthy conditions. The development of hybrid nanostructured materials with a high degree of chemical control and complex engineered surface including biological targeting moieties, allows to specifically bind to a single type of molecule for specific detection, signaling or inactivation processes. Magnetite nanostructures with designed composition and properties are the ones that gather most of the designs as theragnostic agents for their versatility, biocompatibility, facile production and good magnetic performance for remote in vitro and in vivo for biomedical applications. Their superparamagnetic behavior below a critical size of 30 nm has allowed the development of magnetic resonance imaging contrast agents or magnetic hyperthermia nanoprobes approved for clinical uses, establishing an inflection point in the field of magnetite based theragnostic agents.

Keywords: magnetite; superparamagnetism; biodetection; magnetofection; imaging; therapy; tissue engineering

1. Introduction

Magnetism has been technologically exploited for centuries, well before quantum mechanics helped to unveil the fundamental mechanisms governing the behavior of magnetic materials.

Electrical steels, permanents magnets, nickel-iron alloys or soft ferrites mechanized in different configurations just from bulk, ribbon or disks are the enabling materials behind disparate developments like compasses for marine navigation, bulk magnetic separation devices in mining industry, inductive heating in massive foundry industry, sophisticated devices for electric power generation and distribution or communications and information storage in hard disks [1].

The large variety of applications exploiting different aspects of magnetism has permeated our technically developed society in the last decades and follows still an intense evolution by the hand of applications based on magnetic materials tailored at the nanometric scale. In fact, the optimization and maturity of chemical synthetic procedures during the last decades has allowed the development of materials with designed properties which are only observable at the nanoscale such as, surface plasmonic resonance, enhanced and specific catalytic activity, size-dependent fluorescence, superparamagnetism [2], quantum tunneling magnetization [3] or enhanced coercivity [4] that, all combined, open the door to highly interesting biomedical and technological applications.

In addition to their designed properties, magnetic nanoparticles (MNPs) are an intense topic of research in diagnostic, theragnostic and regenerative medicine applications, due to their small size, which is comparable to relevant cell length scales and allows to interact and interfere with biological processes, minimizing adverse effects and opening the way to new diagnostic and therapeutic paradigms [5].

Specifically, superparamagnetic iron oxides nanoparticles (SPIONs) are witnessing a predominant role in nanomedicine developments relaying on their biocompatibility, unbeatable low cost production, physicochemical performance and versatile chemistry that make them almost universally present as a main components in contrast agents for magnetic resonance imaging (MRI), magnetic hyperthermia sources or drug delivery nanoplatforms [6].

It is striking, however, that Nature had incorporated crystalline magnetite nanoparticles (NPs) as a strategy for magnetic guiding in small animals, thousands of years before the recent developments of nanotechnology. Magnetotactic bacteria, bees or pigeons are equipped with magnetic dipolar arrays of small Fe_3O_4 NPs, biologically synthesized in specific vesicles, that serve as natural compasses to orientate in the magnetic field of the Earth. Moreover, magnetite NPs can be found also in humans, when a pathologically altered iron metabolism triggers their synthesis inside ferritin (Fn), a spherical hollow protein in charge of delivering Fe^{3+} to feed our cell biomachinery [7].

Besides its good magnetic performance (Curie temperature well above any biomedical application, large values of initial susceptibility and saturation magnetization) and biocompatibility, the availability of facile wet chemistry techniques to produce superparamagnetic (SPM) cores with well controlled size, shape and composition has promoted magnetite to the most relevant position in the field of nanomedicine for biodetection, imaging and therapy.

In fact, it competes with the most well accepted soft organic compounds, like liposomes or nano-emulsions, fully biocompatible, biodegradable with enhanced ability for encapsulating a variety of hydrophilic or lipophilic drugs [8] that have found approval for clinical uses in a variety of applications as vaccines, antifunghical, anesthetics or antibiotics [9]. Although with a slower pace, a few set of superparamagnetic magnetite NPs have been clinically tested and approved for commercialization as enhanced contrast agents for magnetic resonance imaging (Feridex; Resovist, Ferumoxtran) [10] or magnetic hyperthermia therapies for brain tumor treatment (NanoTherm) [11], establishing an inflection point in the use of inorganic materials as theragnostic agents.

By simple and scalable methods like co-precipitation, hydrothermal or solvothermal decomposition procedures, easy production of spheres, cubes, hexagons, octahedra, hollow spheres, rods, plates or wires can be obtained with controlled size. Combined with surface functionalization procedures, these magnetite NPs can be engineered to produce multifunctional hybrid nanostructures with a designed composition of inorganic/organic/biological shells containing carbon, metal (Au, Ag, Cu, etc.), metal oxides (Ti, Si, Zr, etc.), hydroxides (Al, etc.), organic compounds (polymers like polyacrylic acid (PAA), polyethylene glycol (PEG), etc.), short organic molecules (OAc, dopamine, etc.) and biological moieties (antibodies, aptamers, plasmids, etc.) [12].

This core-shell strategy has given rise to different configurations like single- and multi-core@shell nanoparticles, where magnetite is located in the core (Fe_3O_4@SiO_2; Fe_3O_4@C), in the shell (gelatin-NPs@Fe_3O_4-NPs) or embedded in a polymer matrix (polyester, gelatin magnetic beads). In all cases, the nanostructure inherits a combination of abilities that ensures their multimodal capacities for simultaneous magnetic separation/detection/targeting procedures like contrast agents in magnetic resonance imaging/positron emission tomography (MRI/PET), magnetic hyperthermia (MH)/drug delivery therapeutic agents, among others [12].

Moreover, magnetite based nanostructures can be also included as the magnetic phase in a nanocomposite material like mesoporous silica, biopolymer sponges (chitosan, k-carrageenan, alginate, etc.), porous stiff materials (hydroxyapatite, polycaprolactone, etc.) or hydrogels, allowing to produce magnetic scaffolds for tissue engineering combining all the theragnostic abilities, inherited from magnetite, together with magnetic cell growth stimulation or magnetic external fixation [13].

The list of nanostructured materials containing magnetite NPs is huge, and the applications in nanomedicine cover almost any aspect from detection, diagnosis and therapy to regenerative medicine.

In this work, we present the structure, properties, synthetic procedures and applications emerging from the magnetically intrinsic properties of magnetite nanostructures with tailored configuration, size and shape.

2. Magnetite: Structure and Properties from Bulk to Nanoscale

Magnetite, Fe_3O_4, is an iron oxide compound where iron ions (with valence 3+ and 2+) adjust to the $AB_2O_4 = Fe^{3+}(Fe^{2+}Fe^{3+})O_4$ formulation, arranged in an inverse-spinel crystal structure [14], composed by tetrahedral, A, and octahedral, B, sublattices. The magnetic and electric properties of magnetite arise from the interactions between the Fe^{3+} (d^5) and Fe^{2+} (d^6) ions placed on octahedral positions and Fe^{3+} (d^5) ions on tetrahedral positions. The spinel is a stable crystal structure that accepts the substitution of the A and B lattice locations by a variety of nearly 30 different metal ions with valences ranging from +1 to +6. An example of this stability is the fact that both, natural magnetite is commonly found containing impurity ions (Ti, Al, Mg, and Mn), and substituted ferrites containing transition metals (Co, Mn, Zn) can be easily obtained by wet chemistry procedures [15]. The unit cell in bulk Fe_3O_4 consists in a face centered cubic, fcc, (Fd^{3}m space group) arrangement of O^{2-} ions, in which Fe^{3+} (d^5) cations occupy 1/2 of the tetrahedral interstices, and a 50:50 mixture of Fe^{3+} (d^5) and Fe^{2+} (d^6) cations occupy 1/8 of the octahedral interstices, with a characteristic unit cell parameter ≈8.4 Å (see Figure 1).

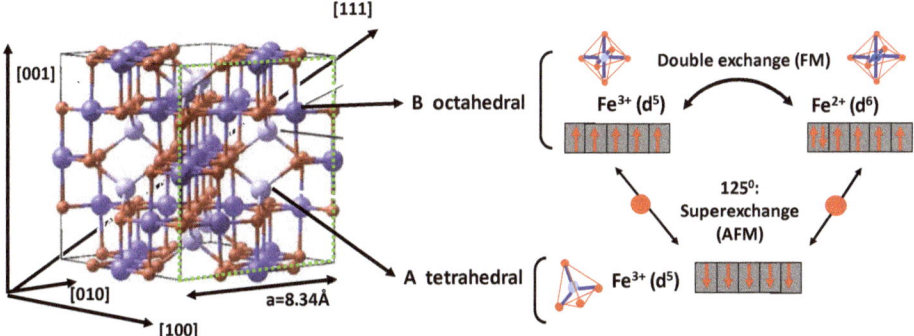

Figure 1. On the left, the inverse spinel structure (crystal structure adapted from [16] (Science Direct, 2016), of Fe_3O_4 is based on a face centered cubic (fcc) arrangement of O^{2-} ions in which Fe^{3+} (d^5) cations occupy 1/2 of the tetrahedral interstices, and a 50:50 mixture of Fe^{3+} (d^5) and Fe^{2+} (d^6) cations occupy 1/8 of the octahedral interstices. On the right, the set of exchange interactions between Fe^{3+} (d^5), Fe^{2+} (d^6) and O^{2-} ions, giving rise to ferrimagnetic ordering.

At temperatures above 118 °K, Fe^{2+} and Fe^{3+} ions are randomly distributed over the octahedral sites allowing electron hopping between them and giving rise to the low electrical resistivity, around 7 mili-Ohm/cm at T_{room}, of magnetite [15]. Below 118 °K, the Fe^{3+} and Fe^{2+} ions become ordered following a cubic to orthorhombic crystallographic transition, as proposed by Verwey [17], where c axis of the new orthorhombic phase is parallel to and slightly smaller than the cube edge of the fcc phase and accompanied by electronic charge ordering of the Fe^{3+} and Fe^{2+} ions on the B sites, which produces a large increase in resistivity [18].

The magnetic ordering in magnetite is dominated by the specific distribution of Fe^{3+} and Fe^{2+} ions on both A and B sites, and the exchange interactions originated when the 3d electron orbital of the Fe ions overlap with the 2p electron orbital of O^{2-} ions, since direct exchange between Fe-Fe interactions are negligible due to the large distance between Fe ions [19]. Fe-O-Fe super-exchange interaction depends on the distance and angle of bonds between the Fe^{3+} and Fe^{2+} and O^{2-} ions and is responsible for antiparallel alignment of the net magnetic moment of A and B sublattices, which gives rise to the ferrimagnetic order in magnetite [15]. As proposed by Neel, Fe^{3+} ions on the oppositely aligned tetrahedral and octahedral cancel each other, and only the remaining magnetic moment of Fe^{2+} ions contributes to the total magnetic moment of magnetite (see Figure 1).

Moreover, the spin magnetic moments, which are tied to their electron orbit by the spin–orbit interaction, orientate themselves into specific directions in the lattice that minimize the crystalline field and give rise to the magnetic anisotropy axes. In magnetite, easy (low-energy), hard (high-energy) and intermediate (medium-energy) magnetocrystalline anisotropy directions are defined by the cubic lattice axes [111], [100] and [110], respectively (see Figure 1) [15]. At low temperatures, 118 °K, the crystallographic transition from cubic to orthorhombic provokes the appearance of a magnetic isotropic point where the anisotropy constant (K1) sign changes from − to +, (K1 = 0) and is known as the Verwey transition.

Compared to other permanent magnetic materials (see Table 1), [20] magnetite shows a low effective magnetocrystalline anisotropy constant, high saturation magnetization per unit mass (M_S~92 emu/g), low coercivity (H_C = 10–40 mT) and high Curie temperature (T_C = 850°) compared to relevant temperatures for biomedical applications, and a molecular magnetic moment of 4.1 μ_{Bohr} (accounting for the larger Fe^{2+} contribution) [15].

Table 1. Bulk magnetocrystalline anisotropy constant, K_{an}, Curie temperature, Tc, for representative magnetic materials. Data compiled from data included in [20].

Material	Fe	Co	Ni	PtFe	Fe₃O₄	γ-Fe₂O₃
K_{an} (kJ/m³)	48	530	4.8	6600	11	4.6
T_C (K)	1043	1388	631	750	858	863

However, besides the specific crystalline structure of different magnetic materials, there is one common fact that affects their main magnetic behavior: size.

In order to accommodate all the magnetic interaction terms (exchange, Zeeman, demagnetizing field and anisotropy) bulk materials attain stability by adopting a magnetic configuration of multidomains separated by domain walls, that minimizes the total magnetic free energy [21]. When preparing small particles with sizes down to the nanometer scale, the balance of magnetic interaction terms changes: the energy cost of introducing domain walls is higher than the reduction of demagnetizing field, the anisotropy energy decreases proportionally to the reduction in volume of the particle, and single domain becomes the most stable magnetic configuration [22]. This multidomain to single domain transition happens for particles with a critical radius in the nanometer scale, (R_C = 10–100 nm), and depends on the material properties as $R_C = 36\sqrt{AK}/\mu_0 M_s^2$ (A, exchange constant, K, anisotropy constant and Ms, saturation magnetization) [23].

Fe₃O₄ NPs undergo a transition from multi- to single-domain magnetic structure 80–90 nm, and by further size reduction, which in magnetite happens between 25 to 30 nm, another transition arises when the total anisotropy energy of the crystallite becomes smaller than thermal energy. This fact originates that, in absence of externally applied magnetic fields, the magnetization (M) spontaneously fluctuates at room temperature by thermal stimulation and, in average, M equals zero. This is the so called superparamagnetic regime, characterized by negligible remanence or coercive forces (Figure 2a) and reversible magnetization with a rapid "on–off" magnetic switching, modulated by the initial magnetic susceptibility (χ_{in}) (in magnetite NPs can range from: χ_{in} = 0.5–1) [24].

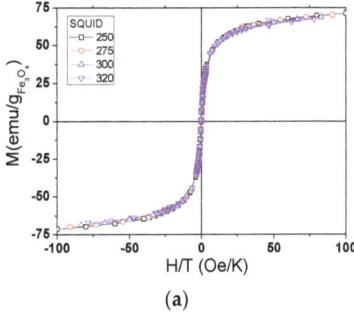 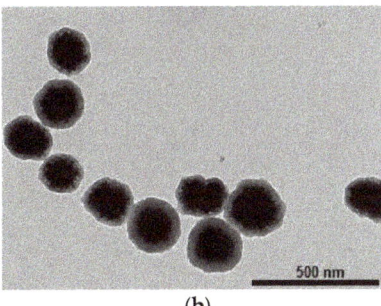

Figure 2. (a) Overlapping into a single curve of magnetization data versus H/T, that correspond to measurements performed corresponding from 250 to 320 K, on a dried sample of SPM multi-core Fe_3O_4@C, showing negligible remanence and coercive forces and (b) Transmission electron microscopy (TEM) micrograph of multi-core Fe_3O_4 @C, with averaged size 187 nm. (Figures reprinted with permission from [25], IEEE, 2016).

Chemical procedures like coprecipitation, thermal decomposition or hydrothermal preparations, are the most used wet chemistry techniques to provide high quality and monodisperse SPIONs with diameters ranging from 10 to 30 nm that have become a standard material as magnetic hyperthermia actuators with high specific absorption rates (SAR) in clinical applications (MAGFORCE-NanoTherm) [11] or as T2 MRI commercial contrast agents (Feridex; Resovist, Ferumoxtran [10]).

In addition, SPM behavior can be preserved in multi-core configurations (see Figure 2b) even though several magnetic cores stand in close contact embedded inside a coating shell (see Figure 2) [25]. These NPs are particularly interesting for those applications that require a high concentration of magnetic material in a small region to ensure an intense magnetic response (i.e., cell isolation purposes). The key procedure consists in coating the single-core magnetite surfaces to avoid exchange interaction between them that may cause exchange bias, commonly resulting in reduced saturation magnetization, low initial magnetic susceptibility or the loss of SPM behavior.

However, associated with the size reduction, the increase of surface-to-volume ratio (typically, for 5 nm NPs, the surface spins represent 30% of total amount of spins [26]), entails the dominant contribution of surface properties, incorporating a crucial problem for magnetic applications: the reduction of saturation magnetization [27]. For very small magnetic NPs, a surface dead magnetic layer appears related to specific features like:

1. The large contribution of surface ions, located on edges or corners, with coordination numbers lower than inner core ions, (see Figure 3) gives rise to an abrupt breakdown of the lattice and magnetic symmetry, which induces changes in magnetic anisotropy at the surface.
2. The chemical environment of the coating shell influences the magnetic properties of the surface ions.
3. The interaction of the surface spins with the inner ones by an exchange bias may lead to some degree of frustration that lowers the total magnetization of the nanoparticle [28].

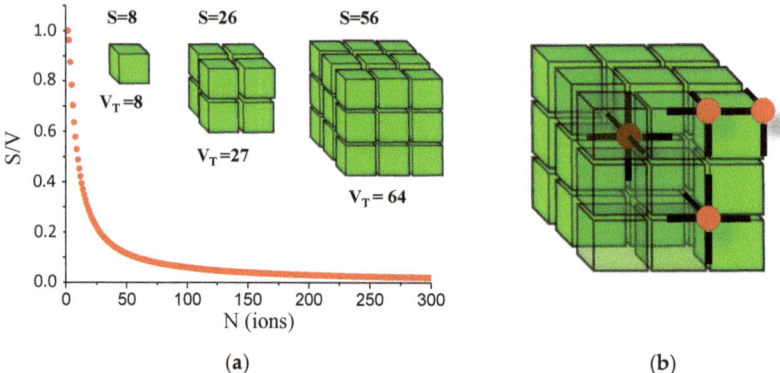

Figure 3. (a) Ratio of surface to volume ions in a cubic lattice, for very small nanoparticles (NPs) surface ions can amount up to large percentages of the totality and (b) corner, edge, surface and inner ions with different coordination numbers.

Although the preservation of optimum magnetic properties in small magnetic particles through the increase of crystalline quality and minimization of surface distortion has witnessed a large effort in chemical approaches in the last years [29], the production of pure colloidal SPIONs remains a challenge. Magnetite cores with a thin overoxidized (Fe^{3+}) surface shell, compositionally close to a maghemite polymorph (γ-Fe_2O_3), are normally obtained and only synthetic procedures driven at high temperatures can improve the purity and crystallinity of colloidal SPIONs with enhanced saturation magnetization (M_S = 70–85 emu/g) [30].

3. Synthetic Procedures of Multifunctional SPM Magnetite Nanostructures

For in vitro or in vivo applications, not only the magnetic core, but also the capping ligands on the surface, are the crucial aspects to ensure an adequate performance of the magnetic nanostructures when they interact with biological media, like fluids or tissues, where they can be critically arrested.

However, besides the efforts devoted to produce multifunctional magnetite nanostructures with high quality, the requirements to ensure a good in vitro and in vivo performance include a biocompatible coating and an adequate solvent dispersant, and for in vitro and in vivo applications is crucial to maintain colloidal stability of the preparations. Therefore, the chemical engineering to prepare SPIONs with several added functionalities requires a hierarchical procedure involving the production of good quality magnetite cores and several functionalization steps to add plasmonic NPs, fluorescent moieties, biological agent or biocompatible coating shells.

3.1. Synthesis of the Magnetic Core. Synthetic Procedures Modulating Size and Shape

With the aim of producing magnetite NPs with exceptional magnetic specifications, high crystalline quality, well-controlled size and shape, and easy procedures, different wet chemistry approaches have been studied based on co-precipitation, thermal decomposition, solvothermal or hydrothermal techniques (summarized in Figure 4). In combination or alone, they can be conveniently modified to produce magnetite NPs with different morphologies (spheres, cubes, hexagons, octahedra, hollow spheres, etc.), high crystalline quality, different architectures of single- or multiple-core configurations [31] or to provide large gram-scale production of NPs [32]. These techniques have allowed the development of SPIONs spanning from 10 nm to several hundreds of nanometers.

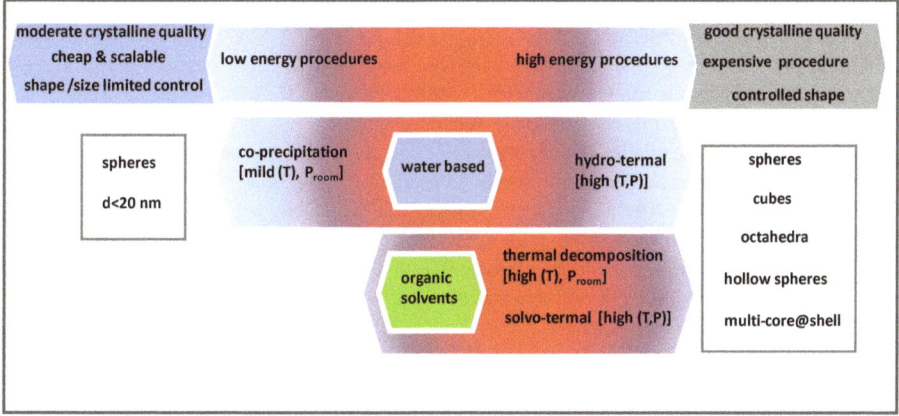

Figure 4. Summary of synthetic routes commonly used to produce superparamagnetic iron oxides nanoparticles (SPIONs).

3.1.1. Precipitation Methods

Precipitation methods of iron salts in a highly basic solution are easy, fast, scalable and can be done at low to moderate temperatures and inert atmosphere. Co-precipitation of two iron Fe^{2+}/Fe^{3+} salt precursors can be easily controlled by experimentally adjusting the Fe^{2+}/Fe^{3+} ions ratio, pH and temperature, providing spherical NPs with a good control of the structural (size, morphology) (see Figure 5a) and magnetic properties but a with wide size distribution. Although its easiness has made this basic method very popular, the ensembles produced in this way inherit a distribution of blocking temperatures, undesired in certain in vivo applications [33] or a distribution of magnetic moments that need to be avoided for magnetic detection kits.

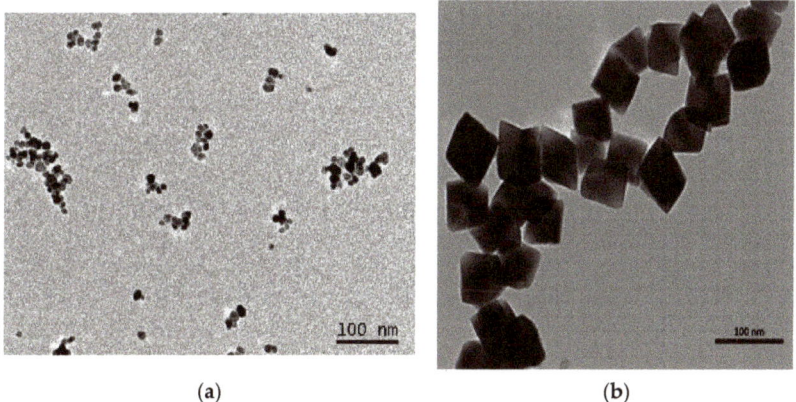

(a)   (b)

Figure 5. TEM image of (a) spherical magnetite NPs coated with citrated and obtained by a coprecipitation method and (b) bare cubic magnetite NPs obtained by a precipitation method.

Related to these needs, optimized co-precipitation procedures have been implemented attending to fundamental chemistry facts: reaction kinetics, atmosphere and temperature control. Following the general theory of nucleation and growth, under the so-called burst nucleation approach, a monodisperse solution of "nuclei" can be obtained by using supersaturated solutions of the precursors to nucleate in a fast and homogenous way. Furtherly, imposing a slow pace at the growth stage, a monodisperse ensemble of NPs can be achieved [34].

In addition, since magnetite easily oxides into hematite (Fe_2O_3), a non-magnetic iron oxide phase, applying inert conditions to the reaction, with a controlled oxygen atmosphere, avoids the formation of Fe_2O_3 and γ-Fe_2O_3, the other ferrimagnetic oxide.

Moreover, crystalline quality can be optimized by supplying energy to facilitate the annealing of the magnetite lattice. A modified technique [35], based on the precipitation of a single iron salt in a basic solution and a free oxygen atmosphere, allows to obtain $Fe(OH)_2$, which after heating at 363 K in a water bath for 2 h, allows the oxidation into Fe_3O_4 to obtain cubic magnetite NPs (see Figure 5b).

The addition of compounds like dextran, polyvinyl alcohol (PVA), PAA, etc., in subsequent step of the reaction ensures protection of the magnetite cores from oxidation, increases biocompatibility and stabilizes the colloidal dispersion.

3.1.2. Thermal Decomposition

Thermal decomposition of organic iron precursor phase in presence of adequate surfactants (fatty acids, oleic acid (OA), oleylamine, etc.), driven in high temperatures, allows to improve the crystalline quality of iron oxide NPs with well controlled morphology, size and narrow distribution (see Figure 6). The reaction temperature is adjusted to the used solvents, which are usually compounds with high boiling points (octylamine, phenyl ether, phenol ether, hexadecanediol, octadecene, etc.).

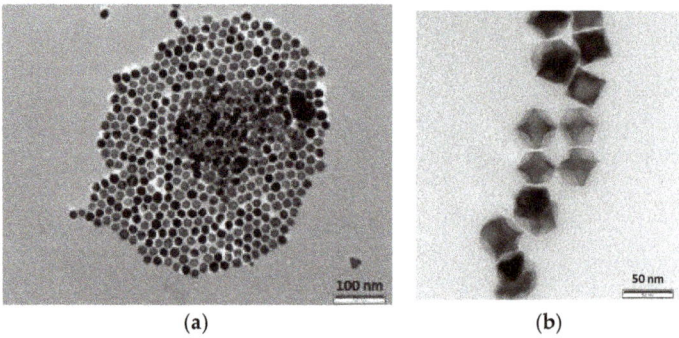

Figure 6. TEM images of (**a**) hydrophobic Fe_3O_4@OA NPs and (**b**) hydrophobic cubic Fe_3O_4@OA NPs, obtained by thermal decomposition method.

The most commonly used iron organic precursors are iron(III) N-nitrosophenylhydroxylamine ($Fe(cup)_3$), iron(III) acetylacetonate ($Fe(acac)_5$), iron pentacarbonyl ($Fe(CO)_5$), which follow different routes: $Fe(cup)_3$ or $Fe(acac)_3$ directly decompose into magnetite/maghemite, while $Fe(CO)_5$ goes through an intermediate step of metal formation and then an oxidation of Fe^0 into magnetite by addition of a mild oxidant [36].

This procedure allows to obtain sophisticated hollow magnetite structures, which in the case of thermal decomposition of iron pentacarbonyl [37] produces in a first stage Fe@Fe_3O_4 structures (see Figure 7a) prior to the final formation of small hollow magnetite spheres (see Figure 6b). Large hollow magnetite spheres (see Figure 7c) can be obtained through the thermal decomposition of ferric chloride hexahydrate ($FeCl_3 \cdot 6H_2O$) [38].

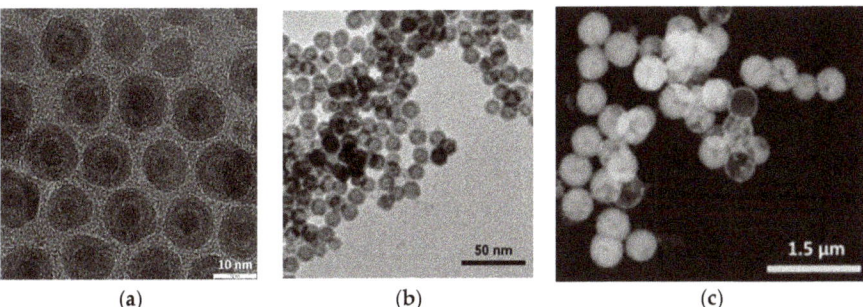

Figure 7. TEM image of (a) Fe@Fe$_3$O$_4$@OA NPs 13 nm, (b) small hollow Fe$_3$O$_4$@OA NPs and (c) STEM of large hollow Fe$_3$O$_4$@OA NPs.

Thermal decomposition is a versatile procedure that allows also to obtain magnetite NPs with a diminished magnetic dead layer [39], different morphologies like spheres [40] or cubes [41], with narrow size distribution and controlled ion substitution with transition metals like Fe, Mn, Co, Ni, or Cr. However, the use on non-polar solvents is a main disadvantage that needs to be overcome by a phase transfer strategy, to change organic-stabilized NPs into water dispersions suitable for biomedical applications.

3.1.3. Hydrothermal Synthesis

Hydrothermal synthesis is a case of solvothermal procedures, that submit the reactants into a stainless-steel autoclave at high pressure and temperatures but using water as solvent. This high energy wet chemistry technique, produces NPs with high crystalline quality and optimum magnetic performances, since lattice formation benefits from the high temperatures (from 355 to 525 K), high vapor pressures (from 0.3 to 4 MPa) and long times (up to 72 h) to which the experimental conditions are subjected. Specifically, a combination of high temperatures, between 355 to 525 K, and prolonged reaction time (24 h), has been studied and successfully applied [42] to produce Fe$_3$O$_4$@OA (see Figure 8) and Fe$_3$O$_4$@PAA coated NPs, with sizes around 20 nm and high yield (nearly 86%), by mixing FeCl$_2$·4H$_2$O and FeCl$_3$·6H$_2$O in a Teflon vessel with either an OA or a PAA solution, respectively. The so obtained NPs show a high degree of crystallinity (see Figure 8) and a saturation magnetization (M_S = 84 emu/g, close to the range of bulk magnetite (M_S~92 emu/g).

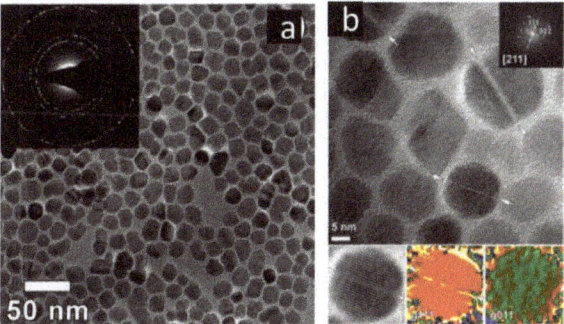

Figure 8. Fe$_3$O$_4$@OA coated NPs developed by hydrothermal method. (a) Low-resolution bright-field TEM images and corresponding ED ring patterns and (b) representative HRTEM image together with Fourier Transform FT pattern (inset). White arrows mark the dimer boundaries. Bottom insets: a filtered HRTEM image of a selected dimer NPs (**left**) and the corresponding GPA images for g1$\bar{1}$1 (**middle**) and g01$\bar{1}$ (**right**) diffraction spots. (Figures reprinted with permission from [42], ACS, 2014.

In another approach, magnetite NPs with rounded cubic shape and 39 nm were obtained by coprecipitation at 343 K of ferrous Fe^{2+} and ferric Fe^{3+} ions by $N(CH_3)_4OH$ solution, and a subsequent Teflon vessel thermal treatment at T = 523 K for 24 h [43]. The improved crystalline and magnetic quality after the annealing at high temperatures was clearly stated by the increase in M_S from 59.8 to 82.5 emu/g.

3.1.4. Solvothermal Procedures

Solvothermal procedures, using organic solvents at high pressure and temperature, open new possibilities to prepare magnetite NPs with complex configurations. Sphere like particles with an average size of 190 nm and containing multiple SPIONs cores closely packed inside a carbon coating shell were prepared using a mixture of ferrocene and acetone and kept at 513 K in a Teflon-lined stainless-steel autoclave for 72 h [44]. By means of chemical control, this solvothermal procedure is suitable to provide NPs with sizes between 100 and 250 nm [45] and morphologically controlled SPM multi-core Fe_3O_4@C spheres (see Figure 9).

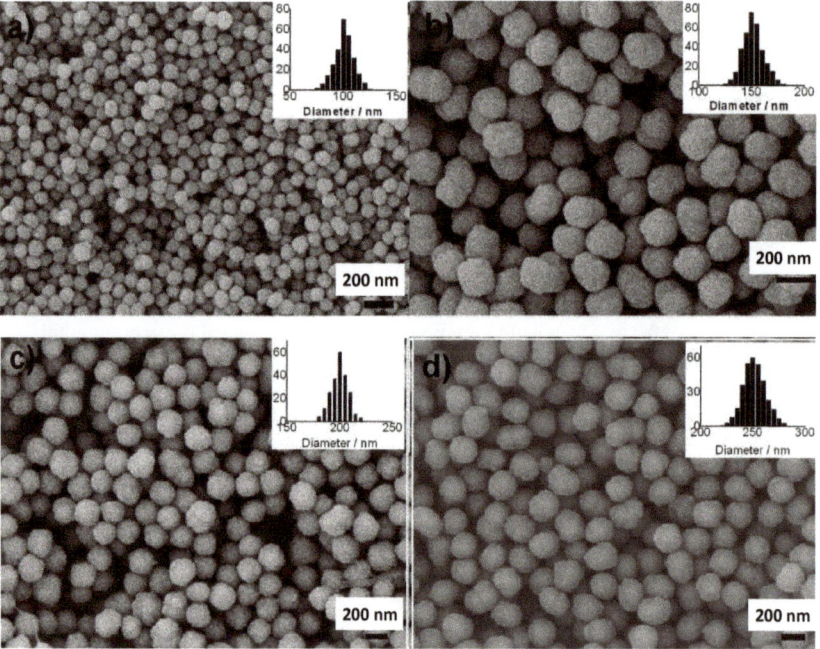

Figure 9. SEM micrographs of SPM multi-core Fe_3O_4@C spheres developed by a solvothermal technique with different amounts of hydrogen peroxide (**a**) 0.50, (**b**) 1.00, (**c**) 1.50, and (**d**) 2.00 mL, ensuring size control (**a**) 100, (**b**) 150, (**c**) 200, and (**d**) 250 nm. (Images reprinted with permission from [45], ACS, 2011).

3.1.5. Biogenic Inspired Procedures

Monodisperse magnetite NPs, with precise shape and size and crystalline quality, appear in magnetotatic bacteria, honeybees, pigeons, reptiles or amphibians. In humans, magnetite NPs can be found and are the signature of diseases in which an altered homeostasis of iron biomineralizes NPs at higher rates (neurological disorders, cancer, etc.). The mechanism of magnetite formation in living organisms (prokaryotes, archaea or eukaryotes) follows three steps: (1) formation of a specific organic reactor matrix (e.g., vesicles, protein cages, etc.) with favorable chemical environment; (2) formation of an intermediate iron compound and (3) conversion of this iron precursor into the magnetite NPs [46].

Compared to synthetic routes that occur at high energy operative conditions, natural magnetite biomineralization strategies occur at soft physiological conditions and are inspiring a new paradigm on green chemistry procedures. One of such strategies is based on the use of hollow Fn cages, an ubiquitous protein present in almost all living organisms that contains toxic Fe^{2+} and transforms it by oxidation into ferryhydrate (FeOOH)—an innocuous iron oxide mineral. In neurological diseases with a biologically altered iron homeostasis, the Fn protein shell transforms its ferryhydrate payload into magnetite NPs by a chemically complex procedure [47].

In a pioneering work [48], empty ferritin (apo-ferritin) was successfully used to synthesize magnetite NPs under high temperature and controlled pH conditions, opening a new bio-mimetic methodology based on the use of hollow biological cavities as templates to perform constrained reactions. Within this approach, cage like structures with sizes in the range from 18 to 500 nm, including virus capsids or ferritins obtained from different animal sources, have been used taking profit from their special characteristics (Fn from Pyrococcus furiosus remains stable above water boiling point) in synthetic procedures, at high reaction temperatures, to produce size controlled magnetite NPs [49,50].

3.2. Surface Functionalization: Core Protection, Colloidal Stability, Biocompatibility and Multifunctional Decoration

Physiological human media (blood, saliva, etc.) are a crowded biochemical environment with a complex machinery in which foreign materials (viruses, bacteria, etc.) are readily recognized and passivated by the immune system (IS) [51]. Therefore, nanoparticles exposed to in vitro or in vivo conditions require a highly engineered surface to protect the magnetite core from possible oxidation into hematite and ensure their magnetic quality, providing colloidal stability by preventing opsonization (unspecific attachment of a protein corona composed of albumin, immunoglobulin, apolipoproteins) [52] and providing abilities for theragnostic functions.

Different capping strategies include the use of small organic molecules, surfactants or active moieties like fluorescent molecules (rhodamine, fluorescein, etc.); natural polysaccharides, such as dextran, artificial block copolymers (poloxamers, poloxamines) or large polymers, like PEG that avoids opsonization [53]; inorganic materials, like amorphous or mesoporous silica and carbon, adding textural properties or thermal insulation; metal NPs (with plasmonic activity) and biological moieties for tagging, penetration or therapeutic abilities (monoclonal antibodies, aptamers, carbohydrates [53] and drugs).

3.2.1. Small Organic Molecules

Small organic molecules, or surfactants, can be anchored easily to magnetite NPs surface, since their hydroxyl groups, Fe-OH, greatly facilitate the anchoring of different compounds: alkoxylanes, carboxylic acids, phosphonic acids, dopamine, etc.

The most popular in situ coating consists in directly adding small biocompatible compounds (amino acid, citric acid, vitamin, cyclodextrin) during core synthesis.

However, additional enhancement of colloidal stability in basic or acidic media, where the organic molecules can decompose, can be achieved by grafting the Fe-OH group surface with silane groups, $Si-OCH_3$, which show good water stability and no cytotoxicity [54,55]. Different silane compounds are available, like 3-aminopropyltriethyloxysilane (APTES) and mercaptopropyltriethoxysilane (MPTES), providing chemical versatility [54] since they incorporate amino and sulfhydryl functional groups which facilitate bioconjugation procedures or drug grafting [55,56].

Phosphonic acid forms strong Fe-O-P bonds, which densely graft the magnetite NPs surface and allow a further combination with polydopamine groups, providing an improved pH and temperature stability [56]. Shahoo et al. have reported an efficient coating of 6–8 nm magnetite NPs, by oleic acid, lauric acid, phosphonic acids (dodecyl-; hexadecyl-) and dihexadecyl-phosphate, concluding that the bonding strengths of alkyl phosphonates and phosphates are stronger than that of carboxylate and proposed them as alternative biocompatible coatings in organic solutions [57].

Oleic acid ($CH_3(CH_2)_7CH = CH(CH_2)_7CO_2H$) provides large colloidal stability to magnetite NPs, but its lipophilic character is a main drawback in biomedical applications (see Figure 10). Its large steric stability, compared to similar compounds like stearic acid ($CH_3(CH_2)_{16}CO_2H$), arises from its cis-double-bond, which forms a kink in the middle of the carbon chain structure [58].

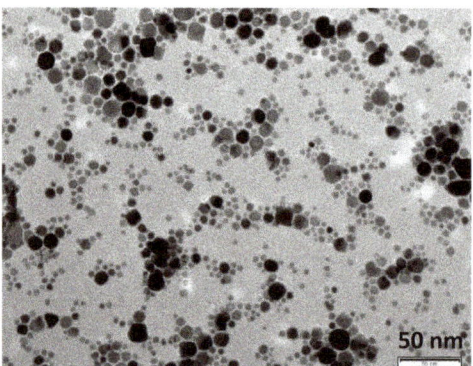

Figure 10. TEM images of magnetite NPs coated with oleic acid.

Moreover, reported by Guardia et al. [59], Fe_3O_4 NPs with sizes from 6 to 17 nm present large saturation magnetization values (M_S from 79 to 84 emu/g at T = 5 K), close to the bulk value (M_S = 92 emu/g), which in contrast to similar bare Fe_3O_4 NPs of 4 nm have only M_S = 50 emu/g. These results point to the role of oleic acid in reducing the spin surface disorder of small magnetite NPs, which is of large interest for the magnetic performance improvement in ultra-small SPIONs.

To enable lipophilic magnetite NPs [33] for biomedical applications which are mainly water based, a phase transfer, like the addition of amphiphilic molecules to the oil-soluble phase is the primary strategy to create a double layer with the hydrophilic segments exposed towards the solvent [60].

Additionally, surfactant exchange can be afforded by replacing the initial one by a new bifunctional surfactant, which has one group capable of binding to the NPs surface with a strong chemical bond and another terminal group that has a polar character and remains exposed to water [60].

Other interesting ability of organic coatings is the protection against degradation in acidic or basic media. Specifically, it has been reported [61] that magnetite coated with bipyridinium, F_3O_4@bipy NPs (13 nm) shows increased water solubility of the ferrofluid up to 300 mg/mL and stability of magnetite in a wide range of pH conditions, from very acidic to very basic ($1 \leq pH \leq 11$), extremely useful for acidic in vivo conditions like in tumor locations, where therapeutic procedures require an extended period of stability of Fe_3O_4 NPs.

3.2.2. Large Polymers

The incorporation of large polymers has been reported to add different advantages like size and shape control in one-pot procedures, enhanced colloidal stability, ability to prevent protein corona formation, biocompatibility and large availability of sites for the bioconjugation of biological moieties (aptamers, antibodies).

Their most remarkable fact is that they offer many repulsive groups balancing the attractive magnetic and Van der Waals interactions that agglomerate magnetite NPs and numerous sites for grafting antibodies, aptamers, etc. Synthetic functional polymers, such as linear or brush structures like, PEG, PVA, polylactic acid (PLA), polyvinilpirrolidone (PVP) or PAA, (see Figure 11) are commonly incorporated by two alternative approaches: grafting from and grafting onto the NPs.

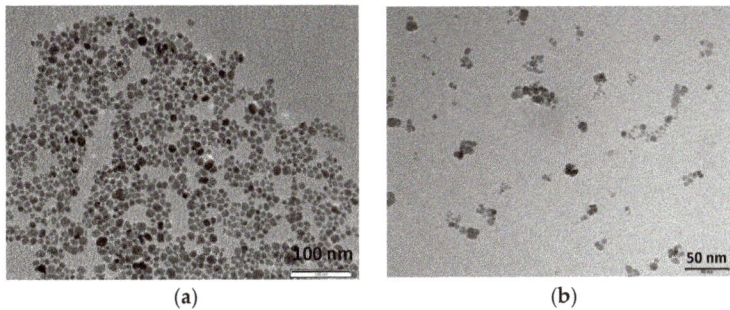

Figure 11. TEM images of magnetite NPs coated with (**a**) aminolauric acid and (**b**) polyacrylic acid (PAA).

Grafting polymers on the NPs' surface, by in situ procedures is the most used strategy, since it allows a strict control of the polymer's architecture and functionality, and although the density of grating is poor, the procedure is easier than a radical polymerization departing from monomer growth, which ensures a dense but uncontrolled coating.

In situ PAA grafting onto Fe_3O_4 NPs by a one-pot method has shown to produce materials with high colloidal stability and versatile surface for grafting biological molecules [62]. Other conventionally prepared one-pot polymer coated NPs include Fe_3O_4@PVP coated nanocrystals [63], with high colloidal stability in 10 different types of organic solvents and aqueous solutions, with pH ranging between 2.0 and 11.0. Generally, polyelectrolyte polymers provide enhanced colloidal stability when grafted onto magnetite NPs, owing to their electrostatic repulsive forces [64].

Other than stability, the incorporation of large polymers can be used to gain size and morphology control. In a one-pot procedure, by adding PVA to an aqueous solution of Fe^{2+}/Fe^{3+} salts with urea at 358 K, nanosized polyhedral particles with an approximated size around 300 nm and modified microspheres, between 100 to 280 nm, could be obtained controlling the polymer concentration [65]. A much more drastic effect on shape control has been shown when two PAA samples with average polymerization degrees of 208 and 126, PAA208 and PAA126, respectively, were used as an additive reactant to produce nanorods and flowerlike magnetite particles, respectively [65].

Besides enhancing colloidal stability, the specific interaction of the coating polymer with the physiological medium is of crucial importance in ensuring biocompatibility, facilitating bioconjugation or avoiding a fast entrapment by the IS. Therefore, taking inspiration from erythrocytes (red blood cells) whose chemical strategy to avoid protein corona formation comprises a protective shell barrier of hydrophilic oligosaccharide groups [66], a neutral electric surface composed of different hydrophilic coating shells (large brushes, densely packed [67]) have been synthetically incorporated and studied [68]. In this context, hydrophilic polymer brushes like linear dextrans and their derivatives, PEG; natural molecules, like polysialic acid, heparin, polysaccharides and artificial block-copolymers, like poloxamers or poloxamines, have shown to act as protein corona evaders [69].

From all these possibilities, PEG coating strategies, known as PEGylation, are the most used for biomedical applications, and their effectiveness in evading the IS depends on their molecular weight and density. PEGylated NPs with different molecules from 2000 and 20,000 g/mol and densities between 0.5 and 50 wt % have been shown to reduce opsonization from 1600 counts per million (cpm), to an almost constant value of 400 cpm, for PEG coating with MW larger than 5000 (g/mol), showing that PEGylation can hinder but not completely stop protein adsorption [67]. Coating density is a key factor in controlling the inter-distance between PEG terminal brushes that below a certain threshold hinder the adsorption of proteins. Above 5% of PEG coating, an inter-distance threshold about 1.0 nm between terminal PEG brushes can be estimated, and small protein adsorption remains constant below 400 cpm [67].

Functional polymers with responsive performance under pH, temperature or light irradiation stimuli are essential to provide controlled drug release [70]. Specifically, thermoresponsive polymer hydrogels like Pluronic, poly-isopropylacrilamide (PNIPAM) and their derivatives (e.g., PNIPAM with chitosan [71]) can be used to expel loaded molecules exploiting their coil-to-globule transition at defined temperatures. These hydrogels, in combination with SPIONs can be heated up by the application of an alternating magnetic field (magnetic hyperthermia) to undergo a controlled network shrinking useful for enhanced drug delivery applications [72].

3.2.3. Inorganic Materials

Inorganic materials are used also to confer core protection; colloidal stability and other functional properties like surface plasmon resonance (metal NPs), thermal isolation (carbon shell), etc. Silica (SiO_2) is one of the most commonly used inorganic coating materials, due to its versatile chemical silanol surface groups (-SiOH), colloidal stability and biocompatibility. The preparation of magnetite NPs coated with silica by sol-gel procedures allows to control the shell thickness [73] and is affordable by the basic hydrolysis of silanes in aqueous solutions of different organosilane compounds (tetraethyl orthosilicate (TEOS), APTES). The reaction between the oxide surface of magnetite and the silica takes places by the OH^- groups [74], and by an adjustment of the amount of added TEOS and the reaction time, the silica shell thickness can be easily tailored. Moreover, different configurations of the silica coated magnetite nanostructures can be achieved following two different routes: Stöber processes generally result into a multi-core coated NPs, while microemulsion processes provide mainly single core-shell NPs [74] (see Figure 12).

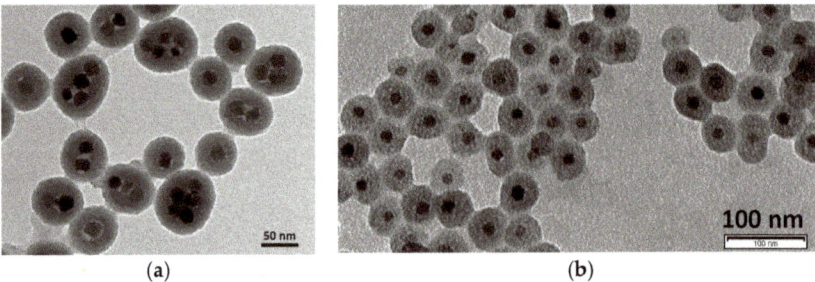

Figure 12. TEM micrographs of silica coated magnetite NPs by (**a**) Stöber processes, which generally result in multi-core coated NPs and (**b**) microemulsion processes, which provide mainly single core-shell NPs.

4. Biomedical Applications Arising from the Tunable Magnetic Properties of Magnetite Nanoparticles

The SPM character, inherent from the magnetite cores, allows to combine several abilities within a single nanostructure that can be triggered externally, under demand, by the application of a remote magnetic field to produce different magnetic responses of biomedical interest (summarized Table 2) like magnetophoresis, hyperthermia, magnetization or magnetic resonance.

Table 2. Summary of biomedical applications based on the combination of SPIONS and magnetic stimulation.

Magnetic Property	Application	Pros/Cons.	Commercial Kit	Toxicity
Magnetophoresis	Cell isolation	- Selective separation of tagged cells without damaging - Unaltered sample fluid after separation - Requires the use of antibodies for selective binding	MACS® Separators, Miltenyi	No in vitro toxicity
	Magnetofection	- Fast/efficient transfection of magnetized agents - Hallbach arrays with permanent magnets are cheap and easy to implement	NONE	No in vitro toxicity
	Magnetic guiding	- Magnetized stents can attract injected magnetic NPs to reduce restenosis - In preclinical stage	NONE	no in vivo toxicity tested in rat
Magnetic detection	Magnetometry SQUID	- Most sensitive magnetometry for iron detection - Expensive devices	NONE	No in vitro toxicity
	GMR sensors	- Detecting surface requires the binding of antibodies - Versatile for microarray detection	NONE	No in vitro toxicity
	Impedance Sensors	- Immunodetection requires the binding of antibodies - Implemented in paper strips kit - Attains detection limits in the clinical range	NONE	No in vitro toxicity
Inductive heating	Hyperthermia cancer treatment	- Selective killing of cancer cells - In clinical use for glioblastoma tumors - Increase of life expectancy 6–13 months	MAGFORCE NanoTherm, (clinical therapy)	NONE
	Thermally Enhanced release of therapeutic agents	- Controlled release by magnetic hyperthermia stimulation - Selective targeting - Under demand dosage - Under study stage	NONE	No in vitro toxicity
	Thermal stimulation	- Allows deep brain stimulation avoiding the implantation of electrodes in brain - In preclinical stage	NONE	no in vivo toxicity tested in mouse
Magneticrelaxation	MRI contrast agents: single (T2)	- MRI contrast enhancement for soft tissues - In clinical use	Ferucarbotran (Resovist®, Bayer Healthcare) (MRI clinical diagnosis)	NONE
	MRI contrast agents: dual(T1/T2)	- Enhanced contrast for soft and hard tissues. - Avoiding the use of Gd for T1 contrast - In preclinical stage	NONE	no in vivo toxicity tested in mouse
Magnetic prototyping	3D magnetic bioprinting	- Bioprinting of tissue or replacements with biologically functional - No need of artificial substrate - Bioprinted functional saliva secretory organoids - Tested ex vivo - Under study stage	NONE	No in vitro and ex vivo toxicity

4.1. Magnetophoresis

Magnetophoresis refers to the controlled motion of SPIONs in a viscous medium induced by the application of an external magnetic field. This useful characteristic can be used to isolate, concentrate and drive magnetically labelled biomarkers or cells, from physiological samples (cerebrospinal fluid (CSF), blood, saliva, cell aspirates, etc.) and for in vivo targeting with the application of an external magnetic gradient. The use of magnetic separation techniques saves energy when exposing analytes to a permanent magnet and includes a high degree of specificity, if magnetic particles are conveniently coated with antibodies that specifically target the desired biomarker. Moreover, extraction of the target can be done, without damaging the rest of the fluid for further analysis.

4.1.1. Cell Isolation

Purification and preconcentration of biomarkers or cells from patient's fluid samples or aspirates are crucial for a successful culture of isolated cells for transplantation or for an accurate high signal-to-noise ratio detection step (magnetic, optical or chemical) without the unspecific interference of other biochemical compounds in the sample [75]. Simple magnetic separation has been described by using cationic liposomes loaded with SPIONs (MCL), which were mixed with bone marrow aspirates under shaking for 1 h and transferred into tissue culture dishes, with a disk-shaped magnet at the bottom. Magnetically labeled cells were subject to the attraction of the magnetic field and 30% of them were isolated. Increased separation effectivity, up to an 85% was afterwards achieved using magneto-liposomes, conjugated with CD105 antibodies [76].

4.1.2. Magnetofection

Magnetofection, consists in the transfection of magnetic therapeutic vectors (plasmids, engineered viruses, etc.) inside cells, forced by a magnetic field, and is becoming a widely used technique in gene therapy which benefits from its higher degree of penetration compared to non-magnetic approaches.

Polyethylenimine-modified SPIONS/pDNA complexes (PEI-SPIONs/pDNA complexes) have been used to rapidly and uniformly distribute on the surface of MG-63 osteoblasts cells, by their incubation under the exposure to a uniform magnetic field enabled by specially designed Hallbach array of permanent magnets. With this homogeneous magnetic exposure, local transfection, without the disruption of the cells' membrane, was obtained, improving the magnetofection efficiency of pDNA into osteoblasts, thereby providing a novel approach for the targeted delivery of therapeutic genes to osteosarcoma tissues as well as a reference for the treatment of other tumors [77].

4.1.3. Magnetic Guiding

Magnetic guiding of MNPs exposed to the application of a magnetic gradient can be used to deliver therapeutic payloads in a precise location with a high degree of specificity. An innovative approach has been studied to reduce the re-stenosis of vasculature after stenting in in vivo experiments by combining stainless steel stents and the use of paclitaxel loaded SPIONs. The stents were magnetized upon the external application of a magnetic field, creating a magnetic field gradient capable to attract the MNPs delivered to the rat via a catheter. Paclitaxel release to the surrounding tissues was effective, reducing therefore restenosis of the vasculature tissue although the dose of paclitaxel-SPIONs was low [78].

4.2. Magnetic Detection

Magnetic detection exploits different aspects of the magnetic properties of both SPIONs and the components of the detecting sensors.

4.2.1. Superconducting Quantum Interference Device

(SQUID) is the most sensitive magnetometer for DC or low frequency measurements. Constituted by superconducting loops containing Josephson junctions, when a current is induced in the SQUID ring by an external magnetic flux, a change in voltage happens across the junction, which generates an output signal from the amplified voltage [79]. Although SQUID has been used to detect ferromagnetic contamination in the lungs or magnetite NPs brain in AD patients in ex vivo conditions [80], it has been applied to susceptibility measurements for in vivo identification of SPIONs loaded on a tumor in the lymph nodes of rats [81]. Moreover, the effectivity of iron quantification by SQUID magnetic relaxometry was successfully used to evaluate SPIONs conjugated to Her2-expressingMCF/Her2-18 cells (breast cancer cells) injected into xenograft MCF7/Her2-18 tumors in nude mice [82]. Brown relaxation of magnetic NPs in liquids has also been exploited to detect biomarkers in liquid-phase immunoassays using SQUID magnetometry of magnetite beads conjugated with biotin, with sizes from 54 to 322 nm, attaining a sensitivity of 5.6×10^{-8} mol/mL [83].

4.2.2. Giant Magnetoresistance (GMR)

Giant Magnetoresistance (GMR) sensors are based on the significant change in electrical resistance of an arrangement of thin-film layers of alternating ferromagnetic and nonmagnetic conducting spacers when they are exposed to an externally applied magnetic field [84]. The variation in magnetoresistance of these spin-dependent sensors decorated with specific antibodies, provides quantitative analysis in combination with MNPs. The main strategy behind several magnetoresistive detectors, consists in attaching MNPs to the analytes, which during the detection procedure remain attached to the sensing surface creating a magnetic disturbance that triggers the change in electrical resistance of the device [85]. GMR detectors have been improved in the last years, being able to respond even upon small variations of magnetic fields, incrementing their sensitivity to detect small concentrations of analytes [84].

Although accurate GMR detection is facilitated by using SPM magnetite beads [86] with a large magnetic moment, a successful strategy using small SPIONs (30 nm) labeled with streptavidin was developed to detect Interleukin-6 (IL-6) antibody and amine modified DNA (deoxyribonucleic acid) oligonucleotide, by functionalizing the surface of the sensor with APTES and Glutathione [87]. This APTES-Glu modification was successfully extended to microarray detection, showing to be a versatile and robust method [87].

4.2.3. Impedance Based Sensor

Emergent strategies are trying to couple lateral flow immunoassay (LFIA) (paper-strips), which stand out for their low-cost, speed, portability and ease of use, with an innovative magnetic detection based on Cu-impedance change in the presence of MNPs [88].

The sensing property relies on the high rate of oscillation of the magnetic moments of the SPIONs that induces localized eddy currents on the surface of the sensor, increasing its electrical radio-frequency impedance, for which no external magnetic field is required. This facile magnetic detection strategy is based on the use of paper-strip immunodetection kits in combination with SPIONS functionalized to specifically bind to prostate-specific antigen PSA. The strips were seeded with capture anti-PSA antibody and anti-IgG (both at a concentration of 1 mg/mL) forming the test and control lines, respectively. PSA standard solutions at known concentrations were submitted to the strip and attached to test line. The subsequent binding of conjugated SPIONs to PSA ensured the magnetic reading and the final determination of analyte concentrations. This facile method allowed to attain a limit of detection within the clinical range of interest around 0.25 ng/mL and a resolution of 50 pg [89].

Further improvements are reported, by using large SPM multi-core carbon coated nanoflowers (Fe_3O_4@C) as LFIA labels that provide a magnetic moment substantially larger than that of single-core SPIONs, allowing for a more sensitive and precise detection [90].

4.3. Inductive Heating

Inductive heating, also known as magnetic hyperthermia, consists in the transformation of electromagnetic energy into heat, when an alternating external magnetic field (f = 3 kHz, 300 MHz) is applied to a magnetic nanoparticle. The temperature rise that is transmitted to the medium, in which the NPs are housed, depends on the magnetic quality of the NPs, the viscosity of the medium and the parameters of the external magnetic field, among others [91]. This externally controlled rise of temperature can be used for killing cancer cells when rising to 315 K, stimulating cell growth for mild thermal increase or triggering release mechanisms for enhanced delivery.

4.3.1. Cancer Hyperthermia Treatment

Through magnetic hyperthermia, cancer treatments can be developed by selectively heating between 314 and 316 K cancerous tissues which are previously loaded with MNPs. In biomedical applications, magnetic exciters are restricted to a safety upper limit of H·f < 4.58 ×10^8 A·m·s^{-1} [92].

This technique benefits from a natural mechanism called enhanced permeation and retention, due to the defects and poor drainage of cancerous tissues that cause the accumulation of NPs inside the damaged tissue [93]. This entrapment of NPs inside the tumor tissue allows the heating and weakening of cancer cells, minimizing side effects in the surrounding healthy cells. It is worth highlighting the development by MagForce [94] of a clinically used magnetic hyperthermia therapy, which combines a magnetic field applicator (100 kHz) and an injectable therapeutic agent consisting in Fe_3O_4@amylosan NPs to treat glioblastoma, an aggressive brain tumor.

Within this commercial solution, even large tumors around 5 cm can be treated by the direct injection with 3 mL of magnetite based ferrofluid, which heats up by the application of the external alternating magnetic fields. This technique has been used in phase II clinical trials in combination with stereotactic radiotherapy and obtained the European approval as a treatment for brain tumors in 2010, after demonstrating its ability to increase life expectancy from 6 to 13 months in patients with glioblastoma multiforme, compared to others treated only with chemotherapy.

4.3.2. Controlled Release

Another therapeutic strategy based on magnetic hyperthermia consists in the thermal stimulation of thermo-active moieties to provoke the release of therapeutic agents (drugs, growth factor, oligomers, etc.) under demand.

One of the most successful drug delivery applications, triggered by magnetic hyperthermia, combines SPIONs with a coating of thermosensitive polymers such as PNIPAM and its derivates. These polymers form hydrogels at room temperature and can allocate molecules acting as drug nanocarriers. When the temperature rises above a critical range (T = 306–313 K), these structures retract and expel all the drug contained within.

Steps are being taken so that this technique meets the essential conditions of an effective tool in precision medicine, temperature control and release time control. In fact, it has already been possible to produce the collapse of 49% of the volume of the therapeutic agent at a temperature of biomedical interest T = 311 K (see Figure 13) [95]. Optimizing the biopolymers mixture (PNIPAM/chitosan), it is even possible to release 70% of the drug housed in a single second [71].

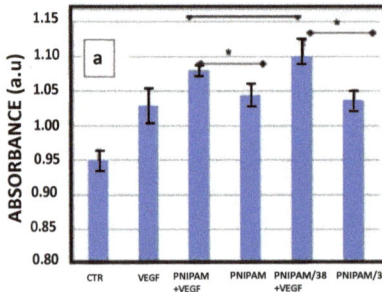 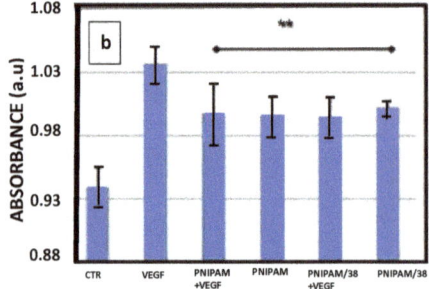

Figure 13. Absorbance measurements performed to address VEGF release for HUVEC cells incubated with PNIPAM (release temperature at 305 K) and PNIPAM/38 (release temperature at 311 K) loaded with VEGF and raised to different temperatures, (**a**) 311 K and (**b**) 293 K. The wells with standard cultural medium with and without VEGF (10 ng/mL) were used as controls. Experiments performed at 311 K show the ability of thermal release of VEGF loaded on PNIPAM based materials. (Images reprinted with permission from [95], Springer, 2014).

Besides drugs, there is a large interest in the controlled release of biological moieties with therapeutic effects for regenerative medicine. Several proteins (recombinant human bone morphogenic proteins, rhBMPs, induce osteogenesis) and growth factors (vascular endothelial growth factor (VEGF)) responsible for the triggering of angiogenesis (process of blood vessel formation) are crucial for ensuring the long-term viability of repaired tissues with functional recovery. Specifically, VEGF is effective only when concentration gradients at physiological levels are generated, and new strategies are needed for an adequate delivery at the site of tissue repair. In this context, the grafting complex-elastin-dendron-VEGF hyperbranched poly(epsilon-lysine) peptides integrating in their core parallel thermoresponsive elastin-like peptide sequences over the surface of Fe_3O_4@PAA NPs (see Figure 14) has been reported [96].

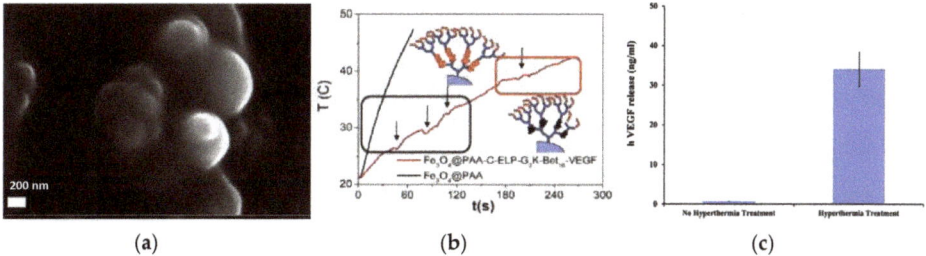

Figure 14. (a) SEM micrograph of Fe3O4@PAA-C-ELP-G3K-Bet16-VEGF, (b) hyperthermia Treatment of Fe_3O_4@PAA and Fe_3O_4@PAA-C-ELP-G3K-Bet16 samples immersed in phosphate buffered saline, pH 7.4, with a volume of 240 µL and a magnetite concentration of 40 µg/µL, and (c) release of hVEGF from Fe3O4@PAA-C-ELP-G3K-Bet16-VEGF after hyperthermia treatment. Negative control shows no hVEGF release after hyperthermia treatment. (Images taken form [96], Elsevier, 2015).

These functionalized SPIONs were able to avidly bind VEGF forming a stable complex. Under the adequate stimulation of the complex Fe_3O_4@PAA-C-ELP-G3K-Bet16-VEGF with a magnetic induction (H = 30 mT, f = 298 kHz), a mild-temperature rise up to 315 K, the range at which the elastin-like peptides collapse provoked the VEGF release in only two minutes after magnetic stimulation without suffering degradation (see Figure 14).

4.3.3. Thermal Stimulation

Additionally, it is worth mentioning a last application of magnetic hyperthermia that has been able to produce DBS (Deep brain stimulation) at the nanometric level in a mouse with induced thermal sensitivity in specific neurons selected by genetic technique. The mouse brain was injected with SPIONs (around 22 nm) and exposed to an external magnetic field which provoked a local increase in temperature. With this procedure, the selective activation of the modified neurons was observed, without any secondary effect in the neighboring neurons, which were preserved practically intact [97].

In another recent study [98], the effect of magnetoelectric particles has been modeled to stimulate the brain of an affected Parkinson's patient by simulating a neural network with electrical levels like those of a healthy person. The simulation estimates optimal values for the design made from 20 nm magnetite NPs, with a concentration of 3×10^6 under the action of an external magnetic field of 300 Oe operating at a frequency 80 Hz. Undoubtedly, these results open the door to the effective development of new innovative and non-invasive DBS methodologies.

4.4. Magnetic Resonance Imaging

Nuclear magnetic resonance (NMR) is a powerful magnetic phenomenon mainly used in clinics for imaging. In contrast to a surface-based sensor like GMR, NMR is capable of sampling an entire volume in a non-invasive way. MRI can be combined with other diagnostic tools, like CT (X-ray computed tomography), PET (positron emission tomography) or US (ultrasound), to obtain more accurate diagnosis, for which multimodal SPIONs can be afforded either combining several agents into a single carrier or by engineering a material which can be active in several modalities [99].

It is a known fact that the magnetic core creates a local magnetic inhomogeneity, which alters the relaxation time of hydrogen protons in the surrounding water molecules. This fact has motivated different studies based on the use of magnetic NPs as dual MRI contrast agents for T1 and T2 relaxation, in order to avoid the conventionally used gadolinium chelates and their potential toxicity.

The strategies developed so far to optimize the magnetic response of magnetite based NPs as MRI contrast agents have been focused in tailoring their architecture: large particles containing several SPM single cores (magnetic beads), hollow magnetite spheres and single core NPs of pure magnetite or doped with transition metals [100].

SPM beads, composed of dozens of SPIONs within a carbon shell [25] and with an approximate diameter around 100 nm (see Figure 15), have been shown to present a large relaxivity (r_2 = 218 mM^{-1} s^{-1}) combined with a negligible thermal rise when tested in magnetic hyperthermia tests (H = 30 mT, f = 293 kHz).

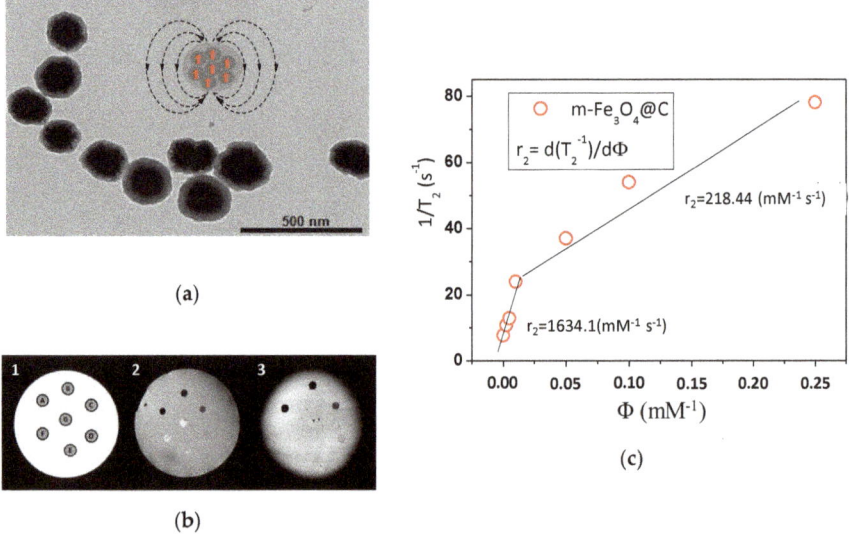

Figure 15. (a) TEM image of multi-Fe$_3$O$_4$@C NPs, (b) scheme of the phantom NPs concentration distribution (b.1): A = 0.25 mg/mL; B = 0.1 mg/mL; C = 0.05 mg/mL; D = 0.025 mg/mL; E = 0.005 mg/mL; F = 0.0025 mg/mL and G = 0 mg/mL; MR T2-weighted image of the agar phantom (b.2); MR T2*-weighted image of the agar phantom (b.2), performed at 9.4 T (BrukerBiospec) on a set of agar phantoms loaded with different concentrations of NPs (0.0025 to 0.25 mM) and (c) relaxivity calculated from T2 MRI relaxation on agar phantoms reprinted with permission from [25], IEEE, 2016.

This combination of enhanced MRI contrast and poor thermomagnetic response offers a potential advantage for using these materials in therapeutic situations, like brain applications, where any temperature increase is highly inadvisable for patients [101]. In this case, despite the high content of magnetic material content in the NPs, the carbon coating shell plays the fundamental role of thermal insulation, which decouples the magnetic activity of the NPs from its thermal response.

Further enhancement of MRI contrast has been achieved by exploring the effect of shape on T2 relaxation mechanisms, using single core magnetite NPs. In this context, water-dispersible polyethylene glycol-phospholipid (PEGphospholipid) coated cubic SIONPs (see Figure 16) showed extremely high r_2 relaxivity (up to 761 mM^{-1} s^{-1}) [102], yielding superior in vivo MRI details. Ascribing this exceptionally high relaxivity to the magnetic shape anisotropy, magnetite NPs with different shapes were studied, from octopod (D = 30 nm, r_2 = 679.3 ± 30 mM^{-1} s^{-1}) [103] to rod-like length of 30–70 nm and diameter of 4–12 nm, seeming to confirm this hypothesis.

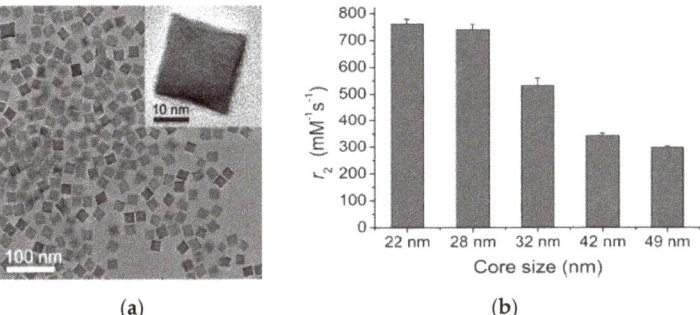

Figure 16. (a) TEM image of coated cubic SPIONs and (b) size dependent r2 relaxivity, reprinted with permission from [102] (ACS, 2012).

Gadolinium, a paramagnetic ion with the largest number of unpaired electrons, is the most effective T1 contrast agent, which has however the main drawback of being toxic. Although it is always used in combination with chelating molecules with the aim of avoiding its potential risk, alternative strategies are seeking to exploit new aspects of SPIONs to produce versatile dual contrast agents, taking advantage of the existing SPION (Ferucarbotran (Resovist®), Bayer Healthcare) clinically approved as MRI contrast agent. Ultra-small magnetite NPs with a diameter around 3.5 nm have been studied as candidates for dual-modal MRI contrast with simultaneous T1/T2 switching, activity [104]. In this study, the observed switching between T1–T2 contrast (see Figure 17) is ascribed to the fact that ultra-small SPIONs are single-dispersed in blood and produce T1 contrast, while after their extravasation and accumulation in the tumoral site, the NPs' self-assembling into larger clusters induces the appearances of T2 contrast modulated by magnetic interactions.

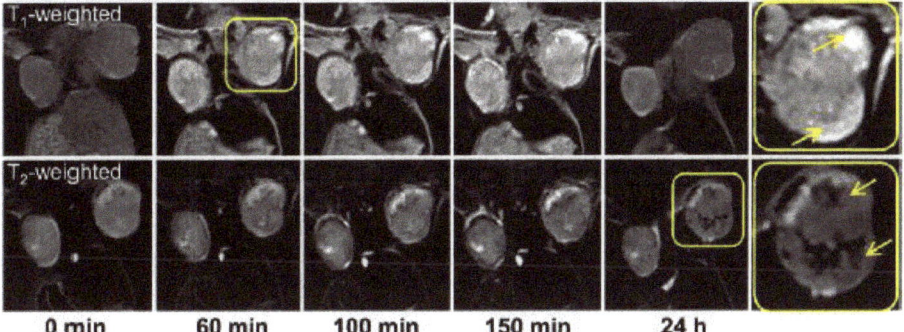

Figure 17. T1- and T2-weighted MRI of a mouse bearing orthotopic 4T1 tumors before and after i.v. administration of ultra-small SPIONs at different time points. Bright contrast with increasing signal in T1-weighted MR images was observed in the tumor, particularly peripheral regions (inset), at early time points (i.e., 5–150 min) resulting from the single-dispersed ultra-small SPIONs, whereas signals in several regions of the tumor turning dark (arrow indicated) were observed in T2-weighted images 24 h after ultra-small SPIONs injection because of ultra-small SPIONs clustering in the tumor interstitials. (Image reprinted with permission from [104], ACS, 2017).

4.5. Magnetic Prototyping of Functional Biological Structures

One of the milestones in regenerative medicine is the fabrication of tissue, replacements or organs with biologically relevant functionality. This emerging field combines multiple strategies arising from different approaches like cell-based therapies, tissue-engineered biomaterials, scaffolds or implantable devices. The exposure of magnetized cells under a three-dimensional (3D) magnetic pattern, known as 3D magnetic bioprinting, allows the prototyping of organelles or autologous implantable biodevices without the need of a material substrate.

Recently a 3D bio-fabrication system, by magnetic 3D bioprinting (M3DB), has been tested to generate innervated saliva secretory (SG) organoids using magnetized neural crest derived mesenchymal stem cells (human dental pulp stem cells (hDPSC). The magnetized cells were spatially arranged with magnet dots to generate 3D spheroids and afterwards cultured with fibroblast growth factor 10 to promote epithelial morphogenesis and neurogenesis. The preformed SG organoids were then transplanted into ex vivo model showing epithelial growth, innervation and production of salivary a-amylase upon FGF10 stimulation [105].

5. Conclusions

Magnetite NPs with superparamagnetic behavior, commonly known as SPIONS, can be easily tailored in nanostructured materials combining functional organic or inorganic matrices (mesoporous or amorphous silica, biocompatible polymers like chitosan, k-carragenan, PNIPAM, PEG, PAA) to incorporate therapeutic or tagging moieties like drugs, aptamers or antibodies.

The list of nanostructured materials containing magnetite NPs is immense, and the applications in nanomedicine cover almost any aspect from diagnosis, therapy or regenerative medicine, since in all cases the nanostructure inherits the intrinsic properties of magnetite that ensure multiple abilities like magnetic separation/detection/targeting, magnetofection, magnetic resonance contrast imaging, magnetic hyperthermia therapy and stimulated delivery, magnetic cell growth stimulation and 3D magnetic prototyping of organelles.

Author Contributions: Conceptualization: Y.P., S.Y.V.; writing: Y.P., M.G.G., L.d.C.A., A.A.P., P.G.A., R.S.G., J.P., C.T., S.Y.V., and J.R.; supervision and group direction: J.R. All authors have read and agreed to the published version of the manuscript.

Funding: This work was supported by the European Commission under (PANA project, Call H2020-NMP-2015-two-stage, Grant 686009; and MADIA project, Call H2020-ICT-2016-1, Grant 732678) and by the Consellería de Educación Program for Reference Research Groups project (GPC2017/015 and the Development of Strategic Grouping in Materials—AEMAT at the University of Santiago de Compostela under Grant No. ED431E2018/08, of the Xunta de Galicia.

Conflicts of Interest: The authors declare no conflict of interest.

References

1. Jacobs, I.S. Role of Magnetism in Technology. *J. Appl. Phys.* **1969**, *40*, 917. [CrossRef]
2. Jacobs, S.; Bean, C.P. Fine Particles, Thin Films and Exchange Anisotropy. In *Magnetism*; Rado, G.T., Suhl, H., Eds.; Academic: New York, NY, USA, 1963; Volume 3, pp. 271–350.
3. Guéron, S.; Deshmukh, M.M.; Myers, E.B.; Ralph, D.C. Tunneling via Individual Electronic States in Ferromagnetic Nanoparticles. *Phys. Rev. Lett.* **1999**, *83*, 4148–4151. [CrossRef]
4. Liou, S.H.; Huang, S.; Klimek, E.; Kirby, R.D.; Yao, Y.D. Enhancement of coercivity in nanometer-size CoPt crystallites. *J. Appl. Phys.* **1999**, *85*, 4334–4336. [CrossRef]
5. Sridhar, S.; Amiji, M.; Shenoy, D.; Nagesha, D.; Weissig, V.; Fu, W. Nanomedicine: A new paradigm in diagnosis and therapy. *Optics East 2005* **2005**, *6008*, 600816. [CrossRef]
6. Piñeiro, Y.; Vargas, Z.; Rivas, J.; López-Quintela, M.A. Iron Oxide based Nanoparticles for Magnetic Hyperthermia Strategies in Biomedical Applications. *Eur. J. Inorg. Chem.* **2015**, *27*, 4495–4509. [CrossRef]
7. Dobson, J. Nanoscale biogenic iron oxides and neurodegenerative disease. *FEBS Lett.* **2001**, *496*, 1–5. [CrossRef]

8. Ramos-Cabrer, P.; Campos, F. Liposomes and nanotechnology in drug development: Focus on neurological targets. *Int. J. Nanomed.* **2013**, *8*, 951–960. [CrossRef]
9. Anselmo, A.C.; Mitragotri, S. Nanoparticles in the clinic. *Bioeng. Transl. Med.* **2016**, *1*, 10–29. [CrossRef]
10. Xiang, Y.; Wang, J. Current status of superparamagnetic iron oxide contrast agents for liver magnetic resonance imaging. *World J. Gastroenterol.* **2015**, *21*, 13400–13402.
11. NanoTherm. Available online: https://www.magforce.com/en/home/our_therapy/ (accessed on 28 July 2019).
12. Vallabani, N.V.S.; Singh, S. Recent advances and future prospects of iron oxide nanoparticles in biomedicine and diagnostics. *Biotech* **2018**, *8*, 279. [CrossRef]
13. Ortolani, A.; Bianchi, M.; Mosca, M.; Caravelli, S.; Fuiano, M.; Marcacci, M.; Russo, A. The prospective opportunities offered by magnetic scaffolds for bone tissue engineering: A review. *Joints* **2016**, *4*, 228–235. [CrossRef] [PubMed]
14. Cornell, R.M.; Schwertmann, U. *The Iron Oxides: Structure, Properties, Reactions, Occurences and Uses*, 2nd ed.; Wiley-VCH: Wienheim, Germany, 2003.
15. Banerjee, S.K.; Moskowitz, B.M. *Magnetite Biomineralization and Magnetoreception in Organisms, a New Biomagnetism*; Kirschvink, J.L., Jones, D.S., MacFadden, B.J., Eds.; Chapter 2: Ferrimagnetic Properties of Magnetite; Springer: New York, NY, USA, 1985.
16. Parkinson, G.S. Iron Oxide Surfaces. *Surface Sci. Rep.* **2016**, *71*, 272–365. [CrossRef]
17. Verwey, E.J.W. Electronic Conduction of Magnetite (Fe_3O_4) and Its Transition Point at Low Temperatures. *Nature* **1939**, *144*, 327–328. [CrossRef]
18. Senn, M.S.; Wright, J.P.; Attfield, J.P. Charge Order and Three-Site Distortions in the Verwey Structure of Magnetite. *Nature* **2012**, *481*, 173–176. [CrossRef]
19. Goodenough, J.B. *Magnetism and the Chemical Bond*; Wiley-Interscience: New York, NY, USA, 1963.
20. Skomski, R.; Sellmeyer, D. *Cap.1, Handbook of Advanced Magnetic Materials*; Sellmeyer, D.J., Liu, Y., Shindo, D., Eds.; Tingshua University Press: New York, NY, USA, 2006.
21. Landau, L.D.; Lifshitz, E. On the theory of the dispersion of magnetic permeability in ferromagnetic bodies. *Phys. Z. Sowjetunion* **1935**, *8*, 153–169.
22. Blundell, S. *Magnetism in Condensed Matter*; Oxford University Press: New York, NY, USA, 2001.
23. Krishnan, K.M. Biomedical Nanomagnetics: A Spin Through Possibilities in Imaging, Diagnostics, and Therapy. *IEEE Trans. Magn.* **2010**, *46*, 2523.
24. Yoon, K.Y.; Xue, Z.; Fei, Y.; Lee, J.H.; Cheng, V.; Bagaria, H.G.; Huh, C.; Bryant, S.L.; Kong, S.D.; Ngo, V.W.; et al. Control of magnetite primary particlesize in aqueous dispersions of nanoclusters for high magnetic susceptibilities. *J. Colloid Interface Sci.* **2015**, *462*, 359–367. [CrossRef]
25. Vargas-Osorio, Z.; Argibay, B.; Piñeiro, Y.; Vázquez-Vázquez, C.; López-Quintela, M.A.; Álvarez-Pérez, M.A.; Sobrino, T.; Campos, F.; Castillo, J.; Rivas, J. Multicore Magnetic Fe3O4@C Beads with Enhanced Magnetic Response for MRI in Brain Biomedical Applications. *IEEE Trans. Magn.* **2016**, *52*, 230604. [CrossRef]
26. Cótica, L.F.; Santos, I.A.; Girotto, E.M.; Ferri, E.V.; Coelho, A.A. Surface spin disorder effects in magnetite and poly(thiophene)-coated magnetite nanoparticles. *J. Appl. Phys.* **2010**, *108*, 064325. [CrossRef]
27. Nedelkoski, Z.; Kepaptsoglou, D.; Lari, L.; Wen, T.; Booth, R.A.; Oberdick, S.D.; Galindo, L.; Ramasse, Q.M.; Evans, R.F.L.; Majetich, S.; et al. Origin of reduced magnetization and domain formation in small magnetite nanoparticles. *Sci. Rep.* **2017**, *7*, 45997. [CrossRef]
28. Fiorani, D. *Surface Effects in Magnetic Nanoparticles*; Fiorani, D., Ed.; Springer: New York, NY, USA, 2005.
29. Lacroix, L.-M.; Lachaize, S.; Falqui, A.; Blon, T.; Carrey, J.; Dumestre, F.; Amiens, C.; Margeat, O.; Chaudret, B.; Lecante, P.; et al. Ultrasmall iron nanoparticles: Effect of size reduction on anisotropy and magnetization. *J. Appl. Phys.* **2008**, *103*, 7. [CrossRef]
30. Park, J.; An, K.J.; Hwang, Y.S.; Park, J.G.; Noh, H.J.; Kim, J.Y.; Park, J.H.; Hwang, N.M.; Hyeon, T. Ultra-large-scale syntheses of monodisperse nanocrystals. *Nat. Mater.* **2004**, *3*, 891–895. [CrossRef] [PubMed]
31. Guardia, P.; Labarta, A.; Batlle, X. Tuning the Size, the Shape, and the Magnetic Properties of Iron Oxide Nanoparticles. *J. Phys. Chem. C* **2011**, *115*, 390–396. [CrossRef]
32. Verma, J.; Lal, S.; van Noorden, C.J.F. Nanoparticles for hyperthermic therapy synthesis strategies and applications in glioblastoma. *Int. J. Nanomed.* **2014**, *9*, 2863–2877.
33. Bañobre-López, M.; Piñeiro Redondo, Y.; López-Quintela, M.A.; Rivas, J. *Handbook of Nanomaterials Properties*; Bhushan, B., Luo, D., Schricker, S., Sigmund, W., Zauscher, S., Eds.; Chapter 15: Magnetic Nanoparticles for Biomedical Applications; Springer-Verlag: Berlin, Germany, 2014.

34. La Mer, V.K.; Dinegar, R.H. Theory, production and mechanism of formation of monodispersed hydrosols. *J. Am. Chem. Soc.* **1950**, *72*, 4847–4854. [CrossRef]
35. Sugimoto, T.; Matijevic, E.J. Formation of uniform spherical magnetite particles by crystallization from ferrous hydroxide gels. *Colloid Interface Sci.* **1980**, *74*, 227–243. [CrossRef]
36. Hyeon, T.; Lee, S.S.; Park, J.; Chung, Y.; Na, H.B. Synthesis of highly crystalline and monodisperse maghemite nanocrystallites without a size-selection process. *J. Am. Chem. Soc.* **2001**, *123*, 12798–12801. [CrossRef]
37. Peng, S.; Sun, S. Synthesis and Characterization of Monodisperse Hollow Fe_3O_4 Nanoparticles. *Angew. Chem.* **2007**, *119*, 4233–4236. [CrossRef]
38. Xiaohui, L.; Guangbin, J.; Yousong, L.; Huang, O.; Yang, Z.; Du, Y. Formation mechanism and magnetic properties of hollow Fe3O4 nanospheres synthesized without any surfactant. *Cryst. Eng. Comm.* **2012**, *14*, 8658–8663.
39. Unni, M.; Uhl, A.M.; Savliwala, S.; Savitzky, B.H.; Dhavalikar, R.; Garraud, N.; Arnold, D.P.; Kourkoutis, L.F.; Andrew, J.S.; Rinaldi, C. Thermal Decomposition Synthesis of Iron Oxide Nanoparticles with Diminished Magnetic Dead Layer by Controlled Addition of Oxygen. *ACS Nano* **2017**, *11*, 2284–2303. [CrossRef]
40. Tong, S.; Quinto, C.A.; Zhang, L.; Mohindra, P.; Bao, G. Size-Dependent Heating of Magnetic Iron Oxide Nanoparticles. *ACS Nano* **2017**, *11*, 6808–6816. [CrossRef] [PubMed]
41. Dokyoon, K.; Nohyun, L.; Mihyun, P.B.; Hyo, K.K.; An Taeghwan, H. Synthesis of Uniform Ferrimagnetic Magnetite Nanocubes. *J. Am. Chem. Soc.* **2009**, *131*, 454–455.
42. Kolen'ko, Y.; Bañobre-López, M.; Rodriguez-Abreu, C.; Carbo-Argibay, E.; Sailsman, A.; Piñeiro-Redondo, Y.; Cerqueira, M.F.; Petrovykh, D.; Kovnir, K.; Lebedev, O.; et al. Large-Scale Synthesis of Colloidal Fe_3O_4 Nanoparticles Exhibiting High Heating Efficiency in Magnetic Hyperthermia. *J. Phys. Chem. C* **2014**, *118*, 8691–8701. [CrossRef]
43. Daou, T.J.; Pourroy, G.; Begin-Colin, S.; Greneche, J.-M.; Ulhaq-Bouillet, C.; Légaré, P.; Bernhardt, P.; Leuvrey, C.; Rogez, G. Hydrothermal Synthesis of Monodisperse Magnetite Nanoparticles. *Chem. Mater.* **2006**, *18*, 4399–4404. [CrossRef]
44. Wang, H.; Sun, Y.B.; Chen, Q.W.; Yu, Y.F.; Cheng, K. Synthesis of carbon-encapsulated superparamagnetic colloidal nanoparticles with magnetic-responsive photonic crystal property. *Dalton Trans.* **2010**, *39*, 9565–9569. [CrossRef]
45. Wang, H.; Chen, Q.W.; Yu, Y.F.; Cheng, K.; Sun, Y.B. Size- and solvent-dependent magnetically responsive optical diffraction of carbon encapsulated superparamagnetic colloidal photonic crystals. *J. Phys. Chem. C* **2011**, *115*, 11427–11434. [CrossRef]
46. Gorobets, O.; Gorobets, S.; Koralewski, M. Physiological origin of biogenic magnetic nanoparticles in health and disease: From bacteria to humans. *Int. J. Nanomed.* **2017**, *12*, 4371–4395. [CrossRef]
47. Uchida, L.; Liepold, O.; Douglas, T. *Protein Cage Magnetic Nanoparticles in Magnetic Nanoparticles from Fabrication to Clinical Applications*; Thanh, N.T.K., Ed.; Taylor and Francis: Boca Raton, FL, USA, 2012; pp. 73–95.
48. Meldrun, F.C.; Wade, V.J.; Nimmo, D.L.; Heywood, B.R.; Mann, S. Synthesis of inorganic nanophase materials in supramolecular protein cages. *Nature* **1991**, *349*, 684–687. [CrossRef]
49. Fantechi, E.; Innocenti, C.; Zanardelli, M.; Fittipaldi, M.; Falvo, E.; Carbo, M.; Shullani, V.; Manelli, C.; Ghelardini, C.; Ferret, A.M.; et al. A smart platform for hyperthermia application in cancer treatment: Cobalt-doped ferrite nanoparticles mineralized in human ferritin cages. *ACS Nano* **2014**, *8*, 4705–4719. [CrossRef]
50. Parker, M.J.; Allen, M.A.; Ramsay, B.; Klem, M.T.; Young, M.; Douglas, T. Expanding the temperature range of biomimetic synthesis using a ferritin from the hyperthermophile pyrococcus furiosus. *Chem. Mat.* **2008**, *20*, 1541–1547. [CrossRef]
51. Lynch, I.; Dawson, K.A. Protein-nanoparticle interactions. *Nanotoday* **2008**, *3*, 40–47. [CrossRef]
52. Barui, A.K.; Oh, J.Y.; Jana, B.; Kim, C.; Ryu, J.-H. Cancer-Targeted Nanomedicine: Overcoming the Barrier of the Protein Corona. *Adv. Therap.* **2019**. [CrossRef]
53. Mosayebi, J.; Kiyasatfar, M.; Laurent, S. Synthesis, Functionalization, and Design of Magnetic Nanoparticles for Theranostic Applications. *Adv. Health Mater.* **2017**, *6*. [CrossRef] [PubMed]
54. Quanguo, H.; Lei, Z.; Wei, W.; Rong, H.; Jingke, H. Preparation and Magnetic comparison of Silane-Functionalized Magnetite Nanoparticles. *Sens. Mater.* **2010**, *22*, 285–295.

55. Mashhadizadeh, M.H.; Amoli-Diva, M. Drug-Carrying Amino Silane Coated Magnetic Nanoparticles as Potential Vehicles for Delivery of Antibiotics. *J. Nanomed. Nanotechnol.* **2012**, *3*, 1000139. [CrossRef]
56. Boyer, C.; Whittaker, M.R.; Bulmus, V.; Liu, J.; Davies, T.P. The design and utility of polymer-stabilized iron-oxide nanoparticles for nanomedicine applications. *NPG Asia Mater.* **2010**, *2*, 23–30. [CrossRef]
57. Sahoo, Y.; Pizem, H.; Fried, T.; Golodnitsky, D.; Burstein, E.; Sukenik, C.N.; Markovich, G. Alkyl Phosphonate/Phosphate Coating on Magnetite Nanoparticles: A Comparison with Fatty Acids. *Langmuir* **2001**, *17*, 7907–7911. [CrossRef]
58. Gupta, A.K.; Gupta, M. Synthesis and surface engineering of iron oxide nanoparticles for biomedical applications. *Biomaterials* **2005**, *26*, 3995–4021. [CrossRef]
59. Guardia, P.; Batlle-Brugal, B.; Roca, A.G.; Iglesias, O.; Morales, M.P.; Serna, C.J.; Labarta, A.; Batlle, X. Surfactant effects in monodisperse magnetite nanoparticles of controlled size. *J. Magn. Magn. Mater.* **2007**, *316*, e756. [CrossRef]
60. Frey, N.A.; Peng, S.; Cheng, K.; Sun, S. Magnetic nanoparticles: Synthesis, functionalization, and applications in bioimaging and magnetic storage. *Chem. Soc. Rev.* **2009**, *38*, 2532–2542. [CrossRef]
61. Fan, J.; Lu, J.; Xu, R.; Jiang, R.; Gao, Y. Use of water-dispersible Fe_2O_3 nanoparticles with narrow size distributions in isolating avidin. *J. Colloid Interface Sci.* **2003**, *266*, 215–218. [CrossRef]
62. Piñeiro-Redondo, Y.; Bañobre-López, M.; Pardiñas-Blanco, I.; Goya, G.; López-Quintela, M.A.; Rivas, J. The influence of colloidal parameters on the specific power absorption of PAA-coated magnetite nanoparticles. *Nanoscale Res. Lett.* **2011**, *6*, 383–389. [CrossRef] [PubMed]
63. Lu, X.; Niu, M.; Qiao, R.; Gao, M. Superdispersible PVP-Coated Fe_3O_4 Nanocrystals Prepared by a "One-Pot" Reaction. *J. Phys. Chem. B* **2008**, *112*, 14390–14394. [CrossRef] [PubMed]
64. Tombácz, E.; Farkas, K.; Földesi, I.; Szekeres, M.; Illés, E.; Tóth, I.Y.; Nesztor, D.; Szabó, T. Polyelectrolyte coating on superparamagnetic iron oxide nanoparticles as interface between magnetic core and biorelevant media. *Interface Focus* **2016**, *6*, 20160068. [CrossRef] [PubMed]
65. Yang, C.; Yan, H. A green and facile approach for synthesis of magnetite nanoparticles with tunable sizes and morphologies. *Mater. Lett.* **2012**, *73*, 129–132. [CrossRef]
66. Mornet, S.; Vasseur, S.; Grasset, F.; Duguet, E. Magnetic nanoparticle design for medical diagnosis and therapy. *J. Mat. Chem.* **2004**, *14*, 2161–2175. [CrossRef]
67. Gref, R.; Luck, M.; Quellec, P.; Marchand, M.; Dellacherie, E.; Harnisch, S.; Blunk, T.; Muller, R.H. 'Stealth' corona-core nanoparticles surface modified by polyethylene glycol (PEG): Influences of the corona (PEG chain length and surface density) and of the core composition on phagocytic uptake and plasma protein adsorption. *Colloids Surf. B* **2000**, *18*, 301–313. [CrossRef]
68. Rahman, M.; Laurent, S.; Tawil, N.; Yahia, L.H.; Mahmoudi, M. *Protein-NP Interactions, the Bio-Nano Interface*; Springer Series in Biophysics; Springer: Berlin/Heidelberg, Germany, 2013; Volume 15, pp. 21–44.
69. Pearson, R.M.; Juettner, V.V.; Hong, S. Biomolecular corona on nanoparticles: A survey of recent literature and its implications in targeted drug delivery. *Front. Chem.* **2014**, *2*, 108. [CrossRef]
70. You, J.O.; Almeda, D.; Ye, G.J.C.; Auguste, D.T. Bioresponsive matrices in drug delivery. *J. Biol. Eng.* **2010**, *4*, 1–15. [CrossRef]
71. Yadavalli, T.; Ramasamy, S.; Chandrasekaran, G.; Michael, I.; Therese, H.A.; Chennakesavulu, R. Dual responsive PNIPAM–chitosan targeted magnetic nanopolymers for targeted drug delivery. *J. Magn. Magn. Mater.* **2015**, *380*, 315–320. [CrossRef]
72. Dionigi, C.; Piñeiro, Y.; Riminucci, A.; Bañobre, M.; Rivas, J.; Dediu, V. Regulating the thermal response of PNIPAM hydrogels by controlling the adsorption of magnetite nanoparticles. *Appl. Phys. A Mater. Sci. Process* **2014**, *114*, 585–590. [CrossRef]
73. Digigow, R.G.; Dechéllez, J.F.; Dietsch, H.; Geissbühler, I.; Vanhecke, D.; Geers, C.; Hirt, A.M.; Rothen-Rutishauer, B. Preparation and characterization of functional silicahybrid magnetic nanoparticles. *J. Magn. Magn. Mater.* **2014**, *362*, 72–79. [CrossRef]
74. Vargas-Osorio, Z.; González-Gómez, M.A.; Piñeiro, Y.; Vázquez-Vázquez, C.; Rodríguez-Abreu, C.; López-Quintela, M.A.; Rivas, J. Novel synthetic routes of large-pore magnetic mesoporous nanocomposites (SBA-15/Fe_3O_4) as potential multifunctional theranostic nanodevices. *J. Mater. Chem. B* **2017**, *5*, 9395–9404. [CrossRef]
75. Ha, Y.; Ko, S.; Kim, I.; Huang, Y.; Mohanty, K.K.; Huh, C.; Maynard, J.A. Recent Advances Incorporating Superparamagnetic Nanoparticles into Immunoassays. *ACS Appl. Nano Mater.* **2018**, *1*, 512–521. [CrossRef]

76. Ito, A.; Hibino, E.; Shimizu, K.; Kobayashi, T.; Yamada, Y.; Hibi, H.; Ueda, M.; Honda, H.J. Magnetic force—Based mesenchymal stem cell expansion using antibody—Conjugated magnetoliposomes. *Biomed. Mater. Res. Part B* **2005**, *75B*, 320–327. [CrossRef]
77. Chao, C.; Jun, W.; Yong, Z.; Cong, L.; Lina, X.; Xin, Z.; Xiaolan, Y.; Ming, L.; Yang, B.; Tingyu, L.; et al. Improving Magnetofection of Magnetic Polyethylenimine Nanoparticles into MG-63 Osteoblasts using a Novel Uniform Magnetic Field. *Nanoscale Res. Lett.* **2019**, *14*, 90.
78. Chorny, M.; Fishbein, I.; Yellen, B.B.; Alferiev, I.S.; Bakay, M.; Ganta, S.; Adamo, R.; Amiji, M.; Friedman, G.; Levy, R.J. Targeting stents with local delivery of paclitaxel-loaded magnetic nanoparticles using uniform fields. *Proc. Natl. Acad. Sci. USA* **2010**, *107*, 8346–8351. [CrossRef]
79. Ryhänen, T.; Seppä, H.; Ilmoniemi, R.; Knuutila, J. SQUID magnetometers for low-frequency applications. *J. Low Temp. Phys.* **1989**, *76*, 287–386. [CrossRef]
80. Pankhurst, Q.; Hautot, D.; Khan, N.; Dobson, J. Increased Levels of Magnetic Iron Compounds in Alzheimer's Disease. *J. Alzheimer's Dis.* **2008**, *13*, 49–52. [CrossRef]
81. Tanaka, S.; Ota, H.; Kondo, Y.; Tamaki, Y.; Kobayashi, S.; Noguchi, S. Detection of magnetic nanoparticles in lymph nodes of rat by high Tc SQUID. *IEEE Trans. Appl. Supercond.* **2003**, *13*, 377–380. [CrossRef]
82. Adolphi, N.L.; Butler, K.S.; Lovato, D.M.; Tessier, T.E.; Trujillo, J.E.; Hathaway, H.J.; Fegan, D.L.; Monson, T.C.; Stevens, T.E.; Huber, D.L.; et al. Imaging of Her2-targeted magnetic nanoparticles for breast cancer detection: Comparison of SQUID-detected magnetic relaxometry and MRI. *Contrast Media Mol. Imaging* **2012**, *7*, 308–319. [CrossRef] [PubMed]
83. Bhuiya, A.K.; Asai, M.; Watanabe, H.; Hirata, T.; Higuchi, Y.; Yoshida, T.; Enpuku, K. Characterization of magnetic markers and sensors for liquid-phase immunoassays using Brownian relaxation. *IEEE Trans. Magn.* **2012**, *48*, 2838–2841. [CrossRef]
84. Cubells-Beltrán, M.D.; Reig, C.; Madrenas, J.; De Marcellis, A.; Santos, J.; Cardoso, S.; Freitas, P.P. Integration of GMR Sensors with Different Technologies. *Sensors* **2016**, *16*, 939. [CrossRef] [PubMed]
85. Osterfeld, S.J.; Yu, H.; Gaster, R.S.; Caramuta, S.; Xu, L.; Han, S.-J.; Hall, E.A.; Wilson, R.J.; Sun, S.; White, R.L.; et al. Multiplex protein assays based on real-time magnetic nanotag sensing. *Proc. Natl. Acad. Sci. USA* **2008**, *105*, 20637–20640. [CrossRef] [PubMed]
86. Chen, Y.T.; Kolhatkar, A.G.; Zenasni, O.; Xu, S.; Lee, T.R. Biosensing Using Magnetic Particle Detection Techniques. *Sensors* **2017**, *17*, 2300. [CrossRef] [PubMed]
87. Wang, W.; Wang, Y.; Tu, L.; Klein, T.; Feng, Y.; Wang, J.P. Surface Modification for Protein and DNA Immobilization onto GMR Biosensor. *IEEE Trans. Magn.* **2013**, *49*, 296–299. [CrossRef]
88. Lago-Cachón, D.; Rivas, M.; Martínez-García, J.C.; García, J.A. Cu impedance-based detection of superparamagnetic nanoparticles. *Nanotechnology* **2013**, *24*, 245501. [CrossRef]
89. Lago-Cachon, D.; Oliveira-Rodriguez, M.; Moyano, A.; Rivas, M.; Blanco-Lopez, M.C.; Martinez-Garcia, J.C.; Salvador, M.; Garcia, J.A. Scanning Magneto-Inductive Sensor for Quantitative Assay of Prostate-Specific Antigen. *IEEE Magn. Lett.* **2017**, *8*, 1–5. [CrossRef]
90. Moyano, A.; Salvador, M.; Martínez, J.C.; Rivas, M.; Blanco-López, M.C.; Gónzalez-Gómez, M.A.; Yáñez, S.; Piñeiro, Y.; Rivas, J. Carbon-coated superparamagnetic nanoflowers as labels in lateral flow imunoassays. In Proceedings of the 10th International Conference on Fine Particle Magnetism, Gijon, Spain, 27–30 May 2019; Book of Abstracts. p. 187.
91. Piñeiro-Redondo, Y.; Vargas-Osorio, Z.; Bañobre-López, M.; Kolen'ko, Y.V.; López-Quintela, M.A.; Rivas, J. Relevant Parameters for Magnetic Hyperthermia in Biological: Applications: Agglomeration, Concentration, and Viscosity. *IEEE Trans. Magn.* **2016**, *52*, 2300704(1-4).
92. Hergt, R.; Andrä, W. *Magnetism in Medicine: A Handbook*, 2nd ed.; Andrä, W., Nowak, H., Eds.; Chapter 4: Magnetic Hyperthermia and Thermoablation; Wiley-VCH: Berlin, Germany, 2007.
93. Minelli, C.; Lowe, S.B.; Stevens, M.S. Engineering Nanocomposite Materials for Cancer therapy. *Small* **2010**, *6*, 2336–2357. [CrossRef]
94. MagForce AG. Available online: https://www.magforce.com/en/home/our_therapy/ (accessed on 29 September 2019).
95. Dionigi, C.; Lungaro, L.; Goranov, V.; Riminucci, A.; Piñeiro-Redondo, Y.; Bañobre-López, M.; Rivas, J.; Dediu, V. Smart magnetic poly(N-isopropylacrylamide) to control the release of bio-active molecules. *J. Mater. Sci. Mater. Electron.* **2014**, *25*, 2365–2371. [CrossRef] [PubMed]

96. Santin, M.; Meikle, S.; Pineiro, Y.; Bañobre Lopez, M.; Rivas, J.; Santin, M. Mild hyperthermia nano-devices based on superparamagnetic nanoparticles conjugated with thermoresponsive poly(epsilon-lysine) dendrons tethered with carboxybetaine. *Acta Biomater.* **2016**, *40*, 235–242.
97. Chen, R.; Romero, G.; Christiansen, M.G.; Mohr, A.; Anikeeva, P. Wireless magnetothermal deep brain stimulation, Sciencexpress. *Science* **2015**, *347*, 1477–1480. [CrossRef]
98. Yue, K.; Guduru, R.; Hong, J.; Llang, P.; Nair, M.; Khizroev, S. Magneto-electric Nanoparticules for Non-Invasive Brain Stimulation. *PLoS ONE* **2012**, *7*, e44040. [CrossRef]
99. Carril, M.; Fernández, I.; Rodriguez, J.; García, I.; Peñadés, S. Gold-coated iron oxide glyconanoparticles for MRI, CT, and US multimodal imaging. *Part. Part. Syst. Charact.* **2014**, *31*, 81–87. [CrossRef]
100. Jang, J.-T.; Nah, H.; Lee, J.-H.; Moon, S.H.; Kim, M.G.; Cheon, J. Critical Enhancements of MRI Contrast and Hyperthermic Effects by Dopant-Controlled Magnetic Nanoparticles. *Angew. Chem.* **2009**, *121*, 1260–1264. [CrossRef]
101. Gupte, A.A.; Shrivastava, D.; Spaniol, M.A.; Abosch, A. MRI-related heating near deep brain stimulation electrodes: More data are needed. *Ster. Funct. Neurosurg.* **2011**, *89*, 131–140. [CrossRef] [PubMed]
102. Lee, N.; Choi, Y.; Lee, Y.; Park, M.; Moon, W.K.; Choi, S.H.; Hyeon, T.; Lee, J. Water-Dispersible Ferrimagnetic Iron Oxide Nanocubes with Extremely High r2 Relaxivity for Highly Sensitive in Vivo MRI of Tumors. *Nano Lett.* **2012**, *12*, 3127–3131. [CrossRef]
103. Zhao, Z.; Zhou, Z.; Bao, J.; Wang, Z.; Hu, J.; Chi, X.; Ni, K.; Wang, R.; Chen, X.; Chen, Z.; et al. Octapod iron oxide nanoparticles as high-performance T2 contrast agents for magnetic resonance imaging. *Nat. Commun.* **2013**, *4*, 2266. [CrossRef]
104. Wang, L.; Huang, J.; Chen, H.; Wu, H.; Xu, Y.; Li, Y.; Yi, H.; Wang, Y.A.; Yang, L.; Mao, H. Exerting Enhanced Permeability and Retention Effect Driven Delivery by Ultrafine Iron Oxide Nanoparticles with T1–T2 Switchable Magnetic Resonance Imaging Contrast. *ACS Nano* **2017**, *11*, 4582–4592. [CrossRef]
105. Adine, C.; Ng, K.K.; Rungarunlert, S.; Souza, G.R.; Ferreira, J.N. Engineering innervated secretory epithelial organoids by magnetic three-dimensional bioprinting for stimulating epithelial growth in salivary glands. *Biomater* **2018**, *180*, 52–66. [CrossRef] [PubMed]

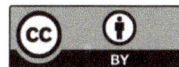

© 2020 by the authors. Licensee MDPI, Basel, Switzerland. This article is an open access article distributed under the terms and conditions of the Creative Commons Attribution (CC BY) license (http://creativecommons.org/licenses/by/4.0/).

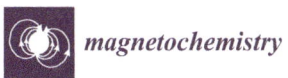

Review

Pharmaceutical Applications of Iron-Oxide Magnetic Nanoparticles

Marcos Luciano Bruschi *[ID] and Lucas de Alcântara Sica de Toledo

Laboratory of Research and Development of Drug Delivery Systems, Department of Pharmacy, State University of Maringa, Av. Colombo, 5790, CEP 87020-900, Maringa 87020-900, PR, Brazil
* Correspondence: mlbruschi@uem.br; Tel.: +55-44-3011-4870

Received: 13 June 2019; Accepted: 20 August 2019; Published: 2 September 2019

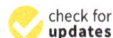

Abstract: Advances of nanotechnology led to the development of nanoparticulate systems with many advantages due to their unique physicochemical properties. The use of iron-oxide magnetic nanoparticles (IOMNPs) in pharmaceutical areas increased in the last few decades. This article reviews the conceptual information about iron oxides, magnetic nanoparticles, methods of IOMNP synthesis, properties useful for pharmaceutical applications, advantages and disadvantages, strategies for nanoparticle assemblies, and uses in the production of drug delivery, hyperthermia, theranostics, photodynamic therapy, and as an antimicrobial. The encapsulation, coating, or dispersion of IOMNPs with biocompatible material(s) can avoid the aggregation, biodegradation, and alterations from the original state and also enable entrapping the bioactive agent on the particle via adsorption or covalent attachment. IOMNPs show great potential for target drug delivery, improving the therapy as a consequence of a higher drug effect using lower concentrations, thus reducing side effects and toxicity. Different methodologies allow IOMNP synthesis, resulting in different structures, sizes, dispersions, and surface modifications. These advantages support their utilization in pharmaceutical applications, and getting suitable drug release control on the target tissues could be beneficial in several clinical situations, such as infections, inflammations, and cancer. However, more toxicological clinical investigations about IOMNPs are necessary.

Keywords: magnetic nanoparticles; iron oxide; pharmaceutics; magnetism; therapy; development; nanotechnology

1. Introduction

In the last few decades, the use of iron-oxide nanoparticles displaying magnetic properties attracted great interest in many application areas, from magnetic recording media to pharmaceutical applications such as therapy and drug delivery [1–14]. Each application of these nanoparticles needs specific and, sometimes, different properties [1,12,15]. For example, temperature control is very important in some applications. Particles should be stable and have a switchable magnetic state to represent bits of information, independent of temperature fluctuations [1].

Furthermore, the biological environment is very important when magnetic nanoparticles are applied in biology, medical diagnosis, and therapy [1,3,4,12]. Dynamic nanoparticle assemblies can also be designed to respond to the environment, such as temperature, pH, magnetic field, light, ultrasound, electric pulses, redox gradients, or enzymatic activity. In this way, "smart" materials can be created by designed synthesis and assembly of nanoparticles. Their surface can receive ligands, and the final structure can display programmed responses to external stimuli for pharmaceutical applications [11]. This is an important strategy to be applied to biosensors, molecular imaging, novel theranostics, and drug delivery systems [11].

Since the early 1960s, metal oxides were used for magnetic separations [3,16]. Specifically, nanoparticles composed of iron oxide attracted great interest for pharmaceutical applications [1,3–6,11,12,17,18]. This mineral compound shows different polymorphic forms, such as hematite, magnetite, and maghemite [19]. Iron-oxide magnetic nanoparticles (IOMNPs) can be obtained via several methods (e.g., co-precipitation, sol–gel, microemulsion, and thermal decomposition), displaying unique electrical, optical, and magnetic properties [3]. Moreover, they are utilized to develop dynamic nanoparticle assemblies for pharmaceutical applications [11].

IOMNPs are chemically and physically stable, biocompatible, and environmentally safe [3,12,13]. The synthesis of these nanoparticles should be well known and controlled, because it is directly related to sizing, shape, coating, and stability [3,12]. Particles showing size higher than 200 nm are easily cleared by the reticuloendothelial system [20,21]. On the other hand, nanoparticles smaller than 8 nm in diameter can be easily excreted from the body through existent pores of the kidney's basal lamina (renal clearance), if surface charge and chemistry are optimized for this excretion pathway [22,23], thereby reducing the blood-circulating time of these nanostructures. A faster clearance may also occur for hydrophobic and negatively charged nanoparticles, which tend to suffer protein opsonization, being quickly recognized by phagocyte cells [24]. Suitable surface-coating of organic and/or inorganic coatings can surpass problems of cell toxicity and oxidation of IOMNPs [6,25]. Moreover, there are important investigations that need to be addressed, such as studies about clinical, biocompatibility, toxicological, and immunological parameters [6].

Recently, the interest for pharmaceutical applications, such as drug delivery, biosensors, theranostics, and antimicrobial agents effective against many bacteria species, increased [11,16,26]. Therefore, the present manuscript provides a review about the state of the art and advances of IOMNPs for pharmaceutical applications. The conceptual information about iron oxides, magnetic nanoparticles, methods of IOMNP synthesis, properties useful for pharmaceutical applications, advantages and disadvantages, dynamic assembly of IOMNPs, and the applications in the production of drug delivery, hyperthermia, theranostics, and as antimicrobials are addressed.

2. Iron Oxides and Nanoparticles

Iron oxides are mineral compounds found abundantly in nature, but they can also be synthesized in the laboratory [3]. They are composed of iron and oxygen, presenting more than one crystal structure and different structural and magnetic properties [27]. Magnetite (Fe_3O_4) is one of the most interesting crystallographic phases of iron oxide, due to its polymorphism and magnetic properties [3]. Moreover, iron (III) oxide (ferric oxide, Fe_2O_3) exhibits four different crystalline polymorphs (α, β, γ, and ε) with unique biochemical, magnetic, catalytic, and other properties. The highly crystalline α-Fe_2O_3 (hematite) and γ-Fe_2O_3 (maghemite) are found in nature, while the forms β-Fe_2O_3 and ε-Fe_2O_3 are generally synthesized. In addition, the amorphous Fe_2O_3 is characterized to have the Fe (III) ions surrounded by an oxygen octahedral, with the symmetry axes randomly orientated in a non-periodic lattice [3,27].

Magnetite, hematite, and maghemite are the main forms of iron oxide, and their structures can be defined according to the close-packed planes of oxygen anions together with iron cations in tetrahedral or octahedral interstitial sites [3,17,27]. Hematite is well known among the iron oxides and shows a weak ferromagnetic or antiferromagnetic behavior at room temperature, but it is paramagnetic above 956 K. Maghemite (γ-Fe_2O_3) is thermally unstable and can be transformed to hematite at higher temperatures. Moreover, maghemite and magnetite (Fe_2O_3) are easily magnetized, displaying high magnetic response when submitted to an external magnetic field [3,27]. They are metastable oxides in an oxidative atmosphere and, thus, they are oxidized to hematite (α-Fe_2O_3) when heated to a temperature above 673 K [28]. The form ε-Fe_2O_3 displays an orthorhombic crystal structure and it can be regarded as a polymorphous intermediate showing similarity to both α-Fe_2O_3 and γ-Fe_2O_3. In addition, its magnetic behavior is not fully understood [3].

In general, iron oxides were shown great interest due to their nanosized form, and these crystalline polymorphs can be suitable for specific pharmaceutical applications. They can generally be synthesized as particulate materials displaying sizes less than 100 nm that can suffer the influence of an external magnetic field and can, thus, be manipulated [11,12,16,27,29,30].

The development of magnetic resonance imaging contributed to the investigation and development of these nanoparticles [31]. Moreover, they were investigated as carriers for active agents for drug targeting [6]. In the last few decades, several studies showed the development of preparations containing IOMNP to be used for in vitro separation, tissue repair, cellular therapy, magnetic separation, magnetic resonance imaging, as spoilers for magnetic resonance spectroscopy, in drug delivery, hyperthermia, sensors for metabolites, and other biomolecules [6,11,12,16,18,30,32–35].

IOMNPs combine chemical accessibility in solution with physical properties of the bulk phase, due to characteristics between the solid and molecular states [36,37]. They show a complex process of synthesis and the obtaining of a monodisperse particle population of suitable size is dependent on the selection of experimental conditions [6,17,21,38]. Therefore, several studies investigated the fluid stability, through the control of particle size, materials, surfactants, and physical behavior [16]. Moreover, the synthesis process selection should consider the reproducibility and scaling up without any complex purification procedure (e.g., ultracentrifugation, size-exclusion chromatography, magnetic filtration, or flow field gradient) [16,38].

Over the last few decades, several IOMNP synthesis methods were investigated using either organic or aqueous phases: synthesis under constrained environment, hydrothermal and high-temperature reactions, sol–gel reactions, polyol method, flow injection, electrochemical, aerosol/vapor, and sonolysis [3,4,16,21]. In this context, the physical, chemical, and biological routes are the main approaches utilized for synthesis of IOMNP [6,17]. Table 1 summarizes the preparation methods of IOMNPs.

Table 1. Summary of preparation methods of iron-oxide magnetic nanoparticles (IOMNPs).

Routes	Methods	References
Physical	Pulsed laser ablation	[6,39–41]
	Pyrolysis	[6]
Chemical	Co-precipitation	[3,6,16,36–38,40–43]
	Microemulsion	[6,37,44]
	Hydrothermal and solvothermal syntheses	[1,3,6,38]
	Thermal decomposition	[6,38]
	Sol–gel synthesis	[3,16,17,21,32,37,38,43–46]
	Sonochemical	[43,47]
	Microwave-assisted synthesis	[6,48]
Biological	Biosynthesis	[6,49]

The synthesis of these nanoparticles into formulations should also be considered. These methodologies aim for the production of IOMNPs with improved characteristics of stability, biocompatibility, high dispersibility, suitable shape, and controlled size [1,3,6,17].

The preparation of IOMNPs in hydrogels, gels, emulsions, or other types of formulations can be accomplished considering several methods: blending, in situ, and grafting onto. These methods are usually employed because they save time and reduce the number of steps. The grafting-onto method is widely used and is the only one that forms covalent bonds between the IOMNPs and the system [50]. Liu and collaborators prepared fiber-like composites of hematite via the in situ addition of an amount of Fe^{+3} into swollen regenerated cellulose [51]. Moreover, via the blending method, the IOMNPs are synthesized separate from the formulation, and then the precipitated and dry particles in the system are dispersed. For example, iron fluid was prepared and added to an n-isopropylacrylamide dispersion to produce a magnetic hydrogel [50,52].

Another important point to be considered during IOMNP preparation for pharmaceutical formulations is that they must exhibit the combined characteristics of high magnetic saturation and a peculiar surface coating of particles [17]. IOMNPs should be nontoxic, biocompatible and, sometimes, must also allow a targetable delivery with particle localization in a specific area [3,13,16,36]. Therefore, it is necessary that the surface of particles displays suitable characteristics to enable their utilization in several in vitro and in vivo applications. However, these characteristics should not affect the stability and magnetization of particles. IOMNPs can be directed to a target site using an external magnetic field. Moreover, they can bind to antibodies, nucleotides, proteins, enzymes, or drugs [38]. Therefore, the surface of these particles could be modified creating new atomic layers of inorganic metallic (e.g., gold), organic polymer, or oxide surfaces (e.g., silica or alumina) [6,17,25,36,53]. Assemblies of IOMNPs are also possible, resulting in nanostructures with physical and chemical properties different from those of both individual IOMNPs and their bulk aggregates. For example, these assembled nanoparticles can be developed to respond to either endogenous or exogenous stimuli [11].

3. Characteristics of IOMNPs for Pharmaceutical Applications

The use of IOMNPs received important attention in bioscience [21]. Their behavior is dependent on temperature, and their uses for pharmaceutical applications should be considered at different temperatures (e.g., body and room temperatures). Pharmaceutical applications require the particles be stable in a physiological environment (aqueous environment and pH ~7) [1,3].

Furthermore, the charge, size, surface chemistry, and both coulombic and steric repulsions of particles are very important variables which are involved in the colloidal stability of IOMNP dispersion [3,13,19,25]. Sometimes, IOMNPs should be protected (encapsulated, coat, or dispersed) with biocompatible polymer(s) in order to avoid aggregation, biodegradation, and alterations from the original structure [3]. This strategy can also enable entrapping the bioactive agent on the particle via adsorption or covalent attachment [3]. Moreover, dynamic assemblies are also possible due to the assistance of surface ligands [11,54].

IOMNP biocompatibility and toxicity are dependent on the nature of the magnetically responsive components of particles. Moreover, iron-oxide nanoparticles such as magnetite (Fe_3O_4) or its oxidized form maghemite (γ-Fe_2O_3) are the most utilized [1]. They must be made of a non-immunogenic and non-toxic material, with size of particle small enough to stay in the circulation after administration and to pass through the thin capillaries of tissues and organs, in order to avoid vessel embolism [1]. Moreover, IOMNPs must show a high magnetization in order to be controlled in the blood and be immobilized just close to the targeted tissue by a magnetic field [1,13].

Size and surface functionality are the two major factors that play an important role for the pharmaceutical applications of IOMNPs [11]. Even without targeting surface ligands, their diameters greatly affect in vivo biodistribution [25]. Nanoparticles displaying diameter greater than 200 nm can easily be cleared by the reticuloendothelial system. However, particles sizing less than 8 nm can easily be excreted from the body through existent pores of the kidney's basal lamina [6], reducing their blood-circulating time. The diameter range of 10–40 nm (including ultra-small IOMNPs) is fundamental for prolonged blood circulation, allowing the nanoparticles to cross capillary walls and often be phagocytized by macrophages trafficking to the lymph nodes and bone marrow [1]. Therefore, the size of IOMNPs enables their lower sedimentation, higher effective surface area (mainly for particles sizing less than 100 nm), and improved tissular diffusion [1,3,13,55].

Furthermore, hydrophobic and negatively charged nanoparticles tend to suffer proteic opsonization and are quickly recognized by phagocytic cells [55], resulting in faster clearance. The success of an IOMNP-based nanosystem is also directly related to the properties of the coating material and the IOMNP limitations can normally be overcome using a suitable surface coating [6,55]. Natural and synthetic polymers, surfactants, gold, silica, and peptides were proposed as coating materials for

IOMNPs [6,25]. Nature, spatial configuration, and shape of the coating play an important role in system performance [6,55].

4. IOMNP Assemblies and Clusters

Over the past two decades, scientists investigated the assembly of nanoparticles to create smart materials for applications in pharmacy [11]. Using nanoarchitectonics, designed nanoparticles can show the ability to change their properties according to the environmental conditions. They can respond to different stimuli from either endogenous (e.g., pH, redox, enzyme) or external (e.g., temperature, light ultrasound and/or magnetic field) sources [56].

The use of IOMNPs in pharmaceutical applications requires their contact with biological fluids (e.g., blood, serum, lymphatic fluid, etc.). Therefore, this contact and their interactions with components of the biological system can adsorb proteins in some degree, resulting in aggregates. As a consequence, a new structure is formed displaying different characteristics (size, aggregation state, interfacial properties, etc.) from individual IOMNPs, affecting IOMNP interaction with cells [57]. Therefore, the formation of clusters and assemblies of IOMNPs can result in structures with physical and chemical properties different from individual nanoparticles and their bulk aggregates, and they can be useful for pharmaceutical applications [11].

In particular, dynamic IOMNP assembly is a type of nanoarchitectonics based on ligand-assisted functional achievement, constituting a strategy to build high-precision materials. IOMNPs can be employed as a substrate to construct responsive assemblies or clusters under the assistance of suitable ligands. In this context, IOMNPs can be utilized as magnetic-force-guided targeting for drug delivery systems due to their magnetic properties [4,58].

Considering their pharmaceutical applications, IOMNPs and their clusters and assemblies must show colloidal stability and biocompatibility in various biological environments [3,12,13,16]. Small molecules, biomacromolecules, and polymers can be utilized as ligands to mediate IOMNP assemblies [7,9,57]. However, small-molecular ligands generally show low stability and biocompatibility, and it is hard to find a small-molecular ligand [11,59].

Polymers are very useful to obtain IOMNP assemblies, and they often can contribute to obtaining smart systems with improved pharmacokinetics with long circulation times, targeting, and controlled release [60].

In this context, the use of stimuli-responsive polymers as ligands to obtain IOMNP assemblies is a good strategy. Temperature-, light-, and pH-sensitive polymers are often used. Considering the biological environment, the pharmaceutical applications generally occur in aqueous medium. IOMNPs show affinity to water; however, the structural alteration of water around interfaces and solutes can increase the intermolecular interactions (hydrophobic interactions) conducing to the assembly [11].

Many types of biomacromolecules can also be utilized to for assembling nanoparticles, such as peptides, polysaccharides (chitosan and dextran), nucleic acids, and proteins. The nanoparticle assemblies using proteins can be based on the modification of substrates on the nanoparticle surface. A protein has multiple binding domains, which can be used for nanoparticle aggregation via crosslinking the corresponding substrates or via binding between antibodies and antigens [11,59].

Table 2 shows a list of ligands utilized for IOMNP assemblies and cluster formation. In addition, clusters of IOMNPs were obtained using silica [61]. Nanochains and nanobundles were fabricated via the simultaneous magnetic assembly of superparamagnetic nanoparticle clusters using an additional layer of ligand (deposited silica) using a sol–gel process. The investigators observed that this magnetically responsive superparamagnetic could lead to applications in the treatment of cancer.

Bioengineered spider silk was used as a ligand for the assembly of IOMNPs. Due to its mechanical properties, biocompatibility, and biodegradability, spider silk enables the fabrication of composite spheres, which can be potentially applied for the therapy of cancer by combined treatment via drug delivery and hyperthermia [62].

Investigations about IOMNP assemblies are based on fundamentals, design, and fabrication. However, the development of several applications of these smart systems is only at the basic stage and their real application to clinical trials is dependent on more studies [11].

Table 2. Examples of biomacromolecules and polymers used as ligands for assembly of iron-oxide magnetic nanoparticles (IOMNPs).

Classification	Ligands	References
Small molecules	Silica	[59,63]
	Dextran	[57]
Biomacromolecules	CXCR4-targeted peptide	[64]
	Biotin–streptavidin	[65]
	Tyrosine kinase and phosphatase	[66]
	Bovine serum albumin	[67]
	Spider silk	[62]
	Nucleic acids	[11]
Polymers	PEG-p(API-Asp)-p(DOPAAsp)-Ce6	[68]
	PVP	[69]
	p(MMA-co-DMA)	[70]
	p(NIPAM-co-AA)	[62]
	VCL-AAEM-VIm	[71]
	PMAA, PNIPAM	[72]
	PHOS-FOL-DOX	[73]
	Poly(allylamine)	[74]
	β-cyclodextrin	[75]
	DMSA, chitosan, PEG, PLGA, PEG-derived phosphine oxide (PO-PEG), PMAO (poly (maleic anhydride-alt-1-octadecene)),	[22,57,76]
	PEG–maleic anhydride	[67]
	PEG–poly(ε-caprolactone)	[77]

CXCR4 = C-X-C chemokine receptor type 4; PEG-p(API-Asp)-p(DOPAAsp)-Ce6 = Poly(ethylene glycol)-poly[1-(3-aminopropyl)imidazole –Aspartate]-poly(Dopamine-Aspartate)-Chlorine6; PVP = Polyvinylpyrrolidone; p(MMA-co-DMA) = Poly(methyl methacrylate-co-dimethylacrylate); p(NIPAM-co-AA) = Poly(N-isopropylacrylamide-co-acrylic acid); VCL-AAEM-VIm = poly(N-vinylcaprolactam-co-acetoacetoxyethyl methacrylate-co-N-vinylimidazole); PMAA = Poly(methacrylic acid); PNIPAM = Poly(N-isopropylacrylamide); PHOS-FOL-DOX = Triblock copolymer [cis-5-norbornene-6-(diethoxyphosphoryl)hexanote]-[norbornene grafted poly(ethyleneglycol)-folate]-[norbornene derived doxorubicin]; DMSA = Dimercaptosuccinic acid; PLGA = poly(lactic-co-glycolic acid).

5. Pharmaceutical Applications

IOMNPs can be used for pharmaceutical applications [1], and the advances in magnetic resonance imaging (MRI), cell separation and detection, tissue repair, magnetic hyperthermia, and drug delivery strongly benefited from employing IOMNPs [11]. These nanoparticles possess very important characteristics, such as superparamagnetism, size, and the possibility of receiving a biocompatible coating. Therefore, ongoing researches are focused on reducing drug concentration, toxicity, and other side effects, and improving the therapy [6,18,21,32].

The pharmaceutical applications of IOMNPs can be classified according to their application inside or outside the body. For external applications, the main use of these nanoparticles is in diagnostic separation, selection, and magnetorelaxometry [1,32]. In this context, they can be administered in a patient for diagnostic applications (nuclear magnetic resonance or magnetic particle imaging), drug delivery, hyperthermia, or as an antimicrobial [1,3,21,78].

5.1. Diagnostic Applications

Magneto-pharmaceuticals are a new class of preparations utilized for clinical diagnosis using the NMR imaging technique. In magnetic resonance imaging (MRI), these formulations must be administered to the patient in order to enhance the image contrast between the normal and diseased tissue and/or indicate the status of organ functions or blood flow [1,32].

Magnetic particle imaging (MPI) is a new, non-invasive, whole-body imaging technique that can detect superparamagnetic iron-oxide nanoparticles similar to those used in MRI. Based on tracer "hot spot" detection instead of providing contrast on MRI scans, MPI is truly quantitative. Without the presence of an endogenous background signal, MPI can also be used in certain tissues where the endogenous MRI signal is too low to provide contrast. Its applications include MPI cell tracking, multiplexed MPI, perfusion and tumor MPI, lung MPI, and functional MPI [8,18].

5.2. Drug Delivery

The research and development of therapeutic drug delivery systems increased with the development of new materials and technologies. The development of biotechnology and the understanding of physiological mechanisms also allowed obtaining more specialized pharmaceutical systems. Therefore, the number of strategies for the development of drug delivery systems showing enhanced properties in relation to modifying and controlling the delivery of active agents increased [32,79].

In this context, nanotechnology is utilized as one of the most common strategies for controlling the drug delivery, and increasing the efficiency, safety, and quality of the systems. Moreover, patient therapy is improved as well.

IOMNPs can be used for controlling the drug delivery [1,6,32,78] and they can enable drug targeting, one of the most important strategies [79]. The application of an external magnetic field together with these nanoparticles and/or magnetizable implants allows the delivery of particles to the desired site, fixing them at the target tissue while the active agent is released, and acting locally (magnetic drug targeting) [32]. This strategy can eliminate side effects and reduce the dosage required.

In this context, IOMNPs are undergoing trials to investigate the possibility that they can be implemented as drug carriers. As the properties of these nanoparticles and the success in delivering active agents are strongly dependent on the composition of the external coating, polymeric layers, capsules, particles, or vesicles were proposed [32]. The modifications of the surface of these particles are generally accomplished using organic polymers and inorganic metals or oxides to make them biocompatible and suitable for further functionalization via the attachment of various bioactive molecules [78].

However, several important criteria should be considered in order for the drug delivery system containing IOMNPs to be effective. The delivery system should be easily dispersed in aqueous media and also provide functional groups, which can be further modified in order to control the drug release or bind targeting units [6,32].

Nanostructured systems composed of a core–shell design are much utilized to attach different drugs to IOMNPs. The core is formed by nanoparticles and the shell represents the surface coating for nanoparticle functionalization. This strategy can improve the system stability, pharmacokinetics, biodistribution, and biocompatibility [6,80].

Synthetic and natural polymers are the most common surface coating used in IOMNPs, due to their capacity to prevent oxidation and confer stability to the nanoparticles. Polyethylene glycol (PEG), poly(vinylpyrrolidone) (PVP), polyvinyl alcohol (PVA), poly(lactic-co-glycolic acid) (PLGA), and chitosan are utilized [17,30,32].

PEG is hydrophilic, uncharged, and biocompatible, and it was utilized for coating the IOMNPs due to non-fouling properties and reduced blood protein opsonization. As a result, the nanoparticles can escape recognition by the immune system, increasing their time in blood circulation and their accumulation in the target cells/tissue [32,79].

PVP and PVA are also water-soluble synthetic polymers, widely used in pharmaceutical applications. Their emulsifying and adhesive properties enable the preparation of hydrogel structures. The hydrogen bonds between the polymer chains can involve the IOMNPs avoiding the agglomeration of nanoparticles [6,29].

A copolymer of polylactic acid and polyglycolic acid (PGA) displayed great potential for use in drug delivery systems [79]. This polymer presents solubility in most of the common solvents and can take different shapes and sizes, enabling the encapsulation of several types of molecules [6]. PLGA microparticles containing co-encapsulated dexamethasone acetate and IOMNPs were developed as one strategy to maintain the particles in the joint cavity via an external magnetic field, controlling the drug release for the treatment of arthritis and osteoarthritis [81].

Chitosan is a natural, biocompatible, biodegradable, and low-toxicity material obtained by chitin deacetylation. Its long chain, generated via the combination of 2-amino-2-deoxy-β-D-glucan with glycosidic linkages, results in a positive charge, driving the systems to the cell membrane which is negatively charged [22]. Therefore, chitosan-coated IOMNPs can display mucoadhesive properties and increase the nanoparticle retention in the target sites [6,82]. The thermal and magnetic properties of IOMNPs are not changed by chitosan coating and, therefore, several systems were developed [6,17]. Chitosan of low molecular weight can protect these nanoparticles from aggregation due to the electrostatic repulsion between the positively charged nanoparticles [83]. However, this polymer shows some limitations as a coating material, due to the partial protonation of its amino groups in water at physiological pH, which reduces chitosan solubility. Chemical changes in chitosan can overcome these problems, making chitosan derivatives more water-soluble [84,85].

IOMNPs can also receive organic surfactants, inorganic compounds, and bioactive molecules on its surface. Organic surfactants are utilized for the functionalization of IOMNPs, mainly when synthesized in organic solutions. Dimercaptosuccinic acid can result in nanoparticles with an anionic surface, avoiding opsonization and clearance by the reticuloendothelial system, reducing the cell toxicity [6]. Oleic acid and trisodium citrate are also capable of stabilizing nanoparticles by creating repulsive forces (mainly steric repulsion) to balance the magnetic and van der Waals attractive forces [86]. Considering that the long hydrocarbon chains of the surfactants can result in hydrophobic nanoparticles, surfactants showing lower values of critical micelle concentrations were used in order to obtain more efficient coatings of the IOMNPs, with improved dispersion capacity in solutions and lower nanoparticle clustering [87].

Inorganic compounds such as carbon, metals, silica, oxides (metal and non-metal), and sulfides were used in IOMNP systems, displaying the advantage of increasing the antioxidant properties of these nanoparticles [1,3,6,37]. SiO_2 can enhance the IOMNP dispersion in solutions, making them more stable and protected in acidic medium [37]. Carbon-based coatings show chemical and thermal stability, good electrical conductivity, and solubility, and they serve as a barrier against IOMNP oxidation [6]. Moreover, the electron transfer between silver and IOMNPs in a nanosystem creates a positively charged silver coating, allowing the conjugation of different antibiotics to the silver-decorated nanoparticles [88]. The use of metal coatings with modifications involving compounds such as thiol can enable their linkage with diverse biomolecules; oxides and sulfides are common in IOMNPs to stabilize the nanosystem and enable good magnetic properties [6].

Considering that the choice of a coating for the IOMNPs must take into account their intrinsic properties and the purpose of the system, ZnO was considered as the most appropriate compound for an anticancer nanosystem due to both its intrinsic anticancer properties and biocompatibility [89].

Peptides, lipids, and proteins are examples of bioactive molecules that can be used in IOMNP-based systems. They should be able to maintain the stability of the nanoparticles and the magnetic properties as well [6]. Human and bovine serum albumin (HSA and BSA) can be attached to IOMNPs via desolvation [90]. IOMNPs coated with BSA show a negatively charged surface that avoids electrostatic interactions with negative biological elements such as plasma and blood cells, thereby maintaining the stability of nanoparticles [91].

As IOMNPs show a greater reactive area than their micrometric counterparts and can cross biological barriers, their use in drug delivery systems is advantageous. Thus, different classes of drugs can be directly bound to these nanoparticles or to core–shell systems [6]. The binding occurs via adsorption, dispersion in the polymer matrix, encapsulation in the nucleus, electrostatic interactions, and/or covalent attachment to the surface, with the aim of improving their pharmacological properties [1,6,12,78]. In this context, IOMNPs were used as carriers of anticancer (e.g., doxorubicin, cetuximab, cytarabine, daunomycin, docetaxel, epirubicin, 5-fluorouracil, gemcitabine, methotrexate, mitoxantrone, paclitaxel, and carmustine), alternative (curcumin, hypericin, propolis, berberine, sanazole, and essential oils), immunosuppressive (e.g., mycophenolate mofetil), anticonvulsant (e.g., phenytoin and 3-mercaptopropionic acid), anti-inflammatory (e.g., ketoprofen, furan-functionalized dexamethasone peptide, and prednisolone), antibiotic (e.g., streptomycin, rifamycin, anthracycline, fluoroquinolone, tetracycline, cephalosporin rifampicin, doxycycline, cefotaxime, ceftriaxone, amikacin, amoxicillin, bacitracin, cefotaxime, erythromycin, gentamicin, kanamycin, neomycin, penicillin, polymyxin, streptomycin, and vancomycin), and antifungal (e.g., nystatin, ketoconazole, amphotericin B) agents [6,92].

5.3. Hyperthermia

When IOMNPs are subjected to an altering current (AC), the magnetic field randomly flips the magnetization direction between the parallel and antiparallel orientations [1,6,29,32]. Magnetic energy can be transmitted to the nanoparticles in the form of heat, and this property can be used in vivo to raise the temperature of tumor tissues. Pathological cells are more sensitive to hyperthermia than healthy ones, leading to their destruction [1,6]. Magnetite cationic liposomal particles and dextran-coated magnetite were shown to be effective for the treatment of tumor cells by hyperthermia [1,16,28].

This strategy is very advantageous due to the magnetic hyperthermia heating the restricted tumor area. In addition, the use of nanometer-size particles (subdomain magnetic particles) is better than using micron-sized particles (multidomain) due to nanoparticles absorbing much more power at tolerable AC magnetic fields [6,32]. Therefore, well-defined synthetic routes are necessary to obtain particles displaying suitable size and shape and, as a consequence, to obtain a rigorous control in temperature [1].

5.4. Antimicrobial Activity

The World Health Organization (WHO) suggested in 1993 some drug use indicators to ease the investigation on drug-prescribing patterns [93]. It would help promote rational drug use, mainly looking to avoid bacterial resistance [94].

However, we saw an over-prescription of antimicrobial medicines during the last three decades; this, together with the global public health concerns regarding bacterial resistance to conventional drugs, shows how fundamental it is to try different types of treatments.

Antimicrobial resistance is an old and huge concern for public health systems, having grown rapidly in recent times, spreading the preoccupation to economics [92,95–97]. The use of gold, silver, aluminum, and iron oxide as antimicrobials was previously proven [29,98–102].

Nanomaterials can show antimicrobial activity via cell membrane damage, releasing toxic metals (which can react with proteins, leading to a loss in protein), and damaging DNA, RNA, and proteins via reactive oxygen species generation. These mechanisms conduce to inhibition or killing of the microorganisms [103].

Therefore, IOMNPs stand out as a possible choice to treat infectious diseases. The use of IOMNPs to oppose microorganism infection is quite relevant when thinking about this resistance. However, it may not overcome all kinds of bacterial resistance [97,104–108].

IOMNPs may act as actual antimicrobial agents, or even in a synergistic way with antimicrobial agents [29,98]. A dosage form containing IOMNPs synergically mixed with streptomycin was already developed; it was prepared in a chitosan-based structure. They performed a modified release from this system, enhancing the base activity of the streptomycin against methicillin-resistant *Staphylococcus aureus* (MRSA) [109]. Moreover, it was observed that a smaller size of the IOMNPs led to higher antimicrobial activity. Thus, it was observed that nanoparticles ranging from 10 to 80 nm in size could penetrate the *Escherichia coli* membrane and cause bacteria inactivation [16,98,110].

IOMNPs exhibit a number of advantages compared to conventional antimicrobial agents: they are less susceptible to bacterial resistance; they may be functionalized to several preferred targets or activities; they may be associated with natural or synthetic drugs; and it is possible to stimulate them with different sources such as heat, pH, magnetic field, light, etc. Nanoparticulate systems can also cross some barriers that the normally employed drugs cannot, such as the blood–brain barrier [16,108,111].

The use of IOMNPs as antimicrobial delivery systems against microorganisms located in different sites with difficult access is important. However, it is important to emphasize that most of the prepared IOMNPs show intrinsic antimicrobial activity without the addition of antibiotics [112].

Moreover, subcellular nanoparticle delivery is an important approach to justify the use of IOMNPs as antimicrobials. These nanoparticles show a high surface-area-to-volume ratio, which results into surfaces with very high free-energy content. In order to decrease this energy and become relatively stable, the surface interacts with possible interactomes present in the cell. The subcellular delivery involving the transfer of various drugs and bio-active molecules (e.g., proteins, peptides, DNAs) through the cell membrane into cells constitutes a very important strategy for antimicrobial applications as well [113].

Once IOMNPs enter the biological environment, they can adsorb surrounding biomolecules, conducing to the formation of a protein corona on the nanoparticle surface. The substances present in the environment where IOMNPs are located (e.g., proteins, metabolites, inorganic salts) and also the nanoparticle shape, size, chargeability, and surface modification can influence the formation of the protein corona [67]. Microorganisms can recognize the protein corona attached to the IOMNPs instead of the nanoparticles themselves. Thus, the destination of nanoparticles in the body and infected sites is dependent on the protein corona, which can also be fabricated by dynamic assemblies [11,77,80]. Protein crowns can determine the endocytosis or adsorption on cell/microorganism membranes, their circulation in the blood, or their maintenance in extracellular tissue for a long time [80,114].

The ability of IOMNPs to adsorb and penetrate into biofilms can be due to their physicochemical characteristics (hydrophobicity, surface charge, and high area ratio by volume) [6]. The antimicrobial activity of the agent erythromycin coupled to IOMNPs against bacterial cultures of *Streptococcus pneumoniae* was improved, and the bacterial viability was diminished in the presence of nanoparticles. Moreover, it was observed that IOMNPs helped erythromycin cross the capsule of the bacterium [115].

The bacteriocin nisin displays a wide spectrum of antimicrobial activity. However, it is commonly inefficient against Gram-negative bacteria. Targeted magnetic nisin-loaded nano-carriers (IOMNPs capped with citric, ascorbic, and gallic acids) were fabricated and tested to overcome the nisin resistance of bacteria. High pulsed electric and electromagnetic fields were applied, and Gram-positive *Bacillus subtilis* and Gram-negative *Escherichia coli* were utilized as cell models. This strategy increased the antimicrobial efficiency of nisin similar to electroporation or magnetic hyperthermia methods, and a synergistic treatment was also shown to be possible [116].

Some explanations for the IOMNP mechanism of action exist. One of them is clarified by the composition. IOMNPs are composed mainly by magnetite and maghemite, which have iron ions (Fe^{2+} and Fe^{3+}). These ions may cause the generation of reactive oxygen species (ROS), specifically superoxide (O^{2-}) and hydroxyl ($-OH$) or hydrogen peroxide (H_2O_2), or even singlet oxygen ($^1O_2$). These radicals may increase the ROS stress inside the microorganism's cells, leading to an inhibition of their growth and multiplication. ROS may damage the DNA in bacteria and also protein production [101,117,118].

A second possible mechanism is that the electrostatic energy of the nanoparticles could be used to bind them to proteins or to the cell membrane, leading to disruption of the essential functions, causing cell death [108,119–123].

Also, IOMNPs may act on the efflux pump of some microorganisms, acting as inhibitors to this pump that aids the cell to eliminate substances that may harm the organism; hence, it could even transport antimicrobial drugs to the outside, leading to a reduction in the drug efficacy [108]. Christena and collaborators prepared magnetic nanoparticles (MNPs) with casein, and they evaluated the inhibition property of the MNPs against the efflux pump of *Pseudomonas aeruginosa* and *Staphylococcus aureus* [124]. They showed that those MNPs were able really inhibit the activity of the efflux pump of those bacteria and, in this sense, would increase the activity of other antimicrobial drugs.

Interestingly, IOMNPs associated with propolis extract (PE) for an intraperiodontal pocket release were shown to be useful for the treatment of periodontal disease [29]. They showed that the incorporation of PE in the formulation containing IOMNPs increased the efficacy of the natural product against *Candida* spp., showing a great synergy between the PE and the IOMNPs.

An extract of *Argemone mexicana*, together with IOMNPs, was evaluated against *Escherichia coli*, *Proteus mirabilis*, and *Bacillus subtilis* [98]. They also stated a good interaction between the IOMNPs and the natural extract for antimicrobial activity.

Not only natural extracts were evaluated with IOMNPs against microorganisms. Maleki and collaborators functionalized IOMNPs with the antimicrobial peptide cecropin mellitin (CM) and evaluated them against *Staphylococcus aureus* and *E. coli* [125]. They also showed that this incorporation presented a synergic interaction.

In this context, IOMNPs can contribute to improving antimicrobial treatments by targeting specific and hard-to-reach sites where pathogens are harbored. Moreover, they can optimize physicochemical characteristics, enabling the clinical use of new antimicrobial agents, or their administration using more convenient routes [103].

5.5. Other Pharmaceutical Applications

Considering the characteristics of IOMNPs, they can also be utilized in the therapy of Alzheimer's disease. Magnetic Fe_3O_4 nanoparticles can interact with lysozyme amyloids in vitro, reducing the amyloid aggregates and promoting depolymerization. The proposed mechanism of the anti-aggregating action of these particles is based on the adsorption and adhesion of lysozyme molecules to the nanoparticles, decreasing the free lysozyme molecular concentration and hampering the nucleation process and fibrillogenesis [126]. However, further investigations are necessary to explore the detailed molecular mechanisms of the anti-amyloidogenic ability of the particles [32].

IOMNPs can deliver photosensitizers in photodynamic therapy (PDT) [32]. The combination of magnetic drug targeting and PDT can be accomplished using dextran coatings to prevent the nanoparticle aggregation and to allow for the linkage of hypericin. This strategy can increase the selectivity and reduce the side effects of PDT, as the therapy occurs only in the site where the IOMNPs are accumulated due to an external magnet, under the influence of a laser [127].

The integration of multiple moieties into a single nano-platform based on IOMNPs for diagnostic and treatment was also proposed. Additionally, IOMNPs can be used to integrate the diagnosis and therapy in one step. Currently, theranostic constitutes an important tendency in research [128]. Considering the unique magnetic properties of IOMNPs, they attracted great interest due to their use as MRI contrasting agents and for the therapy of tumors and other disorders. Cancer magnetic theranostics is attracting increasing interest and can provide a powerful strategy for cancer therapy. Theranostics based on IOMNPs enables tracking the theranostic agent's location, constantly controlling the therapeutic process, and evaluating the efficacy of the treatment [14]. Therefore, it is possible to improve the efficiency and functionality of the therapy [129].

6. Toxicity

Nanotoxicology refers to the study of the potentially harmful effects of nanomaterials on living organisms [21]. Nanoparticles can enter the human body through respiratory inhalation, dermal absorption, or via an oral route. They have nano size and can move across the olfactory mucosa, alveolar membrane, capillary endothelium, and the blood–brain barrier. Therefore, it is very important to understand the potential toxicity associated with IOMNPs, considering the range of surface modifications enabling functionalities of these nanoparticles [21,32,87]. In vitro and in vivo studies on IOMNP toxicity showed some conflicting results [6]. Changes in nanoparticle size and shape were reported as factors inherent to nanosystems able to influence their toxicity. Rod-shaped and nano-sized IOMNPs were shown to be more toxic than sphere-shaped and micrometric particles, respectively [130]. The configuration of the nanosystem can also influence IOMNP toxicity [6].

Furthermore, cell cytotoxicity and genotoxicity may be affected by the surface charge of IOMNPs. Positively charged nanoparticles were shown to be more toxic, because they may undergo nonspecific interactions and adsorptive endocytosis with the negatively charged cell membrane, thus increasing their intracellular accumulation and affecting cell membrane integrity [130]. The influence of other factors (e.g., concentration, form of administration, type of coating, and cell line) may explain the different results for toxicity of these nanoparticles, and they were properly revised in Reference [6].

The mechanisms of IOMNP toxicity for different cell lines are partially explained by the production of reactive oxygen species (ROS), which causes cellular oxidative stress [38,131]. When IOMNPs are taken up by cells via endocytosis, they tend to accumulate in the lysosomes and are degraded to iron ions. These ions would be able to pass through the membranes and reach regions such as the mitochondria and cell nucleus. There, they could react with hydrogen peroxide and oxygen, generating ROS [6].

Iron overload caused by exposure to IOMNPs can also conduce to serious deleterious effects and lead to cell death. Therefore, a high dose of IOMNPs could promote elevated lipid metabolism, breakage of iron homeostasis, and exacerbated loss of liver functions [6]. In contrast, magnetite (Fe_3O_4) was shown to increase the level of lipid peroxidation and decrease the antioxidant enzymes in human lung alveolar epithelial cells (A-549), displaying a concentration-dependent toxicity in vitro [132].

The strategy to coat the surface of IOMNPs is utilized to make these nanoparticles biocompatible and non-toxic, due to the lower number of oxidative sites, with consequently lower DNA damage [20]. To avoid the higher iron intracellular ROS production, coated IOMNPs using lauric acid, a protein corona of BSA, or dextran were developed and were shown to not promote genotoxic effects on human granulosa cells [133]. Polymers (e.g., PLGA) and essential oils (e.g., patchouli essential oil) were shown to reduce the toxic effects of IOMNPs [6].

Therefore, there is an increasing necessity to perform additional tests other than cell viability assays to increase the knowledge about the toxic effects of these IOMNPs.

7. Concluding Remarks

The use of IOMNPs in pharmaceutical areas increased in the last two decades. The uses of these nanoparticles are due to their excellent properties in terms of size, mechanical, optical, and magnetic properties, displaying great potential for pharmaceutical applications. Their surface can be functionalized with targeting ligands, as well as imaging and therapeutic moieties, enabling the development of multifunctional, multimodal nanoagents.

However, these nanoparticles should be stable and have a switchable magnetic state, independent of temperature fluctuations and considering the biological environment. The synthesis process selection should consider the reproducibility and scaling up without any complex purification procedure. Therefore, several synthesis methods were investigated using either organic or aqueous phases, and they are classified into physical, chemical, and biological approaches. Moreover, the synthesis of these nanoparticles into formulations is possible, aiming at the production of more stable, biocompatible, highly dispersible, shape- and size-controlled nanoparticles.

The protection (encapsulation, coating, or dispersion) of IOMNPs with biocompatible materials can avoid their aggregation, biodegradation, and alterations from the original state and also enable entrapping the bioactive agent on the particle via adsorption or covalent attachment. In this context, IOMNPs show great potential for use in nanostructured pharmaceutical systems for target drug delivery, improving the therapy as a consequence of a higher drug effect using lower concentrations, thus reducing side effects and toxicity. Different methodologies of synthesis allowed the preparation of IOMNPs displaying different structures, sizes, dispersions, and surface modifications. These advantages support the utilization of IOMNPs in pharmaceutical applications, and getting suitable drug release control on the target tissues could be beneficial in several clinical situations, such as infections, inflammations, and tumors. However, more toxicological clinical investigations about IOMNPs are necessary, considering their pharmaceutical applications.

Author Contributions: The work was conceptualized, designed, drafted, and revised by M.L.B. and L.d.A.S.d.T.

Funding: This research received no external funding.

Acknowledgments: The authors thank the financial support of the Brazilian funding agencies CNPq (National Counsel of Technological and Scientific Development) and CAPES (Coordination of Improvement of Higher Education Personnel).

Conflicts of Interest: The authors declare no conflicts of interest.

References

1. Akbarzadeh, A.; Samiei, M.; Davaran, S. Magnetic nanoparticles: Preparation, physical properties, and applications in biomedicine. *Nanoscale Res. Lett.* **2012**, *7*, 144. [CrossRef] [PubMed]
2. Feynman, R.P. Plenty of Room at the Bottom. In Proceedings of the APS Annual Meeting, Pasadena, CA, USA, 29 December 1959; Volume 23, pp. 22–36.
3. Campos, E.A.; Pinto, D.V.B.S.; de Oliveira, J.I.S.; da Costa Mattos, E.; de Cássia Lazzarini Dutra, R. Synthesis, Characterization and Applications of Iron Oxide Nanoparticles—A Short Review. *J. Aerosp. Technol. Manag.* **2015**, *7*, 267–276. [CrossRef]
4. Veintemillas-Verdaguer, S.; Serna, C.J.; Morales, M.D.P.; González-Carreño, T.; Tartaj, P. The preparation of magnetic nanoparticles for applications in biomedicine. *J. Phys. D Appl. Phys.* **2003**, *36*, R182.
5. Aftab, S.; Shah, A.; Nadhman, A.; Kurbanoglu, S.; Ozkan, S.A.; Dionysiou, D.D.; Shukla, S.S.; Aminabhavi, T.M. Nanomedicine: An effective tool in cancer therapy. *Int. J. Pharm.* **2018**, *540*, 132–149. [CrossRef]
6. Arias, L.S.; Pessan, J.P.; Vieira, A.P.M.; De Lima, T.M.T.; Delbem, A.C.B.; Monteiro, D.R. Iron Oxide Nanoparticles for Biomedical Applications: A Perspective on Synthesis, Drugs, Antimicrobial Activity, and Toxicity. *Antibiotics* **2018**, *7*, 46. [CrossRef] [PubMed]
7. Bilal, M.; Zhao, Y.; Rasheed, T.; Iqbal, H.M. Magnetic nanoparticles as versatile carriers for enzymes immobilization: A review. *Int. J. Biol. Macromol.* **2018**, *120*, 2530–2544. [CrossRef] [PubMed]
8. Bulte, J.W. Superparamagnetic iron oxides as MPI tracers: A primer and review of early applications. *Adv. Drug Deliv. Rev.* **2019**, *138*, 293–301. [CrossRef] [PubMed]
9. Davaran, S.; Rashidi, M.R.; Hashemi, M. Synthesis and Characterization of Methacrylic Derivatives of 5-Amino Salicylic Acid with PH-Sensitive Swelling Properties. *AAPS PharmSciTech* **2004**, *2*, 80–85. [CrossRef]
10. McCarthy, J.R.; Kelly, K.A.; Sun, E.Y.; Weissleder, R. Targeted delivery of multifunctional magnetic nanoparticles. *Nanomedicine* **2007**, *2*, 153–167. [CrossRef]
11. Lu, J.; Kong, X.; Hyeon, T.; Ling, D.; Li, F. Dynamic Nanoparticle Assemblies for Biomedical Applications. *Adv. Mater.* **2017**, *29*, 1605897.
12. Chen, Y.; Ding, X.; Zhang, Y.; Natalia, A.; Sun, X.; Wang, Z.; Shao, H. Design and synthesis of magnetic nanoparticles for biomedical diagnostics. *Quant. Imaging Med. Surg.* **2018**, *8*, 957–970. [CrossRef] [PubMed]
13. Champagne, P.O.; Westwick, H.; Bouthillier, A.; Sawan, M. Colloidal stability of superparamagnetic iron oxide nanoparticles in the central nervous system: A review. *Nanomedicine* **2018**, *13*, 1385–1400. [CrossRef] [PubMed]
14. Xie, W.; Guo, Z.; Gao, F.; Gao, Q.; Wang, D.; Liaw, B.S.; Cai, Q.; Sun, X.; Wang, X.; Zhao, L. Shape-, size-and structure-controlled synthesis and biocompatibility of iron oxide nanoparticles for magnetic theranostics. *Theranostics* **2018**, *8*, 3284–3307. [CrossRef] [PubMed]

15. Niemirowicz, K.; Markiewicz, K.; Wilczewska, A.; Car, H. Magnetic nanoparticles as new diagnostic tools in medicine. *Adv. Med. Sci.* **2012**, *57*, 196–207. [CrossRef] [PubMed]
16. de Toledo, L.A.S.; Rosseto, H.C.; Bruschi, M.L. Iron oxide magnetic nanoparticles as antimicrobials for therapeutics. *Pharm. Dev. Technol.* **2017**, *23*, 316–323. [CrossRef] [PubMed]
17. Noqta, O.A.; Aziz, A.A.; Usman, I.A.; Bououdina, M. Recent Advances in Iron Oxide Nanoparticles (IONPs): Synthesis and Surface Modification for Biomedical Applications. *J. Supercond. Nov. Magn.* **2019**, *32*, 779–795. [CrossRef]
18. Ling, W.; Wang, M.; Xiong, C.; Xie, D.; Chen, Q.; Chu, X.; Qiu, X.; Li, Y.; Xiao, X. Synthesis, surface modification, and applications of magnetic iron oxide nanoparticles. *J. Mater. Res.* **2019**, *34*, 1828–1844. [CrossRef]
19. Garcell, L.; Morales, M.; Andres-Verges, M.; Tartaj, P.; Serna, C.; Morales, M.D.P. Interfacial and Rheological Characteristics of Maghemite Aqueous Suspensions. *J. Colloid Interface Sci.* **1998**, *205*, 470–475. [CrossRef] [PubMed]
20. Mahmoudi, M.; Sant, S.; Wang, B.; Laurent, S.; Sen, T. Superparamagnetic iron oxide nanoparticles (SPIONs): Development, surface modification and applications in chemotherapy. *Adv. Drug Deliv. Rev.* **2011**, *63*, 24–46. [CrossRef]
21. Assa, F.; Jafarizadeh-Malmiri, H.; Ajamein, H.; Anarjan, N.; Vaghari, H.; Sayyar, Z.; Berenjian, A. A biotechnological perspective on the application of iron oxide nanoparticles. *Nano Res.* **2016**, *9*, 2203–2225. [CrossRef]
22. Banerjee, T.; Mitra, S.; Singh, A.K.; Sharma, R.K.; Maitra, A. Preparation, characterization and biodistribution of ultrafine chitosan nanoparticles. *Int. J. Pharm.* **2002**, *243*, 93–105. [CrossRef]
23. Longmire, M.; Choyke, P.L.; Kobayashi, H. Clearance properties of nano-sized particles and molecules as imaging agents: considerations and caveats. *Nanomedicine* **2008**, *3*, 703–717. [CrossRef] [PubMed]
24. Romberg, B.; Hennink, W.E.; Storm, G. Sheddable Coatings for Long-Circulating Nanoparticles. *Pharm. Res.* **2008**, *25*, 55–71. [CrossRef] [PubMed]
25. Philipse, A.P.; Van Bruggen, M.P.B.; Pathmamanoharan, C. Magnetic silica dispersions: Preparation and stability of surface-modified silica particles with a magnetic core. *Langmuir* **1994**, *10*, 92–99. [CrossRef]
26. Jahangirian, H.; Kalantari, K.; Izadiyan, Z.; Rafiee-Moghaddam, R.; Shameli, K.; Webster, T.J. A review of small molecules and drug delivery applications using gold and iron nanoparticles. *Int. J. Nanomed.* **2019**, *14*, 1633–1657. [CrossRef] [PubMed]
27. MacHala, L.; Tuček, J.; Zbořil, R. Polymorphous Transformations of Nanometric Iron (III) Oxide: A Review. *Chem. Mater.* **2011**, *23*, 3255–3272. [CrossRef]
28. Xu, H.; Wang, X.; Zhang, L. Selective preparation of nanorods and micro-octahedrons of Fe_2O_3 and their catalytic performances for thermal decomposition of ammonium perchlorate. *Powder Technol.* **2008**, *185*, 176–180. [CrossRef]
29. de Alcântara Sica de Toledo, L.; Rosseto, H.C.; Dos Santos, R.S.; Spizzo, F.; Del Bianco, L.; Montanha, M.C.; Esposito, E.; Kimura, E.; Bonfim-Mendonça, P.D.S.; Svidzinski, T.I.E.; et al. Thermal Magnetic Field Activated Propolis Release From Liquid Crystalline System Based on Magnetic Nanoparticles. *AAPS PharmSciTech* **2018**, *19*, 3258–3271. [CrossRef]
30. El-Boubbou, K. Magnetic iron oxide nanoparticles as drug carriers: Clinical relevance. *Nanomedicine* **2018**, *13*, 953–971. [CrossRef]
31. Dadfar, S.M.; Roemhild, K.; Drude, N.I.; Von Stillfried, S.; Knüchel, R.; Kiessling, F.; Lammers, T. Iron oxide nanoparticles: Diagnostic, therapeutic and theranostic applications. *Adv. Drug Deliv. Rev.* **2019**, *138*, 302–325. [CrossRef]
32. Dulińska-Litewka, J.; Łazarczyk, A.; Hałubiec, P.; Szafrański, O.; Karnas, K.; Karewicz, A. Superparamagnetic Iron Oxide Nanoparticles—Current and Prospective Medical Applications. *Materials* **2019**, *12*, 617. [CrossRef] [PubMed]
33. de Souza Ferreira, S.B.; Bruschi, M.L. Improving the Bioavailability of Curcumin: Is Micro/Nanoencapsulation the Key? *Ther. Deliv.* **2019**, *10*, 83–86. [CrossRef] [PubMed]
34. Pinel, S.; Thomas, N.; Boura, C.; Barberi-Heyob, M. Approaches to physical stimulation of metallic nanoparticles for glioblastoma treatment. *Adv. Drug Deliv. Rev.* **2019**, *138*, 344–357. [CrossRef] [PubMed]
35. Jun, Y.W.; Huh, Y.M.; Choi, J.S.; Lee, J.H.; Song, H.T.; Kim, S.; Yoon, S.; Kim, K.S.; Shin, J.S.; Suh, J.S.; et al. Nanoscale Size Effect of Magnetic Nanocrystals and Their Utilization for Cancer Diagnosis via Magnetic Resonance Imaging. *J. Am. Chem. Soc.* **2005**, *127*, 5732–5733. [CrossRef] [PubMed]

36. Nunes, A.C.; Yu, Z.C. Fractionation of a water-based ferrofluid. *J. Magn. Magn. Mater.* **1987**, *65*, 265–268. [CrossRef]
37. Gupta, A.K.; Gupta, M. Synthesis and surface engineering of iron oxide nanoparticles for biomedical applications. *Biomaterials* **2005**, *26*, 3995–4021. [CrossRef] [PubMed]
38. Laurent, S.; Forge, D.; Port, M.; Roch, A.; Robic, C.; Elst, L.V.; Muller, R.N. Magnetic Iron Oxide Nanoparticles: Synthesis, Stabilization, Vectorization, Physicochemical Characterizations, and Biological Applications. *Chem. Rev.* **2008**, *108*, 2064–2110. [CrossRef]
39. Fazio, E.; Santoro, M.; Lentini, G.; Franco, D.; Guglielmino, S.P.P.; Neri, F. Iron oxide nanoparticles prepared by laser ablation: Synthesis, structural properties and antimicrobial activity. *Colloids Surf. A Physicochem. Eng. Asp.* **2016**, *490*, 98–103. [CrossRef]
40. Gupta, R.; Bajpai, A.K. Magnetically Guided Release of Ciprofloxacin from Superparamagnetic Polymer Nanocomposites. *J. Biomater. Sci. Polym. Ed.* **2011**, *22*, 893–918. [CrossRef]
41. Fracasso, G.; Ghigna, P.; Nodari, L.; Agnoli, S.; Badocco, D.; Pastore, P.; Nicolato, E.; Marzola, P.; Mihajlovic, D.; Marković, M.; et al. Nanoaggregates of iron poly-oxo-clusters obtained by laser ablation in aqueous solution of phosphonates. *J. Colloid Interface Sci.* **2018**, *522*, 208–216. [CrossRef]
42. Sun, S.; Zeng, H. Size-Controlled Synthesis of Magnetite Nanoparticles. *J. Am. Chem. Soc.* **2002**, *124*, 8204–8205. [CrossRef] [PubMed]
43. Wu, W.; He, Q.; Jiang, C. Magnetic Iron Oxide Nanoparticles: Synthesis and Surface Functionalization Strategies. *Nanoscale Res. Lett.* **2008**, *3*, 397–415. [CrossRef] [PubMed]
44. Bumajdad, A.; Ali, S.; Mathew, A. Characterization of iron hydroxide/oxide nanoparticles prepared in microemulsions stabilized with cationic/non-ionic surfactant mixtures. *J. Colloid Interface Sci.* **2011**, *355*, 282–292. [CrossRef] [PubMed]
45. Dai, Z.; Meiser, F.; Möhwald, H. Nanoengineering of iron oxide and iron oxide/silica hollow spheres by sequential layering combined with a sol–gel process. *J. Colloid Interface Sci.* **2005**, *288*, 298–300. [CrossRef] [PubMed]
46. Teja, A.S.; Koh, P.Y. Synthesis, properties, and applications of magnetic iron oxide nanoparticles. *Prog. Cryst. Growth Charact. Mater.* **2009**, *55*, 22–45. [CrossRef]
47. Sodipo, B.K.; Aziz, A.A. One minute synthesis of amino-silane functionalized superparamagnetic iron oxide nanoparticles by sonochemical method. *Ultrason. Sonochem.* **2018**, *40*, 837–840. [CrossRef]
48. Osborne, E.A.; Atkins, T.M.; Gilbert, D.A.; Kauzlarich, S.M.; Liu, K.; Louie, A.Y. Rapid microwave-assisted synthesis of dextran-coated iron oxide nanoparticles for magnetic resonance imaging. *Nanotechnology* **2012**, *23*, 215602. [CrossRef]
49. Fatemi, M.; Mollania, N.; Momeni-Moghaddam, M.; Sadeghifar, F.; Momeni-Moghaddam, M. Extracellular biosynthesis of magnetic iron oxide nanoparticles by Bacillus cereus strain HMH1: Characterization and in vitro cytotoxicity analysis on MCF-7 and 3T3 cell lines. *J. Biotechnol.* **2018**, *270*, 1–11. [CrossRef]
50. Helminger, M.; Wu, B.; Kollmann, T.; Benke, D.; Schwahn, D.; Pipich, V.; Faivre, D.; Zahn, D.; Cölfen, H. Synthesis and Characterization of Gelatin-Based Magnetic Hydrogels. *Adv. Funct. Mater.* **2014**, *24*, 3187–3196. [CrossRef]
51. Liu, H.; Wang, C.; Gao, Q.; Liu, X.; Tong, Z. Magnetic hydrogels with supracolloidal structures prepared by suspension polymerization stabilized by Fe_2O_3 nanoparticles. *Acta Biomater.* **2010**, *6*, 275–281. [CrossRef]
52. Shaterabadi, Z.; Nabiyouni, G.; Soleymani, M. High impact of in situ dextran coating on biocompatibility, stability and magnetic properties of iron oxide nanoparticles. *Mater. Sci. Eng. C* **2017**, *75*, 947–956. [CrossRef] [PubMed]
53. Kang, T.; Li, F.; Baik, S.; Shao, W.; Ling, D.; Hyeon, T. Surface design of magnetic nanoparticles for stimuli-responsive cancer imaging and therapy. *Biomaterials* **2017**, *136*, 98–114. [CrossRef] [PubMed]
54. Ulbrich, K.; Holá, K.; Šubr, V.; Bakandritsos, A.; Tuček, J.; Zboril, R. Targeted Drug Delivery with Polymers and Magnetic Nanoparticles: Covalent and Noncovalent Approaches, Release Control, and Clinical Studies. *Chem. Rev.* **2016**, *116*, 5338–5431. [CrossRef] [PubMed]
55. Moghimi, S.M.; Hunter, A.C.; Murray, J.C. Long-circulating and target-specific nanoparticles: Theory to practice. *Pharmacol. Rev.* **2001**, *53*, 283–318. [PubMed]
56. Wang, S.; Huang, P.; Chen, X. Hierarchical Targeting Strategy for Enhanced Tumor Tissue Accumulation/Retention and Cellular Internalization. *Adv. Mater.* **2016**, *28*, 7340–7364. [CrossRef] [PubMed]

57. Gutierrez, L.; De La Cueva, L.; Moros, M.; Mazario, E.; De Bernardo, S.; De La Fuente, J.M.; Morales, M.P.; Salas, G.; Morales, M.D.P. Aggregation effects on the magnetic properties of iron oxide colloids. *Nanotechnology* **2019**, *30*, 112001. [CrossRef]
58. Tartaj, P.; Morales, M.P.; Veintemillas-Verdaguer, S.; Gonzalez-Carreno, T.; Serna, C. *Synthesis, Properties and Biomedical Applications of Magnetic Nanoparticles*; Elsevier: Amsterdam, The Netherlands, 2006.
59. Nel, A.E.; Mädler, L.; Velegol, D.; Xia, T.; Hoek, E.M.V.; Somasundaran, P.; Klaessig, F.; Castranova, V.; Thompson, M. Understanding biophysicochemical interactions at the nano-bio interface. *Nat. Mater.* **2009**, *8*, 543–557. [CrossRef]
60. Kooijmans, S.A.A.; Fliervoet, L.A.L.; Van Der Meel, R.; Fens, M.H.A.M.; Heijnen, H.F.G.; Van Bergen En Henegouwen, P.M.P.; Vader, P.; Schiffelers, R.M. PEGylated and Targeted Extracellular Vesicles Display Enhanced Cell Specificity and Circulation Time. *J. Control. Release* **2016**, *224*, 77–85. [CrossRef]
61. Kralj, S.; Makovec, D. Magnetic Assembly of Superparamagnetic Iron Oxide Nanoparticle Clusters into Nanochains and Nanobundles. *ACS Nano* **2015**, *9*, 9700–9707. [CrossRef]
62. Kucharczyk, K.; Rybka, J.D.; Hilgendorff, M.; Krupinski, M.; Slachcinski, M.; Mackiewicz, A.; Giersig, M.; Dams-Kozlowska, H. Composite spheres made of bioengineered spider silk and iron oxide nanoparticles for theranostics applications. *PLoS ONE* **2019**, *14*, e0219790. [CrossRef]
63. Rittikulsittichai, S.; Kolhatkar, A.; Sarangi, S.; Vorontsova, M.; Vekilov, P.; Brazdeikis, A.; Lee, T.R. Multi-responsive Hybrid Particles: Thermo-, pH-, Photo-, and Magneto-responsive Magnetic Hydrogel Cores with Gold Nanorod Optical Triggers. *Nanoscale* **2016**, *8*, 11851–11861. [CrossRef] [PubMed]
64. Gallo, J.; Kamaly, N.; Lavdas, I.; Stevens, E.; Nguyen, Q.D.; Wylezinska-Arridge, M.; Aboagye, E.O.; Long, N.J. CXCR4-Targeted and MMP-Responsive Iron Oxide Nanoparticles for Enhanced Magnetic Resonance Imaging. *Angew. Chem. Int. Ed.* **2014**, *53*, 9550–9554. [CrossRef] [PubMed]
65. Connolly, S.; Fitzmaurice, D. Programmed Assembly of Gold Nanocrystals in Aqueous Solution. *Adv. Mater.* **1999**, *11*, 1202–1205. [CrossRef]
66. Von Maltzahn, G.; Min, D.H.; Zhang, Y.; Park, J.H.; Harris, T.J.; Sailor, M.; Bhatia, S.N. Nanoparticle Self-Assembly Directed by Antagonistic Kinase and Phosphatase Activities. *Adv. Mater.* **2007**, *19*, 3579–3583. [CrossRef]
67. Wang, S.; Zhang, B.; Su, L.; Nie, W.; Han, D.; Han, G.; Zhang, H.; Chong, C.; Tan, J. Subcellular distributions of iron oxide nanoparticles in rat brains affected by different surface modifications. *J. Biomed. Mater. Res. Part A* **2019**, *107*, 1988–1998. [CrossRef] [PubMed]
68. Ling, D.; Park, W.; Park, S.J.; Lu, Y.; Kim, K.S.; Hackett, M.J.; Kim, B.H.; Yim, H.; Jeon, Y.S.; Na, K.; et al. Multifunctional Tumor pH-Sensitive Self-Assembled Nanoparticles for Bimodal Imaging and Treatment of Resistant Heterogeneous Tumors. *J. Am. Chem. Soc.* **2014**, *136*, 5647–5655. [CrossRef] [PubMed]
69. Jing, Y.; Zhu, Y.; Yang, X.; Shen, J.; Li, C. Ultrasound-Triggered Smart Drug Release from Multifunctional Core–Shell Capsules One-Step Fabricated by Coaxial Electrospray Method. *Langmuir* **2011**, *27*, 1175–1180. [CrossRef]
70. GhavamiNejad, A.; Sasikala, A.R.K.; Unnithan, A.R.; Thomas, R.G.; Jeong, Y.Y.; Vatankhah-Varnoosfaderani, M.; Stadler, F.; Park, C.H.; Kim, C.S. Mussel-Inspired Electrospun Smart Magnetic Nanofibers for Hyperthermic Chemotherapy. *Adv. Funct. Mater.* **2015**, *25*, 2867–2875. [CrossRef]
71. Bhattacharya, S.; Eckert, F.; Boyko, V.; Pich, A. Temperature-, PH-and Magnetic-Field-Sensitive Hybrid Microgels. *Small* **2007**, *3*, 650–657. [CrossRef]
72. Li, J.; Zeng, J.; Du, P.; Liu, L.; Tian, K.; Jia, X.; Zhao, X.; Liu, P. Superparamagnetic Reduction/pH/Temperature Multistimuli-Responsive Nanoparticles for Targeted and Controlled Antitumor Drug Delivery. *Mol. Pharm.* **2015**, *12*, 4188–4199.
73. Rao, N.V.; Ganivada, M.N.; Sarkar, S.; Dinda, H.; Chatterjee, K.; Dalui, T.; Shunmugam, R.; Das Sarma, J. Magnetic Norbornene Polymer as Multiresponsive Nanocarrier for Site Specific Cancer Therapy. *Bioconjug. Chem.* **2014**, *25*, 276–285. [CrossRef] [PubMed]
74. Al-Shakarchi, W.; Alsuraifi, A.; Curtis, A.; Hoskins, C. Dual Acting Polymeric Nano-Aggregates for Liver Cancer Therapy. *Pharmaceutics* **2018**, *10*, 63. [CrossRef] [PubMed]
75. Jeon, H.; Kim, J.; Lee, Y.M.; Kim, J.; Choi, H.W.; Lee, J.; Park, H.; Kang, Y.; Kim, I.S.; Lee, B.H.; et al. Poly-paclitaxel/cyclodextrin-SPION nano-assembly for magnetically guided drug delivery system. *J. Control. Release* **2016**, *231*, 68–76. [CrossRef] [PubMed]

76. Baskaran, M.; Baskaran, P.; Arulsamy, N.; Thyagarajan, B. Preparation and Evaluation of PLGA-Coated Capsaicin Magnetic Nanoparticles. *Pharm. Res.* **2017**, *34*, 1255–1263. [CrossRef] [PubMed]
77. Hannecart, A.; Stanicki, D.; Elst, L.V.; Muller, R.N.; Brûlet, A.; Sandre, O.; Schatz, C.; Lecommandoux, S.; Laurent, S. Embedding of superparamagnetic iron oxide nanoparticles into membranes of well-defined poly(ethylene oxide)-block-poly(ε-caprolactone) nanoscale magnetovesicles as ultrasensitive MRI probes of membrane bio-degradation. *J. Mater. Chem. B* **2019**, *7*, 4692–4705. [CrossRef] [PubMed]
78. Hao, X.; Xu, B.; Chen, H.; Wang, X.; Zhang, J.; Guo, R.; Shi, X.; Cao, X. Stem Cell-Mediated Delivery of Nanogels Loaded with Ultrasmall Iron Oxide Nanoparticles for Enhanced Tumor MR Imaging. *Nanoscale* **2019**, *11*, 4904–4910. [CrossRef]
79. Bruschi, M.L. *Strategies to Modify the Drug Release from Pharmaceutical Systems*; Elsevier: Amsterdam, The Netherlands, 2015. [CrossRef]
80. Li, F.; Liang, Z.; Liu, J.; Sun, J.; Hu, X.; Zhao, M.; Liu, J.; Bai, R.; Kim, D.; Sun, X.; et al. Dynamically Reversible Iron Oxide Nanoparticle Assemblies for Targeted Amplification of T1-Weighted Magnetic Resonance Imaging of Tumors. *Nano Lett.* **2019**, *19*, 4213–4220. [CrossRef]
81. Butoescu, N.; Jordan, O.; Burdet, P.; Stadelmann, P.; Petri-Fink, A.; Hofmann, H.; Doelker, E.; Fink, A. Dexamethasone-containing biodegradable superparamagnetic microparticles for intra-articular administration: Physicochemical and magnetic properties, in vitro and in vivo drug release. *Eur. J. Pharm. Biopharm.* **2009**, *72*, 529–538. [CrossRef]
82. Li, L.; Chen, D.; Zhang, Y.; Deng, Z.; Ren, X.; Meng, X.; Tang, F.; Ren, J.; Zhang, L. Magnetic and fluorescent multifunctional chitosan nanoparticles as a smart drug delivery system. *Nanotechnology* **2007**, *18*, 405102. [CrossRef]
83. Parsian, M.; Unsoy, G.; Mutlu, P.; Yalcin, S.; Tezcaner, A.; Gündüz, U. Loading of Gemcitabine on chitosan magnetic nanoparticles increases the anti-cancer efficacy of the drug. *Eur. J. Pharmacol.* **2016**, *784*, 121–128. [CrossRef]
84. Prabaharan, M. Review Paper: Chitosan Derivatives as Promising Materials for Controlled Drug Delivery. *J. Biomater. Appl.* **2008**, *23*, 5–36. [CrossRef] [PubMed]
85. Saikia, C.; Hussain, A.; Ramteke, A.; Sharma, H.K.; Maji, T.K. Carboxymethyl Starch-Chitosan-Coated Iron Oxide Magnetic Nanoparticles for Controlled Delivery of Isoniazid. *J. Microencapsul.* **2015**, *32*, 29–39. [CrossRef] [PubMed]
86. Soares, P.; Lochte, F.; Echeverria, C.; Pereira, L.C.; Coutinho, J.T.; Ferreira, I.M.; Novo, C.M.; Borges, J.P. Thermal and magnetic properties of iron oxide colloids: Influence of surfactants. *Nanotechnology* **2015**, *26*, 425704. [CrossRef] [PubMed]
87. Luchini, A.; Heenan, R.K.; Paduano, L.; Vitiello, G. Functionalized SPIONs: The surfactant nature modulates the self-assembly and cluster formation. *Phys. Chem. Chem. Phys.* **2016**, *18*, 18441–18449. [CrossRef] [PubMed]
88. Ivashchenko, O.; Lewandowski, M.; Peplińska, B.; Jarek, M.; Nowaczyk, G.; Wiesner, M.; Załęski, K.; Babutina, T.; Warowicka, A.; Jurga, S.; et al. Synthesis and characterization of magnetite/silver/antibiotic nanocomposites for targeted antimicrobial therapy. *Mater. Sci. Eng. C* **2015**, *55*, 343–359. [CrossRef]
89. Bisht, G.; Rayamajhi, S.; Kc, B.; Paudel, S.N.; Karna, D.; Shrestha, B.G. Synthesis, Characterization, and Study of In Vitro Cytotoxicity of ZnO-Fe$_3$O$_4$ Magnetic Composite Nanoparticles in Human Breast Cancer Cell Line (MDA-MB-231) and Mouse Fibroblast (NIH$_3$T$_3$). *Nanoscale Res. Lett.* **2016**, *11*, 537. [CrossRef]
90. Jahanban-Esfahlan, A.; Dastmalchi, S.; Davaran, S. A simple improved desolvation method for the rapid preparation of albumin nanoparticles. *Int. J. Biol. Macromol.* **2016**, *91*, 703–709. [CrossRef]
91. Nosrati, H.; Sefidi, N.; Sharafi, A.; Danafar, H.; Kheiri Manjili, H. Bovine Serum Albumin (BSA) Coated Iron Oxide Magnetic Nanoparticles as Biocompatible Carriers for Curcumin-Anticancer Drug. *Bioorg. Chem.* **2018**, *76*, 501–509. [CrossRef]
92. Alexiou, C.; Schmid, R.J.; Jurgons, R.; Kremer, M.; Wanner, G.; Bergemann, C.; Huenges, E.; Nawroth, T.; Arnold, W.; Parak, F.G. Targeting cancer cells: Magnetic nanoparticles as drug carriers. *Eur. Biophys. J.* **2006**, *35*, 446–450. [CrossRef]
93. World Health Organization. *How to Investigate Drug Use in Health Facilities*; World Health Organization: Geneva, Switzerland, 1993.
94. Cameron, A.; Ewen, M.; Auton, M.; Abegunde, D. *The World Medicines Situation 2011*, 3rd ed.; World Health Organization: Geneva, Switzerland, 2011.

95. Gallo, J.M.; Varkonyi, P.; Hassan, E.E.; Groothius, D.R. Targeting anticancer drugs to the brain: II. Physiological pharmacokinetic model of oxantrazole following intraarterial administration to rat glioma-2 (RG-2) bearing rats. *J. Pharmacokinet. Biopharm.* **1993**, *21*, 575–592. [CrossRef]
96. Willard, M.A.; Kurihara, L.K.; Carpenter, E.E.; Calvin, S.; Harris, V.G. *Encyclopedia of Nanoscience and Nanotechnology*; American Scientific Publishers: Valencia, Spain, 2004.
97. Lima, M.G.; Álvares, J.; Guerra, A.A., Jr.; Costa, E.A.; Guibu, I.A.; Soeiro, O.M.; Leite, S.N.; de Oliveira Karnikowski, M.G.; Costa, K.S.; de Assis Acurcio, F. Indicators related to the rational use of medicines and its associated factors. *Rev. Saúde Pública* **2017**, *51*. [CrossRef] [PubMed]
98. Arokiyaraj, S.; Saravanan, M.; Prakash, N.U.; Arasu, M.V.; Vijayakumar, B.; Vincent, S. Enhanced antibacterial activity of iron oxide magnetic nanoparticles treated with Argemone mexicana L. leaf extract: An in vitro study. *Mater. Res. Bull.* **2013**, *48*, 3323–3327. [CrossRef]
99. Kim, J.S.; Kuk, E.; Yu, K.N.; Kim, J.H.; Park, S.J.; Lee, H.J.; Kim, S.H.; Park, Y.K.; Park, Y.H.; Hwang, C.Y.; et al. Antimicrobial effects of silver nanoparticles. *Nanomed. Nanotechnol. Biol. Med.* **2007**, *3*, 95–101. [CrossRef] [PubMed]
100. Chen, W.Y.; Lin, J.Y.; Chen, W.J.; Luo, L.; Diau, E.W.G.; Chen, Y.C. Functional gold nanoclusters as antimicrobial agents for antibiotic-resistant bacteria. *Nanomedicine* **2010**, *5*, 755–764. [CrossRef] [PubMed]
101. Webster, T.J.T. Bactericidal effect of iron oxide nanoparticles on Staphylococcus aureus. *Int. J. Nanomed.* **2010**, *5*, 277. [CrossRef]
102. Valodkar, M.; Modi, S.; Pal, A.; Thakore, S. Synthesis and anti-bacterial activity of Cu, Ag and Cu–Ag alloy nanoparticles: A green approach. *Mater. Res. Bull.* **2011**, *46*, 384–389. [CrossRef]
103. Rodrigues, G.R.; López-Abarrategui, C.; de la Serna Gómez, I.; Dias, S.C.; Otero-González, A.J.; Franco, O.L. Antimicrobial magnetic nanoparticles based-therapies for controlling infectious diseases. *Int. J. Pharm.* **2019**, *555*, 356–367. [CrossRef]
104. Neu, H.C. The Crisis in Antibiotic Resistance. *Science* **1992**, *257*, 1064–1073. [CrossRef]
105. Kapil, A. The challenge of antibiotic resistance: Need to contemplate. *Indian J. Med. Res.* **2005**, *121*, 83–91.
106. Alanis, A.J. Resistance to Antibiotics: Are We in the Post-Antibiotic Era? *Arch. Med. Res.* **2005**, *36*, 697–705. [CrossRef]
107. Huang, K.S.; Shieh, D.B.; Yeh, C.S.; Wu, P.C.; Cheng, F.Y. Antimicrobial applications of water-dispersible magnetic nanoparticles in biomedicine. *Curr. Med. Chem.* **2014**, *21*, 3312–3322. [CrossRef] [PubMed]
108. Ahmed, K.B.A.; Raman, T.; Veerappan, A. Future prospects of antibacterial metal nanoparticles as enzyme inhibitor. *Mater. Sci. Eng. C* **2016**, *68*, 939–947. [CrossRef] [PubMed]
109. Hussein-Al-Ali, S.H.; El Zowalaty, M.E.; Hussein, M.Z.; Ismail, M.; Webster, T.J. Synthesis, characterization, controlled release, and antibacterial studies of a novel streptomycin chitosan magnetic nanoantibiotic. *Int. J. Nanomed.* **2014**, *9*, 549–557.
110. Lee, C.; Kim, J.Y.; Lee, W.I.; Nelson, K.L.; Yoon, J.; Sedlak, D.L. Bactericidal Effect of Zero-Valent Iron Nanoparticles on Escherichia coli. *Environ. Sci. Technol.* **2008**, *42*, 4927–4933. [CrossRef] [PubMed]
111. Hu, Y.L.; Gao, J.Q. Potential neurotoxicity of nanoparticles. *Int. J. Pharm.* **2010**, *394*, 115–121. [CrossRef] [PubMed]
112. Shekoufeh, B.; Azhar, L.; Lotfipour, F. Magnetic Nanoparticles for Antimicrobial Drug Delivery. *Pharmazie* **2012**, *67*, 817–821. [CrossRef]
113. Xu, Z.P.; Zeng, Q.H.; Lu, G.Q.; Yu, A.B. Inorganic nanoparticles as carriers for efficient cellular delivery. *Chem. Eng. Sci.* **2006**, *61*, 1027–1040. [CrossRef]
114. Hohnholt, M.C.; Geppert, M.; Luther, E.M.; Petters, C.; Bulcke, F.; Dringen, R. Handling of Iron Oxide and Silver Nanoparticles by Astrocytes. *Neurochem. Res.* **2013**, *38*, 227–239. [CrossRef]
115. Aparicio-Caamaño, M.; Carrillo-Morales, M.; Olivares-Trejo, J.J. Iron Oxide Nanoparticle Improve the Antibacterial Activity of Erythromycin. *J. Bacteriol. Parasitol.* **2016**, *7*, 2.
116. Novickij, V.; Stanevičiene, R.; Vepštaite-Monstavičе, I.; Gruškiene, R.; Krivorotova, T.; Sereikaite, J.; Novickij, J.; Serviene, E. Overcoming Antimicrobial Resistance in Bacteria Using Bioactive Magnetic Nanoparticles and Pulsed Electromagnetic Fields. *Front. Microbiol.* **2018**, *8*, 2678. [CrossRef]
117. Sies, H. Oxidative stress: Oxidants and antioxidants. *Exp. Physiol.* **1997**, *82*, 291–295. [CrossRef] [PubMed]
118. Li, Y.; Huang, G.; Zhang, X.; Li, B.; Chen, Y.; Lu, T.; Lu, T.J.; Xu, F. Magnetic Hydrogels and Their Potential Biomedical Applications. *Adv. Funct. Mater.* **2013**, *23*, 660–672. [CrossRef]

119. Stoimenov, P.K.; Klinger, R.L.; Marchin, G.L.; Klabunde, K.J. Metal Oxide Nanoparticles as Bactericidal Agents. *Langmuir* **2002**, *18*, 6679–6686. [CrossRef]
120. Makhluf, S.; Dror, R.; Nitzan, Y.; Abramovich, Y.; Jelinek, R.; Gedanken, A. Microwave-Assisted Synthesis of Nanocrystalline MgO and Its Use as a Bacteriocide. *Adv. Funct. Mater.* **2005**, *15*, 1708–1715. [CrossRef]
121. Thill, A.; Zeyons, O.; Spalla, O.; Chauvat, F.; Rose, J.; Auffan, M. Cytotoxicity of CeO_2 Nanoparticles Physico-Chemical Insight of the Cytotoxicity Mechanism. *Environ. Sci. Technol.* **2006**, *40*, 6151–6156. [CrossRef] [PubMed]
122. Zhang, L.; Jiang, Y.; Ding, Y.; Povey, M.; York, D. Investigation into the Antibacterial Behaviour of Suspensions of ZnO Nanoparticles (ZnO Nanofluids). *J. Nanopart. Res.* **2007**, *9*, 479–489. [CrossRef]
123. Webster, T.J. The Use of Superparamagnetic Nanoparticles. *Int. J. Nanomed.* **2009**, *4*, 145–152. [CrossRef]
124. Christena, L.R.; Mangalagowri, V.; Pradheeba, P.; Ahmed, K.B.A.; Shalini, B.I.S.; Vidyalakshmi, M.; Anbazhagan, V.; Subramanian, N.S. Copper nanoparticles as an efflux pump inhibitor to tackle drug resistant bacteria. *RSC Adv.* **2015**, *5*, 12899–12909. [CrossRef]
125. Maleki, H.; Rai, A.; Pinto, S.; Evangelista, M.; Cardoso, R.M.; Paulo, C.S.O.; Carvalheiro, T.; Paiva, A.; Imani, M.; Simchi, A.A.; et al. High antimicrobial activity and low human cell cytotoxicity of core-shell magnetic nanoparticles functionalized with an antimicrobial peptide. *ACS Appl. Mater. Interfaces* **2016**, *8*, 11366–11378. [CrossRef]
126. Bellova, A.; Bystrenova, E.; Koneracka, M.; Kopcansky, P.; Valle, F.; Tomašovičová, N.; Timko, M.; Bágeľová, J.; Biscarini, F.; Gazova, Z. Effect of Fe_3O_4 magnetic nanoparticles on lysozyme amyloid aggregation. *Nanotechnology* **2010**, *21*, 065103. [CrossRef]
127. Unterweger, H.; Subatzus, D.; Tietze, R.; Janko, C.; Poettler, M.; Stiegelschmitt, A.; Schuster, M.; Maake, C.; Boccaccini, A.R.; Alexiou, C. Hypericin-bearing magnetic iron oxide nanoparticles for selective drug delivery in photodynamic therapy. *Int. J. Nanomed.* **2015**, *10*, 6985–6996. [CrossRef] [PubMed]
128. Gul, S.; Khan, S.B.; Rehman, I.U.; Khan, M.A.; Khan, M.I. A Comprehensive Review of Magnetic Nanomaterials Modern Day Theranostics. *Front. Mater.* **2019**, *6*. [CrossRef]
129. Maboudi, S.; Shojaosadati, S.; Aliakbari, F.; Arpanaei, A. Theranostic magnetite cluster@silica@albumin double-shell particles as suitable carriers for water-insoluble drugs and enhanced T2 MR imaging contrast agents. *Mater. Sci. Eng. C* **2019**, *99*, 1485–1492. [CrossRef] [PubMed]
130. Lee, J.H.; Ju, J.E.; Kim, B.I.; Pak, P.J.; Choi, E.K.; Lee, H.S.; Chung, N. Rod-shaped iron oxide nanoparticles are more toxic than sphere-shaped nanoparticles to murine macrophage cells. *Environ. Toxicol. Chem.* **2014**, *33*, 2759–2766. [CrossRef] [PubMed]
131. Liu, Y.L.; Chen, D.; Shang, P.; Yin, D.C. A review of magnet systems for targeted drug delivery. *J. Control. Release* **2019**, *302*, 90–104. [CrossRef] [PubMed]
132. Dwivedi, S.; Siddiqui, M.A.; Farshori, N.N.; Ahamed, M.; Musarrat, J.; Al-Khedhairy, A.A. Synthesis, characterization and toxicological evaluation of iron oxide nanoparticles in human lung alveolar epithelial cells. *Colloids Surf. B Biointerfaces* **2014**, *122*, 209–215. [CrossRef] [PubMed]
133. Pöttler, M.; Staicu, A.; Zaloga, J.; Unterweger, H.; Weigel, B.; Schreiber, E.; Hofmann, S.; Wiest, I.; Jeschke, U.; Alexiou, C.; et al. Genotoxicity of Superparamagnetic Iron Oxide Nanoparticles in Granulosa Cells. *Int. J. Mol. Sci.* **2015**, *16*, 26280–26290. [CrossRef]

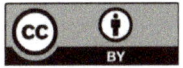

© 2019 by the authors. Licensee MDPI, Basel, Switzerland. This article is an open access article distributed under the terms and conditions of the Creative Commons Attribution (CC BY) license (http://creativecommons.org/licenses/by/4.0/).

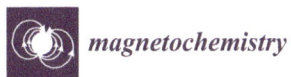

Review

Bio-Catalysis and Biomedical Perspectives of Magnetic Nanoparticles as Versatile Carriers

Muhammad Bilal [1,*], Shahid Mehmood [2], Tahir Rasheed [3] and Hafiz M. N. Iqbal [4,*]

1. School of Life Science and Food Engineering, Huaiyin Institute of Technology, Huaian 223003, China
2. Bio-X Institute, Key Laboratory for the Genetics of Developmental and Neuropsychiatric Disorders (Ministry of Education), Shanghai Jiao Tong University, Shanghai 200030, China
3. School of Chemistry & Chemical Engineering, State Key Laboratory of Metal Matrix Composites, Shanghai Jiao Tong University, Shanghai 200240, China
4. Tecnologico de Monterrey, School of Engineering and Sciences, Campus Monterrey, Ave. Eugenio Garza Sada 2501, Monterrey, N.L. CP 64849, Mexico
* Correspondence: bilaluaf@hotmail.com (M.B.); hafiz.iqbal@itesm.mx or hafiz.iqbal@tec.mx (H.M.N.I.); Tel.: +52-81-8358-2000 (ext. 5679) (H.M.N.I.)

Received: 9 May 2019; Accepted: 27 June 2019; Published: 2 July 2019

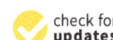

Abstract: In recent years, magnetic nanoparticles (MNPs) have gained increasing attention as versatile carriers because of their unique magnetic properties, biocatalytic functionalities, and capabilities to work at the cellular and molecular level of biological interactions. Moreover, owing to their exceptional functional properties, such as large surface area, large surface-to-volume ratio, and mobility and high mass transference, MNPs have been employed in several applications in different sectors such as supporting matrices for enzymes immobilization and controlled release of drugs in biomedicine. Unlike non-magnetic carriers, MNPs can be easily separated and recovered using an external magnetic field. In addition to their biocompatible microenvironment, the application of MNPs represents a remarkable green chemistry approach. Herein, we focused on state-of-the-art two majorly studied perspectives of MNPs as versatile carriers for (1) matrices for enzymes immobilization, and (2) matrices for controlled drug delivery. Specifically, from the applied perspectives of magnetic nanoparticles, a series of different applications with suitable examples are discussed in detail. The second half is focused on different metal-based magnetic nanoparticles and their exploitation for biomedical purposes.

Keywords: green chemistry; magnetic nanoparticles; enzyme immobilization; controlled drug delivery; supporting materials

---

1. Introduction

Green or sustainable chemistry is the utilization of a set of principles that diminishes the use of toxic substances in the design, manufacture, and application of the chemical product. This fact encouraged the researchers and scientific community to discover simple and effective methods for the separation of homogenous catalysts from the reaction mixture and their subsequent recycling. The use of magnetic nanoparticles (MNPs) as efficient support materials for biocatalyst immobilization has become a theme of considerable interest. A range of attractive properties including high surface area, large surface-to-volume ratio, facile separation using external magnetic fields, and high mass transfer make MNPs ideal candidate for diverse biomedical applications [1,2]. MNPs exhibit their highest performance at sizes typical ranges from 10 to 20 nm due to the occurrence of the superparamagnetism property [3]. Recently, MNPs find potential use in catalysis including nanostructured material-assisted biocatalysts immobilization, biomedicine, target-oriented drug delivery, magnetic resonance imaging

(MRI), microfluidics, nanofluids, optical filters, data storage, and environmental remediation [4]. Herein, we focused on state-of-the-art two majorly studied applications of MNPs as versatile carriers for (1) matrices for enzymes immobilization, and (2) matrices for controlled drug delivery. Following the introduction, the formation and stabilization of magnetic nanoparticles are briefly discussed. From the applied perspectives of magnetic nanoparticles, a series of different applications with suitable examples are discussed in detail. The second half is focused on different metal-based magnetic nanoparticles and their exploitation for biomedical purposes.

2. Magnetic Nanoparticles: Formation and Stabilization

MNPs properties are firmly dependent on formation and construction method. For the synthesis of high-quality nanoparticles, particle-size distribution, particle size, symmetry, and crystallization have been governed with the help of advance colloidal system [5]. All these features of MNPs provide mono-dispersity and homogeneity in the target system. Sometimes, MNP required a stabilizing agent in a competitive environment to avoid from agglomeration, for example, in dipolar conditions, these particles face high surface-to-volume ratio [6]. Currently, there is a variety of nanomaterials available commercially [7]. Therefore, it reduces the effort of nanoparticle researchers and increases productivity. In spite of these facts, more work and experiments are needed to customize, develop, and synthesize purpose-built nanoparticles.

From a material chemistry perspective, the material used for the development of magnetic entity can be originated or constructed from iron (oxides), nickels, and cobalt. Sometimes elements such as strontium, zinc, barium, and zinc can also be conjugated with metals. Generally, MNPs belongs to the nanoalloy and metallic nanomaterials that are coated with specific kind of molecules [8,9]. These modifications make it target specific, enhance the stability, and improve the physiochemical properties (corrosion, oxidation, agglomeration, and toxicity) of nanoparticles [10,11]. Lastly, customized modification of MNPs both core and surface depend upon the system to be applied [12]. For example, agglomeration of MNPs with avidin–biotin (bifunctional linkers) increase the stability up to several months [13], oligos-based modification was used for DNA detection [14,15], modification with iron oxide or ferrites is the potential application for X-ray computed tomography or MRI [16]. Similarly, MNPs were coated with other conjugated molecules such as liposomes, micelles, polymeric coating, and core–shell structures (Figure 1) [17].

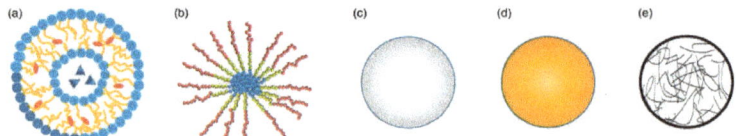

Figure 1. Representative structures of various NPs for drug delivery. (**a**) Liposomes, (**b**) polymeric micelles, (**c**) polymeric nanoparticle, (**d**) gold nanoparticle, and (**e**) nanogel. Reprinted from Wang et al. [17], an open-access article distributed under the terms of the Creative Commons Attribution License (http://creativecommons.org/licenses/by/4.0/). Copyright (2018) the author(s). Published by Informa UK Limited, London, UK, trading as Taylor & Francis Group.

3. Applications of Magnetic Nanoparticles

3.1. Bio-Catalysis Perspectives of Magnetic Nanoparticles

Over the past two decades, a wide variety of nano-carriers has been fabricated and applied as enzymes immobilization supports for diverse applications (Table 1). Among these support materials, MNPs have received substantial attention as versatile carriers, because of their unique physicochemical and magnetic properties, biodegradability, biocompatibility, low cost, and tailor-made surface chemistry. Also, MNPs allow facile, rapid, and efficient biocatalyst separation from the reaction media by using an external magnet [18].

Table 1. Summary of magnetic nanomaterials as versatile carriers for enzymes immobilization, and their applications.

Magnetic Carrier	Name of Enzyme	Immobilization Technique	Improved Properties and Application of Immobilized Enzymes	References
Magnetic graphene oxide	Chloroperoxidase/glucose oxidase	Physical adsorption	Excellent catalytic efficiency, operational durability, and recyclability. Immobilized biocatalyst showed far greater thermal stability compared with the native enzyme. It presented an application in decolorization and degradation of many synthetic dyes from industrial wastewater.	[19]
hydrophobic virus-like organosilica nanoparticles	*Candida antarctica* lipase B	Covalent attachment	Improved pH and thermal resistance High tolerance to organic solvents and long-term storage stability. Efficient esterification reaction of levulinic acid retaining 75.7% of the levulinic acid transformation after 9 continuous biocatalytic cycles.	[20]
Chitosan-cross-linked magnetic nanoparticles	*Candida antarctica* lipase B	Covalent attachment	Superior separation and biocatalytic properties. Excellent storage stability and reusability. Production of bio-based photocurable oligo-esters by the ring opening esterification of polyols and itaconic anhydride.	[21]
Barium ferrite magnetic microparticles	Alcohol oxidase	Covalent attachment	Enhanced thermostability retaining > 65% of the original activity at 45 °C for 24 h. Good catalytic efficacy for oxidizing ethanol and methanol compared with the free enzyme. Recyclability for at three successive batches with 70% activity retention.	[22]
Glutathione-coated gold magnetic nanoparticles	Inulinase	Covalent binding	Enhanced storage and reusability stability. Immobilized biocatalyst preserved about 78% of its original activity after 10 repeated cycles. Improved enzyme performance at acidic pHs (3.0 and 4.0) and high temperature up to 80 °C. Complete hydrolysis of inulin to fructose and glucose.	[23]
Ionic liquid-modified magnetic chitosan composites	Lipase	Adsorption	Elevated catalytic activity (6.72-fold) as compared to the free enzyme Enhanced thermal stability and reusability retaining 92.1% of residual activity after 10 cycles of reuse.	[24]
Fe$_3$O$_4$ magnetic nanoparticles functionalized with wheat gluten hydrolysates	Inulinase	Covalent binding	High activity over a broader pH and temperature ranges, and also exhibited pronounced storage and thermal stability. The inulinase showed 12.3 folds rise in enzyme half-life value at 75 °C Potential recyclability retaining 70% of its preliminary catalytic activity after 12 continuous inulin hydrolysis cycles.	[25]
Functionalized APTMS-magnetite nanoparticles	Cellulase and pectinase	Covalent immobilization	Improved characteristics such as high activities recovery, enhanced temperature stability (2.39-times greater than that to the free enzyme), and reusability for up to 8 continuous cycles in grape juice clarification.	[26]
Chitosan-montmorillonite nanocomposite beads	α-amylase	Cross-linking	High enzyme activity and stability at varying pH and temperature conditions than the free enzyme. Retention of about 53% enzyme relative activity after recycling 5 times	[27]
Chitosan magnetic nanoparticles	Pectinase	Cross-linking	Superior thermal stability than the soluble form of the enzyme. High stabilization retaining 87% of original activity after seven repeated cycles. Excellent durability. Potential apple juice clarification with up to 74% turbidity reduction after 2.5 h of treatment.	[28]
Amino-functionalized magnetic nanoparticle	α-amylase, cellulose, and pectinase	Cross-linking	Increased pH and thermal stability Encouraging enzyme reusability preserving up to 75% of activity after 8 reuse cycles. Clarification of fruit juices. Significant decrease in turbidity.	[29]
Magnetic cornstarch microspheres	Pectinase	Adsorption	Improved pH and thermal stability. Good reusability and operability of the immobilized biocatalyst preserving 60% of its initial activity after 8 reuses in apple juice processing.	[30]
Magnetic Fe$_3$O$_4$@chitosan nanoparticles	Lipase	Covalent immobilization	Immobilized biocatalyst presented more than 50% and 75% residual activity in the pH range 7.0–11.0, and 70 °C. Satisfactory reusability preserving 70% of its original activity after 10 repeated cycles. More than 50% conversion of ascorbic acid was achieved when used for ascorbyl palmitate synthesis in tert-butanol at 50 °C.	[31]

APTMS—3-aminopropyltrimethoxysilane.

3.2. Degradation of Dye Pollutants

Different dyes including acid blue 45, crystal violet, and orange G have shown wider applications in paper, textile, food, and many other industries. However, these dyes and other dyes containing pollutants pose severe threats to human health and aquatic organisms [32]. Due to their high photolytic and chemical stability, these dye pollutants are resilient to classical chemical, physical, and biological treatment methods. Enzymes as biocatalysts can be employed both in free as well as immobilized forms in the treatment of dyes or dyes-harboring industrial wastewater. However, immobilized enzymes present the advantages of durable catalytic stability, easy separation, and recovery, and multiple recycling, which improve the performance and trim-down the overall cost of industrial bioprocess [33–38]. Immobilized enzymes can be developed by different chemical and physical methods, which affect biocatalytic properties of the resulting immobilized system, and hence their applications in explicit processes [39,40].

Reports have shown the fascinating efficiency of chloroperoxidase (CPO) in degrading an array of synthetic dyes. Nevertheless, the lack of durable functioning stability and difficulty in recycling CPO hampered its large-scale application in wastewater bioremediation. To overcome this issue, Gao and coworkers, (2019) co-immobilized CPO and glucose oxidase (GOx) on the surface of magnetic graphene oxide (MGO). The catalytic performance of MGO-GOx-CPO considerably enhanced (96.6%) towards the degradation of orange G relative to MGO-GOx+MGO-CPO (86.2%), presumably because of reduced mass transfer limitation between CPO and H_2O_2 produced from GOx molecules (Figure 2) [19]. Remarkably, MGO-GOx-CPO exhibited its maximum activity at a temperature above 40 °C compared with the optimal temperature of 35 °C for the soluble biocatalyst. It also showed potential repetitive usability retaining ~38.5% of initial activity after six dye-decolorization cycles demonstrating the possibility of co-immobilized CPO and GOx in environmental applications. A peroxidase enzyme isolated and purified from the textile wastewater was immobilized on glutaraldehyde-functionalized Fe_3O_4 MNPs. The MNPs-insolubilized enzyme showed remarkable stability towards a range of pH and temperature perturbations than to the free form of the enzyme. It retained complete catalytic activity following storage at 4 °C and 25 °C for three months, and upon reusing for up to 100 repeated cycles. Moreover, the MNPs-assisted novel peroxidase was effectively used for the decolorization and degradation of industry wastewater containing direct green or reactive red azo dye pollutants in a prototype sequential lab-scale bioreactor [41]. In a recent study, Kashefi and coworkers [42] synthesized the magnetic graphene oxide (MGO) by integrating exclusive GO properties with the superparamagnetic characteristics of the $CuFe_2O_4$ nanoparticles. The amine group on MGO was functionalized chemically modified with 3-amino propyl trimethoxy silane and cross-linked activated with GLU. As-prepared functionalized MGO was utilized to covalently immobilize a laccase enzyme from genetically modified *Aspergillus* and exploited to degrade an azo dye Direct Red 23 using the response surface methodology. Results revealed that the immobilized nanobiocatalyst caused a maximum decolorization efficiency of 95.33% under the optimal conditions—i.e., pH, dye concentration, and enzyme dosage of 4.23, 19.60 mg/L, and 290.23 mg/L—respectively. In conclusion, it can be stated that the superparamagnetic nanomaterials-immobilized enzyme can potentially act as green and environmentally responsive nanobiocatalyst for efficient decolorization purposes [42].

3.3. Fruit Juice Clarification

In recent years, the development of new strategies for fruit juice clarification has gained a great interest in improving the quality of the juices. The turbid and cloudy appearance of the freshly prepared fruit juices resulting from the colloidal dispersion of pectin is one of the major issues in fruit juice processing [43]. Moreover, the presence of starch and other polysaccharides (i.e., cellulose and hemicellulose) tend to settle down during preservation resulting in haziness and poor-quality fruit juice [44]. Current employing microfiltration and ultrafiltration clarification technologies are restricted during the elimination of suspended pulp particles causing membrane fouling and reduce the membrane lifespan [45]. The use of immobilized enzymes has been substantially increased in fruit juice industry to circumvent turbidity, cloudiness, and undesirable haziness accompanied by improving juice yield, quality, and shelf life [46]. Huang et al. [47] designed a biocompatible magnetic chitin nanofiber biocomposite using GLU cross-linker and used as a novel support material for chymotrypsin immobilization with excellent catalytic properties (Figure 3). The GLU-cross-linked insolubilized enzymes exhibited 70.7% of its original activity by incubating at 60 °C for 3 h, whereas the non-immobilized chymotrypsin showed only 29.6% of activity under identical conditions. After storage for 20 days, the immobilized nanobiocatalyst presented 84.9% of the initial activity, as compared to 18.8% for the free enzyme. After enzyme immobilization onto this magnetic nanobiocomposite, the loading capacity of the enzyme was improved up to 6.3-fold following GLU cross-linking. Moreover, the immobilized biocatalyst was easily recovered and recycled from the reaction mixture [47].

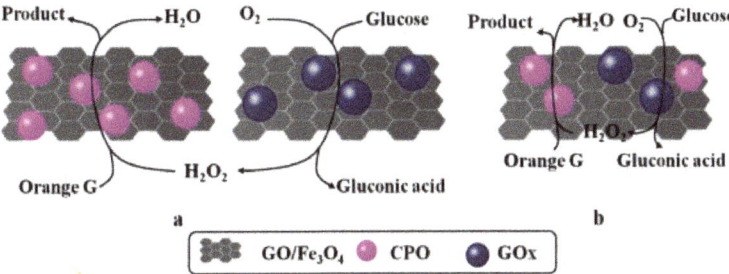

Figure 2. (a) Mass transfer resistance between chloroperoxidase (CPO) and glucose oxidase (GOx) for MGO-GOx+MGO-CPO; (b) no mass transfer resistance between CPO and GOx for MGO-GOx-CPO. Reprinted from Gao et al. [19], with permission from Elsevier. Copyright (2018) Elsevier B.V.

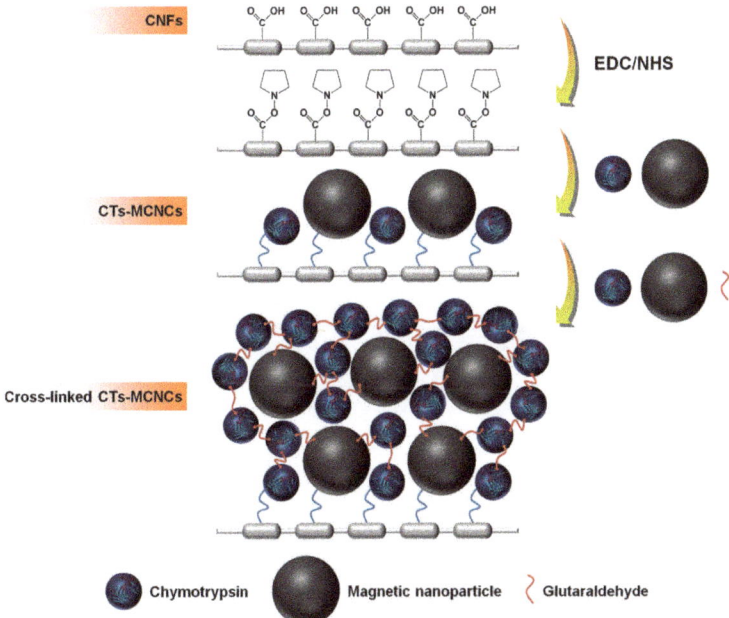

Figure 3. Schematic illustration of the immobilization of chymotrypsin onto the magnetic chitin nanofiber composite. Reprinted from Huang et al. [47], with permission from American Chemical Society. Copyright (2018) American Chemical Society.

Cross-linking agents play a critical role and have a direct effect on activity recovery and functional stability during cross-linking of the enzymes on nano-supports. Glutaraldehyde is considered the preferred cross-linking agent amongst a range of protein cross-linkers due to its cheapness, easy availability, and manipulation and the ability to form covalent bonding with the majority of the enzymes [48]. Nevertheless, some inherent drawbacks are associated with the use of glutaraldehyde as a cross-linker. The use of GLU cross-linker, in some instances, led to complete enzyme deactivation by penetrating into the catalytic site and cross-linking with biocatalytically important amino acids residues due to its small size [49]. Moreover, GLU-assisted cross-linking of enzyme molecules forms enzyme lumps that hinder the active sites resulting in mass transfer resistances and diminished catalytic efficiency [50]. Consequently, polysaccharides-based cross-linkers have gained great attention in the past years for cross-linking of proteins over the use of GLU. Sojitra and coworkers [29] synthesized magnetic tri-enzyme nanobiocatalyst by insolubilizing three enzymes, i.e., α-amylase, pectinase and cellulase onto chitosan MNPs using dextran polyaldehyde as a macromolecular cross-linker and utilized for fruit juice clarification. As compared to the soluble enzyme, the MNPs-immobilized biocatalysts presented more than 2-folds increment in half-life and enhanced tolerance to lower pH. Identical K_m and V_{max} values of the native and immobilized forms of pectinase revealed that conformational flexibility of enzyme was not altered after immobilization. In addition, the magnetic tri-enzyme presented 41%, 53%, and 46% reduction in turbidity for the clarification of apple, pineapple, and grapes juices after 2.5 h treatment. Results revealed that magnetic nanobiocatalysts might be a suitable technology for fruit juice clarification, owing to its possibility to separate enzymes from the reaction mixture and, subsequently, the reutilization of biocatalysts in multiple reaction cycles [29]. A significant improvement in pH and thermal stability of pectinase from *Penicillium oxalicum* F67 has also been achieved by immobilizing enzyme onto magnetic cornstarch microspheres. The resultant biocatalyst displayed about 60% of its preliminary activity after eight successive reuses for apple juice processing [30].

3.4. Biotransformation of Inulin to High Fructose Syrup

Inulin is a polysaccharide made up of fructose monomers and seems to be an abundant source for the production of fructooligosaccharides and fructose syrup in pharmaceutical and food industries. As a low caloric sweetener and prebiotic, fructooligosaccharides possess human health promoting effects such as a reduction in serum triglyceride and cholesterol levels, and significant improvement in the intestinal microbial flora [51,52]. Fructose is an inexpensive, low-calorie, and GRAS-approved sweetener and utilized as a safe alternative sweetener in diabetic patients [53]. Inulinase (EC:3.2.1.7) is well-known hydrolytic biocatalyst that can produce a high level of pure fructose syrup from inulin by a one-step enzymatic process in contrast to uneconomical and hazardous acid hydrolysis, as well as, multi-step enzymatic starch breakdown by glucoamylase, glucose isomerase, α-amylase, and pullulanase [54,55]. Due to lower solubility and high microbial contamination of inulin in the water at room temperature, industrial-scale inulin hydrolysis needs to be executed at elevated temperatures for higher inulin substrate utilization due to the increased solubility [56]. Therefore, thermostable inulinases are desirable biocatalysts for the chemical and food industry. In this context, Torabizadeh and Mahmoudi [25], covalently attached inulinase from *Aspergillus niger* onto wheat gluten hydrolysates (WGHs)-functionalized Fe_3O_4 MNPs in the presence of glutaraldehyde as a cross-linking agent. As-developed inulinase was found to be active over a broader pH and temperature ranges, and also exhibited pronounced storage and thermal stability. The inulinase showed 12.3 folds rise in enzyme half-life value following immobilization on MNPs at 75 °C and retained 70% of its preliminary catalytic activity after 12 continuous inulin hydrolysis cycles [25]. More recently, Mohammadi et al. [23] fabricated unique biocompatible support i.e., glutathione-coated gold MNPs (GSH-AuMNPs) and used for the covalent immobilization of the inulinase enzyme (Figure 4). The resulting magnetically recoverable and solid biocatalyst was applied for efficient biotransformation of inulin to high fructose syrup. After immobilization, the storage stability and reusability of inulinase were considerably improved, and the immobilized biocatalyst preserved about 78% of its original activity after 10 repeated cycles. Immobilization on MNPs improved the enzyme performance at acidic pHs (3.0 and 4.0) and high temperature up to 80 °C. Chromatographic results revealed the complete hydrolysis of inulin and the end-products of both free and immobilized biocatalytic systems only consisted of 98% of fructose and up to 2% of glucose. The findings demonstrated that the magnetic nanomaterials-immobilized inulinase might display a high potential for larger scale synthesis of high fructose syrup and fructooligosaccharides useful for biotechnological, food, and biomedical industries [23].

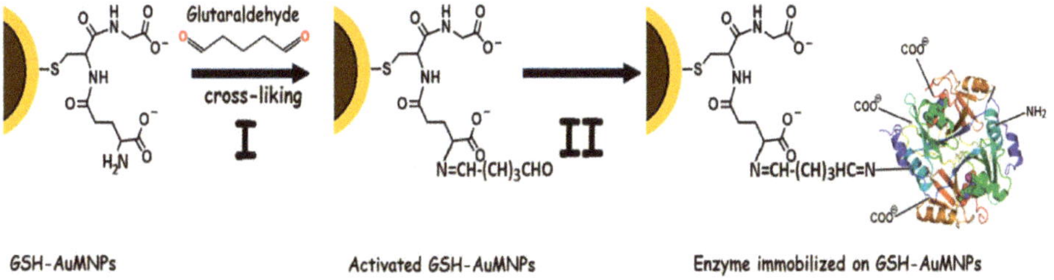

Figure 4. Enzyme immobilization steps including (**I**) cross-linkage of glutathione decorated Fe_3O_4-Au magnetic nanoparticles (GSH-AuMNPs) with GA, and (**II**) enzyme immobilization on GSH-AuMNPs surface. Reprinted from Mohammadi et al. [23], with permission from Elsevier. Copyright (2018) Elsevier B.V.

3.5. Other Applications

In recent years, fabrication of virus-like structured particles has appeared as one of the most creative and state-of-the-art support materials for enzymes immobilization. These novel materials offered a noteworthy biocatalytic platform enabling the durable stability and reusability of the enzymes [57]. For instance, P22 virus-like particles [58], Qβ virus-like particles [59], and cowpea chlorotic mottle virus particles [60,61] have been effectively created and employed for the enzyme immobilization. To date, a range of enzymes has been encapsulated onto these virus-like nano-carriers with the significant activity retention against extreme pH and temperature ranges [57]. For the first time, Jiang and coworkers [20] successfully synthesized hydrophobic virus-like organosilica nanoparticles (VOSNs) with a spherical core (Figure 5A) and employed for the covalent binding of the *Candida antarctica* lipase B (CALB). The synthesized hydrophobic VOSNs secured the active conformation of the CALB from the external hazardous environment because of stronger hydrophobic interfaces between the CALB molecules and VOSNs. As a result, the newly developed CALB@VSNs (Figure 5B) presented superior pH and thermal resistance, high tolerance to organic solvents and long-term storage stability. Under the optimized operating conditions, the CALB@VOSNs efficiently catalyzed the esterification reaction of levulinic acid and n-lauryl alcohol. Interestingly, it maintained 75.7% of the levulinic acid transformation even after nine continuous biocatalytic cycles [20].

Recently, subject to the requisite application, enzymes have been integrated with nanomaterials as immobilization carriers to engineer nano-biocatalysts [62]. Hosseini et al. [21] prepared new nano-magnetic biocatalyst particles following immobilization of CALB onto chitosan-cross-linked MNPs (Figure 6). The as-synthesized CALB-immobilized nanoparticles showed high storage stability and repeatability because of tightly cross-linked chitosan structure and covalent bonding. The newly developed magnetic biocatalyst efficiently catalyzed the ring opening esterification of itaconic anhydride as compared to the free enzyme [21]. In another study, *C. rugosa* lipase (CRL) coupled to new zwitterionic polymer-grafted silica nanoparticles (SNPs-pOD-CRL) displayed substantially improved enzyme–substrate affinity and catalytic performance than soluble enzyme due to the activation of lipase by the hydrophobic alkyl chains of the polymer (Figure 7) [63]. Moreover, a significant increase in thermal stability profile indicates that zwitterionic polymer with shorter alkyl side chains is advantageous to develop thermostable enzymes [63]. Of most recent, Suo et al. [24] developed a novel immobilization strategy to increase the catalytic stability of lipase enzyme. In this method, lipase was adsorbed on ionic liquid (IL) modified magnetic chitosan (MCS) composites and graphene oxide (GO) nanosheets served as shell coating for anchoring the lipase structure (Figure 8) [24]. The GO-shielded novel biocatalytic system sustained 6.72-fold high activity as compared to the free enzyme. In addition, the thermal stability was also enhanced, and the immobilized enzyme retained 92.1% of residual activity after 10 cycles of reuse [24]. Wang et al. [31] synthesized stable magnetic Fe_3O_4@chitosan nanoparticles by an efficient and simple in-situ co-precipitation technique and used to chemically conjugate lipase from *Thermomyces lanuginosus* by covalent immobilization. Besides a broader pH and thermal tolerance, the immobilized lipase also exhibited good reusability maintaining 70% of original activity after 10 reaction batches. The nanobiocatalyst achieved higher than 50% conversion of ascorbic acid when used for ascorbyl palmitate synthesis in tert-butanol at 50 °C [31].

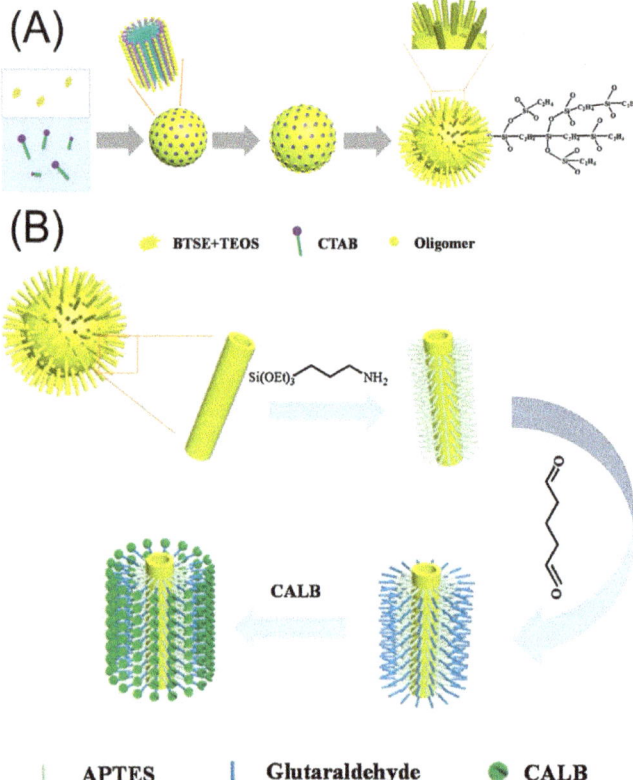

Figure 5. (**A**) Schematic illustration of the formation process of hydrophobic virus-like organosilica nanoparticles VOSNs and (**B**) preparation of the hydrophobic virus-like organosilica nanoparticles immobilized lipase B from *Candida antarctica*. Reprinted from Jiang et al. [20], with permission from Elsevier. Copyright (2019) Elsevier B.V.

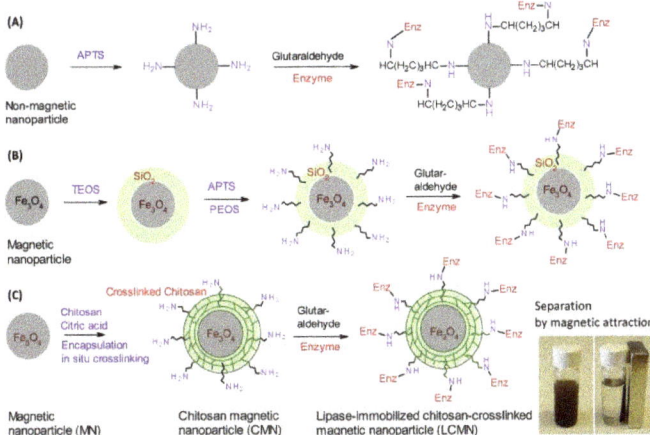

Figure 6. Representative illustrations of enzyme immobilization in the nanoparticle. (**A**) Conventional method using non-magnetic nanoparticle. (**B**) Conventional method using magnetic nanoparticle and organosilane compounds. (**C**) Present study using magnetic nanoparticle and chitosan crosslinked for immobilization of enzyme (lipase). APTS: 3-aminopropyltriethoxysilane, TEOS: tetra-ethoxy silane, PEOS: poly-ethoxysilane. Reprinted from Hosseini et al. [21], with permission from Elsevier. Copyright (2018) Elsevier B.V. (**A**) and (**B**) modified by Hosseini et al. [21] from Kim et al. [62], an open access article distributed under the Creative Commons Attribution License. Copyright (2018) the authors. Licensee MDPI, Basel, Switzerland.

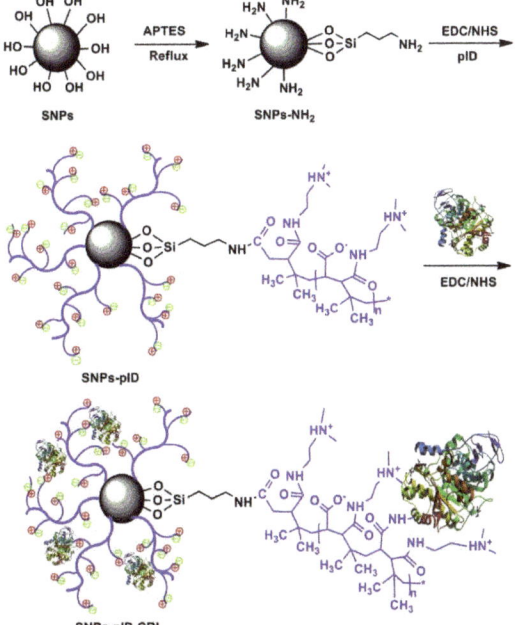

Figure 7. Schematic for the preparation of immobilized lipase on poly(4-((2-(dimethylamino)ethyl) amino)-4-oxobut-2-enoic acid-alt-isobutylene) (pID)-grafted silica nanoparticles. Reprinted from Zhang et al. [63], with permission from Elsevier. Copyright (2019) Elsevier B.V.

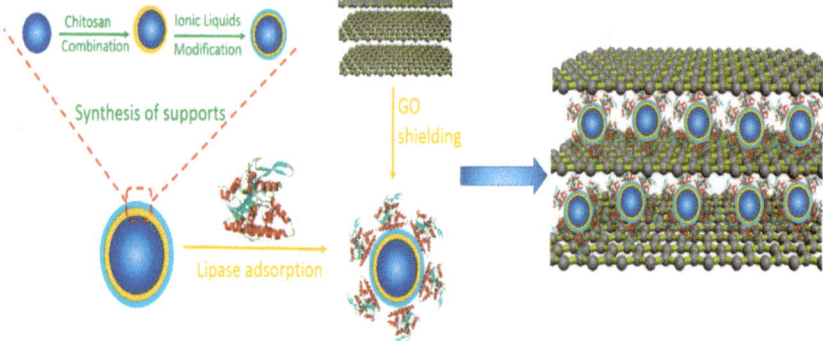

Figure 8. Immobilization of lipase on ionic liquid (IL) modified magnetic chitosan (MCS) composites using graphene oxide (GO) as shell coating. Reprinted from Suo et al. [24], with permission from American Chemical Society. Copyright (2019) American Chemical Society.

4. Biomedical Perspectives of Magnetic Nanomaterials

Magnetic nanoparticles are the most promising area and have a wide range in multi-disciplinary applications because of its unique features such as eco-remediation, biological purification, magnetic fluids, and a number of biomedical applications including hyperthermia mediated cancer treatment, biosensors for disease detection (MRI), and site-specific drug delivery. It varies in size from few to tens of nanometers (nm) [64]. It means MNPs are smaller than a cell (10–100 μm), protein (5–50 nm), gene (2 nm wide and 10–100 nm long), and virus (20–450 nm). Its small size makes enable to get closer to the desired targets. Although, NMPs coated with some biological interacting molecules that enable it to penetrate or tag the biological object [65]. MNPs obey the coulombs law that means it can be deployed by any outward magnetic gradient. These properties of MNPs open up the new site for immobilization or transportation of MNPs into the biological systems including human tissues. Therefore, these particles can act as a protective shield to deliver the variety of drugs especially anticancer, radionuclide entities, and target the hard sites of the human body like brain [66]. Another MNPs advantage is to response against the resonance applied by external system as a result transfer of energy from an excited medium to nanoparticles can be used for detection. For instance, hyperthermia is a nearly acceptable technique that is used for the treatment of cancer along with chemotherapy or radiotherapy, because it induces minimal damage to normal cells. In this technique, particles are used that act as hypothermic mediators [67]. These particles transfer the heat beyond the threshold level that are enough to kill the cells present in the cancer microenvironment. In various envisioned applications of MNPs, the size of the particles play a crucial role in the functionality, for example in various envisioned applications of particles are depends upon the size [68]. The particles have below critical size perform well. These particles are considered as a single functional magnetic domain which shows superparamagnetic properties when exceed the temperature threshold value. Sometime individual particles showed constant paramagnetic behavior and act like gigantic paramagnetic entity. These giant particles have a very quick response to the remnant magnetization or residual magnetization (magnetic force remains after external magnetization removed) and coercive force (the field required to bring the magnetization to zero). These distinctive features of particles make them very strong and potential candidate in biomedical applications [69–71].

Preparation of NPs are usually fall in the inductive method (bottom-up). In this method, NPs are fabricated from an atom level to the molecular level through self-organization pattern. In biomedical applications, core–shell of NPs is from the magnetic origin than make it more stable, compatible, and fast-penetrating through encapsulated with organic or inorganic polymers [72]. These supportive modifications enable them to use in various biomedical applications. Although morbidity rates globally comparatively decrease with the advancement in medical science, cancer is still one of the biggest contributors to increase the mortality rate. Albeit according to the ACS (American Cancer Society) report mortality rate due to cancer decreased in the past few years. This is because of early diagnosis, target specific treatment, and decrease in smoking [73]. The conventional mode of treatment including chemotherapy, radiotherapy, sometimes surgery, and immunotherapy are unable to access and target the core micro tumor environment. Currently, combinatorial therapy also called multimodal treatment in which immunotherapy (relative advance), chemotherapy, and radiotherapy are used in combine fashion to get better results in cancer treatment [74].

Therefore, specific and targeted drug delivery provides a good opportunity to treat diseases. For the drug delivery, small particle (micro or nanoparticles) are being used to get momentous results including: (1) targeting the core area of a diseased body organ; (2) reducing the concentration of drug that is conquered by the surrounding cells of the target area; (3) reducing the maximum uptake of drugs by non-target cells that maximized the efficacy of drugs. Due to these reasons, the NP application graph exponentially increased in previously published articles (Figure 9) [75].

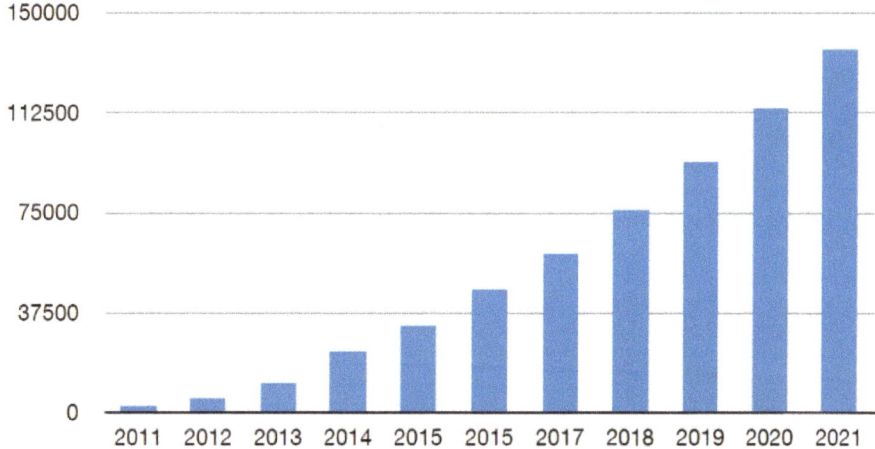

Figure 9. Global market trends for nanotechnology in drug delivery 2011–2021. Adopted from "Market Opportunities in Nanotechnology Drug Delivery". Available at: http://www.cientifica.com/market-opportunities-in-nanotechnology-drug-delivery/. Last accessed 9 May 2019.

NPs can easily internalization in tissue and cells because it can be phagocytosed due to its small size. Magnetic NPs based targeted delivery follows both the pattern of targeting active and passive target delivery. Previously reported that tumor microenvironment is highly permeable and drippy, so it called extravasation as a result of NPs target the tumor passively. These factors combine to enhance the permeability and retention of NPs so this phenomenon is known as enhanced permeation and retention (EPR) [76]. Along with all above-mentioned advantages, NPs have some limitations other than size. The main concern with NPs is the retention time in bloodstream. Therefore, the big problems with passive delivery of conventional NPs are that (i) they only target the reticuloendothelial system or mononuclear phagocyte system (MPS) and related organs including spleen, bone marrow, and liver; and (ii) they are unable to access the other tumor target sites or drug concentration is below the therapeutic level [68,77,78].

Previous studies have shown that in tumor cells were overexpressed different receptors such as G protein-coupled receptor GPR87 (pancreatic cancer) [79], GPR161 (Breast cancer) [80]. Therefore, active targeting vectors have been designed that are delicate to change in temperature, light, sound, magnetism, and pH and mounted it with drugs. Active targeting may be dependent on over-expression of low molecular weight species including Folic acid, sugars, thiamine, hyaluronic acid, transferrin, DNA, etc. [81,82]. There are different types of NPs such as Liposomes, polymeric micelles; polymeric nanoparticle, emulsions, and nanogel are used for specific target delivery. These NPs are different in chemical nature, size, physical properties (light, temperature, pH, electric charge), hydrophobicity, hydrophilicity and pattern of conjugated with drugs (attached, adsorbed, encapsulated) [10]. Hereby, in this section, we mainly address the MNPs.

4.1. Efficacy of Nanoparticles-Based Drug Delivery

With the advancement of drug formulation, the designing of target-specific drugs is always the central and most discussed issue. Nanoparticle-based drug delivery is one of the most considerable and suitable options for target drug delivery. There are several reasons to considering the nanoparticle for a theranostic carrier and agent. Conventional drugs are administered through intravenous or oral dosing. Consequently, these drugs are not always be formulated at optimal dosage. Similarly, sometimes drug formulation is based on degradable biomolecules such as oligos, nucleotides, and proteins. Therefore, these kinds of drugs need an innovative and specifically targeted carrier system that thwarts them from annoying degradation [83,84]. It is reported that drug delivery system is directly linked to the size of particles because the large surface area with small size that enhances the physiochemical properties of particle including bioactivity, solubility, passes the blood–brain barrier (BBB), and crosses the skin endothelial cells [85]. Nanoparticles that are constructed from biodegradable (natural) and non-biodegradable (synthetic) polymers have envisaged the potential customized nanoparticles for drug delivery that help to escape the drugs from the endogenous invasion of enzymes [84]. Another advantage of introducing reliable drug delivery system that increase the sale growth rate of pharmaceutical companies. The state-of-the-art delivery system leads the companies to introduce new drug formulation and minimize the side effects of the drugs. Therefore, these innovative amendments will be valuable for patients [86]. Moreover, this not only increases the company's growth rate but also encourage the innovators to introduce new patents [87]. This nanotechnology will also offer new life to that drugs that are unmarketable due to the high toxicity, low bio absorptivity, etc. (Figure 10) [88,89].

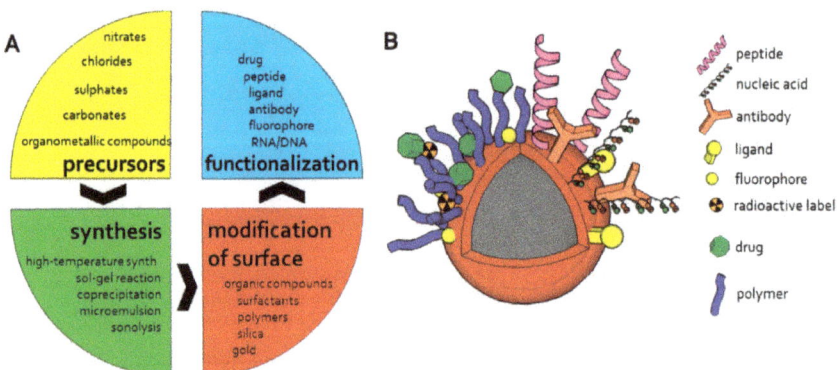

Figure 10. Scheme of magnetic particles design workflow (**A**) and possible modification and functionalization of magnetic particles (**B**). Reprinted from Kudr et al. [89], an open access article distributed under the Creative Commons Attribution License. Copyright (2017) the authors. Licensee MDPI, Basel, Switzerland.

4.2. Iron-Based MNPs for Biomedical Applications

Iron (transition element) is the most important and fourth copious element of earth's crust, as well as, considered as the backbone of modern infrastructure, around the globe. In past years, iron-based nanoparticles were abandoned due to its oxides and other renowned metals including nickel, cobalt, platinum, and gold. Nowadays, the development of iron-based MNPs is a trend in the field of nanoscience. Comparative analysis of ferromagnetic properties of iron with other magnetic material has shown that iron is the leading element for nanoparticles applications. For example, gadolinium has low Curie temperature (Tc), that is below the room temperature and it shows high saturation magnetization (σs) at 0 K. Therefore, it is impractical in most of the experiments. Iron has high enough Tc and σs that are near to the optimum status in most of the experiments. Moreover, iron also shows via magnetocrystalline anisotropy that it was more feasible for work. Superparamagnetic behavior and maximum volume particles of iron at the required temperature is directly linked to magneto-crystalline anisotropy. This means that superparamagnetic behavior is much better and workable than any other metal nanoparticles.

Other than the magnetic feature, momentous features of iron nanoparticles that have been shown that these are less expensive, revealed the adequate biophysical and biochemical stability and compatibility as well as eco-friendly [76,90,91]. Surface modification of the MNPs is an integral part of defining the physiochemical properties and stability as well [92,93]. Surface modification elements should have a strong affinity with iron and also have functional compatibility [94]. Magnetite (Fe_3O_4) nanoparticles have been synthesized through Massart method and co-precipitation. These nanoparticles have varied between 7 to 13 nm in size. Later on, through the chemical alteration of Fe_3O_4 by aeration oxidation process were converted into maghemite (γ-Fe_2O_3) nanoparticles. These nanoparticles have greater biocompatibility, stability in the diverse field, and they demonstrate better heating capability [95]. Maghemite nanoparticles can also be used in ferrofluid that has an immense range of application in biomedicine, such as targeted drug delivery, hyperthermia in tumor treatment, and cell sorting and manipulation [96]. There is a number of methods to be implicated on maghemite nanoparticle synthesis including microemulsion [97], co-precipitation [98], organic decomposition at high temperature [99], and oxidation [100]. Similarly, there are many other ways to synthesize the iron MNPs, but innovative approaches are still needed for commercial production and environmental-friendly nanoparticles [101]. For iron oxide nanoparticles synthesis, sodium oleate, and iron chloride were mixed and add this mixture into cocktail solvent of hexane, ethanol, and water than heat it to get the waxy iron–oleate complex. Afterward, this complex mixed with oleic acid, dissolved into 1-octadecene and heated. Poly(D,L-lactide-co-glycolide) have a wide range of applications in biomedical sciences due to its non-toxic nature, biocompatibility, and bio-resorptive nature [102,103]. Therefore, MNPs-coated with this polymer is very fascinating and catch the attention of biomedical experts. Poly(D, L-lactide-co-glycolide) coated superparamagnetic iron oxide nanoparticles are widely used in MRI as a contrasting agent. For the preparation of this nanoparticle reaction of iron (III) acetylacetonate with 1,2-hexadecanediol, oleic acid, oleylamine, and phenyl at 260 °C in acidic pH [104]. polyethylene glycol (PEG) and polyethyleneimine (PEI) [105–107] coated superparamagnetic iron oxide nanoparticles are synthesized by co-precipitation method and cathodic electrochemical deposition (CED) [108] are a more effective method for this. Nanoparticles coated with PEG-PEI have shown high affinity to bind with DNA phosphate backbone [109].

There are the special amendments that have been occurred according to the area of applications such as improving the molecular images. A distinct group of MNPs having composite with the variety of different metal dopants (trace impurity elements) including M2+, Mn, Zn, Ni, or Co. Metal-doped iron oxides ($MnFe_2O_4$, $FeFe_2O_4$, $CoFe_2O_4$, and $NiFe_2O_4$) based nanoparticles were synthesized at high temperature and reaction occurred between the iron tris-2,4-pentadioate and divalent metal chloride [110,111]. Toxicological analysis of metal-doped nanoparticles has expressed that $MnFe_2O_4$ showed any toxicity in-vitro. While the other Co and Ni toxicity were limiting factors for their use [90]. Finally, the most imperative facet is to construct nanoparticles according to explicit biological applications, for example, magnetic fluid hyperthermia, thermoablation, targeted drug delivery, magnetic separation, and MRI [112].

4.3. Cobalt-Based MNPs for Biomedical Applications

Cobalt-based nanoparticles are rarely used in biomedical science due to their toxicity. However, in some cases, possible modification reduces the toxicity, for example, above-mentioned dopant based MNPs ($CoFe_2O_4$) [112] and metal alloy MNPs ($Fe_{12}Co_{88}$, $Fe_{40}Co_{60}$, and $Fe_{60}Co_{40}$) [112,113]. There is the only way to make it applicable to biological systems. Commercially existing carbon-coated cobalt nanoparticles were functionalized with polyhydroxy-, polyamine-, or PEG2000-functionalized Dendron's or polymers and designed for theoretical biomedical applications as drug carriers [114]. Previous work reported that magnetic cobalt nanoparticle is auspicious material for retinal detachment cure if these nanoparticles were conjugated with poly (dimethylsiloxane), dicobalt octacarbonyl $Co_2(CO)_8$ [115]. Similarly, the above-mentioned application of cobalt that were only testified to repair the detach retina [116]. An altered polyol-process was pragmatic for crystalline cobalt nanoparticles with the possible implication in biomedicine [117].

4.4. Other MNPs for Biomedical Applications

In the traditional point of view refined form of Fe_3O_4 and γ-Fe_2O_3-based superparamagnetic nanoparticles are widely used. Some other materials that have desired features like $Y_3Fe_5O_{12}$, $SrFe_{12}O_{19}$, or $SmCo_5$ were also used [118]. However, the major problem with these materials is they are not prepared by conventional methods. These materials are separated and prepared by advanced methods like submicron particle preparation [119]. Another type of nanoparticle is based on Ni with different chemical modifications. Ni nanocrystals were encapsulated with carbon moieties Ni_3C phase in the core of the nanoparticles [120] and second modification was on the surface by NiO [121]. Similar, EDTA-caped NiO nanoparticles have been prepared by co-precipitation method, while nickel chloride hexahydrate, sodium hydroxide, and EDTA (optionally) served as reagents [89,122].

5. Concluding Remarks and Future Perspectives

Nanomaterials are being widely investigated as a powerful carrier for biomolecules immobilization, therapeutic, and other nanobiomedical applications. Immobilization of enzymes onto nanomaterial is highly encouraging in terms of catalytic activity, enhanced stability, and reusability. Amongst various immobilization techniques, the utilization of NPs is well perceived owing to the high-specific surface area, and thereby high biocatalyst loadings. Particularly, MNPs are becoming increasingly important in the immobilization arena because of their exceptional attributes including biocompatibility, uniform particle size, high surface area to volume ratio, and the recovery of the enzyme using an external magnetic field. Moreover, many MNPs possess noteworthy results in targeted-drug delivery MRI or theranostics. Therefore, MNPs can be anticipated to be the 'material of the future', which will considerably influence all areas of nano-biomedicine. However, despite the tremendous human health-related advantages of nanomaterials, concern has been raised regarding the adverse effects of these nanomaterials. Potential routes for drug delivery are also associated with the possible entry of toxic nanomaterials into the human body. For instance, inhalation-based drug delivery has been widely applied approach for direct delivery of drugs to the bloodstream, and the same route is particularly vulnerable to toxic nanomaterials. Similarly, drug delivery via the olfactory system has also arisen the toxicity issue of nanoparticle via the olfactory system. Therefore, in parallel to extensive research advances on the use of nanoparticles for biomedical purposes, their profound impact on human health also need to be deliberated by the same research. With particular reference to MNPs and their deployment in drug delivery, the following should at least be considered prior to designing MNP-based drug delivery systems. Aiming to uplift the unresolved problems associated to the MNPs based drug delivery, future studies should cover: (1) all types of toxicity issues, i.e., cytotoxicity, hemotoxicity, teratogenicity, and mutagenicity; (2) biocompatibility including cellular-compatibility and hematocompatibility; (3) immunogenicity and mutagenicity; and (4) biodegradation and/or effective release 'removal fate' from the body after targeted delivery. Encapsulation and/or coating of active MNPs using inert materials offer considerable potentialities for future research and could further limit the toxicity of free MNPs.

Author Contributions: Conceptualization, M.B. and H.M.N.I. Literature review, S.M., and T.R.; Writing—Original Draft Preparation, M.B., S.M., T.R., and H.M.N.I.; Figures, M.B. and S.M.; Tables, M.B.; Writing—Review & Editing, M.B., and H.M.N.I.; Revisions & Final editing, M.B. and H.M.N.I.; APC Funding Acquisition, H.M.N.I.

Funding: This research received no external funding. The APC (ID: magnetochemistry-513143) was funded by MDPI, St. Alban-Anlage 66, 4052 Basel, Switzerland.

Acknowledgments: All authors are thankful to their representative universities/institutes for literature services.

Conflicts of Interest: The authors report no conflict of interest in any capacity, i.e., competing or financial.

References

1. Xu, J.; Sun, J.; Wang, Y.; Sheng, J.; Wang, F.; Sun, M. Application of iron magnetic nanoparticles in protein immobilization. *Molecules* **2014**, *19*, 11465–11486. [CrossRef] [PubMed]
2. Bilal, M.; Zhao, Y.; Rasheed, T.; Iqbal, H.M. Magnetic nanoparticles as versatile carriers for enzymes immobilization: A review. *Int. J. Biol. Macromol.* **2018**, *120*, 2530–2544. [CrossRef] [PubMed]
3. Netto, C.G.; Toma, H.E.; Andrade, L.H. Superparamagnetic nanoparticles as versatile carriers and supporting materials for enzymes. *J. Mol. Catal. B Enzym.* **2013**, *85*, 71–92. [CrossRef]
4. Abu-Dief, A.M.; Abdel-Fatah, S.M. Development and functionalization of magnetic nanoparticles as powerful and green catalysts for organic synthesis. *Beni-Suef Univ. J. Basic Appl. Sci.* **2018**, *7*, 55–67. [CrossRef]
5. Jessie, A.; Guillaume, W. Tumor-Targeting Drug-Loaded Particles. U.S. Patent US8043631B2, 3 October 2012.
6. Bazile, D.; Couvreur, P.; Lakkireddy, H.R.; MacKiewicz, N.; Nicolas, J. Functional PLA-PEG Copolymers, the Nanoparticles Thereof, Their Preparation and Use for Targeted Drug Delivery and Imaging. Patent EP2634179A1, 14 June 2016.
7. Laurent, S.; Forge, D.; Port, M.; Roch, A.; Robic, C.; Vander Elst, L.; Muller, R.N. Magnetic iron oxide nanoparticles: Synthesis, stabilization, vectorization, physicochemical characterizations, and biological applications. *Chem. Rev.* **2008**, *108*, 2064–2110. [CrossRef] [PubMed]
8. Taft, D.; Tzannis, S.; Dai, W.-G.; Ottensmann, S.; Bitler, S.; Zheng, Q.; Bell, A. Polymer Formulations for Delivery of Bioactive Materials. U.S. Patent US8784893B2, 14 February 2012.
9. Angelova, A.; Angelov, B.; Drechsler, M.; Lesieur, S. Neurotrophin delivery using nanotechnology. *Drug Discov. Today* **2013**, *18*, 1263–1271. [CrossRef]
10. Martins, P.; Rosa, D.; R Fernandes, A.; Baptista, P.V. Nanoparticle drug delivery systems: Recent patents and applications in nanomedicine. *Recent Pat. Nanomed.* **2013**, *3*, 105–118. [CrossRef]
11. Ako-Adounvo, A.-M.; Marabesi, B.; Lemos, R.C.; Patricia, A.; Karla, P.K. Drug and Gene Delivery Materials and Devices. In *Emerging Nanotechnologies for Diagnostics, Drug Delivery and Medical Devices*; Elsevier: Amsterdam, The Netherlands, 2017; pp. 375–392.
12. Nam, J.-M.; Thaxton, C.S.; Mirkin, C.A. Nanoparticle-based bio-bar codes for the ultrasensitive detection of proteins. *Science* **2003**, *301*, 1884–1886. [CrossRef]
13. Jain, A.; Cheng, K. The principles and applications of avidin-based nanoparticles in drug delivery and diagnosis. *J. Control. Release* **2017**, *245*, 27–40. [CrossRef]
14. Yin, C.; Hong, B.; Gong, Z.; Zhao, H.; Hu, W.; Lu, X.; Li, J.; Li, X.; Yang, Z.; Fan, Q. Fluorescent oligo (p-phenyleneethynylene) contained amphiphiles-encapsulated magnetic nanoparticles for targeted magnetic resonance and two-photon optical imaging in vitro and in vivo. *Nanoscale* **2015**, *7*, 8907–8919. [CrossRef]
15. Bao, G.; Mitragotri, S.; Tong, S. Multifunctional nanoparticles for drug delivery and molecular imaging. *Annu. Rev. Biomed. Eng.* **2013**, *15*, 253–282. [CrossRef]
16. Li, L.; Jiang, W.; Luo, K.; Song, H.; Lan, F.; Wu, Y.; Gu, Z. Superparamagnetic iron oxide nanoparticles as MRI contrast agents for non-invasive stem cell labeling and tracking. *Theranostics* **2013**, *3*, 595. [CrossRef] [PubMed]
17. Wang, J.; Hu, X.; Xiang, D. Nanoparticle drug delivery systems: An excellent carrier for tumor peptide vaccines. *Drug Deliv.* **2018**, *25*, 1319–1327. [CrossRef]
18. Seenuvasan, M.; Kumar, K.; Kumar, M.A.; Iyyappan, J.; Suganthi, J. Response surface estimation and canonical quantification for the pectin degrading Fe_3O_4-SiO_2 nanobiocatalyst fabrication. *Int. J. ChemTech Res.* **2014**, *6*, 3618–3627.

19. Gao, F.; Guo, Y.; Fan, X.; Hu, M.; Li, S.; Zhai, Q.; Jiang, Y.; Wang, X. Enhancing the catalytic performance of chloroperoxidase by co-immobilization with glucose oxidase on magnetic graphene oxide. *Biochem. Eng. J.* **2019**, *143*, 101–109. [CrossRef]
20. Jiang, Y.; Liu, H.; Wang, L.; Zhou, L.; Huang, Z.; Ma, L.; He, Y.; Shi, L.; Gao, J. Virus-like organosilica nanoparticles for lipase immobilization: Characterization and biocatalytic applications. *Biochem. Eng. J.* **2019**, *144*, 125–134. [CrossRef]
21. Hosseini, S.M.; Kim, S.M.; Sayed, M.; Younesi, H.; Bahramifar, N.; Park, J.H.; Pyo, S.-H. Lipase-immobilized chitosan-crosslinked magnetic nanoparticle as a biocatalyst for ring opening esterification of itaconic anhydride. *Biochem. Eng. J.* **2019**, *143*, 141–150. [CrossRef]
22. Mangkorn, N.; Kanokratana, P.; Roongsawang, N.; Laobuthee, A.; Laosiripojana, N.; Champreda, V. Synthesis and characterization of Ogataea thermomethanolica alcohol oxidase immobilized on barium ferrite magnetic microparticles. *J. Biosci. Bioeng.* **2019**, *127*, 265–272. [CrossRef] [PubMed]
23. Mohammadi, M.; Mokarram, R.R.; Ghorbani, M.; Hamishehkar, H. Inulinase immobilized gold-magnetic nanoparticles as a magnetically recyclable biocatalyst for facial and efficient inulin biotransformation to high fructose syrup. *Int. J. Biol. Macromol.* **2019**, *123*, 846–855. [CrossRef]
24. Suo, H.; Xu, L.; Xu, C.; Qiu, X.; Chen, H.; Huang, H.; Hu, Y. Graphene oxide nanosheets shielding of lipase immobilized on magnetic composites for the improvement of enzyme stability. *ACS Sustain. Chem. Eng.* **2019**, *7*, 4486–4494. [CrossRef]
25. Torabizadeh, H.; Mahmoudi, A. Inulin hydrolysis by inulinase immobilized covalently on magnetic nanoparticles prepared with wheat gluten hydrolysates. *Biotechnol. Rep.* **2018**, *17*, 97–103. [CrossRef]
26. Dal Magro, L.; Silveira, V.C.; de Menezes, E.W.; Benvenutti, E.V.; Nicolodi, S.; Hertz, P.F.; Klein, M.P.; Rodrigues, R.C. Magnetic biocatalysts of pectinase and cellulase: Synthesis and characterization of two preparations for application in grape juice clarification. *Int. J. Biol. Macromol.* **2018**, *115*, 35–44. [CrossRef]
27. Mardani, T.; Khiabani, M.S.; Mokarram, R.R.; Hamishehkar, H. Immobilization of α-amylase on chitosan-montmorillonite nanocomposite beads. *Int. J. Biol. Macromol.* **2018**, *120*, 354–360. [CrossRef]
28. Sojitra, U.V.; Nadar, S.S.; Rathod, V.K. Immobilization of pectinase onto chitosan magnetic nanoparticles by macromolecular cross-linker. *Carbohydr. Polym.* **2017**, *157*, 677–685. [CrossRef]
29. Sojitra, U.V.; Nadar, S.S.; Rathod, V.K. A magnetic tri-enzyme nanobiocatalyst for fruit juice clarification. *Food Chem.* **2016**, *213*, 296–305. [CrossRef]
30. Wang, B.; Cheng, F.; Lu, Y.; Ge, W.; Zhang, M.; Yue, B. Immobilization of pectinase from *Penicillium oxalicum* F67 onto magnetic cornstarch microspheres: Characterization and application in juice production. *J. Mol. Catal. B Enzym.* **2013**, *97*, 137–143. [CrossRef]
31. Wang, X.-Y.; Jiang, X.-P.; Li, Y.; Zeng, S.; Zhang, Y.-W. Preparation Fe_3O_4@ chitosan magnetic particles for covalent immobilization of lipase from *Thermomyces lanuginosus*. *Int. J. Biol. Macromol.* **2015**, *75*, 44–50. [CrossRef]
32. Bilal, M.; Rasheed, T.; Iqbal, H.M.; Yan, Y. Peroxidases-assisted removal of environmentally-related hazardous pollutants with reference to the reaction mechanisms of industrial dyes. *Sci. Total Environ.* **2018**, *644*, 1–13. [CrossRef]
33. Rehman, S.; Bhatti, H.N.; Bilal, M.; Asgher, M. Cross-linked enzyme aggregates (CLEAs) of *Pencilluim notatum* lipase enzyme with improved activity, stability and reusability characteristics. *Int. J. Biol. Macromol.* **2016**, *91*, 1161–1169. [CrossRef]
34. Rehman, S.; Wang, P.; Bhatti, H.N.; Bilal, M.; Asgher, M. Improved catalytic properties of *Penicillium notatum* lipase immobilized in nanoscale silicone polymeric films. *Int. J. Biol. Macromol.* **2017**, *97*, 279–286. [CrossRef]
35. Amin, F.; Bhatti, H.N.; Bilal, M.; Asgher, M. Improvement of activity, thermo-stability and fruit juice clarification characteristics of fungal exo-polygalacturonase. *Int. J. Biol. Macromol.* **2017**, *95*, 974–984. [CrossRef]
36. Amin, F.; Bhatti, H.N.; Bilal, M.; Asgher, M. Multiple parameter optimizations for enhanced biosynthesis of exo-polygalacturonase enzyme and its application in fruit juice clarification. *Int. J. Food Eng.* **2017**, *13*. [CrossRef]
37. Asgher, M.; Noreen, S.; Bilal, M. Enhancement of catalytic, reusability, and long-term stability features of *Trametes versicolor* IBL-04 laccase immobilized on different polymers. *Int. J. Biol. Macromol.* **2017**, *95*, 54–62. [CrossRef]

38. Asgher, M.; Noreen, S.; Bilal, M. Enhancing catalytic functionality of *Trametes versicolor* IBL-04 laccase by immobilization on chitosan microspheres. *Chem. Eng. Res. Des.* **2017**, *119*, 1–11. [CrossRef]
39. Bilal, M.; Iqbal, H.M. Chemical, physical, and biological coordination: An interplay between materials and enzymes as potential platforms for immobilization. *Coord. Chem. Rev.* **2019**, *388*, 1–23. [CrossRef]
40. Bilal, M.; Iqbal, H.M. Naturally-derived biopolymers: Potential platforms for enzyme immobilization. *Int. J. Biol. Macromol.* **2019**, *130*, 462–482. [CrossRef]
41. Darwesh, O.M.; Matter, I.A.; Eida, M.F. Development of peroxidase enzyme immobilized magnetic nanoparticles for bioremediation of textile wastewater dye. *J. Environ. Chem. Eng.* **2019**, *7*, 102805. [CrossRef]
42. Kashefi, S.; Borghei, S.M.; Mahmoodi, N.M. Superparamagnetic enzyme-graphene oxide magnetic nanocomposite as an environmentally friendly biocatalyst: Synthesis and biodegradation of dye using response surface methodology. *Microchem. J.* **2019**, *145*, 547–558. [CrossRef]
43. Tapre, A.; Jain, R. Pectinases: Enzymes for fruit processing industry. *Int. Food Res. J.* **2014**, *21*, 447–453.
44. Dal Magro, L.; Hertz, P.F.; Fernandez-Lafuente, R.; Klein, M.P.; Rodrigues, R.C. Preparation and characterization of a Combi-CLEAs from pectinases and cellulases: A potential biocatalyst for grape juice clarification. *RSC Adv.* **2016**, *6*, 27242–27251. [CrossRef]
45. Echavarría, A.; Torras, C.; Pagán, J.; Ibarz, A. Fruit juice processing and membrane technology application. *Food Eng. Rev.* **2011**, *3*, 136–158. [CrossRef]
46. Jiménez-Sánchez, C.; Lozano-Sánchez, J.; Segura-Carretero, A.; Fernández-Gutiérrez, A. Alternatives to conventional thermal treatments in fruit-juice processing. Part 1: Techniques and applications. *Crit. Rev. Food Sci. Nutr.* **2017**, *57*, 501–523. [CrossRef] [PubMed]
47. Huang, W.-C.; Wang, W.; Xue, C.; Mao, X. Effective enzyme immobilization onto a magnetic chitin nanofiber composite. *ACS Sustain. Chem. Eng.* **2018**, *6*, 8118–8124. [CrossRef]
48. Barbosa, O.; Ortiz, C.; Berenguer-Murcia, Á.; Torres, R.; Rodrigues, R.C.; Fernandez-Lafuente, R. Glutaraldehyde in bio-catalysts design: A useful crosslinker and a versatile tool in enzyme immobilization. *RSC Adv.* **2014**, *4*, 1583–1600. [CrossRef]
49. Mateo, C.; Palomo, J.M.; Van Langen, L.M.; Van Rantwijk, F.; Sheldon, R.A. A new, mild cross-linking methodology to prepare cross-linked enzyme aggregates. *Biotechnol. Bioeng.* **2004**, *86*, 273–276. [CrossRef]
50. Zhen, Q.; Wang, M.; Qi, W.; Su, R.; He, Z. Preparation of β-mannanase CLEAs using macromolecular cross-linkers. *Catal. Sci. Technol.* **2013**, *3*, 1937–1941. [CrossRef]
51. Flores-Gallegos, A.C.; Contreras-Esquivel, J.C.; Morlett-Chávez, J.A.; Aguilar, C.N.; Rodríguez-Herrera, R. Comparative study of fungal strains for thermostable inulinase production. *J. Biosci. Bioeng.* **2015**, *119*, 421–426. [CrossRef]
52. Mussatto, S.I.; Aguiar, L.M.; Marinha, M.I.; Jorge, R.C.; Ferreira, E.C. Economic analysis and environmental impact assessment of three different fermentation processes for fructooligosaccharides production. *Bioresour. Technol.* **2015**, *198*, 673–681. [CrossRef]
53. Singh, R.S.; Chauhan, K.; Kennedy, J.F. A panorama of bacterial inulinases: Production, purification, characterization and industrial applications. *Int. J. Biol. Macromol.* **2017**, *96*, 312–322. [CrossRef]
54. Vandamme, E.J.; Derycke, D.G. Microbial inulinases: Fermentation process, properties, and applications. In *Advances in Applied Microbiology*; Elsevier: Amsterdam, The Netherlands, 1983; Volume 29, pp. 139–176.
55. Barthomeuf, C.; Regerat, F.; Pourrat, H. Production of inulinase by a new mold of Penicillium rugulosum. *J. Ferment. Bioeng.* **1991**, *72*, 491–494. [CrossRef]
56. Torabizadeh, H.; Habibi-Rezaei, M.; Safari, M.; Moosavi-Movahedi, A.A.; Sharifizadeh, A.; Azizian, H.; Amanlou, M. Endo-inulinase stabilization by pyridoxal phosphate modification: A kinetics, thermodynamics, and simulation approach. *Appl. Biochem. Biotechnol.* **2011**, *165*, 1661–1673. [CrossRef] [PubMed]
57. Wilkerson, J.W.; Yang, S.-O.; Funk, P.J.; Stanley, S.K.; Bundy, B.C. Nanoreactors: Strategies to encapsulate enzyme biocatalysts in virus-like particles. *New Biotechnol.* **2018**, *44*, 59–63. [CrossRef] [PubMed]
58. Patterson, D.P.; Prevelige, P.E.; Douglas, T. Nanoreactors by programmed enzyme encapsulation inside the capsid of the bacteriophage P22. *ACS Nano* **2012**, *6*, 5000–5009. [CrossRef] [PubMed]
59. Fiedler, J.D.; Brown, S.D.; Lau, J.L.; Finn, M. RNA-directed packaging of enzymes within virus-like particles. *Angew. Chem. Int. Ed.* **2010**, *49*, 9648–9651. [CrossRef] [PubMed]
60. Minten, I.J.; Hendriks, L.J.; Nolte, R.J.; Cornelissen, J.J. Controlled encapsulation of multiple proteins in virus capsids. *J. Am. Chem. Soc.* **2009**, *131*, 17771–17773. [CrossRef] [PubMed]

61. Minten, I.J.; Claessen, V.I.; Blank, K.; Rowan, A.E.; Nolte, R.J.; Cornelissen, J.J. Catalytic capsids: The art of confinement. *Chem. Sci.* **2011**, *2*, 358–362. [CrossRef]
62. Kim, K.; Lee, O.; Lee, E. Nano-immobilized biocatalysts for biodiesel production from renewable and sustainable resources. *Catalysts* **2018**, *8*, 68.
63. Zhang, C.; Liu, Y.; Sun, Y. Lipase immobilized to a short alkyl chain-containing zwitterionic polymer grafted on silica nanoparticles: Moderate activation and significant increase of thermal stability. *Biochem. Eng. J.* **2019**, *146*, 124–131. [CrossRef]
64. Frimpong, R.A.; Hilt, J.Z. Magnetic nanoparticles in biomedicine: Synthesis, functionalization and applications. *Nanomedicine* **2010**, *5*, 1401–1414. [CrossRef] [PubMed]
65. Bárcena, C.; Sra, A.K.; Gao, J. Applications of magnetic nanoparticles in biomedicine. In *Nanoscale Magnetic Materials and Applications*; Springer: New York, NY, USA, 2009; pp. 591–626.
66. Pankhurst, Q.A.; Connolly, J.; Jones, S.; Dobson, J. Applications of magnetic nanoparticles in biomedicine. *J. Phys. D Appl. Phys.* **2003**, *36*, R167. [CrossRef]
67. Jha, S.; Sharma, P.K.; Malviya, R. Hyperthermia: Role and risk factor for cancer treatment. *Achiev. Life Sci.* **2016**, *10*, 161–167. [CrossRef]
68. Neuberger, T.; Schöpf, B.; Hofmann, H.; Hofmann, M.; Von Rechenberg, B. Superparamagnetic nanoparticles for biomedical applications: Possibilities and limitations of a new drug delivery system. *J. Magn. Magn. Mater.* **2005**, *293*, 483–496. [CrossRef]
69. Huber, D.L. Synthesis, properties, and applications of iron nanoparticles. *Small* **2005**, *1*, 482–501. [CrossRef] [PubMed]
70. Bomatí-Miguel, O.; Morales, M.P.; Tartaj, P.; Ruiz-Cabello, J.; Bonville, P.; Santos, M.; Zhao, X.; Veintemillas-Verdaguer, S. Fe-based nanoparticulate metallic alloys as contrast agents for magnetic resonance imaging. *Biomaterials* **2005**, *26*, 5695–5703. [CrossRef] [PubMed]
71. Lee, C.M.; Jeong, H.J.; Kim, E.M.; Kim, D.W.; Lim, S.T.; Kim, H.T.; Park, I.K.; Jeong, Y.Y.; Kim, J.W.; Sohn, M.H. Superparamagnetic iron oxide nanoparticles as a dual imaging probe for targeting hepatocytes in vivo. *Magn. Reson. Med. Off. J. Int. Soc. Magn. Reson. Med.* **2009**, *62*, 1440–1446. [CrossRef]
72. Yean, S.; Cong, L.; Yavuz, C.T.; Mayo, J.; Yu, W.; Kan, A.; Colvin, V.; Tomson, M. Effect of magnetite particle size on adsorption and desorption of arsenite and arsenate. *J. Mater. Res.* **2005**, *20*, 3255–3264. [CrossRef]
73. Yokoyama, T.; Masuda, H.; Suzuki, M.; Ehara, K.; Nogi, K.; Fuji, M.; Fukui, T.; Suzuki, H.; Tatami, J.; Hayashi, K. Basic properties and measuring methods of nanoparticles. In *Nanoparticle Technology Handbook*; Elsevier: Amsterdam, The Netherlands, 2008; pp. 3–48.
74. Wiekhorst, F.; Seliger, C.; Jurgons, R.; Steinhoff, U.; Eberbeck, D.; Trahms, L.; Alexiou, C. Quantification of magnetic nanoparticles by magnetorelaxometry and comparison to histology after magnetic drug targeting. *J. Nanosci. Nanotechnol.* **2006**, *6*, 3222–3225. [CrossRef]
75. Namdeo, M.; Saxena, S.; Tankhiwale, R.; Bajpai, M.; Mohan, Y.; Bajpai, S. Magnetic nanoparticles for drug delivery applications. *J. Nanosci. Nanotechnol.* **2008**, *8*, 3247–3271. [CrossRef]
76. Lu, A.H.; Salabas, E.E.; Schüth, F. Magnetic nanoparticles: Synthesis, protection, functionalization, and application. *Angew. Chem. Int. Ed.* **2007**, *46*, 1222–1244. [CrossRef]
77. Arruebo, M.; Galán, M.; Navascués, N.; Téllez, C.; Marquina, C.; Ibarra, M.R.; Santamaría, J. Development of magnetic nanostructured silica-based materials as potential vectors for drug-delivery applications. *Chem. Mater.* **2006**, *18*, 1911–1919. [CrossRef]
78. Rosengart, A.J.; Kaminski, M.D.; Chen, H.; Caviness, P.L.; Ebner, A.D.; Ritter, J.A. Magnetizable implants and functionalized magnetic carriers: A novel approach for noninvasive yet targeted drug delivery. *J. Magn. Magn. Mater.* **2005**, *293*, 633–638. [CrossRef]
79. Wang, L.; Zhou, W.; Zhong, Y.; Huo, Y.; Fan, P.; Zhan, S.; Xiao, J.; Jin, X.; Gou, S.; Yin, T. Overexpression of G protein-coupled receptor GPR87 promotes pancreatic cancer aggressiveness and activates NF-κB signaling pathway. *Mol. Cancer* **2017**, *16*, 61. [CrossRef] [PubMed]
80. Blake, A.; Dragan, M.; Tirona, R.G.; Hardy, D.B.; Brackstone, M.; Tuck, A.B.; Babwah, A.V.; Bhattacharya, M. G protein-coupled KISS1 receptor is overexpressed in triple negative breast cancer and promotes drug resistance. *Sci. Rep.* **2017**, *7*, 46525. [CrossRef] [PubMed]
81. Boyd, B. *Drug Delivery Report Autumn/Winter*; PharmaVentures Ltd.: Oxford, UK, 2005.
82. Tomalia, D.A. Birth of a new macromolecular architecture: Dendrimers as quantized building blocks for nanoscale synthetic polymer chemistry. *Prog. Polym. Sci.* **2005**, *30*, 294–324. [CrossRef]

83. Vo, T.N.; Kasper, F.K.; Mikos, A.G. Strategies for controlled delivery of growth factors and cells for bone regeneration. *Adv. Drug Deliv. Rev.* **2012**, *64*, 1292–1309. [CrossRef] [PubMed]
84. Zhang, J.; Saltzman, M. Engineering biodegradable nanoparticles for drug and gene delivery. *Chem. Eng. Prog.* **2013**, *109*, 25. [PubMed]
85. Kohane, D.S. Microparticles and nanoparticles for drug delivery. *Biotechnol. Bioeng.* **2007**, *96*, 203–209. [CrossRef] [PubMed]
86. D. Friedman, A.; E. Claypool, S.; Liu, R. The smart targeting of nanoparticles. *Curr. Pharm. Des.* **2013**, *19*, 6315–6329. [CrossRef]
87. Osakwe, O.; Rizvi, S.A. *Social Aspects of Drug Discovery, Development and Commercialization*; Academic Press: San Diego, CA, USA, 2016.
88. Onoue, S.; Yamada, S.; Chan, H.-K. Nanodrugs: Pharmacokinetics and safety. *Int. J. Nanomed.* **2014**, *9*, 1025. [CrossRef]
89. Kudr, J.; Haddad, Y.; Richtera, L.; Heger, Z.; Cernak, M.; Adam, V.; Zitka, O. Magnetic nanoparticles: From design and synthesis to real world applications. *Nanomaterials* **2017**, *7*, 243. [CrossRef]
90. Sun, C.; Lee, J.S.; Zhang, M. Magnetic nanoparticles in MR imaging and drug delivery. *Adv. Drug Deliv. Rev.* **2008**, *60*, 1252–1265. [CrossRef] [PubMed]
91. Skalickova, S.; Nejdl, L.; Kudr, J.; Ruttkay-Nedecky, B.; Jimenez Jimenez, A.; Kopel, P.; Kremplova, M.; Masarik, M.; Stiborova, M.; Eckschlager, T. Fluorescence characterization of gold modified liposomes with antisense N-myc DNA bound to the magnetisable particles with encapsulated anticancer drugs (doxorubicin, ellipticine and etoposide). *Sensors* **2016**, *16*, 290. [CrossRef] [PubMed]
92. Mahmoudi, M.; Sant, S.; Wang, B.; Laurent, S.; Sen, T. Superparamagnetic iron oxide nanoparticles (SPIONs): Development, surface modification and applications in chemotherapy. *Adv. Drug Deliv. Rev.* **2011**, *63*, 24–46. [CrossRef] [PubMed]
93. Gupta, A.K.; Gupta, M. Synthesis and surface engineering of iron oxide nanoparticles for biomedical applications. *Biomaterials* **2005**, *26*, 3995–4021. [CrossRef] [PubMed]
94. McCarthy, J.R.; Weissleder, R. Multifunctional magnetic nanoparticles for targeted imaging and therapy. *Adv. Drug Deliv. Rev.* **2008**, *60*, 1241–1251. [CrossRef] [PubMed]
95. Heger, Z.; Zitka, J.; Cernei, N.; Krizkova, S.; Sztalmachova, M.; Kopel, P.; Masarik, M.; Hodek, P.; Zitka, O.; Adam, V. 3D-printed biosensor with poly (dimethylsiloxane) reservoir for magnetic separation and quantum dots-based immunolabeling of metallothionein. *Electrophoresis* **2015**, *36*, 1256–1264. [CrossRef] [PubMed]
96. Zitka, O.; Cernei, N.; Heger, Z.; Matousek, M.; Kopel, P.; Kynicky, J.; Masarik, M.; Kizek, R.; Adam, V. Microfluidic chip coupled with modified paramagnetic particles for sarcosine isolation in urine. *Electrophoresis* **2013**, *34*, 2639–2647. [CrossRef] [PubMed]
97. Pileni, M.P. Magnetic fluids: Fabrication, magnetic properties, and organization of nanocrystals. *Adv. Funct. Mater.* **2001**, *11*, 323–336. [CrossRef]
98. Tartaj, P.; del Puerto Morales, M.; Veintemillas-Verdaguer, S.; González-Carreño, T.; Serna, C.J. The preparation of magnetic nanoparticles for applications in biomedicine. *J. Phys. D Appl. Phys.* **2003**, *36*, R182. [CrossRef]
99. Sun, Y.-k.; Ma, M.; Zhang, Y.; Gu, N. Synthesis of nanometer-size maghemite particles from magnetite. *Colloids Surf. A Physicochem. Eng. Asp.* **2004**, *245*, 15–19. [CrossRef]
100. Ma, M.; Zhang, Y.; Yu, W.; Shen, H.-Y.; Zhang, H.-Q.; Gu, N. Preparation and characterization of magnetite nanoparticles coated by amino silane. *Colloids Surf. A Physicochem. Eng. Asp.* **2003**, *212*, 219–226. [CrossRef]
101. Park, J.; An, K.; Hwang, Y.; Park, J.-G.; Noh, H.-J.; Kim, J.-Y.; Park, J.-H.; Hwang, N.-M.; Hyeon, T. Ultra-large-scale syntheses of monodisperse nanocrystals. *Nat. Mater.* **2004**, *3*, 891. [CrossRef] [PubMed]
102. Zitka, O.; Krizkova, S.; Krejcova, L.; Hynek, D.; Gumulec, J.; Masarik, M.; Sochor, J.; Adam, V.; Hubalek, J.; Trnkova, L. Microfluidic tool based on the antibody-modified paramagnetic particles for detection of 8-hydroxy-2′-deoxyguanosine in urine of prostate cancer patients. *Electrophoresis* **2011**, *32*, 3207–3220. [CrossRef] [PubMed]
103. Kang, B.J.; Jeun, M.; Jang, G.H.; Song, S.H.; Jeong, I.G.; Kim, C.-S.; Searson, P.C.; Lee, K.H. Diagnosis of prostate cancer via nanotechnological approach. *Int. J. Nanomed.* **2015**, *10*, 6555.
104. Patel, D.; Moon, J.Y.; Chang, Y.; Kim, T.J.; Lee, G.H. Poly (D, L-lactide-co-glycolide) coated superparamagnetic iron oxide nanoparticles: Synthesis, characterization and in vivo study as MRI contrast agent. *Colloids Surf. A Physicochem. Eng. Asp.* **2008**, *313*, 91–94. [CrossRef]

105. Prabha, G.; Raj, V. Formation and characterization of β-cyclodextrin (β-CD)–polyethyleneglycol (PEG)–polyethyleneimine (PEI) coated Fe₃O₄ nanoparticles for loading and releasing 5-Fluorouracil drug. *Biomed. Pharmacother.* **2016**, *80*, 173–182. [CrossRef] [PubMed]
106. Karimzadeh, I.; Aghazadeh, M.; Doroudi, T.; Ganjali, M.R.; Kolivand, P.H. Superparamagnetic iron oxide (Fe₃O₄) nanoparticles coated with PEG/PEI for biomedical applications: A facile and scalable preparation route based on the cathodic electrochemical deposition method. *Adv. Phys. Chem.* **2017**, *2017*. [CrossRef]
107. Li, J.; Zheng, L.; Cai, H.; Sun, W.; Shen, M.; Zhang, G.; Shi, X. Polyethyleneimine-mediated synthesis of folic acid-targeted iron oxide nanoparticles for in vivo tumor MR imaging. *Biomaterials* **2013**, *34*, 8382–8392. [CrossRef]
108. Rodrigo, M.A.M.; Krejcova, L.; Kudr, J.; Cernei, N.; Kopel, P.; Richtera, L.; Moulick, A.; Hynek, D.; Adam, V.; Stiborova, M. Fully automated two-step assay for detection of metallothionein through magnetic isolation using functionalized γ-Fe₂O₃ particles. *J. Chromatogr. B* **2016**, *1039*, 17–27. [CrossRef]
109. Jian, P.; Fen, Z.; Lu, L.; Liang, T.; Li, Y.; Wei, C.; Hui, L.; TANG, J.-b.; WU, L.-x. Preparation and characterization of PEG-PEI/Fe₃O₄ nano-magnetic fluid by co-precipitation method. *Trans. Nonferrous Metals Soc. China* **2008**, *18*, 393–398.
110. Lee, J.-H.; Huh, Y.-M.; Jun, Y.-W.; Seo, J.-W.; Jang, J.-T.; Song, H.-T.; Kim, S.; Cho, E.-J.; Yoon, H.-G.; Suh, J.-S. Artificially engineered magnetic nanoparticles for ultra-sensitive molecular imaging. *Nat. Med.* **2007**, *13*, 95. [CrossRef] [PubMed]
111. Kim, J.; Lee, N.; Hyeon, T. Recent development of nanoparticles for molecular imaging. *Philos. Trans. R. Soc. A Math. Phys. Eng. Sci.* **2017**, *375*, 20170022. [CrossRef]
112. Dutz, S.; Clement, J.H.; Eberbeck, D.; Gelbrich, T.; Hergt, R.; Müller, R.; Wotschadlo, J.; Zeisberger, M. Ferrofluids of magnetic multicore nanoparticles for biomedical applications. *J. Magn. Magn. Mater.* **2009**, *321*, 1501–1504. [CrossRef]
113. Seo, W.S.; Lee, J.H.; Sun, X.; Suzuki, Y.; Mann, D.; Liu, Z.; Terashima, M.; Yang, P.C.; McConnell, M.V.; Nishimura, D.G. FeCo/graphitic-shell nanocrystals as advanced magnetic-resonance-imaging and near-infrared agents. *Nat. Mater.* **2006**, *5*, 971. [CrossRef] [PubMed]
114. Kainz, Q.M.; Fernandes, S.; Eichenseer, C.M.; Besostri, F.; Körner, H.; Müller, R.; Reiser, O. Synthesis of functionalized, dispersible carbon-coated cobalt nanoparticles for potential biomedical applications. *Faraday Discuss.* **2015**, *175*, 27–40. [CrossRef] [PubMed]
115. Stevenson, J.; Rutnakornpituk, M.; Vadala, M.; Esker, A.; Charles, S.; Wells, S.; Dailey, J.; Riffle, J. Magnetic cobalt dispersions in poly (dimethylsiloxane) fluids. *J. Magn. Magn. Mater.* **2001**, *225*, 47–58. [CrossRef]
116. Rutnakornpituk, M.; Baranauskas, V.; Riffle, J.; Connolly, J.; St Pierre, T.; Dailey, J. Polysiloxane fluid dispersions of cobalt nanoparticles in silica spheres for use in ophthalmic applications. *Eur. Cells Mater* **2002**, *3*, 102–105.
117. Osorio-Cantillo, C.; Santiago-Miranda, A.; Perales-Perez, O.; Xin, Y. Size-and phase-controlled synthesis of cobalt nanoparticles for potential biomedical applications. *J. Appl. Phys.* **2012**, *111*, 07B324. [CrossRef]
118. Joubert, J. Magnetic micro composites as vectors for bioactive agents: The state of art. *Anales de Quimica* **1997**, *93*, 70–76.
119. Grasset, F.; Mornet, S.; Demourgues, A.; Portier, J.; Bonnet, J.; Vekris, A.; Duguet, E. Synthesis, magnetic properties, surface modification and cytotoxicity evaluation of Y₃Fe₅₋ₓAlₓO₁₂ (0 ≤ x ≤ 2) garnet submicron particles for biomedical applications. *J. Magn. Magn. Mater.* **2001**, *234*, 409–418. [CrossRef]
120. Rinaldi-Montes, N.; Gorria, P.; Martínez-Blanco, D.; Amghouz, Z.; Fuertes, A.B.; Barquín, L.F.; de Pedro, I.; Olivi, L.; Blanco, J.A. Unravelling the onset of the exchange bias effect in Ni (core)@ NiO (shell) nanoparticles embedded in a mesoporous carbon matrix. *J. Mater. Chem. C* **2015**, *3*, 5674–5682. [CrossRef]
121. Zhou, W.; Zheng, K.; He, L.; Wang, R.; Guo, L.; Chen, C.; Han, X.; Zhang, Z. Ni/Ni3C core–shell nanochains and its magnetic properties: One-step synthesis at low temperature. *Nano Lett.* **2008**, *8*, 1147–1152. [CrossRef] [PubMed]
122. Rahal, H.; Awad, R.; Abdel-Gaber, A.; Bakeer, D. Synthesis, characterization, and magnetic properties of pure and EDTA-capped NiO nanosized particles. *J. Nanomater.* **2017**, *2017*. [CrossRef]

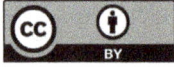

© 2019 by the authors. Licensee MDPI, Basel, Switzerland. This article is an open access article distributed under the terms and conditions of the Creative Commons Attribution (CC BY) license (http://creativecommons.org/licenses/by/4.0/).

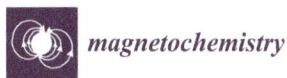

Review

Principles of Magnetic Hyperthermia: A Focus on Using Multifunctional Hybrid Magnetic Nanoparticles

Ihab M. Obaidat [1,*], Venkatesha Narayanaswamy [2], Sulaiman Alaabed [2], Sangaraju Sambasivam [1] and Chandu V. V. Muralee Gopi [3]

1. Department of Physics, United Arab Emirates University, Al-Ain 15551, UAE; sambaphy@gmail.com
2. Department of Geology, United Arab Emirates University, Al-Ain 15551, UAE; venkateshnrn@gmail.com (V.N.); s.alaabed@uaeu.ac.ae (S.A.)
3. School of Electrical and Computer Engineering, Pusan National University, Busan 46241, Korea; naga5673@gmail.com
* Correspondence: iobaidat@uaeu.ac.ae; Tel.: +971(3)-7136321; Fax: +971(3)-7136944

Received: 11 October 2019; Accepted: 29 November 2019; Published: 6 December 2019

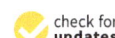

Abstract: Hyperthermia is a noninvasive method that uses heat for cancer therapy where high temperatures have a damaging effect on tumor cells. However, large amounts of heat need to be delivered, which could have negative effects on healthy tissues. Thus, to minimize the negative side effects on healthy cells, a large amount of heat must be delivered only to the tumor cells. Magnetic hyperthermia (MH) uses magnetic nanoparticles particles (MNPs) that are exposed to alternating magnetic field (AMF) to generate heat in local regions (tissues or cells). This cancer therapy method has several advantages, such as (a) it is noninvasive, thus requiring surgery, and (b) it is local, and thus does not damage health cells. However, there are several issues that need to achieved: (a) the MNPs should be biocompatible, biodegradable, with good colloidal stability (b) the MNPs should be successfully delivered to the tumor cells, (c) the MNPs should be used with small amounts and thus MNPs with large heat generation capabilities are required, (d) the AMF used to heat the MNPs should meet safety conditions with limited frequency and amplitude ranges, (e) the changes of temperature should be traced at the cellular level with accurate and noninvasive techniques, (f) factors affecting heat transport from the MNPs to the cells must be understood, and (g) the effect of temperature on the biological mechanisms of cells should be clearly understood. Thus, in this multidisciplinary field, research is needed to investigate these issues. In this report, we shed some light on the principles of heat generation by MNPs in AMF, the limitations and challenges of MH, and the applications of MH using multifunctional hybrid MNPs.

Keywords: magnetic hyperthermia; cancer; nanoparticles; magnetic relaxation; magnetic anisotropy; heat generation; multifunctional nanoparticles; graphene oxide; photothermal therapy

---

1. Introduction

1.1. Effects and Categories of Hyperthermia

Hyperthermia which is the treating of diseases by heating was known since the ancient era [1]. Increasing the temperature of cells above 41 °C is known to cause some effects in the membrane and interior of the cell, such as (a) increasing the fluidity and permeability of the cell membrane, (b) slowing down of the mechanisms of synthesis of nucleic acid and protein, (c) inducing protein denaturation and agglomeration, and (d) damaging the tumor vasculature resulting in a decrease of blood flow [2].

Hyperthermia is divided into three main categories depending on the size of the cancer region being treated [3–5]: whole-body, regional, and local hyperthermia. In the whole-body hyperthermia approach, heat is applied to the whole body in several ways such as using hot water blankets, electric blankets and hot wax. In the regional hyperthermia method, heat is applied to a whole organ or region of the body using external arrays of applicators, and regional perfusion. In local hyperthermia, heat is applied to small tumor regions using electromagnetic waves such as radio waves, microwaves, and ultrasound, which are generated by applicators that are placed at the surface or under skin of superficial cancer or implanted inside the targeted region. In these methods, the temperature must be increased between 41 °C and 45 °C. Each one of these has its negatives. Some of these negatives [2,6] are in all these techniques: (a) heat is applied to the healthy cells in addition to the unhealthy ones which could cause negative side effects, (b) temperature control and measurement at the cell level is difficult, (c) the applied heat is not uniform through the targeted region, and (d) the amount of heat delivered is small. In local hyperthermia, there is a better control on the area exposed to heat and a better heat uniformity. However, local hyperthermia sufferers from two main drawbacks: (a) it is highly invasive for deep cancer regions and (b) the small penetration depth, which is approximately a few centimeters. These drawbacks of local hyperthermia make it better used for small and superficial cancer regions. Nanotechnology can help in eliminating these two negatives of local hyperthermia. Using local hyperthermia with magnetic nanoparticles (MNPs) that are delivered only to the cancer cells and heated externally by an alternating magnetic field (AMF) makes it a noninvasive method, minimizes the side effects and allows for targeting deep cancer cells [5].

Note that for practical applications of MH, the MNPs should have narrow size distribution. Particles with considerably different sizes will result in inhomogeneous heat generation in tissues. This means that while the heat generated through the whole tissue is still below the required value, some parts in the tissue might get overheated causing negative side effects. Also, note that for in vivo hyperthermia experiments, it is difficult to measure the temperature of deep parts of the targeted body. In addition, measuring the temperature at the cell level is not yet permitted. For in vivo experiments, the MNPs can be injected directly in the tumor region or through blood (intravenous administration). In the latter case, two main issues should be resolved; (a) the MNP concentration should be large enough to generate the required amount of heat, and (b) the size of the MNPs to be used should be between 5 nm and 100 nm. If the size of MNPs is less than 5 nm, they will be eliminated through the kidney, whereas particles larger than 100 nm will be cleared by macrophages and moved to the liver [7]. The blood circulation time will thus be minimized and thus the chances for particles to reach the targeted region with enough concentration will be reduced. Additionally, note that Brownian relaxation (will be discussed later) is prevented or minimized in vitro and in vivo experiments when the MNPs are placed in cells or on their membranes. Thus, Neel relaxation will dominate. Thus, hyperthermia measurements are important not only in aqueous suspension, but also in media that is similar to the targeted tissue [8]. In addition, for in vivo experiments, reasonable data is obtained only when the frequency and amplitude of the AMF satisfy the safety criteria.

Several review papers and books discussed the physics and application of MH using MNPs [9–21]. In this report, we present the principles of MH and the physics of heat generation. We also discuss how to measure the power dissipation using calorimetry methods. We also discuss the multifunctional applications of MNPs.

1.2. Magnetic Nanoparticles for Local Hyperthermia

The magnetic properties of MNPs are determined by two main features: (a) finite-size effects and (b) surface effects [16]. Finite-size effects are related to the structure of the NP (single-domain or multidomain). On the other hand, surface effects result from several effects such as the symmetry breaking of the crystal structure at the surface of the particle, dangling bonds, oxidation, and surface stain. The role of surface effects increases as the particle size decreases. This is the case because the ratio of the number of surface atoms to the core atoms increases as the particle size decreases. Due to size-effects and surface effects, magnetic properties of MNPs, such as magnetic moment per atom, saturation magnetization, magnetic anisotropy, coercivity, and Curie temperature, can differ from those of a bulk material [16,22]. The preferred size of the MNPs in most medical applications, is between 10 and 50 nm. Usually, MNPs become single domain particles and display superparamagnetic behavior above a certain temperature called the blocking temperature. In the superparamagnetic state, a nanoparticle has a large magnetic moment and behaves like a giant paramagnetic atom with a fast response to applied magnetic fields with almost zero magnetic reminiscence and coercivity. For MH applications, MNPs must possess large saturation magnetization: M_s values that will generate large amount of heat in the tumor cells under the application of AMF. In addition, large M_s values allow for more control on the movement of the MNPs in the blood using external magnetic field [23]. In addition to the requirement of large M_s, MNPs should be superparamagnetic to achieve good colloidal stability. In the absence of an applied magnetic field, the MNPs in superparamagnetic state lose their magnetism at temperatures above the blocking temperature. This guarantees that the particles will not aggregate and thus they will maintain their colloidal stability. In addition, the interparticle (dipolar) interactions between MNPs decrease with the decrease of the size of particles. This can be understood since the dipole–dipole interaction energy scales as r^6 (r is the interparticle distance). Thus, the small dipolar interactions will result in minimizing the particle aggregation in the existence of applied magnetic field. However, it is important to understand that these two conditions on MNPs (with large M_s and superparamagnetic) should not be isolated from other factors that affect heat generation. For example, heating power was found to be maximized in large ferromagnetic NPs with low anisotropy [23]. Also, the optimum size for the maximum power loss was found to vary with the amplitude of the applied magnetic field [24] and frequency as well. Therefore, several experimental conditions should be considered before we can decide on the choice between superparamagnetic and larger ferromagnetic NPs for MH.

Iron oxide nanoparticles (IONPs), such as magnetite (Fe_3O_4) and maghemite (γ-Fe_2O_3), have good magnetic properties [25,26] that can be tuned by (a) changing synthesis methods, (b) changing the shape and size, (c) modifying the surface structure, (d) and synthesizing core–shell structures with tunable interface exchange anisotropy. The IONPs are good candidates for hyperthermia applications [25,27] due to (a) the ease of synthesis with small sizes and well controlled size distribution, (b) their biocompatibility, and (c) their biodegradability. Although the IONPs are degraded in human body, iron atoms are released. The metabolic mechanisms in humans can manage the released iron atoms by storing or transferring them [28,29].

2. Heat Generation

2.1. Magnetic Relaxation Processes

Magnetocrystalline (or magnetic) anisotropy in magnetic materials results from the spin-orbital interactions of the electrons. The magnetic anisotropy is responsible for keeping the magnetic moments in a particular direction. Atomic orbitals mainly have nonspherical shapes, and thus they tend to align in a specific crystallographic direction. This preferred direction is called the easy direction. In magnetic materials with large magnetic anisotropy the atomic spin and the orbital angular moments are strongly coupled and thus the magnetization prefers to align along the easy direction. Energy (called the anisotropy energy) is needed to rotate the magnetization away from the easy direction. For uniaxial anisotropy, the anisotropy energy per particle is given by [30]

$$E = K\,V\,\sin^2\theta + higher\ order\ terms \quad (1)$$

Here, K is the anisotropy constant (it includes all sources of anisotropy and has a unit of J/m^3), V is the magnetic volume of the particle, and θ is the angle between the particle magnetization and the easy magnetization axis. The higher order terms are very small compared with the first term, and thus can be ignored. In this case, there is only one easy axis with two energy minima separated by the energy maximum, KV.

From Equation (1), we can see that the anisotropy energy is directly proportional to the particle size and to the anisotropy constant. For a fixed K, when the particle size, V decreases the anisotropy energy, E decreases. When V gets very small (reaching the single magnetic domain region), E (which holds the magnetic moment of the particle along the easy axis) might become smaller than the thermal energy, $E_{th} = k_B T$ (k_B is the Boltzmann constant). The particle magnetic moment thus starts to flip freely and randomly in all directions leading to zero net magnetization (in the absence of an external magnetic field). When a magnetic field is applied, energy is given to the particles which will force the magnetic moments of the particles to align along the field direction away from the easy axis. When the field is removed (as with AMF), the magnetic moments will return back (relax) and align along the easy axis. Thus, the gained energy by the applied magnetic field will be lost as heat. If the applied field is AMF, this aligning and relaxation of moments processes will continue, and thus heat will be generated as long as the AMF is applied.

When the orientation of the particle itself is not allowed to change (no physical rotation) during the flipping of its magnetic moment, then the relaxation time of the moment of the particle is called the Néel relaxation time, τ_N and is given by [15,31–33]

$$\tau_N = \frac{\tau_0}{2} \sqrt{\frac{\pi k_B T}{K_{eff} V}} \exp\left(\frac{K_{eff} V}{k_B T}\right) \qquad (2)$$

where K_{eff} is the effective magnetic anisotropy and the factor $\tau_0 \approx 10^{-13}$–10^{-9} s [10,34].

In a magnetic measurement, we call τ_m the measurement time. When the magnetization of a MNP is measured, where $\tau_m \gg \tau_N$, the magnetic moment of the MNP will flip several times (randomly) during the measurement giving zero average magnetization. In this case, the MNP is said to be in the superparamagnetic state. On the other hand, when $\tau_m \ll \tau_N$ the magnetic moment of the particle will not have enough time to flip during the measurement and thus the moment will be blocked at the initial non-zero value at the beginning of the measurement. In this case, the NP is said to be in the blocked state. When $\tau_m = \tau_N$, a transition between the superparamagnetic state and the blocked state occurs [30]. Therefore, at T_b, the Néel relaxation time will be equal to the measurement time, $\tau_N = \tau_m$. In the superparamagnetic state, no magnetization appears when applied magnetic field is zero.

In magnetization experiments the measurement time is usually kept constant while the temperature is varied. In such case the transition between superparamagnetic and blocked states is obtained as a function of temperature. The temperature at which this transition occurs is called the blocking temperature, T_b. In addition to its dependence on the particle size and magnetic anisotropy, the blocking temperature also depends on other factors such as particle-particle interactions. When the MNPs are exposed to a magnetic field, their magnetic moments will be forced to align along the magnetic field direction. If the particles can (physically) rotate and their magnetic anisotropy is large enough, the magnetic field might be successful in causing the particles to physically rotate by pinning their moments. Once the field is removed, the particles will start rotating again and the magnetic moments will relax. This relaxation of magnetic moments is called the Brownian relaxation mechanism, τ_B and is given by [15,31,35]

$$\tau_B = \frac{3 V_H \eta}{k_B T} \qquad (3)$$

where η is the viscosity of the liquid containing the particles and V_H is the hydrodynamic volume of the particle. The hydrodynamic volume includes the magnetic volume and the attached layers on the surface. These attached layers are due to particle coating, absorbed surfactants or interaction with the fluid. Therefore, V_H is larger than the original volume of the particle, V. The physical rotation of the MNPs will cause friction between the particles and the medium in which they exist and heat will be generated. This generated heat will depend on the hydrodynamic volume and the viscosity of the medium.

If both moments relaxation processes exist, the effective magnetic relaxation time, τ_{eff} is then given by

$$\frac{1}{\tau_{eff}} = \frac{1}{\tau_N} + \frac{1}{\tau_B} \qquad (4)$$

As evident from Equation (4), the effective relaxation time, τ_{eff}, is determined by the shorter relaxation time (τ_N or τ_B). For large particles in low viscosity medium, Brownian relaxation mechanism dominates while for small particles in high viscous medium Néel relaxation mechanism dominates. For MNPs with an average size smaller than 15 nm, τ_N is smaller than τ_B, and therefore τ_{eff} is dominated by τ_N, whereas for MNPs with average size larger than 15 nm, τ_B is smaller than τ_N, and therefore τ_{eff} is dominated by τ_B [31]. In in vivo MH experiments, both of these mechanisms are expected to contribute in generating heat. It is important to realize that Equations (3) and (4) were derived for single-domain and identical particles (same size and shape) that are isolated from each other (non-interacting particles). In addition, Equations (1) and (2) are valid for zero (or very small) applied magnetic field. If the applied field is not zero, then Zeeman energy should be included [15].

2.2. Power Loss in MNPs in AMF

For efficient in vivo hyperthermia experiment, we need to generate large SAR values while maintaining safety conditions. Safety conditions include (a) the use of minimum amounts of MNPs and (b) the use of an AMF that will not cause negative side effects due to the induced eddy currents in living tissues. To satisfy the first condition, we need to produce MNPs with optimal magnetic properties that will lead to large heat generation at low concentrations. These properties include saturation magnetization and effective magnetic anisotropy. These properties depend on the size, size distribution, interparticle interactions, particle composition, particle shape, and structure such as MNPs with single magnetic core or MNPs with magnetic core and magnetic shell (called bimagnetic core–shell particles). To satisfy the second condition an AMF with will defined range of intensity and frequency is needed.

In an adiabatic process, the internal energy of a magnetic system is equal to the magnetic work done on it [35]:

$$U = -\mu_0 \oint M dH \qquad (5)$$

During a complete magnetic field cycle, the power dissipation in the magnetic system is equal to the internal energy divided by the time field cycle. Thus, during several field cycles the power dissipation, is equal to internal energy multiplied by the frequency:

$$P = Uf \qquad (6)$$

The power dissipated in superparamagnetic NPs, due to the application of an AMF of maximum strength H_o and frequency f ($\omega = 2\pi f$), was suggested to depend on magnetic moment relaxations and is given by [35]

$$P(f, H) = Uf = \pi \mu_0 \chi'' H_o^2 f \qquad (7)$$

where μ_0 is the permeability of free space and χ'' is the imaginary part of the susceptibility χ ($\chi = \chi' - i\chi''$). In the linear response theory (LRT) the magnetization, M is assumed to have linear relation with the applied magnetic field, H, and thus χ remains constant with increasing H ($M = \chi H$). The LRT can be applied for very small magnetic fields. Therefore, it can be stated that the LRT is valid in the superparamagnetic regime where $H_{max} < k_B T / \mu_0 M_s V$ and when the magnetization of MNPs is linearly proportional to the applied magnetic field. Therefore, in the LRT the magnetic fields should be much smaller than the saturation field (the field required to produce saturation magnetization) of the MNPs ($H_{max} \ll H_K$). Here, H_{max} is the amplitude of the AMF and H_K is the anisotropy field [23].

Thus, when the LRT is assumed, the real part (in-phase component) of the magnetic susceptibility, χ' is given by

$$\chi' = \chi_0 \frac{1}{1 + (2\pi f \tau_{eff})^2} \tag{8}$$

The imaginary part (out-of-phase component) of the susceptibility, χ'' is given by [36,37]

$$\chi'' = \chi_0 \frac{2\pi f \tau_{eff}}{1 + (2\pi f \tau_{eff})^2} \tag{9}$$

The initial constant susceptibility χ_0 is given by

$$\chi_0 = \frac{\mu_0 M_s^2 V}{k_B T} \tag{10}$$

The heating efficiency is represented by the specific absorption rate (SAR) which is also referred to as the specific loss power (SLP). SAR is measured in watts per gram and is given by [38]

$$SAR(f, H) = \frac{P(f, H)}{\rho} = \frac{\pi \mu_0 \chi'' H^2 f}{\rho} \tag{11}$$

where ρ is the mass density of the magnetic material.

In order for the MNPs to have a practical safe application in MH the MNPs should produce large SAR values. This is needed because of two reasons: (a) for safety measures, the MNPs should be used in small concentrations, and (b) in living organs, the water-based medium around the cells absorb a lot of the heat generated by the MNPs. In Rosensweig's theory or LRT, the heat generation of the MNPs depends on several factors such as: strength and frequency of the applied magnetic field, the solvent viscosity, the size of the particles, the saturation magnetization and the magnetic anisotropy of the MNPs. For safety requirements, the strength and frequency of the AMF cannot have any value for applications on living organs. This is because eddy currents are induced in a conductor due to an AMF and thus produce heating in the conductor. As water is a conductor, in human body eddy currents can be induced under an AMF which could result in damaging effect. In general, the parameters that determine the heat generation in MH using MNPs can be classified into two categories: intrinsic and extrinsic parameters. Intrinsic parameters are related to properties of the single isolated MNP. Magnetic anisotropy, size, composition, structure, magnetization, and shape are examples of intrinsic parameters. On the other hand, extrinsic parameters are related to effects that have to do with environment of the MNPs such as the parameters of the AMF (frequency, strength, homogeneity, ...), the distance between the MNPs (concentration or agglomeration), the viscosity of the medium, and electric conducting properties of the tissues. In the following sections, we will focus on one intrinsic parameter which is the anisotropy and on two extrinsic parameters which are the agglomeration parameter and the AMF parameters (frequency and amplitude).

3. Intrinsic Parameters

3.1. Overview of Intrinsic Parameters

Intrinsic parameters include, structure, composition, phase (crystalline or amorphous), shape, size distribution, magnetization, and magnetic anisotropy. Several actions can affect the intrinsic parameters of MNPs such as doping [39–41], surface and interface effects [26,42]. Under an AMF, heat generation by MNPs is determined by hysteresis loss and relaxation effects [43]. Magnetic hysteresis loss occurs in large MNPs with more than one magnetic domain. Domain wall motion due to the applied magnetic field will cause heat loss [44]. These large MNPs will always display magnetic hysteresis regardless if the applied magnetic field is constant (DC) or is AMF. In small MNPs with single magnetic domain (these are called superparamagnetic nanoparticles), heat loss is caused by magnetic relaxation processes. In these small MNPs no magnetic hysteresis is displayed in DC applied magnetic field. However, when these MNPs are placed in an AMF magnetic hysteresis will be displayed due to Brownian and Neel relaxation processes.

In addition to the MNPs volume and the viscosity of the medium in which they exist, Brownian and Neel relaxation processes are determined also by the magnetocrystalline anisotropy of the material. This type of anisotropy determines along which direction the magnetic moments of the material tend to align. However, SAR values depend not only on the magnetocrystalline anisotropy, but on the effective anisotropy which is the net magnetic anisotropy of the MNP.

3.2. The Effective Magnetic Anisotropy

To minimize the negative side effects, the dosage of MNPs required for MH treatment should be reduced. Thus, it becomes necessary to use MNPs with the best heating capability. Magnetic anisotropy is an important intrinsic parameter of MNPs that can be tuned to vary the heating efficiency. However, tuning the magnetic anisotropy of MNPs is a challenging task. The effective anisotropy has four main components: (a) the magnetocrystalline anisotropy, (b) shape anisotropy, (c) surface anisotropy, and (d) exchange anisotropy at the interface of core–shell MNPs. All these types can be tuned. The magnetocrystalline anisotropy can be modified by doping the iron oxides with other elements [41]. The shape anisotropy can be changed by changing the shape of the MNPs from spherical to cubic or other shapes [45–47]. Surface anisotropy which results from surface spin effects can be modified by coating the MNPs [48].

The magnetic anisotropy of MNPs can be varied by synthesizing particles with bimagnetic core–shell phases [49,50]. Theses bimagnetic core–shell MNPs with two different magnetic phases exhibit very interesting properties [51,52]. The magnetic properties (including magnetic anisotropy) of the bimagnetic core–shell MNPs can be tailored by manipulating the interfacial exchange interaction between the core and shell phases [48,53]. This can be achieved by several ways: (a) selecting of the many possible combinations of the core–shell phases, (b) controlling core and shell dimensions [54], and (c) by controlling the interface quality [55–57]. Exchange coupling at the core–shell interface of the MNPs could result in extremely large SAR values [41]. Large number of reports discussed the exchange bias in MNPs with bimagnetic core–shell structures [58–60]. However, the origin of the exchange bias is not fully understood. One of the interesting models reported to describe the exchange bias in bimagnetic materials is based on the existence of interfacial spin-glass-like structures. The interfacial spin-glass-like structures prevent the direct exchange coupling of the core and shell moments.

Low symmetry near the surface causes large contribution to the local magnetic anisotropy, resulting in spin canting [61]. Lattice mismatching between the shell and core materials in the core–shell MNPs could result in large degree of interfacial structural disorder. The smaller the core diameter, the larger is the interfacial structural disorder [62]. This is suggested to case also at the core–shell interface where interfacial canted spins can freeze into spin-glass-structures. Randomly spread spin-glass-like phases at the interfaces of bimagnetic layered and core–shell interfaces were suggested to significantly influence the exchange bias effect [58,63,64].

4. Extrinsic Parameters

4.1. Parameters of the AMF

In all types of experimental methods (which will be discussed in the next section), a source of AMF is needed to heat the MNPs. Heat will be conducted to targeted cells through the living tissues. This displays the necessity to understand such heat conduction and to accurately monitor the changes in the target temperature. The AMF is usually generated using a solenoid [65] or Helmholtz coil [66]. The coil diameter is determined by the sample size. The sample is insulated from the coil by vacuum or a material that has low thermal conductivity and is placed at the center of the coil where the field is most homogeneous. The well-controlled cooling process of the coil is an important task to maintain during the experiment. If the coil becomes very hot, indirect heating of the sample by the heat irradiated from the hot coil itself will occur. On the other hand, if the coil is cold, the sample might get cooled by the coil [67]. If one of these processes occurs, the SAR data will not be reliable. For effective cooling, the coils are usually made of copper tubes to allow cooling water to go through the wire.

As discussed in the previous section, the SAR values depend on the frequency, f, and amplitude, H_o, of the AMF. In theory, large amount of heat can be generated by increasing these two parameters. However, practically this is not possible due to two main reasons: (a) difficulties in designing equipment needed to generate large frequency and high field and (b) increased harm to healthy cells due to induced eddy currents at high f and H_o. The frequency of AMF that will cause reasonable heating in MH is limited within the range of 50 kHz < f < 1 MHz. Above 1 MHz, negative physiological reposes might occur [21]. On the other hand, the field amplitude is limited to H_o < 15 kA/m, which is based on estimation of the heat dissipation by the induced eddy current [21]. Several safety conditions in terms of the product $H_o f$ were suggested [68]. One of these safety conditions is called Atkinson–Brezovich limit of $H_o f < 4.85 \times 10^8$ Am^{-1}s^{-1} (6×10^6 Oe Hz) [69], which was suggested based on real tests on patients who were exposed to AMF for a duration that exceeds 1 h. The value of the product $H_o f$ at which the patents started feeling considerable discomfort was found to be 4.85×10^8 Am^{-1}s^{-1}. Another safety condition was suggested to be $H_o f < 5 \times 10^9$ Am^{-1}s^{-1} (6.25×10^7 Oe Hz) [69]. This limit is 10 times greater than the Atkinson–Brezovich limit and was suggested to be applied to small regions of the body of patients whose lives might be in jeopardy. A third safety condition was suggested to be $H_o f < 2 \times 10^8$ Am^{-1}s^{-1} [70]. This limit is based on a simulation study of the heat resulted from the electromagnetic field distribution in a model of human body. As can be realized that none of these limits is based on real measurements of the effect of the AMF parameters on the functions of cells, and thus further research is needed. Based on Atkinson–Brezovich limit, if the frequency of the AMF is fixed at 100 kHz (which is very suitable for medical applications), H_o must have values be between 4.85×10^3 Am^{-1} (60 Oe) and 50×10^3 Am^{-1} (625 Oe) [71].

4.2. Role of Interparticle Interactions on the Heating Efficiency

The dipolar interaction is a long range interaction where the interaction energy is proportional to $1/r^6$, where r is the interparticle distance. Therefore, dipolar interactions between MNPs decrease strongly with increasing the interparticle distance. This means that particles with small concentrations will experience small dipolar interactions. Strong dipolar interactions are expected to have an impact on the magnetic relaxations of MNPs, and thus on their heating efficiency in the existence of an AMF. In clinical treatments using MH, the concentrations of MNPs is 112 mg Fe/mL, while in MH experiments the concentrations used are much smaller, usually between 0.1 and 30 mg/mL [72–83]. The high concentration of MNPs in clinical treatments result in smaller interparticle distances and thus large dipolar interactions that could lead to agglomerations or aggregates. The agglomerations could have a negative influence on the heating efficiency of the MNPs due to hindered relaxation processes [31,73]. Although several theoretical and experimental studies were conducted to reveal the role of dipolar interactions on heating efficiency in MH, there is no complete understanding of this topic yet due to contradiction results that could have several sources [24,84–86]. By calculating $\omega\tau$ in some conflicting reports [31], the authors suggested that MNP concentration always suppresses the relaxation time. However, this reduction in relaxation time could have opposite effects on SAR depending on whether the value of $\omega\tau > 1$ or $\omega\tau < 1$. They suggested that when $\omega\tau < 1$, SAR decreases as the relaxation time and τ decreases, whereas for $\omega\tau > 1$, SAR increases as τ decreases.

4.3. Beyond the LRT

LRT is only applicable at very small applied magnetic fields. Therefore, for MNPs with low anisotropy energies the LRT will not be applicable where the magnetization saturation is reached at small magnetic fields. In such case, the Stoner–Wohlfarth model is an option. The standard Stoner–Wohlfarth model is applicable when $T = 0$ (or in the limit of infinite frequency). If the magnetization of the MNPs needs to flip direction between the two equilibrium positions (potential wells) it must overcome the energy barrier between the potential wells. Since $T = 0$, thermal energy cannot provide such energy. Thus, the applied magnetic field will provide the needed energy. Researchers investigated a modification to Stoner–Wohlfarth model where thermal activation of magnetization and the sweeping rate of the AMF were included [23]. The role of frequency and finite temperature on the areas of hysteresis loops and coercivity were studied where analytical formulas for such dependence were obtained. In other studies, the dynamics of rotatable MNPs in aqueous phase (which resembles the cytoplasm) were studied in a large AMF using numerical simulations [87,88].

Monodisperse spheroidal MNPs with non-magnetic surfactant layers were considered. The MNPs were considered to be uniformly dispersed with no aggregation due to the absence of dipolar interactions. A two-level approximation was used where thermal activation causes reversals between two meta-stable directions. The outcomes of the study could not be explained by the conventional models that consider a linear response of thermodynamic equilibrium states ($H_0 = 0$, $T \neq 0$) or the Stoner–Wohlfarth model of magnetic field-driven reversals ($H_0 \neq 0$, $T = 0$).

In MH experiments, the MNPs are dispersed in a liquid medium. The application of an AMF will result in complex dynamics of MNPs in such viscous liquid. These complex dynamics are ignored in the conventional LRT causing oversimplification of the real situation. Stochastic equations of motion were used to study the dynamics of an assembly of MNPs dispersed in a viscous Liquid [89]. It was found that SAR values of an assembly of MNPs in a liquid can be considerably enhanced by selecting a suitable mode of magnetization oscillations. For H_0 = 200–300 Oe and f = 300–500 kHz, with magnetic parameters typical for iron oxides, the SAR values can be of the order of 1 kW/g. This result clearly displays the significant difference between the magnetic dynamics of MNPs dispersed in a viscous liquid from that of immobilized MNPs in a solid matrix.

Uniaxial superparamagnetic particles suspended in a viscous fluid and subjected to an AMF were studied [90]. Néel and Brownian magnetic relaxations were considered. Significant contribution to the full magnetic response of the particles (and thus to the specific loss power) was obtained due to the viscous losses because of the particle motion in the fluid; a modification to the conventional LRT, where the field-dependent Brownian relaxation time is suggested to replace the field-independent one.

In [23], the authors reported three types of theories can be used to describe hysteresis loops of MNPs: the LRT, equilibrium functions, and theories based on Stoner–Wohlfarth model. Limitations and domains of validity of each theory were discussed. The authors proposed that the separation between "hysteresis losses" and "relaxation losses" is artificial and not correct. The LRT was shown to be pertinent only for MNPs with strong anisotropy. Theories based on Stoner–Wohlfarth model should be used for particles with small anisotropy. On the other hand, the LRT including Brownian motion was suggested to be valid only for small magnetic fields [23,91].

5. Experimental and Theoretical Limitations in the Determination of SAR

There are two main experimental approaches that can be used to measure SAR. The first approach is based on the magnetic properties of MNPs, whereas the second method is based on their thermodynamic (calorimetric) properties. In a recent review [92], the experimental methods to measure SAR were discussed along with the possible uncertainties. Comparison between magnetic methods and calorimetric methods were also discussed. Here, we focus on the calorimetric methods.

Thermodynamic properties of MNPs (or any material) are not easy to be measured since they should be done in thermal equilibrium. To minimize external heat transfer, measurements of heating power of MNPs should be done in adiabatic conditions which are not easy to achieve. Most of calorimetric experiments using MNPs are done in nonadiabatic conditions, and thus result in appreciable errors [92–94]. Thus, there are always some inaccuracies in such measurements and results should be carefully discussed.

However, because of the difficulty to build efficient adiabatic measurement systems and because the measurements in such systems are time-consuming, the SAR measurements are usually conducted in nonadiabatic conditions which results in some errors. It was suggested that accurate SAR measurements can be made using nonadiabatic conditions by using suitable experimental and analytical methods where heat losses from the nonadiabatic setup are accounted for [94]. Possible sources of the inaccuracy in in nonadiabatic SAR measurement are (a) the spatial inhomogeneity of temperature in the sample where the location of the thermal probe in the sample becomes important, (b) the delaying of heating since it takes some time for the heating curve to take off after the start of the heating process, (c) the change of heat capacity with temperature, (d) the inhomogeneity of the magnetic field through the volume of the sample, and (e) heating due to the experimental set-up itself (peripheral heating) and not due to heated MNPs.

In calorimetric experiments, an AMF is applied to the sample of MNPs and the variation of temperature is measured with time. The SAR is usually obtained from the initial slope of the (temperature–time curve) measured data using this equation.

The induced increase in the temperature of the water dispersion enables us to calculate SAR using Equation (12),

$$SAR\ (W/g) = \frac{C}{m_{MNP}} \frac{dT}{dt} \qquad (12)$$

where C (in J/K) is the heat capacity of the sample (which includes the MNPs and the suspending medium), m_{MNP} is the mass (in g) of the MNPs in the sample, and $\frac{dT}{dt}$ is the initial slope of the temperature–time curve. The heat capacity of the sample is the sum of the specific heat multiplied by the mass of the components of the sample. For example, if the MNPs are suspended in water, the heat capacity of the sample will be $C = c_{MNP} m_{MNP} + c_{water} m_{water}$, where c_{MNP} and c_{water} are the specific heat values for the MNPs and the water, respectively, and m_{water} is the mass of the water in the sample [95]. The rationale behind the use of the "initial slope" method relies on three assumptions at the very initial stage of heating (a) heat transfer between the sample and the environment does not exist yet and thus adiabatic conditions are applicable, (b) temperature variations within the sample are very small and thus can be ignored, and (c) constant temperature approximations of heat transport properties results in very small errors and thus can be valid [96–99].

This "initial slope" method depends only on the initial temperature changes and ignores the entire heating curve and thus it does not display the entire temperature dependence of SAR [100]. In addition, it was shown that fluctuations and non-linear temperature rise can occur in the initial heating stage [96,101], which contradicts the main assumption of the initial slope method. This commonly used initial slope method was suggested to underestimate values by up to 25% [94]. The full-curve fit method was found to improve upon the "initial slope" method, but underestimation by up to 10% could result. A third method, the "corrected slope" method [94], was found to be the most accurate method. More details about several proposed methods to calculate SAR from heating data can be found in [92,94,101]. In [98], the validity of measured trends of SAR values with varied experimental conditions was discussed. The SAR values for obtained for magnetic nanoparticles depends on the geometry, saturation magnetization, coating used for functionalization, and parameters of ac magnetic field used for the measurements.

SAR values for of several ferrite nanoparticle systems are listed in Table 1.

Table 1. Specific absorption rate (SAR) values of ferrite nanoparticles with respect to size, shape, surface coating, and parameters used for obtaining hyperthermia measurements.

Shape & Size (nm)	Material	Coating	(kA/m) Field	Frequency (kHz)	(W/g) SAR	Reference
Octahedral-43	Fe_3O_4	CTAB	63	358	2483	[102]
Rings-73	Fe_3O_4	mPEG	35	400	2213	[103]
Disc-225	Fe_3O_4	CTAB	47.8	488	5000	[104]
Cubes-19	Fe_3O_4	PEG	29	520	2452	[48]
Sphere-14	$MnFe_2O_4$	GO	60	240	1588	[105]
Core–shell	$CoFe_2O_4$@$MnFe_2O_4$	DMSA	37.3	500	2250	[41]
Nanoclusters-33	Fe_3O_4	PMA	23.8	302	253	[106]
Sphere-45	Fe_3O_4	GO	32.5	400	5160	[107]
Sphere-45	Fe_3O_4	PVP	32.5	400	1100	[107]

6. Thermometry in Magnetic Hyperthermia

For in vivo hyperthermia, the temperature of the targeted tissue or cells must be measured accurately using noninvasive methods. Tracking the temperature change in the tissue is important during the whole hyperthermia experiment, because a large increase in the temperature could cause damage to healthy cells. On the other hand, low temperatures of the tissue will not result in the required amount of heat to kill tumor cells. Several thermometry methods in magnetic hyperthermia are being investigated. The most used thermometry method is based on optical fibers. This method is being used mainly in hyperthermia in aqueous suspension and in vitro experiments. This method has two main limitations: (a) it cannot provide a detailed scan of temperature within the sample because the dimensions of the fiber tip are larger (~200 μm) [67], and (b) it is an invasive technique which is not preferred for in vivo applications. Noninvasive thermometry methods that depend on optical properties were investigated [108,109]. However, as these methods depend on properties of the light they face the limitation of short penetration depth into tissues. One of the good noninvasive thermometry method is based on magnetic resonance imaging (MRI) technique [110]. When conducting the magnetic hyperthermia treatment, the tumor tissue is placed at the center of the coil generating the AMF, whereas MRI thermometry requires the placement of the tumor tissue at the center of the MRI cavity. However, MRI uses high constant magnetic field (usually 3 T), which can pin the magnetic moments of MNPs and prevent them from rotating while they are exposed also to the AMF of hyperthermia. This will lead to a narrow dynamic hysteresis loops and thus will slow down heat generation of the MNPs in the hyperthermia process [111,112]. Thus, MRI thermometry might not be the optimum choice of thermometry in hyperthermia treatment. Several other noninvasive methods which depend on the magnetic response of MNPs to the applied magnetic field were proposed [113–122]. In these methods, the temperature-dependent of coercively [117,123], the temperature-dependent of magnetization, and the higher-order harmonics of the magnetization of MNPs were used as temperature sensors. In these noninvasive methods, the MNPs will do the heating and at the same time will work as a temperature probe.

7. Multifunctional Hybrid Magnetic Nanoparticles for hyperthermia Based Biomedical Applications

Magnetic nanoparticles with efficient heating capacity are subjected to intense research for various thermal based in vivo and in vitro studies for biomedical applications [124,125]. There are numerous reports of the detailed investigations for the applications of magnetic nanoparticles for magnetic imaging guided hyperthermia, magnetic actuated drug delivery, thermal cancer therapy, and biofilm eradication [126]. Magnetic nanoparticle when combined with materials like graphene oxide (GO), photoactive materials, mesoporous silica nanoparticles, and polymeric nanoparticles results in hybrid materials with multifunctionality [126–128]. Schematic representation of various phenomena involved in magnetic hyperthermia, thermosensitive drug delivery, and biomedical applications using magnetic nanoparticles are shown in Figure 1 [129].

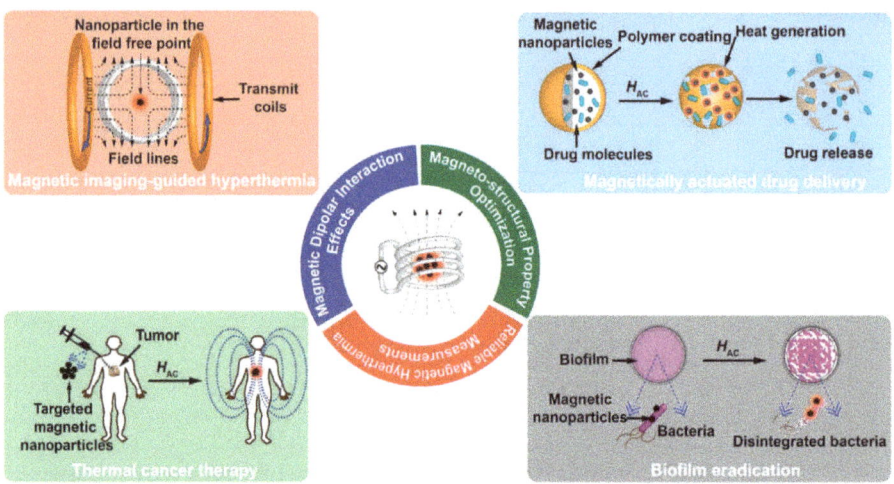

Figure 1. Schematic illustration of multifunctional ability of magnetic nanoparticles for various types of biomedical magnetic hyperthermia applications and parameters affecting the efficiency of magnetic hyperthermia treatment (reproduced with permission from Science Direct 2016) [129].

7.1. Graphene oxide-Fe$_3$O$_4$ Nanocomposites for Hyperthermia

Graphene oxide-Fe$_3$O$_4$ nanoparticle-based nanocomposites are widely investigated for various biomedical applications like drug delivery, magnetic hyperthermia, and MRI (Magnetic Resonance Imaging) contrast agents [130]. The unique chemical and physical properties of graphene oxide-based nanocomposites enable designing nanocomposites as per the requirement of physiological system. The presence of –OH, –COOH, and –CHO functional groups renders the easy attachment and release of various anticancer drugs [131]. The anticancer drugs usually delivered using graphene oxide-based composites as carrier vehicle, by change of pH or local heating via hyperthermia [132]. There are various studies where graphene oxide-based composites are considered for diagnosis and treatment of cancer. The first comprehensive report of graphene oxide-ferrite nanocomposite for magnetic hyperthermia was reported by Peng et al. [105]. They have reported the synthesis of hydrophobic ferrite nanoparticles attached to GO sheets using oleylamine as intermediary resulting in water dispersible MFNPs/GO nanocomposites. MGONCs-4 and MGONCs-4-PEG water dispersions were subjected to ac magnetic field, time-dependent temperature curves of MGONCs-4 and MGONCs-4-PEG were shown in Figure 2. From the magneto thermic data, it is evident that the heating rate of MGONCs-4-PEG was relatively lower than MGONCs-4. The difference in the heating rate could be explained by the presence of long-chain polyethylene glycol (PEG) which significantly altered the heating conduction. The field-dependent SAR values (Figure 2c) showed that the calculated SAR value of MGONCs-4 was greater than that of MGONCs-4-PEG. The SAR values of MGONCs-4 and MGONCs-4-PEG are 1541.6 and 1108.9 Wg^{-1} respectively. This finding is in good agreement with the other reported surface coating effects in which the heating capability would be hindered as the surface coating increases due to the suppression of the Brownian relaxation processes [133].

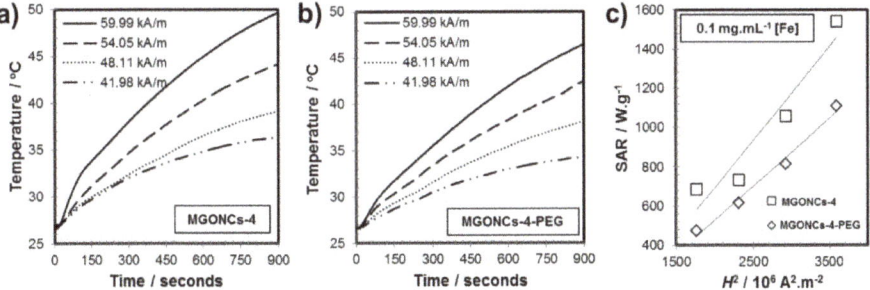

Figure 2. Magneto thermic data of water dispersions of (**a**) MGONCs-4 and (**b**) MGONCs-4-PEG treated with alternating magnetic field (AMF) (41.98–59.99 kAm^{-1}) at 240 kHz frequency. (**c**) Field-dependent SAR values of nanocomposite dispersions (reproduced with permission from Wiley Online Library 2012) [105].

Sugumaran et al. reported a GO-iron oxide-based nanocomposite system consisting of 45 nm nanoparticles grafted on GO sheet with very high SAR value [107]. They were able to achieve a SAR value of 5020 Wg^{-1} with alternating magnetic field of 400 kHz and 32.5 kAm^{-1}. Peng et al. have also studied the T$_2$-weighted MR imaging contrast enhancing ability of GO-ferrite nanocomposites. GO-ferrite nanoparticle system showed a high T$_2$ relaxation rate as 64.47 s^{-1} (with r$_2$ relaxivity value of 256.2 Fe mM^{-1} s^{-1}) with the MGONCs-4 with the iron concentration as low as 0.25 mM Fe. These results suggested that the presence of the aggregation of MFNPs on GO could provide additional enhancement of relaxation of water protons. The aggregation effect on relaxation process observed is further confirmed by the other reports [134]. The aggregation of ferrite nanoparticles leads to higher magnetic inhomogeneity in the water dispersion which causes the decrease in the transverse relaxivity of water protons. The graphene oxide framework of the composite provides an addition advantage of attaching water insoluble anticancer drugs and releasing them at the site of interest.

Sugumaran et al. have reported an in vivo magnetic hyperthermia studies for targeting of tumor bearing mouse model using PEGylated GO-IONPs [107]. Tumors were induced in mice by injecting 4T1 cancer cells into the mammary pads of mice. The mice with tumor volumes of approximately 100 mm^3 were treated with PEGylated GO-IONPs (Fe dose of 1 mg/cm^3) with PBS, PEG-GO-IONP under magnetic field. Mice tumors are subjected to AMF with 400 kHz frequency and a magnetic field of 32 kA/m for 10 min. Body weights and tumor volumes subjected to various conditions are shown in Figure 3. The mice injected with PBS or PEG-GO-IONP alone without AMF application and mice subjected to AMF alone, failed to suppress the growth of 4T1 tumor. The test group significantly inhibited the 4T1 tumor growth, indicating that the antitumor efficacies of PEG-GO-IONP mediated magnetic hyperthermia treatment were greater than that of either PEG-GO-IONP or AMF alone. The tumor treated under ac magnetic field with PEG-GO-IONP completely disappeared. In addition, no body weight loss (Figure 3d) was observed in the PEG-GO-NP-mediated magnetic hyperthermia treatment, indicating the relative safety of the treatment and tolerability of the administered dosage.

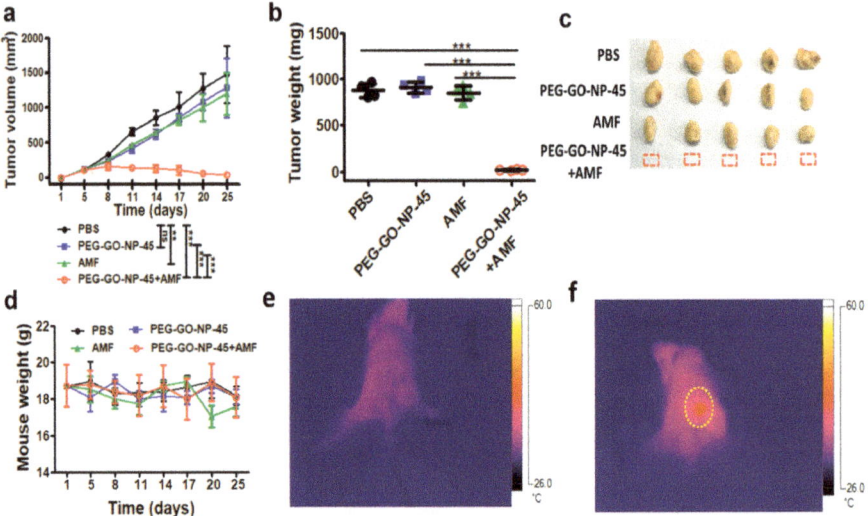

Figure 3. (**a**) Tumor volume versus days after the treatment with GO-NP and AMF. (**b**) Weights and (**c**) photographs of excised tumors at the end point for different treatment groups. (Tumor completely disappeared after hyperthermia treatment with PEG-GO-NP-45.) (**d**) Mouse weight after the treatments. Thermal images showing the temperature at the site of tumor and entire body of mouse during hyperthermia treatment: (**e**) control and (**f**) PEG-GO-NP-45+AMF (reproduced with permission from American Chemical Society 2019) [107].

7.2. Magnetic Nanogels for Thermosensitive Drug Delivery

Thermosensitive drug delivery agents are polymeric micelles which are synthesized using thermo-responsive polymers. These magnanogels are formulated using self-assembly process of amphiphilic block-copolymer [135]. Magnanogels are class of thermosensitive materials which are activated by ac magnetic field, formulation of these nanoparticles was reported in detail by several studies [136,137]. Nanogels are used in various biomedical applications like drug delivery systems, analytical and diagnostic devices, and thermal therapy [138]. These nanocarries are functionalized with target specific molecules, enabling differentiation between normal and tumor tissues [139]. Advances in material fabrication and designing enables to use of thermosensitive nanocarriers for controlled drug delivery in the future.

Nanogels were prepared in a batch reactor by conventional precipitation radical copolymerization of oligo(ethylene glycol) methyl ether methacrylate in water, without using any surfactants [140]. Magnetic nanoparticles were synthesized by chemical coprecipitation of ferrous and ferric ions in basic medium. To synthesize the magnanogel, a known quantity of nanogel is taken and pH is adjusted to 3.0 and magnetic nanoparticles are added drop wise into the nanogel solution under stirring at room temperature. The anticancer drug doxorubicin is attached to magnanogel in HEPS buffer solution under stirring for 24 h. The schematic of anticancer drug delivery using magnanogels is explained in Figure 4.

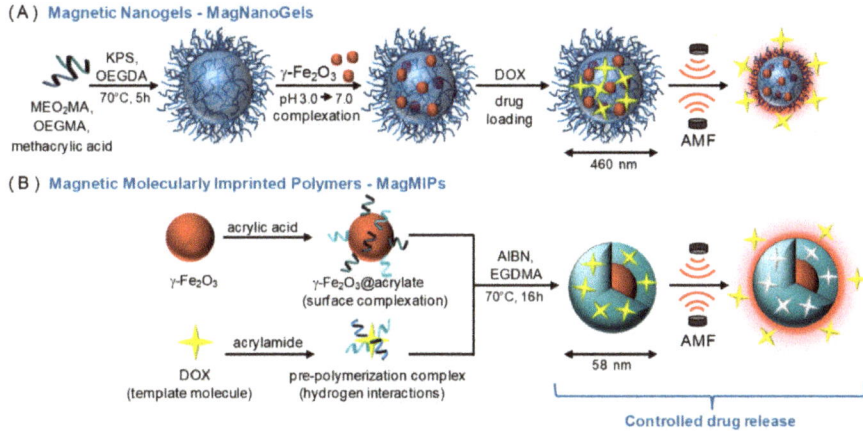

Figure 4. (**A**) Schematic illustration of the synthesis of magnanogels by radical copolymerization and post-assembly of MNPs inside nanogels and (**B**) synthesis of MagMIPs by grafting of acrylic acid compound in the surface of MNPs and the growth of the polymer in the presence of DOX for imprinting polymerization. Loading and release of DOX under an AMF (reproduced with permission from MDPI (open access) 2018) [141].

Intracellular DOX release experiments using magnanoels is reported by Esther et al. [140]. DOX release is stimulated by change of pH (internal stimulus) and externally applied AMF (external stimulus). DOX release is highly pH sensitive at pH 7.5 25% of DOX is released after 4 h whereas at pH 5.0 the release of DOX is increased to 96%. These results are in good agreement with other reported results of pH-sensitive nanogels functionalized with carboxylic acid groups [142,143]. Under the same pH conditions DOX release increased under ac magnetic field of 335 kHz and 12.0 kAm^{-1}. These studies demonstrate that ac magnetic field helps in remotely trigger DOX release without macroscopic heating. The diameter of the magnanogels decreases under ac magnetic field due to the generated magnetic heat. The shrinkage facilitates the release of DOX at the site of interest. They have also studied in vitro DOX release in cancer cells (PC-3) using DOX-magnanogels. PC-3 cancer cells were treated with 15 and 10 pg of DOX-magnogels and DOX-Magnetic nanoparticles. The studies showed that the internalization did not cause any toxic cellular response, demonstrating the biocompatible nature of both nanogels and nanoparticles without DOX. Confocal images of cancer cells treated with DOX encapsulated magnanogels and magnetic nanoparticles were shown in Figure 5b. Cell viability was more impacted by the internalization of the magnanogels containing DOX than magnetic nanoparticles associated with DOX. These results confirm that the payload is continuously released from magnanogels, but can be delivered in larger amounts under AMF. By contrast, when DOX is bonded to the MIP, DOX is inactive. Internalization and DOX release experiments using magnanogels showed the efficiency under AMF due to local heating of the magnetic nanoparticles.

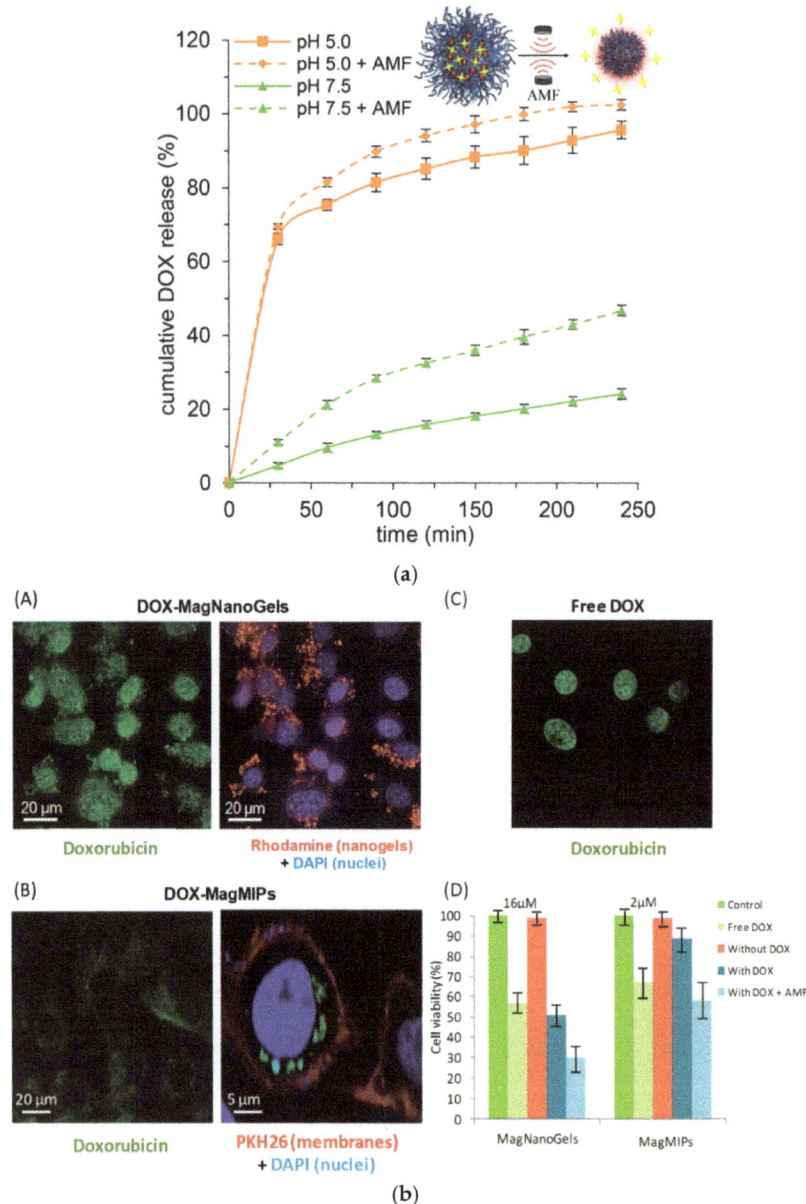

Figure 5. (**a**) DOX release profile (%) versus time under physiological conditions (pH 7.5, 0.1 M HEPES sodium) and acidic (pH 5.0, 0.05 M citric acid and 0.1 M sodium phosphate) at 37 °C without and with an AMF. (**b**) Confocal imaging of tumor cells (PC-3) having internalized: (A) Magnanogels and (B) DOX-MagMIPs nanoparticles. (C) Cells incubated for 2 h with free DOX (D) Cell viabilities for free DOX, DOX-magnanogels, and DOX-magnetic nanoparticles (reproduced with permission from American Chemical Society 2017) [140].

7.3. Magnetic Mesoporus Silica Nanoparticles for High Dose Delivery of Anticancer Drugs

Mesoporous silica nanoparticles (MSNs) have some unique advantage of large pore volume with uniform mesoporosity, biocompatibility, and biodegradation [144,145]. This unique property of silica nanoparticles renders high drug loading capacity. Conventional MSNs can load 200–300 mg of anticancer drug per 1 g of silica. However, MSNs with hollow core–mesoporous shell structure can achieve 1 g drug per 1 g silica [144,146]. Physical entrapment of anticancer drugs due to the hallow core–shell geometry prevents uncontrolled burst release or poor drug loading [147]. In addition, functionalization of MSNs with materials, such as magnetic nanoparticles, luminescent materials and polymers introduces the multifunctional modality of targeted dug delivery and imaging. The polymers attached to the core–shell nanoparticles act as thermosensitive gatekeepers for opening the pores and release the drug using ac magnetic field. Thamos et al. has reported a nanomotor based on MSPs with zinc doped ferrite nanoparticles in silica matrix [148]. These MSNPs were coated with temperature-sensitive copolymer of poly-ethyleneimine and n-isopropylacrylamide which acts as a gatekeeper and retains DOX into the polymer shell linked by electrostatic forces or hydrogen bonds [149]. Once these nanomotors are administrated into cancer cells motors were activated by applying ac magnetic field. This study shows that the polymer can be used as a gatekeeper for controlled drug delivery along with the thermic effect of magnetic nanoparticles. The schematic illustration of mesoporous silica-based nanomotors for drug delivery is shown in Figure 6.

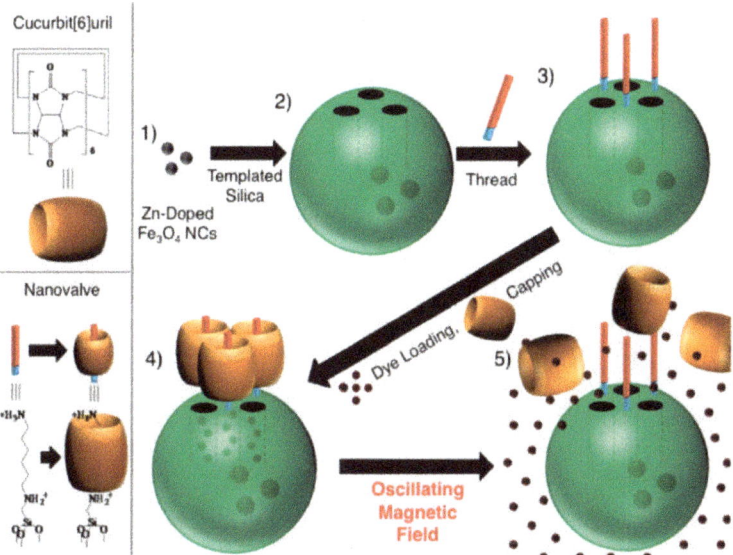

Figure 6. ZnNCs (1) are synthetically positioned at the core of the mesoporous silica nanoparticles (2). The base of the molecular machine is then attached to the nanoparticle surface (3). Drug is loaded into the particle and capped (4) to complete the system. Release can be realized using remote heating via the introduction of an oscillating magnetic field (5) (reproduced with permission from American Chemical Society 2010) [148].

Lee et al. has reported the synthesis of multifunctional nanocontainer with iron oxide and mesoporus silica and cyclodextran as gatekeeper [150]. They have estimated the pore size of the using Brunauer–Emmett–Teller (BET) nitrogen adsorption–desorption isotherms and Barrett–Joyner–Halenda (BJH). The pore diameter obtained is 2.5 nm and pore volume is 1.756 $cm^3 g^{-1}$. Eduardo et al. reported the use of magnetic mesoporous core shell nanoparticles coated with thermoresponsive polymer (TRP) for in vitro drug release using magnetic field, the schematic illustration of the same is provided in

Figure 7 [151]. Magnetic nanoparticles used in this study were synthesized by simple coprecipitation method and stabilized by exadecyltrimethylammonium bromide (CTAB) in water medium. The surfaces of the nanoparticles were functionalized with polymerizable groups with 3-tris(trimethylsiloxy) prpyl methacrylate. The polymer shell has a lower critical solution temperature of 42 °C, which can be adjusted by altering the ratio between monomers. Below critical solution temperature the polymer chains forms a mesh which is useful to block the pores of mesoporous silica, which in turn helps hold the drug. Upon magnetic field treatment the polymer surface collapses and triggers drug release [152].

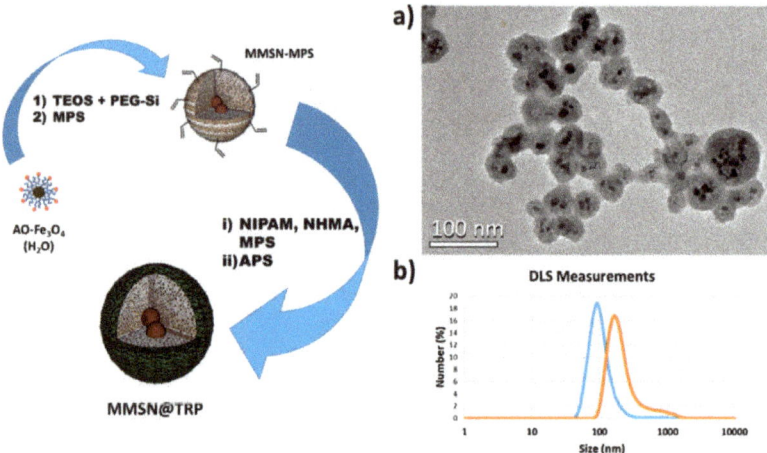

Figure 7. Schematic of the synthesis method of MMSN@TRP (thermo responsive polymer). (**a**) TEM image of the MMSNs coated with TRP (**b**) hydrodynamic size of the precursor (MMSN-nanoparticles, blue line) and the final nanocarrier (MMSN@TRP, orange line) (reproduced with permission from American Chemical Society 2018) [151].

7.4. Multifunctional Drug Delivery Agents Through Magnetic and Photothermal Therapy

Photoactive multifunctional magnetic nanoparticles are designed for the synergistic therapy of controlled drug release, magnetic hyperthermia, and photothermal therapy [153,154]. The combination of magnetic nanoparticles and photothermal agents can be directed magnetically to the site of interest (tumor), and their distribution in tumors and other organs can be imaged through MPI [155]. The controlled clustering of magnetic nanoparticles along with photothermal agents increases the molar adsorption coefficient in the near infrared region. The conversion efficiency of near-infrared (NIR) light energy into heat is also high for magnetic photothermal hybrid nanoparticles. The multifunctional magnetic composite consists of quantum dots as local photothermal generators and magnetic mesoporous silica nanoparticles (MMSN) or CQDs as drug carriers and magnetic nanoparticles as thermal seeds. The schematic illustration of hybrid composites for dual therapy is shown in Figure 8.

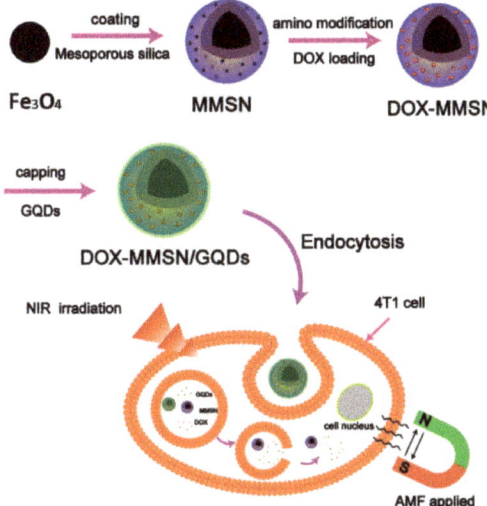

Figure 8. Schematic illustration of the synthesis of the DOX MMSN/GQDs nanoparticles and synergistic therapy combined with controlled drug release using magnetic hyperthermia and photothermal therapy (reproduced with permission from Wiley Online Library 2017) [156].

Yan et al. reported gold nanoshell-coated ferrite nanomicelles for MRI and light-induced drug delivery and photothermal therapy [157]. Nanomicelles possess improved drug loading capacity and good response to magnetic field for targeting the tumor. Nanomicelles show surface plasmon absorbance in the near infrared region (808 nm). Cancer cells incubated with gold-coated nanomicelles show good biocompatibility, and when treated with NIR and magnetic field they showed significant cytotoxicity. The thermal effects are synergic in nature. Heating profile and DOX releasing behavior is shown in Figure 9.

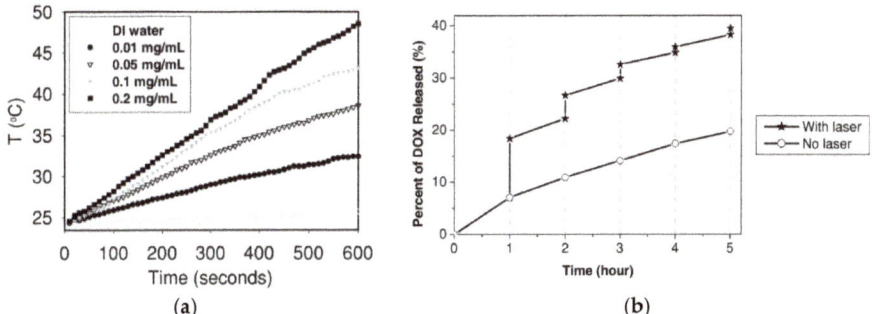

Figure 9. (a) Temperature elevation in aqueous solutions containing CDF-Au-shell nanomicelles of different concentrations under night-infrared (NIR) laser irradiation (808 nm, 2 W) measured every 10 s using a digital thermometer, over a period of 10 min. (b) NIR-triggered release of DOX from CDF-Au-shell nanomicelles. (Reproduced with permission from Wiley Online Library 2013) [157].

Yoa et al. has reported the drug release behavior under the stimuli of magnetic hyperthermia and photothermal effect using magnetic mesoporous silica nanoparticles (MMSN/GQDs). Fe_3O_4 nanoparticles are prepared and encapsulated by mesoporous silica matrix to obtain Fe_3O_4/SiO_2 (MMSN). MMSN nanoparticles are spherical and the particles size is estimated to be approximately 100 nm. The obtained nanoparticles were modified with amino groups and GQDs with hydroxyl, epoxy, and carboxyl groups are used to cap the outlets of mesoporous channels for the formation of the DOX-MMSN/GQDs nanoparticles. GQDs prevent the DOX from leaking and uncontrolled burst of DOX at the site of off target. This is unique composite which can be used for the delivery of both water soluble and insoluble drug together. The organic nature of GQD frame work enables to attach water insoluble anticancer drugs. The magnetic and photo thermic heating efficiency of the MMSN/GQDs nanoparticles is shown in Figure 10. Temperature of the MMSN/GQDs suspension increased rapidly under AMF, and the temperature increase rate is concentration dependent. The specific absorption rate (SAR) value of the MMSN/GQDs nanoparticles was calculated as ~44 Wg^{-1}. MMSN/GQDs suspensions were irradiated under NIR laser irradiation (λ = 808 nm, 2.5 Wcm^{-2}). It visually confirmed the rapid temperature increase for the MMSN/GQDs suspension by NIR irradiation. MMSN/GQDs nanoparticles have the advantage of producing heat by dual methods that can be used for increasing the temperature in physiological systems, which helps kill cancer cells.

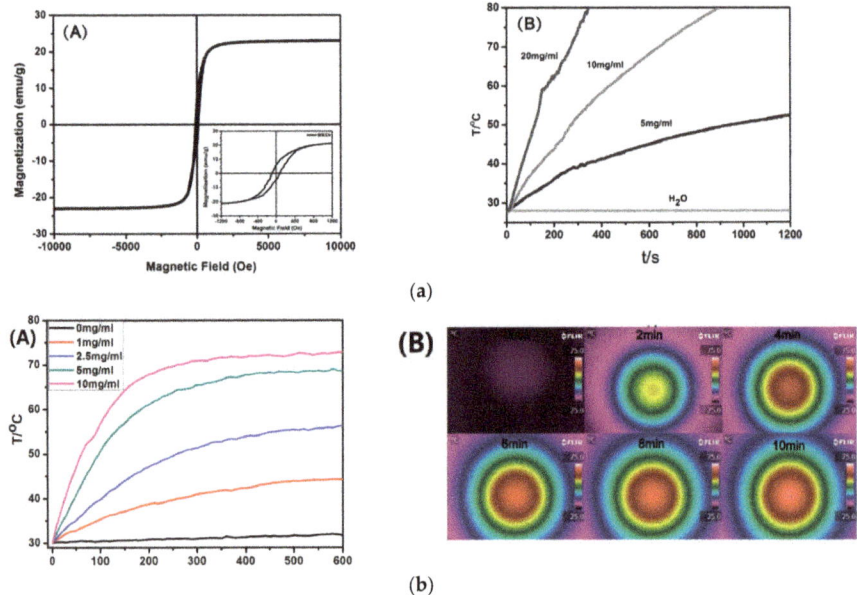

Figure 10. (a) (A) The magnetization curve of the MMSN/GQDs nanoparticles measured at 298 K. (B) Magnetic heating curves of the H$_2$O and MMSN/GQDs suspensions under an alternating magnetic field with a magnetic field strength of 180 G and frequency of 409 kHz. (b) (A) Photothermal heating curves of MMSN/GQDs suspension evaluated by 808 nm laser irradiation (2.5 Wcm^{-2}). (B) The infrared thermal images of the MMSN/GQDs suspension at a concentration of 10 mg mL^{-1} with 808 nm laser irradiation (reproduced with permission from Wiley Online Library 2017) [156].

Shawei et al. reported a multifunctional NaYF$_4$:Yb,Er@PE$_3$@Fe$_3$O$_4$ nanocomposite with superparamagnetic and photothermal performance. The multicomponent hybrid nanoparticles were synthesized by layer-by-layer self-assemble method. Compared to bare Fe$_3$O$_4$ nanoparticles, the multifunctional nanocomposites exhibited enhanced absorption at 808 nm and showed improved near-infrared photothermal effect. The fluorescent imaging sensitivity is increased when it is combined with magnetic field. The in vivo images of the mouse 4T1 breast cancer cells treated with hybrid nanoparticles in the presence of magnetic field and without magnetic field are shown in Figure 11a. The fluorescence images taken without magnetic field shows weak luminescent signals, whereas in the case magnetic field treated cells the up conversion signals are observed from the 4T1 cells. This demonstrates that the application of magnetic field for targeted drug delivery enhanced synergistic imaging sensitivity. Photothermal therapy ability of the NaYF$_4$:Yb,Er@PE$_3$@Fe$_3$O$_4$ nanocomposites for killing 4T1 cancer cells is shown in Figure 11b. The cell viability results show that hybrid nanocomposite treated with external magnetic field is highly effective for killing of cancer cells. The reasons might be cancer cells were pushed close to the photothermal agents under the external magnetic field.

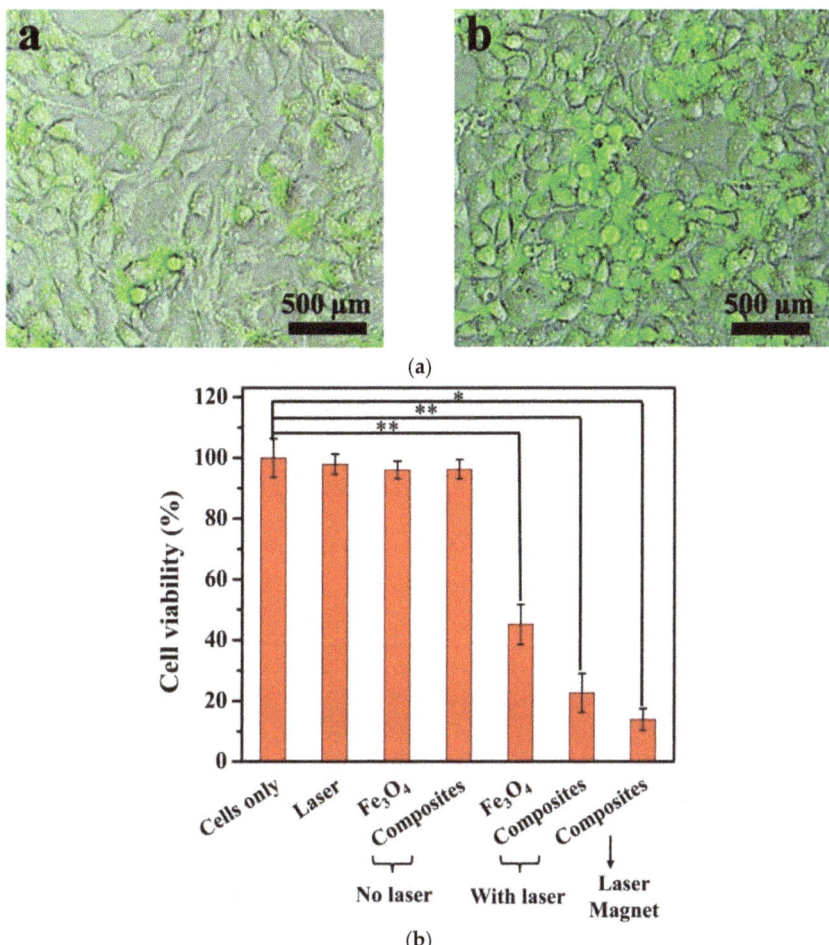

Figure 11. (a) The fluorescence images of 4T1 cells after incubating with NaYF$_4$: Yb, Er@PE$_3$@Fe$_3$O$_4$ nanocomposites (A) without or (B) with external magnetic field. (b) Viabilities of the mouse 4T1 breast cancer cells treated with hybrid nanoparticles under various conditions. Error bars were based on standard deviations, * $p < 0.05$ and ** $p < 0.01$. (Reproduced with permission from Royal Society of Chemistry 2019) [158].

7.5. Magnetic Particle Imaging and Hyperthermia in Vivo Applications

Magnetic particle imaging (MPI) is a new tomographic technique developed in the early 2000 [159]. MPI is tracer tracking technique that allows tracking and quantification of the signal from tracer magnetic nanoparticles [160]. MPI gives quantitative 3D information of the region of the interest with high spatial and temporal resolution which helps in real-time high resolution in vivo imaging. As a tracer tracking technique MPI may lead to the new possibility of 3D in vivo real-time imaging which will be of great help for real time treatment and imaging [161], human scanners will become available in a few years. The tracer used in the MPI imaging is usually superparamagnetic nanoparticles; this also adds additional advantage as iron oxide nanoparticles are well investigated for MRI contrast agents and their behavior in physiological environments is thoroughly understood [162]. Image-guided treatment of tumors enables physicians to localize the treatment with great precision and minimal damage to the healthy tissue. More details of the instrumentation and working principles can be found in the recently published review reports [9].

Tay et al. has reported the in vivo studies of magnetic hyperthermia treatment and magnetic particle image-guided modality [163]. This study demonstrated theranostic investigation of quantitative MP image-guided treatment using spatial localization of magnetic hyperthermia to arbitrarily selected organs. This addresses a key challenge of conventional magnetic hyperthermia affecting off-target organs causing collateral heat damage. Superparamagnetic iron oxide nanoparticles were injected to the tumor site and subjected to ac magnetic field. During MPI scan, negligible heating was observed in the mouse when it is subjected low frequency (20 kHz). During a high-frequency (354 kHz) heating scan without MPI gradients, all in vivo locations with nanoparticles heat up, damaging the healthy liver. When the MPI gradients are used, only the tumor is heated while the liver is spared. Dual tumor mouse was used to demonstrate arbitrary user-control of which tumor to heat. Only the bottom tumor heated up while the top tumor was spared. Only the top tumor heated up while the bottom tumor was spared, demonstrating arbitrary control of the site of heating just by shifting the MPI field-free line. The results shown in Figure 12 for the experimental MPI guided hyperthermia confirm that localization is achieved in vivo. A control mouse with saline instead of SPIONs was also subjected to the same uniform AMF but showed no increase in tumor and liver temperatures, verifying that this indiscriminate heating is not a result of nonspecific SAR from AMF interacting with biological tissue. These studies show that, with MPI gradients, the user can arbitrarily control the location of heating. With guidance from the initial MPI image, the treatment planning can design a heating to avoid collateral damage to healthy tissue.

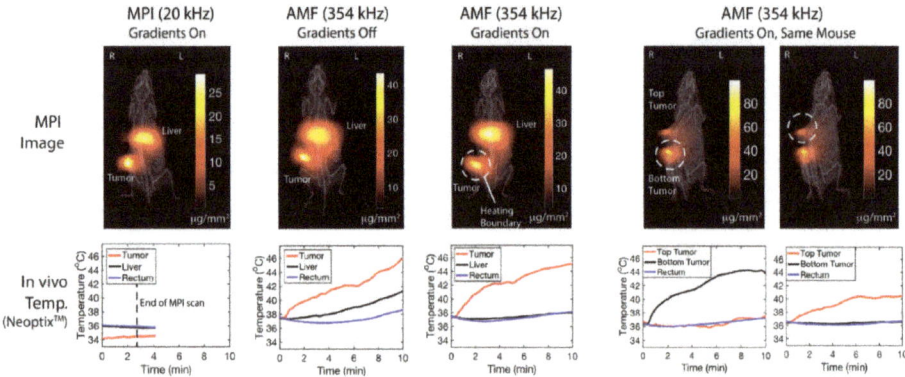

Figure 12. In vivo experimental demonstration of localization of magnetic hyperthermia. All in vivo local temperatures were measured by Neoptix fiber optic temperature sensors (reproduced with permission from American Chemical Society 2018) [163].

8. Synthesis of IONPs

It is well known that MNP synthesis method has a significant role in determining MNP magnetic properties, and thus their SAR values [164]. However, the synthesis mechanisms needed to produce well controlled magnetic properties are not well established. Here, we present several synthesis methods that are currently being used to produce IONPs. Various approaches such as wet chemical [165–167], template-directed [168,169], microemulsion [170–172], thermal decomposition [172,173], solvothermal method [174,175], solid state [176,177], deposition method [178], spray pyrolysis [179,180], self-assembly [181], physical, and lithographic [182,183] techniques have been extensively used for the synthesis of a wide variety of magnetic nanoparticles including iron oxide, metal, metal alloys and core–shell and composites structures. However, a comprehensive review of various synthetic techniques, and we will give a short description of only those methods that offer excellent size and shape control.

8.1. Thermal Decomposition

This method of synthesis involves the chemical decomposition of the substance at elevated temperature. During this method the breaking of the chemical bond takes place. This method of synthesis for magnetic nanostructures mostly use organometallic compounds such as acetylacetonates in organic solvents (benzyl ether, ethylenediamine, and carbonyls) with surfactants such as oleic acid, oleylamine, polyvinyl pyrrolidone (PVP), cetyltrimethyl ammonium bromide (CTAB), and hexadecylamine. In this method the composition of various precursors that are involved in the reaction determine the final size and morphology of the magnetic nanostructures. Peng et al. and co-workers used the thermal decomposition approach for controlled synthesis (in term of size and shape) of magnetic oxide [184]. Using this method, nanocrystals with very narrow-sized distribution (4–45 nm) could be synthesized along with the excellent control of morphology (spherical particles, cubes). When thermal decomposition method is used, iron oxide nano particles with excellent control of size, morphology and good crystallinity have been resultantly fabricated by Alivisatos and co-workers [185]. The preparation of magnetic nanoparticles for applications in biomedicine have fabricated maghemite nanocrystals with size of 3–9 nm by thermal decomposition of FeCup3 (Cup: N-nitrosophenylhydroxylamine) at 250–300 °C, as shown in Figure 13. Recently, Sun and Zeng et al. [186] have demonstrated the fabrication of monodisperse magnetite nanoparticles with size ranges of 2–20 nm by decomposition of iron (III) acetyl acetone at 260 °C in the presence of benzyl ether, oleic acid, and oleyl amine. In a more recent study, Nogues and co-workers have synthesized highly mono disperse cubic and spherical maghemite (Fe_2O_3) nanocrystals by using thermal decomposition method [187], as shown in Figure 14. The ratio of precursors and the thermal decomposition time can be used to achieve size and morphology controlled nanocrystals.

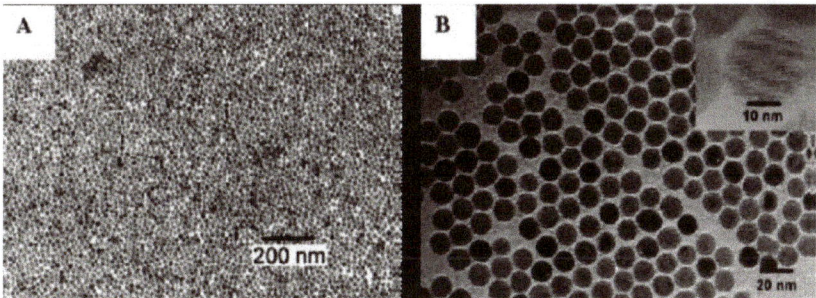

Figure 13. Maghemite nanoparticles prepared by thermal decomposition of Iron precursors: (**A**) FeCup$_3$ and (**B**) Fe(CO)$_5$ (reproduced with permission from American Chemical Society 1999) [185].

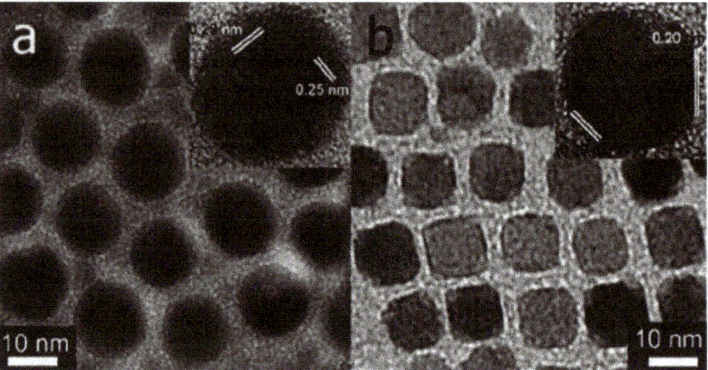

Figure 14. High-resolution TEM images showing the monodisperse (**a**) nanosphere and (**b**) nanocubes achieved by thermal decomposition method (reproduced with permission from American Chemical Society 2006) [187].

Nogues et al. showed that short decomposition duration (2–4 h) resulted in spherical whereas longer duration (10–12 h) resulted in cubic morphology. The technique of thermal decomposition was not only used for synthesis of metal oxide magnetic nanocrystals but metal magnetic nanoparticles of transition metals (Co, Ni, and Fe) were also synthesized through introducing a reducing agent into a hot solution of metal precursor and surfactant [26]. With precise control of the temperature and ratio of metal precursor to surfactant, MNPs with the control size and shape were synthesized.

8.2. Hydrothermal Synthesis

Another important chemical synthesis technique that involves the use of liquid–solid–solution (LSS) reaction and gives excellent control over the size and shape of the MNPs is the hydrothermal synthesis. This method involves the synthesis of MNPs from high boiling point aqueous solution at high vapor pressure. It is a unique approach for the fabrication of metal, metal oxide [188,189], rare earth transition metal magnetic nanocrystals [190], semiconducting [191], dielectric, rare earth fluorescent, and polymeric [192]. This synthetic technique involved the fabrication of magnetic metallic nanocrystals at different reactions conditions. The reaction strategy is based upon the phase separation which occurs at the interface of solid–liquid–solution phases present in the reaction. For example, the fabrication of monodisperse (6, 10 and 12 nm) Fe_3O_4 and MFe_2O_4 nanocrystals is demonstrated by Sun et al. and co-worker [193]. Wuwei and co-worker have synthesized oblique and truncated nanocubes of α-Fe_2O_3 by one step facile hydrothermal method. This group studied the effect of volume ratio of oleylamine and acetylacetone for the fabrication of α-Fe_2O_3 with two different morphologies as shown in Figure 15. The synthesize magnetic nanoparticles were used for photocatalytic degradation of organic dye, and it was observed that truncated nanocubes possess much higher photocatalytic degradation activity as compared to oblique nanocubes [194].

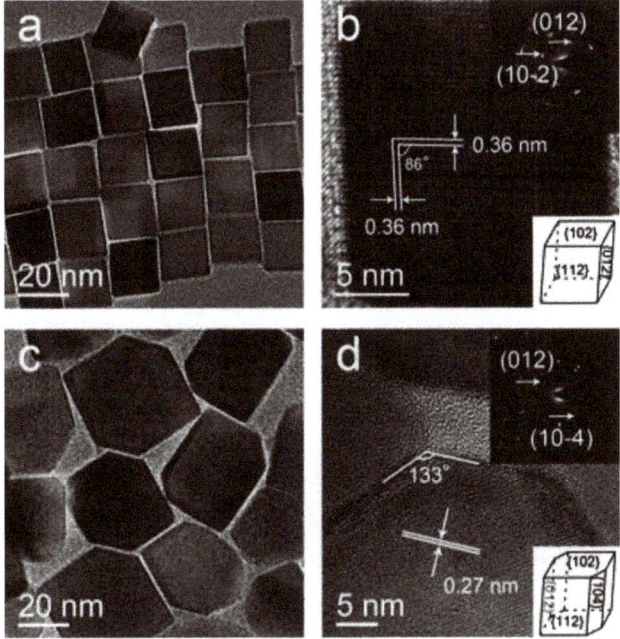

Figure 15. (a) TEM image of oblique nanocubes, (b) HRTEM image, FFT pattern and geometrical model of oblique nanocubes, (c) TEM image of truncated nanocubes, and (d) HRTEM image, FFT pattern and geometrical model of truncated nanocubes (reproduced with permission from Royal Society of Chemistry 2013) [194].

The mechanism of formation of the α-Fe$_2$O$_3$ nanoparticles with oblique and truncated morphology is given below in Figure 16. The main cause of formation of two different morphologies is the presence of oleic acid. The presence of oleic acid led to the formation of oblique nanocubes, whereas truncated nanocubes are formed in the absence of oleic acid.

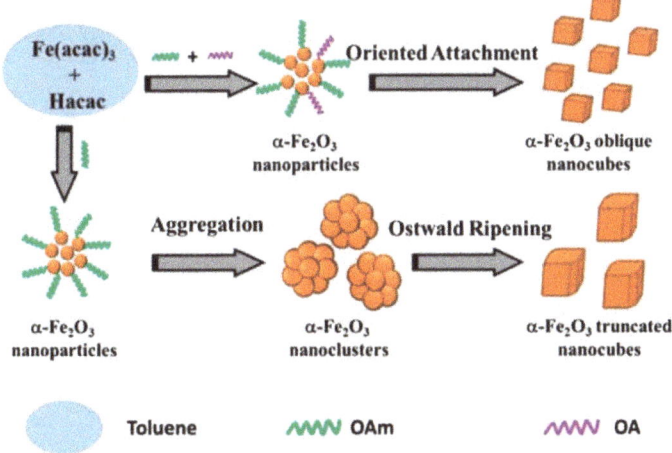

Figure 16. Mechanism of formation of oblique and truncated nanocubes (reproduced with permission from Royal Society of Chemistry 2013) [194].

Zeng et al. have synthesized novel Fe$_3$O$_4$ nanoprism by a hydrothermal process using oleylamine (OAm) both as surfactant and reducing agent. The synthesized Fe$_3$O$_4$ exposed two kinds of crystal planes (111) and (220), as shown in Figure 17 [195].

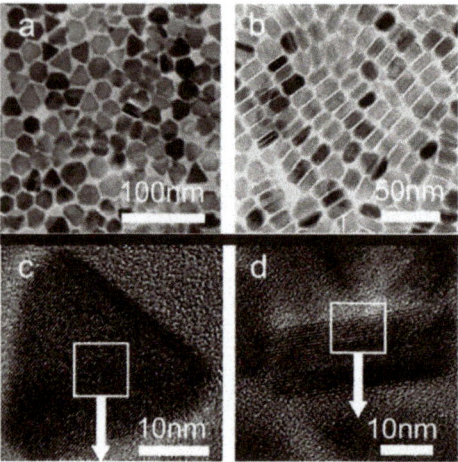

Figure 17. TEM images of Fe$_3$O$_4$ nanoprisms (**a**) lying flat and (**b**) self- assembled on the substrates (**c**), and (**d**) HRTEM images of Fe$_3$O$_4$ nanoprisms with a spacing of 0.301 nm (reproduced with permission from Royal Society of Chemistry 2010) [195].

They experimentally proved the crystal plane dependent electrochemical activities of nanoprism as clear from Figure 18b. Oleylamine was found to plays key role in the formation of different planes Fe$_3$O$_4$ nanoprism, because the amine group of oleylamine absorb at certain planes and slows their growth while allowing the growth of other planes leading to different morphology.

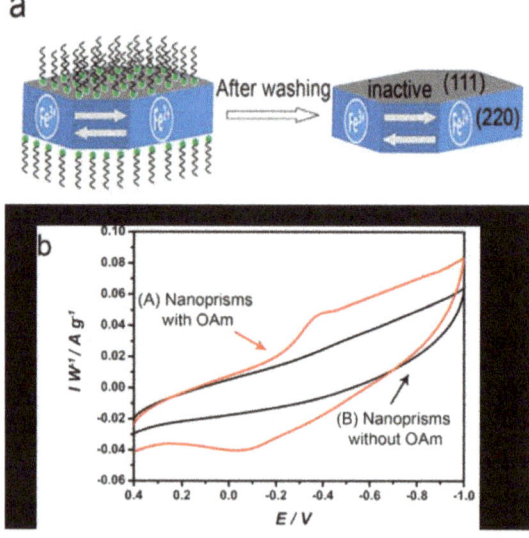

Figure 18. (**a**) Schematic illustration of Fe$_3$O$_4$ nanoprisms redox reaction. (**b**) Cyclic voltammograms of electrodes made of (A) Fe$_3$O$_4$ nanoprism with OAm (B) Fe$_3$O$_4$ nanoprisms without OAm in 1 M Na$_2$SO$_3$ (reproduced with permission from Wiley Online Library 2006) [195].

8.3. Microwave-Assisted Synthesis

Microwave-assisted method is a chemical method that use microwave radiation for heating materials containing electrical charges for instance polar molecule in the solvent or charge ion in the solid. Compared with other heating methods, microwave-assisted solution fabrication methods have got more focus of research because of rapid processing, high reaction rate, reduce reaction time, and high yield of product. Wang reported the synthesis of cubical spinal MFe_2O_4 (M = Co, Mn, Ni) high crystalline structure in a short time of just 10 min by exposure the precursors to microwave radiation [196] shown in Figure 19; they also used the microwave radiations for the synthesis of magnetite (Fe_3O_4) and hematite (α-Fe_2O_3), and used $FeCl_3$, polyethylene glycol, and $N_2H_4 \cdot H_2O$ as precursors, finding that the amount of $N_2H_4 \cdot H_2O$ has a key role in controlling the final phase of Fe_3O_4 [197].

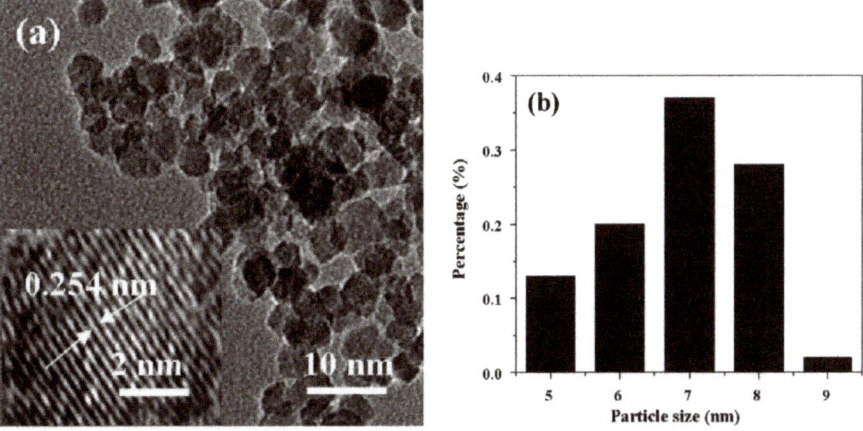

Figure 19. (a) TEM image of the $MnFe_2O_4$ and (b) the histogram showing particle size (reproduced with permission from Springer 2007) [197].

8.4. Template Assisted Fabrication

Another fabrication method used for the synthesis of MNPs is the template-assisted fabrication [198]. The active template-based synthesis involves the growth of the nuclei at the holes and defects of the template. Subsequently, the growth of the nuclei at the pre-formed template yields the desired morphology of the nanostructures. So through proper selection of base template, the size and shape of the MNPs can be controlled. This technique has two important advantages over the chemical routes:

(i) Template use in the fabrication process determines the final size and morphology of the nanostructures.
(ii) Complex nanostructures such as nanobarcodes (segmented nanorods) nanoprism, nanocubes hexagons, and octahedrons MNPs can be fabricated in an easy manner, with full control on size and morphology.

However, this method has also some drawback. It is a multistep process, first requiring the fabrication base templates and then the subsequent deposition of magnetic material within the template. In the following discussion, we will highlight important recent progress that has been done in the template-assisted synthesis of complex magnetic nanostructures. Mirkin et al. have demonstrated the synthesis of nanobarcodes (segmented nanowires with excellent control of composition along the length) of metals and polymers magnetic and non-magnetic materials. They demonstrated the fabrication of two component rod structure that was made by deposition of hydrophilic Au block and hydrophobic Polypyrrole block on anodic alumina oxide template. Due to the difference in the diameter of hydrophilic Au and hydrophobic Polypyrrole these sections were assembled in unique and exclusive pseudo-conical shape with three-dimensional bundle- and tubular-shaped structure as shown in Figure 20 [199].

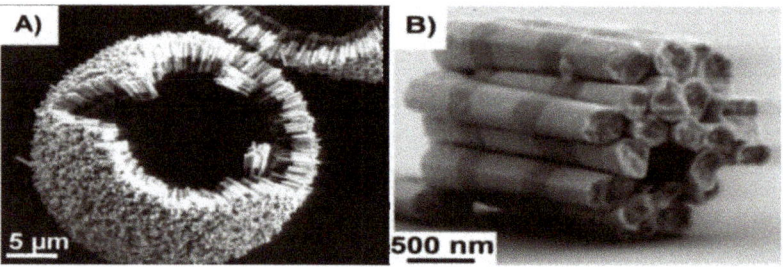

Figure 20. (A) SEM image of self-assembly of Au-Polypyrrole rods into a tubular shape. (B) SEM image showing the alignment of the ferromagnetic portion in a bundle of Au–Ni rods (reproduced with permission from Wiley Online Library 2006) [199].

8.5. Sol–Gel Method

The sol–gel process is a versatile chemical approach for the synthesis of nanoparticles with precise shapes and size. Sol–gel synthetic strategy makes use of a gelling agent to form a homogeneous gel where a metal salt is stirred [200]. This process involves the hydroxylation and condensation of metal precursors in solution to form a colloid. Sol–gel method provides a wide range of synthesis temperature, for instance, we managed to obtain nearly monodispersed α-Fe$_2$O$_3$, γ-Fe$_2$O$_3$ and Fe$_3$O$_4$ with same procedure and same starting reagent through a medium temperature sol–gel route [201]. Uniquely, the formation of different final iron oxide structures is only dependent on the drying process (Figure 21). The size displayed by TEM revealed that 4.9 nm of Fe$_3$O$_4$ nanoparticles are obtained by the centrifugation of sol, whereas slight increment in size of γ-Fe$_2$O$_3$ was formed when xerogel was heated at 150 °C. Yet, directly drying of wet Fe$_3$O$_4$ gel at 150 °C without the formation of xerogel first allowed phase transformation to 10.1 nm α-Fe$_2$O$_3$ [201].

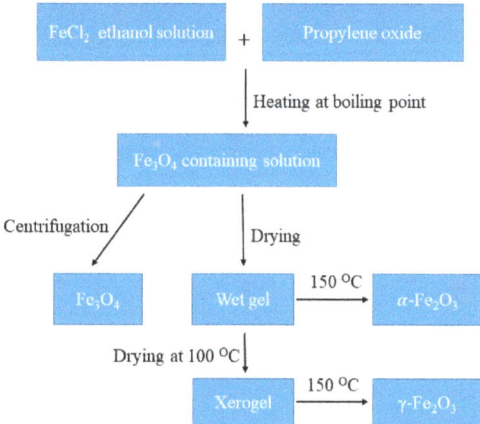

Figure 21. Scheme flow for the preparation of α-Fe$_2$O$_3$, γ-Fe$_2$O$_3$ and Fe$_3$O$_4$ nanoparticles (reproduced with permission from Science Direct 2013) [201].

The sizes of obtained magnetite nanoparticles are readily tailored by longer annealing temperature range under vacuum environment. The magnetic behavior, particle size and crystallinity of magnetite nanoparticles is very sensitive to the annealing temperature where these physico-chemical properties increase as annealing temperature was adjusted from 200 °C to 400 °C [202]. Combination of microwave heating with this route provides a fast and energy efficient synthesis methodology to metal oxide nanoparticles [203]. The reaction mixture of Fe(acec)$_3$ that dissolved in benzyl alcohol was heated at 170 °C by exposure to microwave radiation for 12 min and accomplished to yield 5–6 nm of nanoparticles [204].

8.6. Synthesis of GO-Fe$_3$O$_4$ Nanocomposite

8.6.1. Coprecipitation Method

Graphene oxide was synthesized by well-known Hummers method [205]. To synthesize the GO-Fe$_3$O$_4$ composite, a weighed amount of as-synthesized graphene oxide, prepared by Hummers method, was dispersed in distilled water by sonication. An aqueous solution containing FeCl$_3$ and FeCl$_2$.4H$_2$O was then added into the graphene oxide dispersion kept under constant stirring. After 2 h of stirring, CH$_3$NH$_2$ was added drop wise into the dispersion to precipitate Fe$_3$O$_4$ nanoparticles [206].

8.6.2. Organometallic Decomposition and Ligand Exchange Method

Ferrite nanoparticles with high saturation magnetization, narrow size distribution, and better shape control is achieved by organometallic decomposition method. Nanoparticles synthesized by organometallic decomposition method are not dispersible in water and they are functionalized with biocompatible molecules for further use. GO–nanoparticle composites were synthesized using emulsification process, the details of which are described in Figure 22. The particles are coated with GO and PEG which improves water dispersibility and biocompatibility of PEG-coated particles is well recorded.

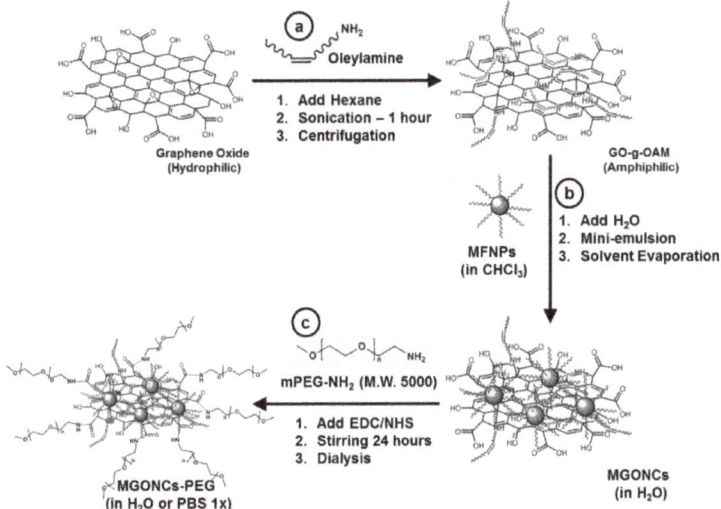

Figure 22. Schematic illustration of the formation of (**a**) amphiphilic graphene oxide sheets (GO-g-OAM), (**b**) water-dispersible NP/GO nanocomposite (MGONC), and (**c**) PEGylation of MGONC (reproduced with permission from Wiley Online Library 2012) [105].

8.7. Cytotoxicity of Ferrite Nanoparticles

The cytotoxicity of the ferrite nanoparticles is thoroughly studied and there are numerous reports of cytotoxicity of ferrite nanoparticles functionalized with various polymeric coatings [207,208]. Ferrite nanoparticles are usually functionalized with chitosan, polyethylene glycol, and graphene oxide [209].

Iron oxide NPs coated with different substances have shown variable cell viability results [210]. There are various in vitro methods, and the LDH, MTT and MTS assays are most widely used for assessment of nanoparticles cytotoxicity [211]. Magnetic iron oxide NPs have been observed to accumulate in the liver, spleen, lungs, and brain after inhalation, showing its ability to cross the blood–brain barrier [212].

9. Conclusions

MH is a cancer therapy method which involves delivering MNPs to the tumor cells and heating them by applying AMF. The world is witnessing great progress in understanding the principles and applications of this noninvasive and localized therapy technique. In this report, we discussed the basic principles of MH using MNPs. The basics of heat generation under an AMF were discussed. Some of the extrinsic and intrinsic parameters that influence heat generation by MNPs were explained. Calorimetric measurements were introduced along with the sources of errors. Several synthesis methods of MNPs where presented. The interesting features of multifunctional hybrid MNPs were also introduced.

Author Contributions: All authors I.M.O., V.N., S.A., S.S. and C.V.V.M.G. contributed equally in the preparation of this review article, including writing—original draft preparation and writing—review and editing.

Funding: This work was financially supported by the UAEU Program for Advanced Research (UPAR) under the Grant no. 31S312.

Conflicts of Interest: The authors declare no conflicts of interest.

References

1. Dou, Y.; Hynynen, K.; Allen, C. To heat or not to heat: Challenges with clinical translation of thermosensitive liposomes. *J. Control Release* **2017**, *249*, 63–73. [CrossRef] [PubMed]
2. Mallory, M.; Gogineni, E.; Jones, G.C.; Greer, L.; Simone, C.B. Therapeutic hyperthermia: The old, the new, and the upcoming. *Crit. Rev. Oncol. Hematol.* **2016**, *97*, 56–64. [CrossRef] [PubMed]
3. Fratila, R.; Fuente, J. *Nanomaterials for Magnetic and Optical Hyperthermia Applications*, 1st ed.; Elsevier: Amsterdam, The Nederland, 2019; pp. 1–10. ISBN 978-0-12-813928-8.
4. Pérez-Hernández, M. Chapter 8—Mechanisms of Cell Death Induced by Optical Hyperthermia. In *Nanomaterials for Magnetic and Optical Hyperthermia Applications*; Micro and Nano Technologies; Fratila, R.M., De La Fuente, J.M., Eds.; Elsevier: Amsterdam, The Netherlands, 2019; pp. 201–228. ISBN 978-0-12-813928-8.
5. Dhavalikar, R.; Bohórquez, A.C.; Rinaldi, C. Chapter 10—Image-Guided Thermal Therapy Using Magnetic Particle Imaging and Magnetic Fluid Hyperthermia. In *Nanomaterials for Magnetic and Optical Hyperthermia Applications*; Micro and Nano Technologies; Fratila, R.M., De La Fuente, J.M., Eds.; Elsevier: Amsterdam, The Netherlands, 2019; pp. 265–286. ISBN 978-0-12-813928-8.
6. Beik, J.; Abed, Z.; Ghoreishi, F.S.; Hosseini-Nami, S.; Mehrzadi, S.; Shakeri-Zadeh, A.; Kamrava, S.K. Nanotechnology in hyperthermia cancer therapy: From fundamental principles to advanced applications. *J. Control Release* **2016**, *235*, 205–221. [CrossRef] [PubMed]
7. Ito, M.; Hiramatsu, H.; Kobayashi, K.; Suzue, K.; Kawahata, M.; Hioki, K.; Ueyama, Y.; Koyanagi, Y.; Sugamura, K.; Tsuji, K.; et al. NOD/SCID/gamma(c)(null) mouse: An excellent recipient mouse model for engraftment of human cells. *Blood* **2002**, *100*, 3175–3182. [CrossRef]
8. Di Corato, R.; Espinosa, A.; Lartigue, L.; Tharaud, M.; Chat, S.; Pellegrino, T.; Ménager, C.; Gazeau, F.; Wilhelm, C. Magnetic hyperthermia efficiency in the cellular environment for different nanoparticle designs. *Biomaterials* **2014**, *35*, 6400–6411. [CrossRef]
9. Fratila, R.M.; Fuente, J.M.D.L. *Nanomaterials for Magnetic and Optical Hyperthermia Applications*; Elsevier: Amsterdam, The Netherlands, 2018; ISBN 978-0-12-813929-5.
10. Laurent, S.; Dutz, S.; Häfeli, U.O.; Mahmoudi, M. Magnetic fluid hyperthermia: Focus on superparamagnetic iron oxide nanoparticles. *Adv. Colloid Interface Sci.* **2011**, *166*, 8–23. [CrossRef]
11. Kumar, C.S.S.R.; Mohammad, F. Magnetic nanomaterials for hyperthermia-based therapy and controlled drug delivery. *Adv. Drug Deliv. Rev.* **2011**, *63*, 789–808. [CrossRef]

12. Hergt, R.; Dutz, S.; Müller, R.; Zeisberger, M. Magnetic particle hyperthermia: Nanoparticle magnetism and materials development for cancer therapy. *J. Phys. Condens. Matter* **2006**, *18*, S2919–S2934. [CrossRef]
13. Vallejo-Fernandez, G.; Whear, O.; Roca, A.G.; Hussain, S.; Timmis, J.; Patel, V.; Grady, K. Mechanisms of hyperthermia in magnetic nanoparticles. *J. Phys. D Appl. Phys.* **2013**, *46*, 312001. [CrossRef]
14. Piñeiro, Y.; Vargas, Z.; Rivas, J.; López-Quintela, M.A. Iron Oxide Based Nanoparticles for Magnetic Hyperthermia Strategies in Biological Applications. *Eur. J. Inorganic Chem.* **2015**, *2015*, 4495–4509.
15. Dennis, C.L.; Ivkov, R. Physics of heat generation using magnetic nanoparticles for hyperthermia. *Int. J. Hyperth.* **2013**, *29*, 715–729. [CrossRef] [PubMed]
16. Obaidat, I.M.; Issa, B.; Haik, Y. Magnetic Properties of Magnetic Nanoparticles for Efficient Hyperthermia. *Nanomaterials* **2015**, *5*, 63–89. [CrossRef] [PubMed]
17. Périgo, E.A.; Hemery, G.; Sandre, O.; Ortega, D.; Garaio, E.; Plazaola, F.; Teran, F.J. Fundamentals and advances in magnetic hyperthermia. *Appl. Phys. Rev.* **2015**, *2*, 041302. [CrossRef]
18. Mahmoudi, K.; Bouras, A.; Bozec, D.; Ivkov, R.; Hadjipanayis, C. Magnetic hyperthermia therapy for the treatment of glioblastoma: A review of the therapy's history, efficacy and application in humans. *Int. J. Hyperth.* **2018**, *34*, 1316–1328. [CrossRef]
19. Angelakeris, M. Magnetic nanoparticles: A multifunctional vehicle for modern theranostics. *Biochim. Biophys. Acta Gen. Subj.* **2017**, *1861*, 1642–1651. [CrossRef]
20. Spirou, S.V.; Costa Lima, S.A.; Bouziotis, P.; Vranješ-Djurić, S.; Efthimiadou, E.K.; Laurenzana, A.; Barbosa, A.I.; Garcia-Alonso, I.; Jones, C.; Jankovic, D.; et al. Recommendations for in Vitro and In Vivo Testing of Magnetic Nanoparticle Hyperthermia Combined with Radiation Therapy. *Nanomaterials* **2018**, *8*, 306. [CrossRef]
21. Spirou, S.V.; Basini, M.; Lascialfari, A.; Sangregorio, C.; Innocenti, C. Magnetic Hyperthermia and Radiation Therapy: Radiobiological Principles and Current Practice. *Nanomaterials* **2018**, *8*, 401. [CrossRef]
22. Issa, B.; Obaidat, I.M.; Albiss, B.A.; Haik, Y. Magnetic nanoparticles: Surface effects and properties related to biomedicine applications. *Int. J. Mol. Sci.* **2013**, *14*, 21266–21305. [CrossRef]
23. Carrey, J.; Mehdaoui, B.; Respaud, M. Simple models for dynamic hysteresis loop calculations of magnetic single-domain nanoparticles: Application to magnetic hyperthermia optimization. *J. Appl. Phys.* **2011**, *109*, 083921. [CrossRef]
24. Mehdaoui, B.; Meffre, A.; Carrey, J.; Lachaize, S.; Lacroix, L.-M.; Gougeon, M.; Chaudret, B.; Respaud, M. Optimal Size of Nanoparticles for Magnetic Hyperthermia: A Combined Theoretical and Experimental Study. *Adv. Funct. Mater.* **2011**, *21*, 4573–4581. [CrossRef]
25. Colombo, M.; Carregal-Romero, S.; Casula, M.F.; Gutiérrez, L.; Morales, M.P.; Boehm, I.; Heverhagen, J.T.; Prosperi, D.; Parak, W.J. Biological applications of magnetic nanoparticles. *Chem. Soc. Rev.* **2012**, *41*, 4306–4334. [CrossRef] [PubMed]
26. Obaidat, I.M.; Nayek, C.; Manna, K.; Bhattacharjee, G.; Al-Omari, I.A.; Gismelseed, A. Investigating Exchange Bias and Coercivity in Fe_3O_4–γ-Fe_2O_3 Core–Shell Nanoparticles of Fixed Core Diameter and Variable Shell Thicknesses. *Nanomaterials* **2017**, *7*, 415. [CrossRef] [PubMed]
27. Obaidat, I.M.; Nayek, C.; Manna, K. Investigating the Role of Shell Thickness and Field Cooling on Saturation Magnetization and Its Temperature Dependence in $Fe3O_4$/γ-Fe_2O_3 Core/Shell Nanoparticles. *Appl. Sci.* **2017**, *7*, 1269. [CrossRef]
28. Rachakatla, R.S.; Balivada, S.; Seo, G.-M.; Myers, C.B.; Wang, H.; Samarakoon, T.N.; Dani, R.; Pyle, M.; Kroh, F.O.; Walker, B.; et al. Attenuation of mouse melanoma by A/C magnetic field after delivery of bi-magnetic nanoparticles by neural progenitor cells. *ACS Nano* **2010**, *4*, 7093–7104. [CrossRef]
29. Ruiz, A.; Gutiérrez, L.; Cáceres-Vélez, P.R.; Santos, D.; Chaves, S.B.; Fascineli, M.L.; Garcia, M.P.; Azevedo, R.B.; Morales, M.P. Biotransformation of magnetic nanoparticles as a function of coating in a rat model. *Nanoscale* **2015**, *7*, 16321–16329. [CrossRef]
30. Guimarães, A.P. The Basis of Nanomagnetism. In *Principles of Nanomagnetism*; NanoScience and Technology; Guimarães, A.P., Ed.; Springer International Publishing: Cham, Switzerland, 2017; pp. 1–23, ISBN 978-3-319-59409-5.
31. Deatsch, A.E.; Evans, B.A. Heating efficiency in magnetic nanoparticle hyperthermia. *J. Magn. Magn. Mater.* **2014**, *354*, 163–172. [CrossRef]
32. Brown, W.F. Thermal Fluctuations of a Single-Domain Particle. *Phys. Rev.* **1963**, *130*, 1677–1686. [CrossRef]
33. Néel, L. Théorie du traînage magnétique des substances massives dans le domaine de Rayleigh. *J. Phys. Radium* **1950**, *11*, 49–61. [CrossRef]

34. Leslie-Pelecky, D.L.; Rieke, R.D. Magnetic Properties of Nanostructured Materials. *Chem. Mater.* **1996**, *8*, 1770–1783. [CrossRef]
35. Rosensweig, R.E. Heating magnetic fluid with alternating magnetic field. *J. Magn. Magn. Mater.* **2002**, *252*, 370–374. [CrossRef]
36. Delaunay, L.; Neveu, S.; Noyel, G.; Monin, J. A new spectrometric method, using a magneto-optical effect, to study magnetic liquids. *J. Magn. Magn. Mater.* **1995**, *149*, L239–L245. [CrossRef]
37. Glöckl, G.; Hergt, R.; Zeisberger, M.; Dutz, S.; Nagel, S.; Weitschies, W. The effect of field parameters, nanoparticle properties and immobilization on the specific heating power in magnetic particle hyperthermia. *J. Phys. Condens. Matter* **2006**, *18*, S2935–S2949. [CrossRef]
38. Hergt, R.; Dutz, S. Magnetic particle hyperthermia—Biophysical limitations of a visionary tumour therapy. *J. Magn. Magn. Mater.* **2007**, *311*, 187–192. [CrossRef]
39. Moroz, P.; Jones, S.K.; Gray, B.N. Magnetically mediated hyperthermia: Current status and future directions. *Int. J. Hyperth.* **2002**, *18*, 267–284. [CrossRef]
40. Fantechi, E.; Innocenti, C.; Albino, M.; Lottini, E.; Sangregorio, C. Influence of cobalt doping on the hyperthermic efficiency of magnetite nanoparticles. *J. Magn. Magn. Mater.* **2015**, *380*, 365–371. [CrossRef]
41. Lee, J.-H.; Jang, J.-T.; Choi, J.-S.; Moon, S.H.; Noh, S.-H.; Kim, J.-W.; Kim, J.-G.; Kim, I.-S.; Park, K.I.; Cheon, J. Exchange-coupled magnetic nanoparticles for efficient heat induction. *Nat. Nanotechnol.* **2011**, *6*, 418–422. [CrossRef]
42. Obaidat, I.M.; Mohite, V.; Issa, B.; Tit, N.; Haik, Y. Predicting a major role of surface spins in the magnetic properties of ferrite nanoparticles. *Cryst. Res. Technol.* **2009**, *44*, 489–494. [CrossRef]
43. Cotin, G.; Perton, F.; Blanco-Andujar, C.; Pichon, B.; Mertz, D.; Bégin-Colin, S. Chapter 2—Design of Anisotropic Iron-Oxide-Based Nanoparticles for Magnetic Hyperthermia. In *Nanomaterials for Magnetic and Optical Hyperthermia Applications*; Micro and Nano Technologies; Fratila, R.M., De La Fuente, J.M., Eds.; Elsevier: Amsterdam, The Netherlands, 2019; pp. 41–60. ISBN 978-0-12-813928-8.
44. Cullity, B.D.; Graham, C.D. *Introduction to Magnetic Materials*; Wiley: Hoboken IEEE Press: Chichester, UK, 2009; ISBN 978-0-471-47741-9.
45. Guardia, P.; Di Corato, R.; Lartigue, L.; Wilhelm, C.; Espinosa, A.; Garcia-Hernandez, M.; Gazeau, F.; Manna, L.; Pellegrino, T. Water-Soluble Iron Oxide Nanocubes with High Values of Specific Absorption Rate for Cancer Cell Hyperthermia Treatment. *ACS Nano* **2012**, *6*, 3080–3091. [CrossRef]
46. Martinez-Boubeta, C.; Simeonidis, K.; Makridis, A.; Angelakeris, M.; Iglesias, O.; Guardia, P.; Cabot, A.; Yedra, L.; Estrade, S.; Peiro, F.; et al. Learning from Nature to Improve the Heat Generation of Iron-Oxide Nanoparticles for Magnetic Hyperthermia Applications. *Sci. Rep.* **2013**. [CrossRef]
47. Usov, N.A.; Nesmeyanov, M.S.; Gubanova, E.M.; Epshtein, N.B. Heating ability of magnetic nanoparticles with cubic and combined anisotropy. *Beilstein J. Nanotechnol.* **2019**, *10*, 305–314. [CrossRef]
48. Nayek, C.; Manna, K.; Bhattacharjee, G.; Murugavel, P.; Obaidat, I. Investigating Size- and Temperature-Dependent Coercivity and Saturation Magnetization in PEG Coated Fe_3O_4 Nanoparticles. *Magnetochemistry* **2017**, *3*, 19. [CrossRef]
49. Liu, W.; Zhong, W.; Du, Y.W. Magnetic nanoparticles with core/shell structures. *J. NanoSci. Nanotechnol.* **2008**, *8*, 2781–2792. [CrossRef] [PubMed]
50. Venkatesha, N.; Qurishi, Y.; Atreya, H.S.; Srivastava, C. Effect of core–shell nanoparticle geometry on the enhancement of the proton relaxivity value in a nuclear magnetic resonance experiment. *RSC Adv.* **2016**, *6*, 64605–64610. [CrossRef]
51. Obaidat, I.M.; Haik, Y.; Mohite, V.; Issa, B.; Tit, N. Peculiar Magnetic Properties of MnZnGdFeO Nanoparticles. *Adv. Sci. Lett.* **2009**, *2*, 60–64. [CrossRef]
52. Venkatesha, N.; Pudakalakatti, S.M.; Qurishi, Y.; Atreya, H.S.; Srivastava, C. $MnFe_2O_4$–Fe_3O_4 core–shell nanoparticles as a potential contrast agent for magnetic resonance imaging. *RSC Adv.* **2015**, *5*, 97807–97815. [CrossRef]
53. Mandal, S.; Chaudhuri, K. Engineered magnetic core shell nanoprobes: Synthesis and applications to cancer imaging and therapeutics. *World J. Biol. Chem.* **2016**, *7*, 158–167. [CrossRef] [PubMed]
54. Sun, X.; Huls, N.F.; Sigdel, A.; Sun, S. Tuning exchange bias in core/shell FeO/Fe_3O_4 nanoparticles. *Nano Lett.* **2012**, *12*, 246–251. [CrossRef]

55. Nayek, C.; Al-Akhras, M.-A.; Narayanaswamy, V.; Khaleel, A.; Al-Omari, I.A.; Rusydi, A.; Obaidat, I.M. Role of Shell Thickness and Applied Field on The Magnetic Anisotropy and Temperature Dependence of Coercivity in Fe_3O_4 -Fe_2O_3 Core/shell Nanoparticles. *Mater. Express* **2019**, *9*, 2158–5849. [CrossRef]
56. Thomas, S.; Reethu, K.; Thanveer, T.; Myint, M.T.Z.; Al-Harthi, S.H. Effect of shell thickness on the exchange bias blocking temperature and coercivity in Co-CoO core-shell nanoparticles. *J. Appl. Phys.* **2017**, *122*, 063902. [CrossRef]
57. Dimitriadis, V.; Kechrakos, D.; Chubykalo-Fesenko, O.; Tsiantos, V. Shape-dependent exchange bias effect in magnetic nanoparticles with core-shell morphology. *Phys. Rev. B* **2015**, *92*, 064420. [CrossRef]
58. Nogués, J.; Sort, J.; Langlais, V.; Skumryev, V.; Suriñach, S.; Muñoz, J.S.; Baró, M.D. Exchange bias in nanostructures. *Phys. Rep.* **2005**, *422*, 65–117. [CrossRef]
59. López-Ortega, A.; Estrader, M.; Salazar-Alvarez, G.; Roca, A.G.; Nogués, J. Applications of exchange coupled bi-magnetic hard/soft and soft/hard magnetic core/shell nanoparticles. *Phys. Rep.* **2015**, *553*, 1–32. [CrossRef]
60. Phan, M.-H.; Alonso, J.; Khurshid, H.; Lampen-Kelley, P.; Chandra, S.; Stojak Repa, K.; Nemati, Z.; Das, R.; Iglesias, Ó.; Srikanth, H. Exchange Bias Effects in Iron Oxide-Based Nanoparticle Systems. *Nanomaterials* **2016**, *6*, 221. [CrossRef] [PubMed]
61. Desautels, R.D.; Skoropata, E.; Chen, Y.-Y.; Ouyang, H.; Freeland, J.W.; van Lierop, J. Tuning the surface magnetism of γ-Fe2O3 nanoparticles with a Cu shell. *Appl. Phys. Lett.* **2011**, *99*, 262501. [CrossRef]
62. Rostamnejadi, A.; Venkatesan, M.; Alaria, J.; Boese, M.; Kameli, P.; Salamati, H.; Coey, J.M.D. Conventional and inverse magnetocaloric effects in La0.45Sr0.55MnO3 nanoparticles. *J. Appl. Phys.* **2011**, *110*, 043905. [CrossRef]
63. Batlle, X.; Labarta, A. Finite-size effects in fine particles: Magnetic and transport properties. *J. Phys. D Appl. Phys.* **2002**. [CrossRef]
64. Ho, C.-H.; Lai, C.-H. Size-Dependent Magnetic Properties of PtMn Nanoparticles. *IEEE Trans. Magn.* **2006**, *42*, 3069–3071. [CrossRef]
65. Zhao, Q.; Wang, L.; Cheng, R.; Mao, L.; Arnold, R.D.; Howerth, E.W.; Chen, Z.G.; Platt, S. Magnetic Nanoparticle-Based Hyperthermia for Head & Neck Cancer in Mouse Models. *Theranostics* **2012**, *2*, 113–121.
66. Nieskoski, M.D.; Trembly, B.S. Comparison of a single optimized coil and a Helmholtz pair for magnetic nanoparticle hyperthermia. *IEEE Trans. Biomed. Eng.* **2014**, *61*, 1642–1650. [CrossRef]
67. Cabrera, D.; Rubia-Rodríguez, I.; Garaio, E.; Plazaola, F.; Dupré, L.; Farrow, N.; Terán, F.J.; Ortega, D. Chapter 5—Instrumentation for Magnetic Hyperthermia. In *Nanomaterials for Magnetic and Optical Hyperthermia Applications*; Micro and Nano Technologies; Fratila, R.M., De La Fuente, J.M., Eds.; Elsevier: Amsterdam, The Netherlands, 2019; pp. 111–138. ISBN 978-0-12-813928-8.
68. Mamiya, H.; Jeyadevan, B. Chapter 1—Design Criteria of Thermal Seeds for Magnetic Fluid Hyperthermia—From Magnetic Physics Point of View. In *Nanomaterials for Magnetic and Optical Hyperthermia Applications*; Micro and Nano Technologies; Fratila, R.M., De La Fuente, J.M., Eds.; Elsevier: Amsterdam, The Netherlands, 2019; pp. 13–39. ISBN 978-0-12-813928-8.
69. Hergt, R.; Hiergeist, R.; Hilger, I.; Kaiser, W.A.; Boguslavsky, Y.; Margel, S.; Richter, U. Maghemite nanoparticles with very high AC-losses for application in RF-magnetic hyperthermia. *J. Magn. Magn. Mater.* **2004**, *270*, 345–357. [CrossRef]
70. Dössel, O.; Bohnert, J. Safety considerations for magnetic fields of 10 mT to 100 mT amplitude in the frequency range of 10 kHz to 100 kHz for magnetic particle imaging. *Biomed. Tech. (Berl)* **2013**, *58*, 611–621. [CrossRef] [PubMed]
71. Kita, E.; Oda, T.; Kayano, T.; Sato, S.; Minagawa, M.; Yanagihara, H.; Kishimoto, M.; Mitsumata, C.; Hashimoto, S.; Yamada, K.; et al. Ferromagnetic nanoparticles for magnetic hyperthermia and thermoablation therapy. *J. Phys. D Appl. Phys.* **2010**, *43*, 474011. [CrossRef]
72. Lemal, P.; Balog, S.; Geers, C.; Taladriz-Blanco, P.; Palumbo, A.; Hirt, A.M.; Rothen-Rutishauser, B.; Petri-Fink, A. Heating behavior of magnetic iron oxide nanoparticles at clinically relevant concentration. *J. Magn. Magn. Mater.* **2019**, *474*, 637–642. [CrossRef]
73. Ovejero, J.G.; Cabrera, D.; Carrey, J.; Valdivielso, T.; Salas, G.; Teran, F.J. Effects of inter- and intra-aggregate magnetic dipolar interactions on the magnetic heating efficiency of iron oxide nanoparticles. *Phys. Chem. Chem. Phys.* **2016**, *18*, 10954–10963. [CrossRef]

74. Narayanaswamy, V.; Obaidat, I.M.; Latiyan, S.; Jain, S.; Nayek, C.; Goankar, S.; AL-Akhras, M.-A.; Al-Omari, I.A. Role of interface quality in iron oxide core/shell nanoparticles on heating efficiency and transverse relaxivity. *Mater. Express* **2019**, *2158–5849*. [CrossRef]
75. Narayanaswamy, V.; Obaidat, I.M.; Kamzin, A.S.; Latiyan, S.; Jain, S.; Kumar, H.; Srivastava, C.; Alaabed, S.; Issa, B. Synthesis of Graphene Oxide-Fe$_3$O$_4$ Based Nanocomposites Using the Mechanochemical Method and in Vitro Magnetic Hyperthermia. *Int. J. Mol. Sci.* **2019**, *20*, 3368. [CrossRef]
76. Espinosa, A.; Di Corato, R.; Kolosnjaj-Tabi, J.; Flaud, P.; Pellegrino, T.; Wilhelm, C. Duality of Iron Oxide Nanoparticles in Cancer Therapy: Amplification of Heating Efficiency by Magnetic Hyperthermia and Photothermal Bimodal Treatment. *ACS Nano* **2016**, *10*, 2436–2446. [CrossRef]
77. Kandasamy, G.; Sudame, A.; Bhati, P.; Chakrabarty, A.; Maity, D. Systematic investigations on heating effects of carboxyl-amine functionalized superparamagnetic iron oxide nanoparticles (SPIONs) based ferrofluids for in vitro cancer hyperthermia therapy. *J. Mol. Liq.* **2018**, *256*, 224–237. [CrossRef]
78. de la Presa, P.; Luengo, Y.; Velasco, V.; Morales, M.P.; Iglesias, M.; Veintemillas-Verdaguer, S.; Crespo, P.; Hernando, A. Particle Interactions in Liquid Magnetic Colloids by Zero Field Cooled Measurements: Effects on Heating Efficiency. *J. Phys. Chem. C* **2015**, *119*, 11022–11030. [CrossRef]
79. Blanco-Andujar, C.; Ortega, D.; Southern, P.; Nesbitt, S.A.; Thanh, N.T.K.; Pankhurst, Q.A. Real-time tracking of delayed-onset cellular apoptosis induced by intracellular magnetic hyperthermia. *Nanomedicine (Lond)* **2016**, *11*, 121–136. [CrossRef]
80. Wan, J.; Yuan, R.; Zhang, C.; Wu, N.; Yan, F.; Yu, S.; Chen, K. Stable and Biocompatible Colloidal Dispersions of Superparamagnetic Iron Oxide Nanoparticles with Minimum Aggregation for Biomedical Applications. *J. Phys. Chem. C* **2016**, *120*, 23799–23806. [CrossRef]
81. Shetake, N.G.; Kumar, A.; Gaikwad, S.; Ray, P.; Desai, S.; Ningthoujam, R.S.; Vatsa, R.K.; Pandey, B.N. Magnetic nanoparticle-mediated hyperthermia therapy induces tumour growth inhibition by apoptosis and Hsp90/AKT modulation. *Int. J. Hyperth.* **2015**, *31*, 909–919. [CrossRef] [PubMed]
82. Sakellari, D.; Brintakis, K.; Kostopoulou, A.; Myrovali, E.; Simeonidis, K.; Lappas, A.; Angelakeris, M. Ferrimagnetic nanocrystal assemblies as versatile magnetic particle hyperthermia mediators. *Mater. Sci. Eng. C Mater. Biol. Appl.* **2016**, *58*, 187–193. [CrossRef] [PubMed]
83. Mendo, S.G.; Alves, A.F.; Ferreira, L.P.; Cruz, M.M.; Mendonça, M.H.; Godinho, M.; Carvalho, M.D. Hyperthermia studies of ferrite nanoparticles synthesized in the presence of cotton. *New J. Chem.* **2015**, *39*, 7182–7193. [CrossRef]
84. Burrows, F.; Parker, C.; Evans, R.F.L.; Hancock, Y.; Hovorka, O.; Chantrell, R.W. Energy losses in interacting fine-particle magnetic composites. *J. Phys. D Appl. Phys.* **2010**, *43*, 474010. [CrossRef]
85. Tan, R.P.; Carrey, J.; Respaud, M. Magnetic hyperthermia properties of nanoparticles inside lysosomes using kinetic Monte Carlo simulations: Influence of key parameters and dipolar interactions, and evidence for strong spatial variation of heating power. *Phys. Rev. B* **2014**, *90*, 214421. [CrossRef]
86. Coral, D.F.; Mendoza Zélis, P.; Marciello, M.; Morales, M.d.P.; Craievich, A.; Sánchez, F.H.; Fernández van Raap, M.B. Effect of Nanoclustering and Dipolar Interactions in Heat Generation for Magnetic Hyperthermia. *Langmuir* **2016**, *32*, 1201–1213. [CrossRef]
87. Mamiya, H. Recent Advances in Understanding Magnetic Nanoparticles in AC Magnetic Fields and Optimal Design for Targeted Hyperthermia. Available online: https://www.hindawi.com/journals/jnm/2013/752973/ (accessed on 10 October 2019).
88. Mamiya, H.; Jeyadevan, B. Hyperthermic effects of dissipative structures of magnetic nanoparticles in large alternating magnetic fields. *Sci. Rep.* **2011**, *1*, 157. [CrossRef]
89. Usov, N.A. Low frequency hysteresis loops of superparamagnetic nanoparticles with uniaxial anisotropy. *J. Appl. Phys.* **2010**, *107*, 123909. [CrossRef]
90. Raikher, Y.L.; Stepanov, V.I. Physical aspects of magnetic hyperthermia: Low-frequency ac field absorption in a magnetic colloid. *J. Magne. Magn. Mater.* **2014**, *368*, 421–427. [CrossRef]
91. Raikher, Y.; Stepanov, V. Absorption of AC field energy in a suspension of magnetic dipoles. *J. Magn. Magn. Mater.* **2008**, *320*, 2692–2695. [CrossRef]
92. Andreu, I.; Natividad, E. Accuracy of available methods for quantifying the heat power generation of nanoparticles for magnetic hyperthermia. *Int. J. Hyperth.* **2013**, *29*, 739–751. [CrossRef]

93. Drayton, A.; Zehner, J.; Timmis, J.; Patel, V.; Vallejo-Fernandez, G.; O'Grady, K. A comparative measurement technique of nanoparticle heating for magnetic hyperthermia applications. *J. Phys. D Appl. Phys.* **2017**, *50*, 495003. [CrossRef]
94. Wildeboer, R.R.; Southern, P.; Pankhurst, Q.A. On the reliable measurement of specific absorption rates and intrinsic loss parameters in magnetic hyperthermia materials. *J. Phys. D Appl. Phys.* **2014**, *47*, 495003. [CrossRef]
95. Lemal, P.; Geers, C.; Rothen-Rutishauser, B.; Lattuada, M.; Petri-Fink, A. Measuring the heating power of magnetic nanoparticles: An overview of currently used methods. *Mater. Today Proc.* **2017**, *4*, S107–S117. [CrossRef]
96. Bordelon, D.E.; Cornejo, C.; Grüttner, C.; Westphal, F.; DeWeese, T.L.; Ivkov, R. Magnetic nanoparticle heating efficiency reveals magneto-structural differences when characterized with wide ranging and high amplitude alternating magnetic fields. *J. Appl. Phys.* **2011**, *109*, 124904. [CrossRef]
97. Verde, E.L.; Landi, G.T.; Carrião, M.S.; Drummond, A.L.; Gomes, J.A.; Vieira, E.D.; Sousa, M.H.; Bakuzis, A.F. Field dependent transition to the non-linear regime in magnetic hyperthermia experiments: Comparison between maghemite, copper, zinc, nickel and cobalt ferrite nanoparticles of similar sizes. *Aip Adv.* **2012**, *2*, 032120. [CrossRef]
98. Soetaert, F.; Kandala, S.K.; Bakuzis, A.; Ivkov, R. Experimental estimation and analysis of variance of the measured loss power of magnetic nanoparticles. *Sci. Rep.* **2017**, *7*, 6661. [CrossRef]
99. Natividad, E.; Castro, M.; Mediano, A. Adiabatic vs. non-adiabatic determination of specific absorption rate of ferrofluids. *J. Magn. Magn. Mater.* **2009**, *321*, 1497–1500. [CrossRef]
100. Landi, G.T. Simple models for the heating curve in magnetic hyperthermia experiments. *J. Magn. Magn. Mater.* **2013**, *326*, 14–21. [CrossRef]
101. Wang, S.-Y.; Huang, S.; Borca-Tasciuc, D.-A. Potential Sources of Errors in Measuring and Evaluating the Specific Loss Power of Magnetic Nanoparticles in an Alternating Magnetic Field. *IEEE Trans. Magn.* **2013**, *49*, 255–262. [CrossRef]
102. Lv, Y.; Yang, Y.; Fang, J.; Zhang, H.; Peng, E.; Liu, X.; Xiao, W.; Ding, J. Size dependent magnetic hyperthermia of octahedral Fe3O4 nanoparticles. *RSC Adv.* **2015**, *5*, 76764–76771. [CrossRef]
103. Liu, X.L.; Yang, Y.; Ng, C.T.; Zhao, L.Y.; Zhang, Y.; Bay, B.H.; Fan, H.M.; Ding, J. Magnetic vortex nanorings: A new class of hyperthermia agent for highly efficient in vivo regression of tumors. *Adv. Mater. Weinh.* **2015**, *27*, 1939–1944. [CrossRef] [PubMed]
104. Yang, Y.; Liu, X.; Lv, Y.; Herng, T.S.; Xu, X.; Xia, W.; Zhang, T.; Fang, J.; Xiao, W.; Ding, J. Orientation Mediated Enhancement on Magnetic Hyperthermia of Fe3O4 Nanodisc. *Adv. Funct. Mater.* **2015**, *25*, 812–820. [CrossRef]
105. Peng, E.; Choo, E.S.G.; Chandrasekharan, P.; Yang, C.-T.; Ding, J.; Chuang, K.-H.; Xue, J.M. Synthesis of Manganese Ferrite/Graphene Oxide Nanocomposites for Biomedical Applications. *Small* **2012**, *8*, 3620–3630. [CrossRef]
106. Niculaes, D.; Lak, A.; Anyfantis, G.C.; Marras, S.; Laslett, O.; Avugadda, S.K.; Cassani, M.; Serantes, D.; Hovorka, O.; Chantrell, R.; et al. Asymmetric Assembling of Iron Oxide Nanocubes for Improving Magnetic Hyperthermia Performance. *ACS Nano* **2017**, *11*, 12121–12133. [CrossRef]
107. Sugumaran, P.J.; Liu, X.-L.; Herng, T.S.; Peng, E.; Ding, J. GO-Functionalized Large Magnetic Iron Oxide Nanoparticles with Enhanced Colloidal Stability and Hyperthermia Performance. *ACS Appl. Mater. Interfaces* **2019**, *11*, 22703–22713. [CrossRef]
108. Zhu, M.; Wu, L.; Rao, F.; Song, Z.; Ren, K.; Ji, X.; Song, S.; Yao, D.; Feng, S. Uniform Ti-doped Sb2Te3 materials for high-speed phase change memory applications. *Appl. Phys. Lett.* **2014**, *104*, 053119. [CrossRef]
109. Ortgies, D.H.; de la Cueva, L.; del Rosal, B.; Sanz-Rodríguez, F.; Fernández, N.; Iglesias-de la Cruz, M.C.; Salas, G.; Cabrera, D.; Teran, F.J.; Jaque, D.; et al. In Vivo Deep Tissue Fluorescence and Magnetic Imaging Employing Hybrid Nanostructures. *ACS Appl. Mater. Interfaces* **2016**, *8*, 1406–1414. [CrossRef]
110. Rieke, V.; Pauly, K.B. MR thermometry. *J. Magn. Reson. Imaging* **2008**, *27*, 376–390. [CrossRef]
111. Dhavalikar, R.; Rinaldi, C. Theoretical Predictions for Spatially-Focused Heating of Magnetic Nanoparticles Guided by Magnetic Particle Imaging Field Gradients. *J. Magn. Magn. Mater.* **2016**, *419*, 267–273. [CrossRef] [PubMed]
112. Murase, K.; Takata, H.; Takeuchi, Y.; Saito, S. Control of the temperature rise in magnetic hyperthermia with use of an external static magnetic field. *Phys. Med.* **2013**, *29*, 624–630. [CrossRef] [PubMed]

113. Barati, M.R.; Selomulya, C.; Sandeman, K.G.; Suzuki, K. Extraordinary induction heating effect near the first order Curie transition. *Appl. Phys. Lett.* **2014**, *105*, 162412. [CrossRef]
114. Rauwerdink, A.M.; Hansen, E.W.; Weaver, J.B. Nanoparticle temperature estimation in combined ac and dc magnetic fields. *Phys. Med. Biol.* **2009**, *54*, L51–L55. [CrossRef]
115. Weaver, J.B.; Rauwerdink, A.M.; Hansen, E.W. Magnetic nanoparticle temperature estimation. *Med. Phys.* **2009**, *36*, 1822–1829. [CrossRef]
116. Zhong, J.; Liu, W.; Du, Z.; César de Morais, P.; Xiang, Q.; Xie, Q. A noninvasive, remote and precise method for temperature and concentration estimation using magnetic nanoparticles. *Nanotechnology* **2012**, *23*, 075703. [CrossRef]
117. Akin, Y.; Obaidat, I.M.; Issa, B.; Haik, Y. Ni1-x Crx alloy for self controlled magnetic hyperthermia. *Cryst. Res. Technol.* **2009**, *44*, 386–390. [CrossRef]
118. Zhong, J.; Dieckhoff, J.; Schilling, M.; Ludwig, F. Influence of static magnetic field strength on the temperature resolution of a magnetic nanoparticle thermometer. *J. Appl. Phys.* **2016**, *120*, 143902. [CrossRef]
119. Garaio, E.; Collantes, J.-M.; Garcia, J.A.; Plazaola, F.; Sandre, O. Harmonic phases of the nanoparticle magnetization: An intrinsic temperature probe. *Appl. Phys. Lett.* **2015**, *107*, 123103. [CrossRef]
120. Garaio, E.; Collantes, J.M.; Plazaola, F.; Garcia, J.A.; Castellanos-Rubio, I. A multifrequency eletromagnetic applicator with an integrated AC magnetometer for magnetic hyperthermia experiments. *Meas. Sci. Technol.* **2014**, *25*, 115702. [CrossRef]
121. Connord, V.; Mehdaoui, B.; Tan, R.P.; Carrey, J.; Respaud, M. An air-cooled Litz wire coil for measuring the high frequency hysteresis loops of magnetic samples–a useful setup for magnetic hyperthermia applications. *Rev. Sci. Instrum.* **2014**, *85*, 093904. [CrossRef] [PubMed]
122. Garaio, E.; Sandre, O.; Collantes, J.-M.; Garcia, J.A.; Mornet, S.; Plazaola, F. Specific absorption rate dependence on temperature in magnetic field hyperthermia measured by dynamic hysteresis losses (ac magnetometry). *Nanotechnology* **2015**, *26*, 015704. [CrossRef] [PubMed]
123. Hildebrandt, B.; Wust, P.; Ahlers, O.; Dieing, A.; Sreenivasa, G.; Kerner, T.; Felix, R.; Riess, H. The cellular and molecular basis of hyperthermia. *Crit. Rev. Oncol. Hematol.* **2002**, *43*, 33–56. [CrossRef]
124. Chang, D.; Lim, M.; Goos, J.A.C.M.; Qiao, R.; Ng, Y.Y.; Mansfeld, F.M.; Jackson, M.; Davis, T.P.; Kavallaris, M. Biologically Targeted Magnetic Hyperthermia: Potential and Limitations. *Front. Pharm.* **2018**, *9*. [CrossRef] [PubMed]
125. Chang, L.; Liu, X.L.; Di Fan, D.; Miao, Y.Q.; Zhang, H.; Ma, H.P.; Liu, Q.Y.; Ma, P.; Xue, W.M.; Luo, Y.E.; et al. The efficiency of magnetic hyperthermia and in vivo histocompatibility for human-like collagen protein-coated magnetic nanoparticles. *Int. J. Nanomed.* **2016**, *11*, 1175–1185.
126. Dutz, S.; Hergt, R.; Mürbe, J.; Töpfer, J.; Müller, R.; Zeisberger, M.; Andrä, W.; Bellemann, M.E. Magnetic Nanoparticles for Biomedical Heating Applications. *Z. Phys. Chem.* **2006**, *220*, 145–151. [CrossRef]
127. Long, N.V.; Yang, Y.; Teranishi, T.; Thi, C.; Cao, Y.; Nogami, M. Biomedical Applications of Advanced Multifunctional Magnetic Nanoparticles. *J. Nanosci. Nanotechnol.* **2015**, *15*, 10091–10107. [CrossRef]
128. Kim, D.; Shin, K.; Kwon, S.; Hyeon, T. Synthesis and Biomedical Applications of Multifunctional Nanoparticles. *Adv. Mater.* **2018**, *30*, 1802309. [CrossRef]
129. Abenojar, E.C.; Wickramasinghe, S.; Bas-Concepcion, J.; Samia, A.C.S. Structural effects on the magnetic hyperthermia properties of iron oxide nanoparticles. *Prog. Nat. Sci. Mater. Int.* **2016**, *26*, 440–448. [CrossRef]
130. Chung, C.; Kim, Y.-K.; Shin, D.; Ryoo, S.-R.; Hong, B.H.; Min, D.-H. Biomedical Applications of Graphene and Graphene Oxide. *Acc. Chem. Res.* **2013**, *46*, 2211–2224. [CrossRef]
131. Dembereldorj, U.; Kim, M.; Kim, S.; Ganbold, E.-O.; Lee, S.Y.; Joo, S.-W. A spatiotemporal anticancer drug release platform of PEGylated graphene oxide triggered by glutathione in vitro and in vivo. *J. Mater. Chem.* **2012**, *22*, 23845–23851. [CrossRef]
132. Liu, J.; Cui, L.; Losic, D. Graphene and graphene oxide as new nanocarriers for drug delivery applications. *Acta Biomater.* **2013**, *9*, 9243–9257. [CrossRef] [PubMed]
133. Liu, X.L.; Fan, H.M.; Yi, J.B.; Yang, Y.; Choo, E.S.G.; Xue, J.M.; Fan, D.D.; Ding, J. Optimization of surface coating on Fe3O4 nanoparticles for high performance magnetic hyperthermia agents. *J. Mater. Chem.* **2012**, *22*, 8235–8244. [CrossRef]
134. Venkatesha, N.; Qurishi, Y.; Atreya, H.S.; Srivastava, C. ZnO coated $CoFe_2O_4$ nanoparticles for multimodal bio-imaging. *RSC Adv.* **2016**, *6*, 18843–18851. [CrossRef]

135. Sundar, S.; Chen, Y.; Tong, Y.W. Delivery of therapeutics and molecules using self-assembled peptides. *Curr. Med. Chem.* **2014**, *21*, 2469–2479. [CrossRef]
136. Mazzotta, E.; Tavano, L.; Muzzalupo, R. Thermo-Sensitive Vesicles in Controlled Drug Delivery for Chemotherapy. *Pharmaceutics* **2018**, *10*, 150. [CrossRef]
137. Bi, H.; Xue, J.; Jiang, H.; Gao, S.; Yang, D.; Fang, Y.; Shi, K. Current developments in drug delivery with thermosensitive liposomes. *Asian J. Pharm. Sci.* **2019**, *14*, 365–379. [CrossRef]
138. Yadav, H.K.; Halabi, N.A.A.; Alsalloum, G.A. Nanogels as Novel Drug Delivery Systems—A Review. *J. Pharm. Pharm. Res.* **2017**, *1*, 1–8.
139. Blackburn, W.H.; Dickerson, E.B.; Smith, M.H.; McDonald, J.F.; Lyon, L.A. Peptide-Functionalized Nanogels for Targeted siRNA Delivery. *Bioconjug. Chem.* **2009**, *20*, 960–968. [CrossRef]
140. Cazares-Cortes, E.; Espinosa, A.; Guigner, J.-M.; Michel, A.; Griffete, N.; Wilhelm, C.; Ménager, C. Doxorubicin Intracellular Remote Release from Biocompatible Oligo(ethylene glycol) Methyl Ether Methacrylate-Based Magnetic Nanogels Triggered by Magnetic Hyperthermia. *ACS Appl. Mater. Interfaces* **2017**, *9*, 25775–25788. [CrossRef]
141. Cazares-Cortes, E.; Nerantzaki, M.; Fresnais, J.; Wilhelm, C.; Griffete, N.; Ménager, C. Magnetic Nanoparticles Create Hot Spots in Polymer Matrix for Controlled Drug Release. *Nanomaterials* **2018**, *8*, 850. [CrossRef] [PubMed]
142. Eslami, P.; Rossi, F.; Fedeli, S. Hybrid Nanogels: Stealth and Biocompatible Structures for Drug Delivery Applications. *Pharmaceutics* **2019**, *11*, 71. [CrossRef] [PubMed]
143. Oh, J.K.; Drumright, R.; Siegwart, D.J.; Matyjaszewski, K. The development of microgels/nanogels for drug delivery applications. *Prog. Polym. Sci.* **2008**, *33*, 448–477. [CrossRef]
144. Bharti, C.; Nagaich, U.; Pal, A.K.; Gulati, N. Mesoporous silica nanoparticles in target drug delivery system: A review. *Int. J. Pharm. Investig.* **2015**, *5*, 124–133. [CrossRef]
145. Wang, Y.; Zhao, Q.; Han, N.; Bai, L.; Li, J.; Liu, J.; Che, E.; Hu, L.; Zhang, Q.; Jiang, T.; et al. Mesoporous silica nanoparticles in drug delivery and biomedical applications. *Nanomedicine* **2015**, *11*, 313–327. [CrossRef]
146. Jafari, S.; Derakhshankhah, H.; Alaei, L.; Fattahi, A.; Varnamkhasti, B.S.; Saboury, A.A. Mesoporous silica nanoparticles for therapeutic/diagnostic applications. *Biomed. Pharmacother.* **2019**, *109*, 1100–1111. [CrossRef]
147. Mura, S.; Nicolas, J.; Couvreur, P. Stimuli-responsive nanocarriers for drug delivery. *Nat. Mater.* **2013**, *12*, 991–1003. [CrossRef]
148. Thomas, C.R.; Ferris, D.P.; Lee, J.-H.; Choi, E.; Cho, M.H.; Kim, E.S.; Stoddart, J.F.; Shin, J.-S.; Cheon, J.; Zink, J.I. Noninvasive Remote-Controlled Release of Drug Molecules in Vitro Using Magnetic Actuation of Mechanized Nanoparticles. *J. Am. Chem. Soc.* **2010**, *132*, 10623–10625. [CrossRef]
149. Coll, C.; Mondragón, L.; Martínez-Máñez, R.; Sancenón, F.; Marcos, M.D.; Soto, J.; Amorós, P.; Pérez-Payá, E. Enzyme-mediated controlled release systems by anchoring peptide sequences on mesoporous silica supports. *Angew. Chem. Int. Ed. Engl.* **2011**, *50*, 2138–2140. [CrossRef]
150. Lee, J.; Kim, H.; Kim, S.; Lee, H.; Kim, J.; Kim, N.; Park, H.J.; Choi, E.K.; Lee, J.S.; Kim, C. A multifunctional mesoporous nanocontainer with an iron oxide core and a cyclodextrin gatekeeper for an efficient theranostic platform. *J. Mater. Chem.* **2012**, *22*, 14061–14067. [CrossRef]
151. Guisasola, E.; Asín, L.; Beola, L.; de la Fuente, J.M.; Baeza, A.; Vallet-Regí, M. Beyond Traditional Hyperthermia: In Vivo Cancer Treatment with Magnetic-Responsive Mesoporous Silica Nanocarriers. *ACS Appl. Mater. Interfaces* **2018**, *10*, 12518–12525. [CrossRef] [PubMed]
152. Gandhi, A.; Paul, A.; Sen, S.O.; Sen, K.K. Studies on thermoresponsive polymers: Phase behaviour, drug delivery and biomedical applications. *Asian J. Pharm. Sci.* **2015**, *10*, 99–107. [CrossRef]
153. Cheng, L.; Yang, K.; Li, Y.; Zeng, X.; Shao, M.; Lee, S.-T.; Liu, Z. Multifunctional nanoparticles for upconversion luminescence/MR multimodal imaging and magnetically targeted photothermal therapy. *Biomaterials* **2012**, *33*, 2215–2222. [CrossRef] [PubMed]
154. Park, H.; Yang, J.; Seo, S.; Kim, K.; Suh, J.; Kim, D.; Haam, S.; Yoo, K.-H. Multifunctional nanoparticles for photothermally controlled drug delivery and magnetic resonance imaging enhancement. *Small* **2008**, *4*, 192–196. [CrossRef] [PubMed]
155. Ma, X.; Tao, H.; Yang, K.; Feng, L.; Cheng, L.; Shi, X.; Li, Y.; Guo, L.; Liu, Z. A functionalized graphene oxide-iron oxide nanocomposite for magnetically targeted drug delivery, photothermal therapy, and magnetic resonance imaging. *Nano Res.* **2012**, *5*, 199–212. [CrossRef]

156. Yao, X.; Niu, X.; Ma, K.; Huang, P.; Grothe, J.; Kaskel, S.; Zhu, Y. Graphene Quantum Dots-Capped Magnetic Mesoporous Silica Nanoparticles as a Multifunctional Platform for Controlled Drug Delivery, Magnetic Hyperthermia, and Photothermal Therapy. *Small* **2017**, *13*, 1602225. [CrossRef]
157. Ma, Y.; Liang, X.; Tong, S.; Bao, G.; Ren, Q.; Dai, Z. Gold Nanoshell Nanomicelles for Potential Magnetic Resonance Imaging, Light-Triggered Drug Release, and Photothermal Therapy. *Adv. Funct. Mater.* **2013**, *23*, 815–822. [CrossRef]
158. Fu, S.; Ding, Y.; Cong, T.; Yang, X.; Hong, X.; Yu, B.; Li, Y.; Liu, Y. Multifunctional $NaYF_4$:Yb,Er@PE_3@Fe_3O_4 nanocomposites for magnetic-field-assisted upconversion imaging guided photothermal therapy of cancer cells. *Dalton Trans.* **2019**, *48*, 12850–12857. [CrossRef]
159. Buzug, T.M.; Bringout, G.; Erbe, M.; Gräfe, K.; Graeser, M.; Grüttner, M.; Halkola, A.; Sattel, T.F.; Tenner, W.; Wojtczyk, H.; et al. Magnetic particle imaging: Introduction to imaging and hardware realization. *Z Med. Phys.* **2012**, *22*, 323–334. [CrossRef]
160. Lim, J.-W.; Son, S.U.; Lim, E.-K. *Recent Advances in Bioimaging for Cancer Research. State of the Art Nano-Bioimaging*; Ghamsari, M.S., Ed.; IntechOpen: London, UK, 2018; pp. 11–33.
161. Wu, L.C.; Zhang, Y.; Steinberg, G.; Qu, H.; Huang, S.; Cheng, M.; Bliss, T.; Du, F.; Rao, J.; Song, G.; et al. A Review of Magnetic Particle Imaging and Perspectives on Neuroimaging. *Am. J. Neuroradiol.* **2019**, *40*, 206–212. [CrossRef]
162. Reddy, L.H.; Arias, J.L.; Nicolas, J.; Couvreur, P. Magnetic Nanoparticles: Design and Characterization, Toxicity and Biocompatibility, Pharmaceutical and Biomedical Applications. *Chem. Rev.* **2012**, *112*, 5818–5878. [CrossRef] [PubMed]
163. Tay, Z.W.; Chandrasekharan, P.; Chiu-Lam, A.; Hensley, D.W.; Dhavalikar, R.; Zhou, X.Y.; Yu, E.Y.; Goodwill, P.W.; Zheng, B.; Rinaldi, C.; et al. Magnetic Particle Imaging-Guided Heating in Vivo Using Gradient Fields for Arbitrary Localization of Magnetic Hyperthermia Therapy. *ACS Nano* **2018**, *12*, 3699–3713. [CrossRef] [PubMed]
164. Basly, B.; Popa, G.; Fleutot, S.; Pichon, B.P.; Garofalo, A.; Ghobril, C.; Billotey, C.; Berniard, A.; Bonazza, P.; Martinez, H.; et al. Effect of the nanoparticle synthesis method on dendronized iron oxides as MRI contrast agents. *Dalton Trans.* **2013**, *42*, 2146–2157. [CrossRef] [PubMed]
165. Sun, J.; Zhou, S.; Hou, P.; Yang, Y.; Weng, J.; Li, X.; Li, M. Synthesis and characterization of biocompatible Fe_3O_4 nanoparticles. *J. Biomed. Mater. Res. A* **2007**, *80*, 333–341. [CrossRef]
166. Liu, Z.; Zhang, D.; Han, S.; Li, C.; Lei, B.; Lu, W.; Fang, J.; Zhou, C. Single Crystalline Magnetite Nanotubes. *J. Am. Chem. Soc.* **2005**, *127*, 6–7. [CrossRef]
167. Zhong, Z.; Lin, M.; Ng, V.; Ng, G.X.B.; Foo, Y.; Gedanken, A. A Versatile Wet-Chemical Method for Synthesis of One-Dimensional Ferric and Other Transition Metal Oxides. *Chem. Mater.* **2006**, *18*, 6031–6036. [CrossRef]
168. Jiao, F.; Jumas, J.-C.; Womes, M.; Chadwick, A.V.; Harrison, A.; Bruce, P.G. Synthesis of Ordered Mesoporous Fe_3O_4 and γ-Fe_2O_3 with Crystalline Walls Using Post-Template Reduction/Oxidation. *J. Am. Chem. Soc.* **2006**, *128*, 12905–12909. [CrossRef]
169. Du, N.; Xu, Y.; Zhang, H.; Zhai, C.; Yang, D. Selective Synthesis of Fe_2O_3 and Fe_3O_4 Nanowires Via a Single Precursor: A General Method for Metal Oxide Nanowires. *Nanoscale Res. Lett.* **2010**, *5*, 1295–1300. [CrossRef]
170. Wang, G.; Wang, C.; Dou, W.; Ma, Q.; Yuan, P.; Su, X. The synthesis of magnetic and fluorescent bi-functional silica composite nanoparticles via reverse microemulsion method. *J. Fluoresc.* **2009**, *19*, 939–946. [CrossRef]
171. Jin, J.; Ohkoshi, S.; Hashimoto, K. Giant Coercive Field of Nanometer- Sized Iron Oxide. *Adv. Mater.* **2004**, *16*, 48–51. [CrossRef]
172. Han, Y.C.; Cha, H.G.; Kim, C.W.; Kim, Y.H.; Kang, Y.S. Synthesis of Highly Magnetized Iron Nanoparticles by a Solventless Thermal Decomposition Method. *J. Phys. Chem. C* **2007**, *111*, 6275–6280. [CrossRef]
173. Sun, S.; Zeng, H. Size-controlled synthesis of magnetite nanoparticles. *J. Am. Chem. Soc.* **2002**, *124*, 8204–8205. [CrossRef] [PubMed]
174. Ai, L.; Zhang, C.; Chen, Z. Removal of methylene blue from aqueous solution by a solvothermal-synthesized graphene/magnetite composite. *J. Hazard. Mater.* **2011**, *192*, 1515–1524. [CrossRef] [PubMed]
175. Kang, M. Synthesis of Fe/TiO_2 photocatalyst with nanometer size by solvothermal method and the effect of H2O addition on structural stability and photodecomposition of methanol. *J. Mol. Catal. A Chem.* **2003**, *197*, 173–183. [CrossRef]
176. Park, J.; An, K.; Hwang, Y.; Park, J.-G.; Noh, H.-J.; Kim, J.-Y.; Park, J.-H.; Hwang, N.-M.; Hyeon, T. Ultra-large-scale syntheses of monodisperse nanocrystals. *Nat. Mater.* **2004**, *3*, 891–895. [CrossRef]

177. Teja, A.; Koh, P.Y. Synthesis, properties, and applications of magnetic iron oxide nanoparticles. *Prog. Cryst. Growth Charact. Mater.* **2009**, *55*, 22–45. [CrossRef]
178. Guo, Q.; Teng, X.; Rahman, S.; Yang, H. Patterned Langmuir–Blodgett Films of Monodisperse Nanoparticles of Iron Oxide Using Soft Lithography. *J. Am. Chem. Soc.* **2003**, *125*, 630–631. [CrossRef]
179. Taniguchi, I. Powder properties of partially substituted $LiM_xMn_{2-x}O_4$ (M=Al, Cr, Fe and Co) synthesized by ultrasonic spray pyrolysis. *Mater. Chem. Phys.* **2005**, *92*, 172–179. [CrossRef]
180. Dosev, D.; Nichkova, M.; Dumas, R.K.; Gee, S.J.; Hammock, B.D.; Liu, K.; Kennedy, I.M. Magnetic/luminescent core/shell particles synthesized by spray pyrolysis and their application in immunoassays with internal standard. *Nanotechnology* **2007**, *18*, 055102. [CrossRef]
181. Polshettiwar, V.; Baruwati, B.; Varma, R.S. Self-Assembly of Metal Oxides into Three-Dimensional Nanostructures: Synthesis and Application in Catalysis. *ACS Nano* **2009**, *3*, 728–736. [CrossRef]
182. Jia, C.-J.; Sun, L.-D.; Luo, F.; Han, X.-D.; Heyderman, L.J.; Yan, Z.-G.; Yan, C.-H.; Zheng, K.; Zhang, Z.; Takano, M.; et al. Large-Scale Synthesis of Single-Crystalline Iron Oxide Magnetic Nanorings. *J. Am. Chem. Soc.* **2008**, *130*, 16968–16977. [CrossRef] [PubMed]
183. Li, Z.; Wei, L.; Gao, M.Y.; Lei, H. One-Pot Reaction to Synthesize Biocompatible Magnetite Nanoparticles. *Adv. Mater.* **2005**, *17*, 1001–1005. [CrossRef]
184. Jana, N.R.; Chen, Y.; Peng, X. Size- and Shape-Controlled Magnetic (Cr, Mn, Fe, Co, Ni) Oxide Nanocrystals via a Simple and General Approach. *Chem. Mater.* **2004**, *16*, 3931–3935. [CrossRef]
185. Rockenberger, J.; Scher, E.C.; Alivisatos, A.P. A New Nonhydrolytic Single-Precursor Approach to Surfactant-Capped Nanocrystals of Transition Metal Oxides. *J. Am. Chem. Soc.* **1999**, *121*, 11595–11596. [CrossRef]
186. Zeng, H.; Li, J.; Liu, J.P.; Wang, Z.L.; Sun, S. Exchange-coupled nanocomposite magnets by nanoparticle self-assembly. *Nature* **2002**, *420*, 395–398. [CrossRef]
187. Salazar-Alvarez, G.; Qin, J.; Šepelák, V.; Bergmann, I.; Vasilakaki, M.; Trohidou, K.N.; Ardisson, J.D.; Macedo, W.A.A.; Mikhaylova, M.; Muhammed, M.; et al. Cubic versus Spherical Magnetic Nanoparticles: The Role of Surface Anisotropy. *J. Am. Chem. Soc.* **2008**, *130*, 13234–13239. [CrossRef]
188. Hayashi, H.; Hakuta, Y. Hydrothermal Synthesis of Metal Oxide Nanoparticles in Supercritical Water. *Materials* **2010**, *3*, 3794–3817. [CrossRef]
189. Yu, J.; Yu, X. Hydrothermal Synthesis and Photocatalytic Activity of Zinc Oxide Hollow Spheres. *Environ. Sci. Technol.* **2008**, *42*, 4902–4907. [CrossRef]
190. Yang, T.; Li, Y.; Zhu, M.; Huang, J.; Jin, H.; Hu, Y. Room-temperature ferromagnetic Mn-doped ZnO nanocrystal synthesized by hydrothermal method under high magnetic field. *Mater. Sci. Eng. B-Adv. Funct. Solid-State Mater.* **2010**, *170*, 129–132. [CrossRef]
191. Hu, J.; Bando, Y. Growth and Optical Properties of Single-Crystal Tubular ZnO Whiskers. *Appl. Phys. Lett.* **2003**, *82*, 1401–1403. [CrossRef]
192. Wang, X.; Zhuang, J.; Peng, Q.; Li, Y. A general strategy for nanocrystal synthesis. *Nature* **2005**, *437*, 121–124. [CrossRef] [PubMed]
193. Sun, S.; Zeng, H.; Robinson, D.B.; Raoux, S.; Rice, P.M.; Wang, S.X.; Li, G. Monodisperse MFe_2O_4 (M = Fe, Co, Mn) Nanoparticles. *J. Am. Chem. Soc.* **2004**, *126*, 273–279. [CrossRef] [PubMed]
194. Wu, W.; Hao, R.; Liu, F.; Su, X.; Hou, Y. Single-crystalline α-Fe_2O_3 nanostructures: Controlled synthesis and high-index plane-enhanced photodegradation by visible light. *J. Mater. Chem. A* **2013**, *1*, 6888–6894. [CrossRef]
195. Zeng, Y.; Hao, R.; Xing, B.; Hou, Y.; Xu, Z. One-pot synthesis of Fe_3O_4 nanoprisms with controlled electrochemical properties. *Chem. Commun.* **2010**, *46*, 3920–3922. [CrossRef] [PubMed]
196. Weiwei, W. Microwave-induced polyol-process synthesis of $M^{II}Fe_2O_4$ (M = Mn, Co) nanoparticles and magnetic property. *Mater. Chem. Phys.* **2008**, *108*, 227–231.
197. Wang, W.-W.; Zhu, Y.-J.; Ruan, M.-L. Microwave-assisted synthesis and magnetic property of magnetite and hematite nanoparticles. *J. Nanopart. Res.* **2007**, *9*, 419–426. [CrossRef]
198. Sander, D.; Oka, H.; Corbetta, M.; Stepanyuk, V.; Kirschner, J. New insights into nano-magnetism by spin-polarized scanning tunneling microscopy. *J. Electron. Spectrosc. Relat. Phenom.* **2013**, *189*, 206–215. [CrossRef]
199. Hurst, S.J.; Payne, E.K.; Qin, L.; Mirkin, C.A. Multisegmented one-dimensional nanorods prepared by hard-template synthetic methods. *Angew. Chem. Int. Ed. Engl.* **2006**, *45*, 2672–2692. [CrossRef]

200. Lam, T.; Pouliot, P.; Avti, P.K.; Lesage, F.; Kakkar, A.K. Superparamagnetic iron oxide based nanoprobes for imaging and theranostics. *Adv. Colloid Interface Sci.* **2013**, *199–200*, 95–113. [CrossRef]
201. Cui, H.; Liu, Y.; Ren, W. Structure switch between alpha-Fe_2O_3, gamma-Fe_2O_3 and Fe_3O_4 during the large scale and low temperature sol-gel synthesis of nearly monodispersed iron oxide nanoparticles. *Adv. Powder Technol.* **2013**, *24*, 93–97. [CrossRef]
202. Xu, J.; Yang, H.; Fu, W.; Du, K.; Sui, Y.; Chen, J.; Yi, Z.; Li, M.; Zou, G. Preparation and Magnetic Properties of Magnetite Nanoparticles by Sol–Gel Method. *J. Magn. Magn. Mater.* **2010**, *309*, 307–311. [CrossRef]
203. Bilecka, I.; Elser, P.; Niederberger, M. Kinetic and Thermodynamic Aspects in the Microwave-Assisted Synthesis of ZnO Nanoparticles in Benzyl Alcohol. *ACS Nano* **2009**, *3*, 467–477. [CrossRef] [PubMed]
204. Bilecka, I.; Kubli, M.; Amstad, E.; Niederberger, M. Simultaneous formation of ferrite nanocrystals and deposition of thin films via a microwave-assisted nonaqueous sol–gel process. *J. Sol. Gel Sci. Technol.* **2011**, *57*, 313–322. [CrossRef]
205. Marcano, D.C.; Kosynkin, D.V.; Berlin, J.M.; Sinitskii, A.; Sun, Z.; Slesarev, A.; Alemany, L.B.; Lu, W.; Tour, J.M. Improved Synthesis of Graphene Oxide. *ACS Nano* **2010**, *4*, 4806–4814. [CrossRef]
206. Venkatesha, N.; Poojar, P.; Qurishi, Y.; Geethanath, S.; Srivastava, C. Graphene oxide-Fe_3O_4 nanoparticle composite with high transverse proton relaxivity value for magnetic resonance imaging. *J. Appl. Phys.* **2015**, *117*, 154702. [CrossRef]
207. Kumar, V.; Sharma, N.; Maitra, S.S. In vitro and in vivo toxicity assessment of nanoparticles. *Int. Nano Lett.* **2017**, *7*, 243–256. [CrossRef]
208. Khalili Fard, J.; Jafari, S.; Eghbal, M.A. A Review of Molecular Mechanisms Involved in Toxicity of Nanoparticles. *Adv. Pharm. Bull.* **2015**, *5*, 447–454. [CrossRef]
209. Demirer, G.S.; Okur, A.C.; Kizilel, S. Synthesis and design of biologically inspired biocompatible iron oxide nanoparticles for biomedical applications. *J. Mater. Chem. B* **2015**, *3*, 7831–7849. [CrossRef]
210. Zahraei, M.; Marciello, M.; Lazaro-Carrillo, A.; Villanueva, A.; Herranz, F.; Talelli, M.; Costo, R.; Monshi, A.; Shahbazi-Gahrouei, D.; Amirnasr, M.; et al. Versatile theranostics agents designed by coating ferrite nanoparticles with biocompatible polymers. *Nanotechnology* **2016**, *27*, 255702. [CrossRef]
211. Aslantürk, Ö.S. In Vitro Cytotoxicity and Cell Viability Assays: Principles, Advantages, and Disadvantages. In *Genotoxicity A Predictable Risk to Our Actual World*; Larramendy, M., Ed.; IntechOpen: London, UK, 2018; pp. 1–17.
212. Pasukonienė, V.; Mlynska, A.; Steponkienė, S.; Poderys, V.; Matulionytė, M.; Karabanovas, V.; Statkutė, U.; Purvinienė, R.; Kraśko, J.A.; Jagminas, A.; et al. Accumulation and biological effects of cobalt ferrite nanoparticles in human pancreatic and ovarian cancer cells. *Medicina* **2014**, *50*, 237–244. [CrossRef]

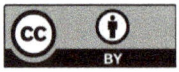

© 2019 by the authors. Licensee MDPI, Basel, Switzerland. This article is an open access article distributed under the terms and conditions of the Creative Commons Attribution (CC BY) license (http://creativecommons.org/licenses/by/4.0/).

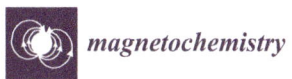

Review

Implication of Magnetic Nanoparticles in Cancer Detection, Screening and Treatment

Oana Hosu [†], Mihaela Tertis [†] and Cecilia Cristea *

Department of Analytical Chemistry, Faculty of Pharmacy, Iuliu Hațieganu University of Medicine and Pharmacy, 4 Pasteur Street, 400349 Cluj-Napoca, Romania; hosuoanaalexandra@gmail.com (O.H.); mihaela.tertis@umfcluj.ro (M.T.)
* Correspondence: ccristea@umfcluj.ro; Tel.: +40-721-375789
† These authors contributed equally to this work.

Received: 30 August 2019; Accepted: 27 September 2019; Published: 1 October 2019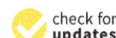

Abstract: During the last few decades, magnetic nanoparticles have been evaluated as promising materials in the field of cancer detection, screening, and treatment. Early diagnosis and screening of cancer may be achieved using magnetic nanoparticles either within the magnetic resonance imaging technique and/or sensing systems. These sensors are designed to selectively detect specific biomarkers, compounds that can be related to the onset or evolution of cancer, during and after the treatment of this widespread disease. Some of the particular properties of magnetic nanoparticles are extensively exploited in cancer therapy as drug delivery agents to selectively target the envisaged location by tailored in vivo manipulation using an external magnetic field. Furthermore, individualized treatment with antineoplastic drugs may be combined with magnetic resonance imaging to achieve an efficient therapy. This review summarizes the studies about the implications of magnetic nanoparticles in cancer diagnosis, treatment and drug delivery as well as prospects for future development and challenges of magnetic nanoparticles in the field of oncology.

Keywords: magnetic nanoparticles (MNPs); cancer biomarkers; MNPs synthesis; MNPs functionalization; sensors; cancer detection; cancer treatment; cancer screening; magnetic/targeted drug delivery

---

1. Introduction

Material science has gained particular attention in the scientific field since the discovery of nanomaterials. In fact, nanotechnology emerged in this field of research as dealing with the fabrication of materials and technologies at length scales between 1 and 100 nm and integrating these nanoscale materials as building blocks of novel structures and devices. Furthermore, nanotechnology can offer benefits to medical applications like early diagnosis and monitoring, and due to the enhanced biocompatibility of new materials can give access to imaging and therapeutic purposes, playing an important role in disease treatment and targeted drug delivery [1].

One of the possible applications could be imagined for cancer prevention, diagnosis, and treatment where new nanomaterials could have a tremendous impact. Cancer, as defined by the World Health Organization (WHO) "is a generic term for a large group of diseases characterized by the growth of abnormal cells beyond their usual boundaries that can then invade adjoining parts of the body and/or spread to other organs" [2]. The WHO statistics show that cancer is the second leading cause of worldwide deaths and a prognostic of 29.5 million deaths was estimated by 2040. Several types of cancer are commonly found in both men and women such as lung and colorectal cancer. Stomach, liver and prostate cancers are the most common among men, while women are more likely to develop thyroid, breast, or cervical cancers.

In order to prevent metastasis, early stage cancer diagnosis is of high interest and challenging as symptoms appear only in advanced cancer stages. For this, highly accurate, fast, robust and non-invasive or minimal invasive procedures are of great importance.

In this regard, nanomaterials have already showed their medical usefulness in imaging technology applied for tumor target and visualization, allowing for early diagnosis of cancer. Another biomedicine application of nanomaterials is targeted drug delivery, where intelligent nanocarriers could improve the therapy efficacy by tailored transport of anticancer drugs to a well-established place where their release takes place without harming healthy cells.

Magnetic nanoparticles (MNPs) have recently contributed to important development in oncology presenting major implications in cancer diagnosis, cancer screening, targeted drug delivery and cancer treatment. MNPs are widely applied in tumor targeting since tumor imaging technology opened the possibility for early detection of this wide-spread disease. Due to their magnetism in particular, MNPs (especially superparamagnetic iron oxide nanoparticles, so called SPIONs) have been mostly used as contrast agents in cancer screening for magnetic resonance imaging (MRI), in magneto-acoustic tomography (MAT), computed tomography (CT) and near-infrared (NIR) imaging. Moreover, drug delivery is also a hard to ignore application where the use of MNPs as drug agents (carriers) for in vivo targeted specific location can be performed by applying an external magnetic field (EMF). The specificity of MNPs is generally obtained by their functionalization with antibodies for target cells together with chemotherapeutic drugs. MNPs can be also applied in cancer treatment through magnetically induced hyperthermia (MHT), photodynamic therapy (PDT) and photothermal therapy (PTT). All these individual strategies are used in oncology, but the best therapeutic effect is usually assured by combining them since the modular design enables MNPs to perform multiple functions simultaneously. For example, MRI (Figure 1A) could be applied for early diagnosis of cancer, thus the individualized treatment (chemotherapy) may be combined with MRI, in order to achieve better and faster results [3–6].

The synthesis protocol influences the final properties of MNPs. The most important properties of MNPs that can be exploited for medical applications are superparamagnetism, high magnetic moment, magnetocaloric effect, small particle size and large specific surface area that can be easily functionalized [7–12]. The magnetic properties are related to the core of the MNPs; therefore, the superparamagnetism effect depends on the nanoparticle size and is generally observed for the MNPs with the size dimension up to 100 nm. These particles are magnetized when an EMF is applied and lose their magnetization in the absence of the field, therefore, preventing the MNPs clustering [8,9]. Magnetocaloric effect is an important property of some MNPs that are able switch their temperature depending on the existence of the EMF [11]. This feature combined with a large surface-to-volume ratio allows the efficient heat exchange with the environment, making possible the latest cancer therapy strategy, namely hyperthermia [8].

The special properties of MNPs are fully exploited in cell labeling and targeted drug delivery systems (Figure 1B), wherein the in vivo transportation of the drugs to the specific target is performed using a magnetic field positioned properly and outside the body [4,5]. MNPs may be considered a kind of intelligent magnetic material since they absorb the heat generated by the electromagnetic wave in the alternating magnetic field [3]. As already mentioned, a great advantage of MNPs is their small size, which is less or comparable to biological entities ranging from several nanometers in the case of genes and proteins, to hundreds of nanometers (viruses) up to 100 µm (cells). Such small dimensions allow for their good diffusion and distribution in tissues exactly or in the vicinity of the targeted sites [6]. Moreover, various processes to improve the magnetic properties of MNPs as well as to predict their in vivo behavior could be adjusted by modulating parameters such as size, composition, morphology or surface functionalization [5]. The most commonly used MNPs, iron oxide nanoparticles and in particular magnetite (Fe_3O_4) and its oxidized form maghemite (γ-Fe_2O_3) have attracted attention mainly due to their biocompatibility, low toxicity and cost, facile preparation, as well as their specific optical and magnetic properties that can be exploited in microsystems and medical devices' fabrication [3–5].

Furthermore, MNPs applications in the field of cancer biomedicine are related to their use in MRI as contrast agents and in cancer thermotherapy, or so called hyperthermia [13], as heating mediators (Figure 1C). Additionally, novel applications of MNPs as platforms of immobilization of antibodies or aptamers for biosensors development have been proposed [14]. Affinity ligands (aptamers, hEGF, folic acid, lectin) can be immobilized at the MNPs surface to orderly direct them in the vicinity of tumors, thus enabling the MNPs to accumulate in a specific location of cells or tissues (Figure 1F) [15]. Significant progress in gene delivery and therapy has been made when a viral vector carrying a gene attached to the MNPs surface was performed. By this, rectification of genetic disorders can be enabled by gene transfection and expression with the complementary gene carried by the virus-attached MNPs [16]. This procedure is called magnetic transfection or magnetofection gene therapy and has aimed to cure lung, gastrointestinal and blood malignancies; future adaptation to non-viral transfection of biomolecules (e.g. DNA, siRNA) is yet to be envisaged.

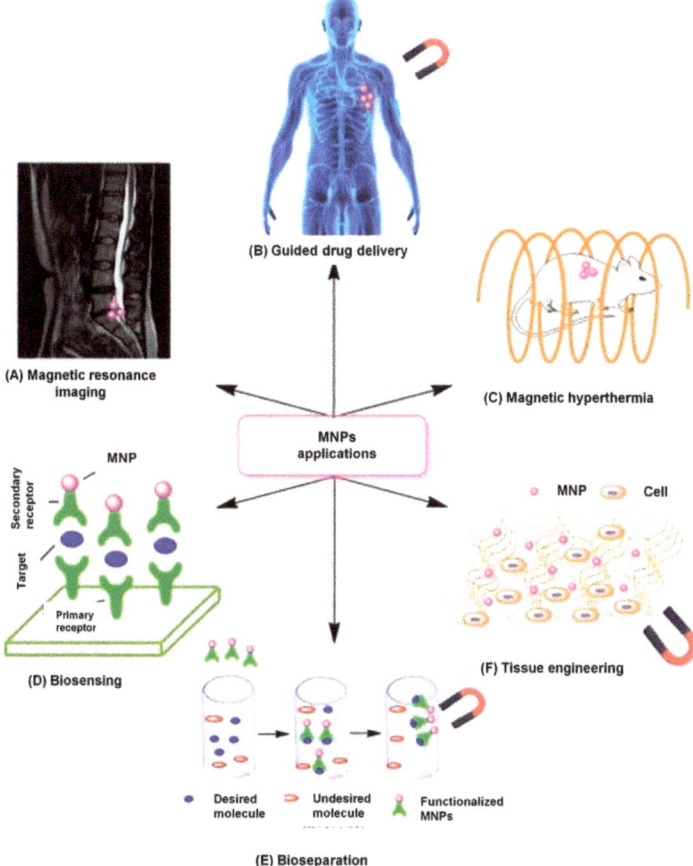

Figure 1. Schematic representation of possible applications of MNPs in biomedicine: (**A**) magnetic resonance imaging, (**B**) guided/targeted drug delivery, (**C**) magnetic hyperthermia, (**D**) biosensing, (**E**) bioseparation, and (**F**) tissue engineering. Reproduced with permission from Elsevier [17].

Therefore, these strategies combined with targeted drug delivery and magnetic hyperthermia enables a synergetic effect in the efficient treatment of cancer.

MNPs could also be used for the early detection and diagnosis of cancer being building blocks of electrochemical immunoassays.

The multi-functional properties of MNPs have made them the ideal material for several applications in cancer detection, screening and treatment for: MRI, hyperthermia, drug carriers, tissue repairs, immunoassay and biosensors.

There are several reviews and book chapters describing the advances and applications of MNPs [17–25]; this paper aims to summarize and underline the latest findings in the field focusing on synthesis, functionalization and application of MNPs in cancer biomedicine. Cancer detection, screening and treatment within the MNPs use is presented starting with biosensing technologies, followed by the visualization of tumors within imaging techniques and the treatment of tumors through targeted delivery approaches, and lastly by hyperthermia and photodynamic therapy. Some of these applications will be detailed in the next subchapters. Finally, future perspectives and challenges yet to be solved will be presented.

2. Synthesis and Characterization of Magnetic Nanoparticles

Several ways to synthesize MNPs were proposed by researchers; many of them offer special features like shape control, monodispersity and stability and preparation on a large scale like sol-gel procedure, hydrothermal synthesis or co-precipitation. New and innovative methods were addressed: sonolysis and biosynthesis, thermal decomposition, and microemulsion [26]. Choosing the best synthesis method depends mainly on the nature of MNPs one wishes to obtain. Depending on their composition, MNPs could be classified in:

- iron oxide nanoparticles or oxides (ferrites): hematite (α-Fe_2O_3), maghemite (γ-Fe_2O_3) and magnetite (Fe_3O_4); their involvement in biomedical application is based on their easy surface modification with various compounds for increased stability in aqueous media (e.g. surfactants, silica) [27];
- metallic nanoparticles with only a metallic core: more suitable for biomedical applications due to their higher magnetic moment compared to oxides; reported drawbacks are pyrophoric property, and presence of high reactivity to oxidizing agents;
- shell-based ferrites: chemically inert MNPs core covered by a silica shell for further functionalization through covalent bonding;
- shell-based metallic nanoparticles: metallic core covered by a shell made of polymers, precious metals or modified surfactants [27].

Table 1 describes several methods for the synthesis of MNPs [25].

Table 1. Different methods for MNPs preparation.

Methods	Details	Ref.
Co-precipitation	—the most facile and efficient method for MNPs synthesis; —iron oxides nanoparticles obtained from Fe^{2+}/Fe^{3+} salts aqueous solutions; —several parameters need to be well established like pH, Fe^{2+}/Fe^{3+} ratio, temperature, nature of the solvent, etc;	[27]
Thermal and Hydrothermal Decomposition	—synthesis in aqueous media at high pressure and high temperature; —improves the nucleation rate and speed up the growth of the new particles; —hydrolysis and oxidation reaction are the most commonly used; —another route is neutralization of hybrid metal hydroxides; —advantage: generates particles of small diameter size;	[28]

Table 1. Cont.

Methods	Details	Ref.
Sol-Gel Processes	—hydroxylation and condensation reactions generate a sol of nanoparticles; —condensation reaction of sol generates a three-dimensional network gel of metal oxide; —crystallization form of the gel can be obtained by temperature-controlled treatment; —several parameters need to be well established like pH, concentration of salts precursors and ratio, temperature, nature of the solvent, etc; —surfactants addition influences the synthesis of the 3D gel structure; —major drawback: coagulation of the gels may occur;	[26]
Microemulsion and Inverse Micelles	—specific synthesis of MFe_2O_4-type MNPs, where M could be Mn, Co, Ni, Cu, Zn, Mg, or Cd, etc., important magnetic materials for electronic applications; —the size and shape of the MFe_2O_4 can be easily tailored depending on the parameters applied; —major drawbacks: harsh experimental conditions (narrow working window, high solvent consumption), low yield of nanoparticles;	[29]
Biosynthesis	—environment friendly method which generates biocompatible MNPs; —biosynthesis of MNPs can be performed using reducing agents such as plant phytochemicals, microbial enzymes, bacteria and magnetotactic bacteria; —major drawbacks: the mechanism of biological synthesis has not been yet clearly elucidated; parameters cannot be modulated for shape- and size-controlled synthesis of the nanoparticles;	[30]
Sonolysis	—high intensity ultrasound-based method; —oscillating cavities of different size can be achieved by the commutative expansive and compressive acoustic waves; —when the oscillating cavities grow to a certain size, the ultrasonic energy can be accumulated by them; —advantage: mild experimental conditions (pressure, temperature or reaction time);	[31]
Spray/laser Pyrolysis	—nucleation of the particles occurs through condensation after spraying an iron salt solution into a hot air or a laser beam; —temperature assisted decomposition of the formed particles is usually followed; —advantage: effective production of small particle size (5–60 nm); —major drawbacks: sophisticated and expensive equipment, oxygen or other gaseous interferences;	[32]

New methods of producing MNPs which try to overcome the drawbacks of the established ones are periodically reported; however, for mass production of highly controlled features, MNPs, co-precipitation and thermal/hydrothermal decomposition remain the most secure and easy to use methods.

3. Functionalization and Stabilization of Magnetic Nanoparticles

Due to the fact that biomedical applications usually need special requirements to control the MNPs' interfaces, the functionalization of MNPs surfaces is a way of tailoring their properties. Functionalization is a useful process for enhancing the colloidal stability in complex biological environments which affect the molecular recognition. Stabilizers that prevent aggregation are generally surfactants (sodium oleate, sodium carboxymethylcellulose) or either synthetic polymers like poly(ethylene-covinyl acetate), poly(lactic-co-glycolic acid), poly(vinylpyrrolidone), polyethylene-imine, or natural ones like chitosan, gelatin, and dextran [27].

To enhance the stabilization in non-aqueous solvents, MNPs are usually covered by a hydrocarbon layer. By contrast, biomedical applications require MNPs with hydrophilic and biocompatible properties [33]. Ligand addition, ligand exchange and hydrophilic silica coating are the three most important methods for surface functionalization; organic and inorganic coatings will increase the stabilization and the resistance towards oxidation in the water or humid air [28].

For example, the process of binding different molecules at MNPs' surfaces could be easily explained by the presence of hydroxyl groups of nanoparticles obtained by co-precipitation [34] which can be negatively or positively charged depending on the pH of the media. Although, non-peptizable particles can be synthesized at pH 7.5 when OH– ligands are free of charge, ligands still remain attached to the MNPs when the pH is kept in the range 6–10. Therefore, biomolecules can be further attached to the free hydroxyl groups at the surface of the particles. A possible biomedical application of these hydrophilic particles is represented by targeted drug delivery.

Different modifications that could be performed at MNPs surface were already revised in several papers [18,35,36] and schematically represented in Figure 2a. Furthermore, a summary of types, shapes and functionalities that have been explored for MNPs in order to be used as carriers for drug delivery in cancer therapy, together with illustrations of biophysicochemical properties, is presented in Figure 2b.

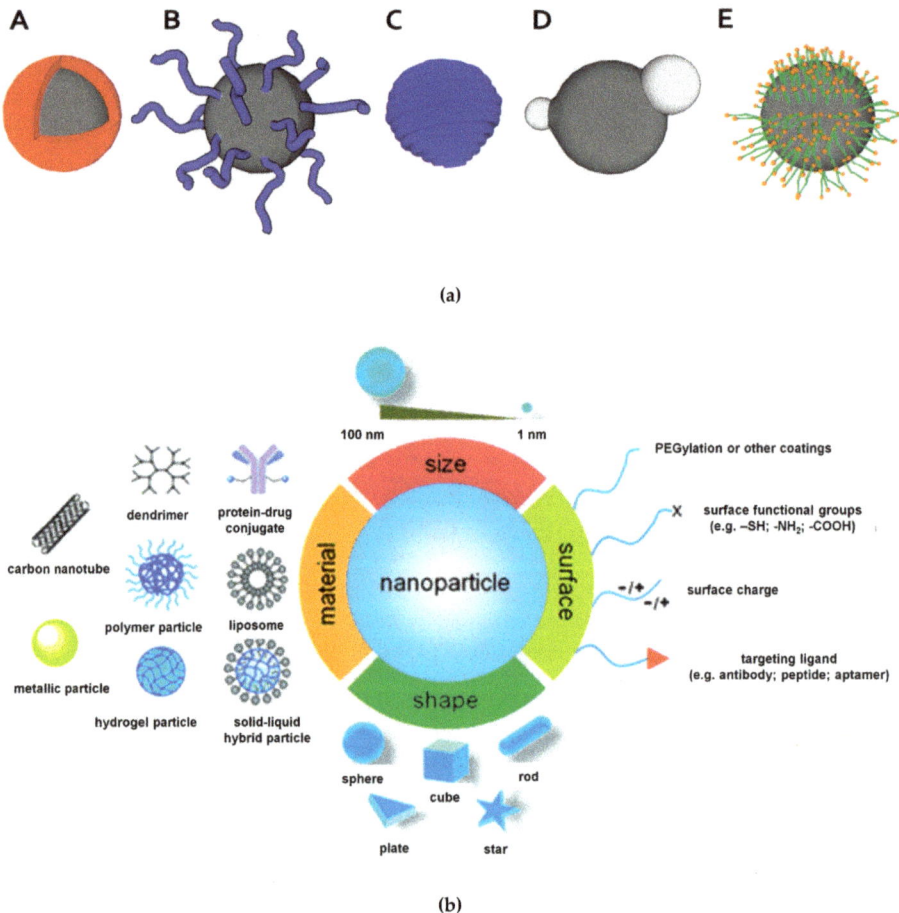

Figure 2. (a) Different types of modification of magnetic nanoparticles (MNPs): (A) MNPs type core-shell; (B) MNPs modified with polymers; (C) MNPs entrapped in polymeric films; (D) heterodimer MNPs; (E) MNPs modified with lipids mono- and bi-layers. Reproduced with permission from MDPI (open access) [35]; (b) A summary of nanoparticles that have been explored as carriers for drug delivery in cancer therapy, together with illustrations of biophysicochemical properties. Reproduced with permission from Wiley Online Library [37].

The surface modification is extremely important when MNPs are used as drug carriers due to their low drug-loading capacity and fast clearance from blood fluids. There are three approaches to overcome these drawbacks. The first approach is based on conjugation of MNPs with drugs followed by surface modification with various polymers. The next two approaches use the modification of

MNPs with a pro-drug–polymer composite or either the adsorption of the drugs on the MNPs modified with polymers.

Polyethylene glycol (PEG), a frequently used polymer, is an interesting material since it owns two end-hydroxyl functional groups available for different reactions. PEG has also been used for drug conjugation, enhancing the drug solubility and bioavailability. PEG-MNPs were investigated as highly biocompatible drug carriers for antitumor medicines as curcumin [38] and doxorubicine (DOX) [34]. MNPs modified with dextrane was able to efficiently entrap indomethacine, an antiinflamatory drug, as reported by C. Jin et al. [39].

The magnetic properties of MNPs based on magnetite may decrease when subjected to acidic pH (<4) due to the fact that Fe^{2+} is easily oxidized to Fe^{3+}. To answer this, coating protocols with inert oxides (e.g. silica, alumina) have been applied for enhanced magnetism stability [40]. The use of silica (SiO_2) as protecting material for Fe_3O_4 is justified by its special properties namely chemical and magnetic stability and suitability for surface functionalization. Moreover, besides preventing degradation of MNPs, silanol groups (-SiOH) can be used as anchoring sites for further modification. Applications of silica-based MNPs are mainly reported as drug carriers, and in the field of electronics, paints, or catalysis etc.

Besides silica, decoration of MNPs with noble metals (gold or silver) enables new properties such as optical properties and enhanced bioaffinity, biocompatibility, chemical and physical properties, without affecting the magnetic features of the core. Thus, gold nanoparticles (AuNPs) are widely used for surface coverage of Fe_3O_4; several papers report the application of AuNPs@Fe_3O_4 in electrochemical (bio)sensing, separation of biological structures, targeted delivery of drugs and bioimaging [7].

4. Applications of Magnetic Nanoparticles in Cancer Biomedicine

4.1. Cancer Biomarker Detection Using Magnetic Nanoparticles

4.1.1. Biomolecules Conjugation

In the field of cancer biosensing based on MNPs, one important step in the biosensors' development is represented by the immobilization of specific biological elements at the functionalized MNPs. Cancer biomarkers are molecules or structures involved in disease development and evolution that can offer a prognostic concerning cancer prevalence and outcome [41]. Therefore, the detection of these molecules, which can range from small elements (peptides, aptamers, DNA) to high-weighted proteins, is of crucial importance [42].

The functionalized MNPs' surface offers linker groups to allow the binding event with the complementary biomolecules. Different bioconjugation strategies include physical interactions (e.g., electrostatic interaction, hydrophilic-hydrophobic, affinity interactions) and chemical interactions (e.g., covalent bonds) for easy immobilization on MNPs or transducers [43]. Some specific interactions between protein and their recognition elements, like biotin-avidin and antigen-antibody linking systems, have proven their utility in the design of biosensors [20].

4.1.2. Bioseparation

MNPs play a significant role in bioanalysis as biological separation represents a cost-effective and fast alternative to traditional separation methods (centrifugation and filtration) [18]. Therefore, functionalized MNPs interact with the complementary target from the pristine mixture and upon conjugation the as-formed composites can be manipulated by applying an EMF, allowing for efficient bioseparation (Figure 1E). Various types of biomolecules and cells were separated and purified using this technique as bacteria, viruses, tumor cells, T cells, monocytes [17,18].

4.1.3. Biosensing

The as-conjugated MNPs with the specific biomarkers are further used in the final step: the sensing approach. In the last decades, cancer biomarkers detection has gained significant attention and development.

Various promising sensing methods to detect the level of cancer biomarkers in plasma, blood or diseased tissues have been developed: electrophoresis, optical methods (fluorescence, electrochemiluminescence, colorimetric assay, surface plasmon resonance (SPR), surface-enhanced Raman spectroscopy (SERS), etc), immunological methods (enzyme-linked immunosorbent assay (ELISA), polymerase chain reaction (PCR), etc), microcantilevers, electrochemical assay, and others [44,45]. Biosensing events may be outlined through different labelling approaches, depending on the method (fluorescent labels, electroactive molecules, enzymes, and nano-/micro-particles, etc). Two major strategies of the integration of MNPs in the design of biosensing systems are represented by direct labelling and indirect labelling.

In the first approach, direct labelling, MNPs could be immobilized at the transducing element by affinity recognition reactions between complementary DNA sequences or streptavidin-biotin. For example, the sensor surface is modified with the magnetic particles functionalized with single-stranded DNA as capture probe, the hybridization reaction will occur as the complementary oligonucleotides are put in contact with the sensor and a physical or/and chemical response will be generated.

In the second approach, indirect labelling, the principle resembles ELISA, namely sandwich immunoassays. For example, primary antibodies complementary to the target protein are immobilized at the sensing surface followed by the affinity reaction with the solution containing the biomarker. Next, the secondary biotin-labelled antibodies are introduced into the system to enable the affinity reaction when the streptavidin-labelled MNPs solution is put in contact with the sensor surface [18]. For a more comprehensive description, we categorize the sensing approaches for cancer detection according to the detection principle as follows: electrochemical, optical, and magnetic. Inside each subsection, different detection strategies are detailed if available.

In the last decades, electrochemical biosensors have gained much attention for cancer biomarkers detection mainly due to their high accuracy and sensitivity, multiplexing and cost-effective features, and selectivity in challenging the matrix without requiring multiple sample treatments or complex protocols [46]. Currently, a wide range of analytical techniques has been integrated for the development of multiplexed immunosensing systems for cancer biomarkers. Electrochemical immunosensors have received great interest due to their high sensitivity provided by coupling the immunochemical affinity reaction (antigen-antibody) with the particular features of multifunctional electrode transduction elements [41,47].

An example of a MNPs-based sandwich immunoassay for the electrochemical determination of cancer antigen 153 (CA153) is detailed [48]. The sensing system uses disposable screen-printed carbon-based electrodes functionalized with graphene oxide (GO) and peroxidase-like magnetic silica nanoparticles/GO composites acting as labels. Firstly, the silica MNPs were functionalized with azide groups to enable the acetylene-functionalized GO via click chemistry for labelling purposes, then a monoclonal anti-CA153 antibody was immobilized at the GO-modified screen-printed carbon electrodes. The immunoassay exhibited a broad linear range (10^{-3} - 200 U/mL) for the determination of the cancer antigen and a limit of detection (LOD) of 2.8×10^{-4} U/mL. Another example involves the use of AuNPs-modified porous paper acting as a working electrode (Au-PWE) which is further functionalized with 1-azido undecan-11-thiol [49]. A click reaction enables the conjugation of the alkyne end-terminated capture antibody. Azide-functionalized sphere-like peroxidase magnetic silica ($Fe_3O_4@SiO_2$) nanoparticles were prepared to couple alkynylated peroxidase and secondary antibodies as detection label tags in the presence of hydrogen peroxide and thionine. A sandwich immunosensor was developed for the simultaneous electrochemical detection of carcinoembryonic antigen (CEA) and alpha-fetoprotein (AFP), by the aid of multi-labelled AuNPs as signalling probes [50]. The experimental setup was fabricated by means of AuNPs conjugated with thionine and ferrocene as probes and MNPs as immobilization surface for both specific antibodies under application of an EMF. The magnetoimmunosensor enabled the simultaneous detection in the linear range of 0.05–120 ng/mL with a LOD of 0.012 ng/mL for CEA, and 0.05–100 ng/mL with a LOD of 0.018 ng/mL for AFP (S/N = 3), respectively.

Biotin-streptavidin affinity reaction is one of the most used reactions in the design of immunoassays. Guerrero and co-workers developed a new strategy for the detection of IL-13Rα2 from cells lysates and from tumor tissues extracts (sample amount 0.5 µg) by an integrated electrochemical immunosensor [51]. To this, modified screen-printed electrodes with diazonium salts and hybrid composite based on multi-walled carbon nanotubes (MWCNTs) and graphene quantum dots (GQDs) were employed as advanced nanocarriers of several enzymes and an antibodies detector to achieve signal amplification. The sensor showed a time-response of approximately 2 h and enabled the determination of IL-13Rα2 down to 0.8 ng/mL (linear range 2.7 - 100 ng/mL).

Given the knowledge gained in the last decades, aptasensing bioassays have attracted great interest because of aptamers' ability to selectively and moreover specifically bind their target with high affinity [52]. To that end, Tian et al. designed an electrochemical aptasensor for MCF-7 circulating tumor cells (CTCs). The strategy was to use an EMF to perform a preliminary pre-concentration and separation step by inserting a magnet inside the glassy carbon electrode setup. Furthermore, an electrode modifier based on rGO/MoS$_2$ hybrid material combined with bi-nanozyme/aptamer-functionalized Fe$_3$O$_4$NPs accounts for signal generation and enrichment (Figure 3). The proposed electrochemical biosensor was able to detect MCF-7 in the linear range from 15 to 45 cells/mL with a LOD of 6 cells/mL, presenting good reproducibility and stability parameters [53].

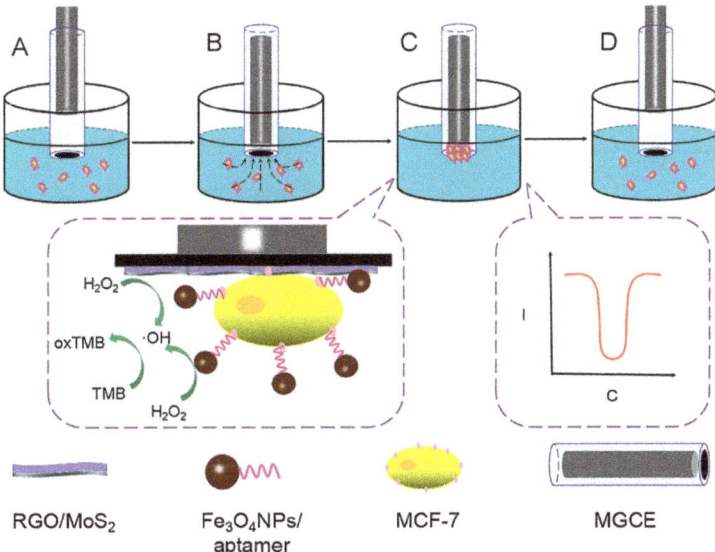

Figure 3. Schematic representation of bi-nanozyme/aptamer-functionalized MNPs for circulating tumor cells (CTCs) determination. Reproduced with permission from Elsevier [53].

Optical techniques supply the most diverse class of biosensors due to the plethora of optical processes that can be followed during the detection step such as absorption, fluorescence, phosphorescence, refraction, dispersion, and others [45]. These methods showed promising results for use in point-of-care (POC) early cancer diagnostics and imaging, due to the fact they are fast and the signal can be often easily be seen by the naked eye (e.g., colorimetric assays), however, sometimes optical techniques require more specialized instrumentation or personnel (e.g., SPR, SERS) [44,54].

Xu and co-workers designed a DNA-based MNPs (DNA/dextran/PAA/Fe$_3$O$_4$ NPs) sensor working as a signal-off fluorescent assay for the sensitive determination of p53 protein expression [55]. The fluorescent sensor showed a dose-response in the linear range from 50 pM to 2 nM and detected p53 low to 8 pM (LOD). The use of MNPs allows for sensitive analysis of real samples with minimum sample treatment steps and simple instrumentation. Another MNPs-based optical sensor is described for tumour biomarker anterior gradient homolog 2 (AGR2) by means of ultraviolet–visible (UV–Vis) spectrophotometric measurements [56]. The as proposed aptasensor, which requires 3.5 h for the overall sensing operational steps and low sample volumes (20 µL), showed a LOD of 6.6 pM (linear detection range over 10–1280 pM). The synergistic effect of combining the properties of MNPs with AuNPs can be also seen in the next example.

A mucin-1 (MUC1) optical electrochemiluminescence (ECL) sensor was developed based on a sandwich-type assay and hybrid materials of luminol-decorated gold-functionalized MNPs (Lu–AuNPs@Fe$_3$O$_4$) [57]. The MNPs were functionalized with the synthesized ECL label via electrostatic interaction to allow the formation of the composite Lu–AuNPs@Fe$_3$O$_4$. The sensor was applied for the MUC1 quantification in a wide linear range from 10 fg/mL to 10 ng/mL and a very low LOD of 4.5 fg/mL MUC1 was obtained. The concept of signal enhanced Fe$_3$O$_4$ nanozyme was first introduced by Li and co-workers in a photoelectrochemical (PEC) immunoassay for highly sensitive determination of prostate-specific antigen (PSA) [58]. The *his*-Fe$_3$O$_4$@nanozyme allow for signal amplification much higher than that of catalytic-induced activity of the natural enzyme HRP, and hence, with lower cost fabrication, ease of preparation and modification (Figure 4). The combination of the PEC enhanced features of the ZnIn$_2$S$_4$/ZnO-NRs/indium tin oxide photoelectrode and the highly effective *his*-Fe$_3$O$_4$@nanozyme enabled the determination of PSA down to fg/mL range (LOD = 18 fg/mL).

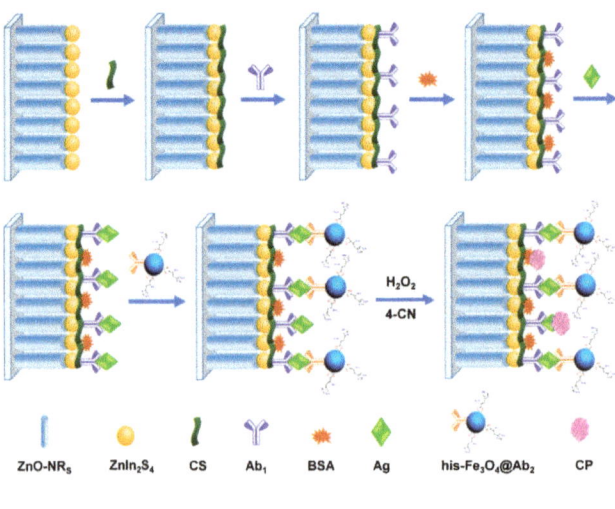

(a)

Figure 4. *Cont.*

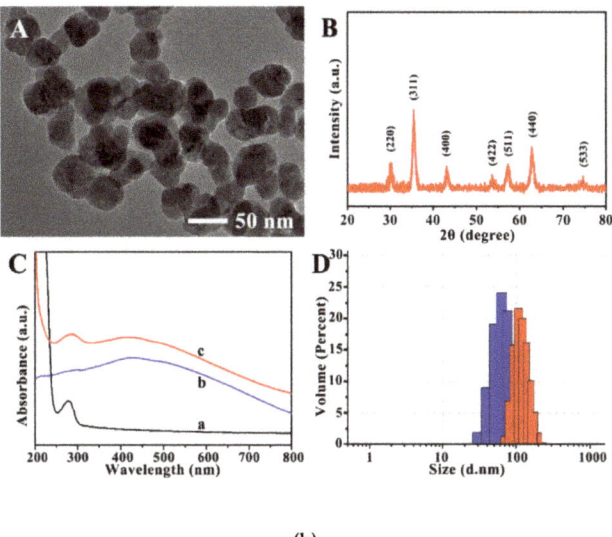

(b)

Figure 4. (a) Schematic representation of the photoelectrochemical (PEC) immunoassay design by means of high-activity Fe_3O_4 nanozyme as signal amplifier. (b) Transmission electron microscope (TEM) image (A) and X-ray diffraction (XRD) pattern (B) of the *his*-Fe_3O_4 nanoparticles; (C) ultraviolet–visible (UV–vis) absorption spectra of Ab2 (black), *his*-Fe_3O_4 (blue), and *his*-Fe_3O_4@Ab2 (red). (D) Hydrodynamic-size distribution of the *his*-Fe_3O_4 nanoparticles before (blue) and after (red) Ab2 modification. Reproduced with permission from Elsevier [58].

Another nanohybrid composite that showed high catalytic effect was developed starting from Fe_3O_4 MNPs and platinum nanoparticles (PtNPs), simultaneously entrapped in the framework of GO [59]. The results showed a 30-fold increase of the maximal reaction velocity (V_{max}) compared to the one obtained without GO within the colorimetric induced response of the peroxidase substrate, 3,3′,5,5′-tetramethylbenzidine (TMB). The sensor enabled fast quantification in the timeframe of 5 minutes of clinically important breast tumour cells. Gui et al. developed a charge-coupled device (CCD)-based reader to quantitatively measure the fluorescence signal of quantum dots (QDs) immobilized on lateral flow test strips for cytotoxin-associated protein (CagA) detection, which is commonly over-expressed in gastric carcinoma [60]. The sensor showed possible POC applications for CagA detection with a LOD of 20 pg/mL.

However, oftentimes sophisticated instrumentation for optical methods restricts their use for POC development in determining tumour biomarkers in real scenarios for early stage cancer diagnosis. Given this, colorimetric approaches are the most sensitive and widely employed methods due to their main advantages as simplicity, possibility for miniaturization and development of POC devices, and low costs. For example, Peng et al. proposed a magnetic colorimetric immunoassay (CIA) for human interleukin-6 (IL-6) based on Cerium oxide NPs (CeNPs)-labelling approach to enable the oxidation catalysis of the substrate into a stable yellow product [61]. Studies showed that IL-6 is overexpressed in breast and prostate cancer [62,63]. Spectrophotometric measurements showed a curve dose response in the range of 0.0001–10 ng/mL toward IL-6 and a LOD of 0.04 pg/mL was obtained. A colorimetric sandwich immunosensor based on a reverse strategy for PSA detection in biological fluids is presented [64]. To this end, hybrid nanostructured composite based on MNPs and AuNPs was synthesized and further used for the functionalization with both capture antibody (anti-PSA) and detection antibody (catalase/anti-PSA), respectively. Next, the signal generation and amplification for PSA assessment was realised by the aid of functional catalase/anti-PSA/AuNPs as enzymatic catalyst and anti-PSA-conjugated/MNPs as an optical generator. Despite classical colorimetric immunosensors, the reverse CIA technique revealed the remained quantity of H_2O_2 in the substrate after its depletion by the labelled-catalase. Under the optimal conditions, the immunoassay was applied for PSA sensing down to 0.03 ng/mL (S/N = 3) in a broad range of 0.05–20 ng/mL PSA.

There is a plethora of magnetic detection techniques exploited to determine the magnetic response of MNPs such as, spintronic sensors based on giant magnetoresistance (GMR), tunnel magnetoresistance (TMR), and planar Hall effect (PHE) sensors, superconducting quantum interference devices (SQUIDs), atomic magnetometers (AMs), nuclear magnetic resonance (NMR) systems, fluxgate sensors, Faraday induction coil sensors, diamond magnetometers, and domain wall-based sensors [20]. Compared to electrochemical or optical methods, the magnetic sensing techniques have proven superior performances for biomarker detection, providing high sensitivity (increased signal-to-noise ratio), high stability (fluorescent labelling presents no photo-bleaching) and feasibility for POC development [18].

The biosensing principle of magnetic sensors lies in magnetic field alterations that occur after interacting with the magnetic field of the MNPs. Therefore, a current or resistance difference of the magneto-resistive MNPs-functionalized sensor will be generated [17]. For example, DNA hybridization events can be monitored by the magnetic turbulence detected by the magnetic sensor by indirect approaches using affinity reactions (streptavidin-biotin or complementary DNA receptors) (Figure 5) [65].

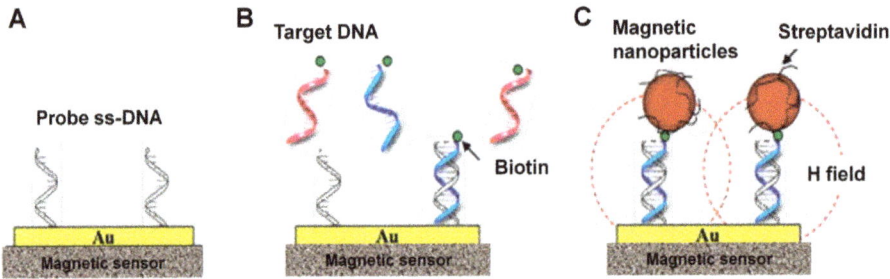

Figure 5. Schematic representation of magnetic biosensor. (**A**) Immobilization of single-stranded DNA with known sequence. (**B**) Hybridization of complementary target DNA. (**C**) Capture of MNPs via streptavidin–biotin interaction. The resistance of the sensor is altered by the magnetic field generated from immobilized MNPs. Reproduced with permission from SAGE Journals (open access) [65].

The design of a lateral-flow immunoassay based on a magnetoresistive sensor combined with MNPs acting as labels is described [66]. The magnetic signal generated by the MNPs within the spin valves biosensor exhibited a detection limit of 5.5 ng/mL of the human chorionic gonadotropin hormone. Spintronic sensors and immunosensors based on giant magnetoresistance principle have also been developed. A magentosensor for S100β biomarker detection was prepared using 300 nm MNPs for signal generation and enabled a LOD of 27 pg/mL [67]. A Hall-based magnetic transduction system was applied for the sensing of a 35-base DNA-strand for a pathogenic target [68].

LOD of 364 pM and high selectivity for target DNA was obtained by optical microscopy detection using a DNA-based Hall magnetometer sensor by the aid of MNPs of 350 nm [67]. This novel strategy allows the simultaneous ultrasensitive detection (fM) of up to eight cancer biomarkers from the cytokines class with signal amplification accomplished through MNPs of about 50 nm in diameter.

Table 2. Sensors for diagnosis and monitoring of biomarkers involved in cancer based on MNPs.

Target	Type of assay	Detection method	LOD	Sample	Ref
AFP	Label-free immunosensor based on graphite electrode modified with Fe_3O_4-ε-PL-Hep nanoparticles with anti-biofouling and anticoagulating MNPs	Electrochemical	72 pg/mL	Blood	[69]
AGR2	Optical aptasensor based on MNPs	UV-Vis spectroscopy	6.6 pM	Cell culture	[56]
ERα	Sandwich immunoassay based on SPCEs modified HOOC-MNPs and HRP as label	Electrochemical	19 pg/mL	Serum and cell lysate	[70]
D556 CTCs	Polyethyleneglycol-block-ally lglycidy lether copolymer coated iron oxide nanoparticles conjugated with transferrin	Flow cytometry	-	Cell culture and blood	[71]
IL-13Rα2	Disposable detection system based on a hybrid nanomaterial composed of MWCNTs and graphene quantum dots and enzyme label	Electrochemical	0.8 ng/mL	Cell lysate and extracts from tumor tissues	[51]
p53PE	DNA sensors based on DNA functionalized MNPs	Fluorescence	8 pM	Serum	[55]
CagA	CCD-based reader combined with CdS quantum dot-labeled lateral flow strips	Fluorescence	20 pg/mL	-	[60]
LNCaP	Sandwich-based magnetic DNA sensor	Piezoelectric	0.4 ng/mL	Cell culture	[65]
αvβ3 TM	Nanohybrid composite based on MNPs and platinum nanoparticles simultaneously immobilized in the framework of GO	Colorimetric	-	Cell culture	[59]
hCG	Lateral-flow magnetoresistive immunoassays based on MNPs	Magnetoresistive sensor	5.5 ng/mL	Serum	[66]
S100β	Magnetosensor based on GMR	Optical	27 pg/mL	Serum	[67]
CEA	Sandwich immunoassay based on carbon fiber microelectrode modified with thionine-doped magnetic gold nanospheres as labels and HRP as enhancer	Electrochemical	10 pg/mL	Serum	[72]
TNF-α	Hall-based magnetic transduction platform 35-base pathogenic DNA target	Fluorescence	5.7 pM	Serum	[68]
IL-6	Colorimetric immunoassay based on CeNPs	Colorimetric	40 fg/mL	Serum	[61]
	Sandwich-based label free magnetoimmunosensor based on ProteinG-functionalized MNPs	Electrochemical	0.3 pg/mL	Serum	[73]
MUC1	Sandwich immunosensor based on a multifunctional hybrid materials of luminol-decorated gold-functionalized MNPs	Electrochemiluminescence	4.5 fg/mL	-	[57]
	Sandwich immunoassay using graphite SPEs modified with MNPs functionalized with ProteinG and HRP as label	Electrochemical	1.34 ng/mL	Serum	[74]

Table 2. Cont.

Target	Type of assay	Detection method	LOD	Sample	Ref
PSA	Sandwich-type immunoassay; primary Ab immobilized on MNPs; secondary Ab labelled with HRP	Electrochemical	0.5 ng/mL	Serum	[75]
PSA	PEC-based immunoassay based on $ZnIn_2S_4/ZnO$-NRs/ITO photoelectrode	UV-Vis spectroscopy	18 fg/mL	-	[58]
	Sandwich-type colorimetric immunoassay based on a reverse strategy based on two nanostructures including MNPs and AuNPs	Colorimetric	30 pg/mL	Serum	[64]
CA 15-3	Sandwich immunoassay built on carbon-based SPE modified with graphene oxide and peroxidase-like silica MNPs/GO composites as labels	Electrochemical	2.8×10^{-4} U/mL	Serum	[48]
	Sandwich assay; capture aptamer/Ab immobilized on MNPs modified with Protein-G and streptavidin; Detection aptamer / Ab labelled with AP	Electrochemical	0.07 nM (aptasensor) 0.19 nM (immunosensor)	Serum	[76]
	Label-free immunoassay; aptamer immobilized on AuNPs modified graphite and Au SPEs	Electrochemical	0.95 ng/mL	Serum	[77]
CEA AFP	Sandwich immunoassay based on azide-functionalized sphere-like peroxidase silica MNPs and alkynylated peroxidase as label	Electrochemical	12 pg/mL 18 pg/mL	Serum	[50]
MCF-7 CTCs	Aptamer-functionalized cytosensor based on MNPs nanozyme and rGO/molybdenum disulfide immobilized on magnetic glassy carbon electrode	Electrochemical	6 cells/mL	Cell culture	[53]
PSA CA125 CEA	Nanoroughened, biotin-doped polypyrrole immunosensor based on MNPs with HRP as label	Electrochemical and colorimetric	0.7 pg/mL 0.005 U/mL 0.8 pg/mL	Plasma	[78]
CA15-3 CA 125 CA19-9	Sandwich immunoassay; primary Ab immobilized on MNPs; secondary Ab labelled with PAMAM dendrimer-metal sulfide QD	Electrochemical	$5\,10^{-3}$ U/mL	Serum	[79]

AFP: alpha-fetoprotein; AGR2: anterior gradient homolog 2; CA15-3: cancer antigen 153; CEA: carcinoembryonic antigen; hCG: human chorionic gonadotropin hormone; IL-6: Interleukin 6; ITO: indium tin oxide; LNCaP: human prostate cancer cells; CagA: cytotoxin-associated protein; D556 CTCs: Circulating D556 tumor cells; p53PE: p53 protein expression; $\alpha v \beta 3$ TM: integrin $\alpha v \beta 3$ tumor marker; PSA: prostate specific antigen; SPCEs: screen-printed carbon electrodes; TNF-α tumor necrosis factor alpha; PAMAM: methoxy-PEGylated poly(amidoamine).

The applications of MNPs used in several sensing approaches based on electrochemical, optical and magnetic readout of cancer biomarkers are summarized in Table 2 presenting the type of assay, detection method, LOD, and the type of tested real samples.

4.2. Cancer Screening Using Magnetic Nanoparticles

Magnetic Resonance Imaging (MRI)

MRI is an intense used method for cancer screening during and after chemotherapy. Despite common imaging techniques which require ionization radiation, MRI uses the magnetic properties of ions for projecting the image. When no magnetic moment is applied, protons have a randomized orientation whereas a parallel or anti-parallel arrangement occurs once the magnetic field is on. Contrast agents including those based on MNPs are used to enhance the quality of MRI images [80]. The development of reactive MNPs and magnetic colloidal particles for immobilization and easy magnetic separation of biomolecules is of great importance for early detection of diseases and consequently in therapy management and treatment of cancer in early stages. Thus, chitosan-stabilized magnetite nanoparticles were synthesized and successfully applied as negative contrast agents in MRI which further led to several biomedical applications [4].

Iron oxide MNPs are widely used in cancer screening and treatment because of their multiple advantages extensively discussed in the introduction of which we emphasize the ease distribution and functionalization. The most common functionalization of Fe_3O_4 particles consists in coating with antibodies. This strategy has been extensively applied for cell separation, recognition, and early diagnosis of malignancies. However, the biomedical use of Fe_3O_4 is restricted by the reduced biocompatibility, the remediation of this aspect being achieved by preliminary functionalization with natural compounds presenting high biocompatibility, blood compatibility, as well as microbial degradability. Therefore, a combination of magnetic Fe_3O_4 core particles and α-ketoglutarate chitosan shells (Fe_3O_4@KCTS) was applied for cancer screening through direct multi-labeling with different antibodies to sort lymphatic endothelial cells [81]. As noticed in Figure 6, firstly, the magnetic core was coated with α-ketoglutarate chitosan (KCTS) to enable the formation of Fe_3O_4@KCTS core-shell MNPs, followed by an activation step of the –COOH functional groups via NHS/EDC chemistry. Next, the covalent immobilization of two complementary antibodies for lymphatic endothelial cells, anti-Lyve-1 antibody and anti-podplanin antibody were bound at the Fe_3O_4@KCTS MNPs. A dual-targeting magnetic nanoprobe was obtained and injected into the tail vein of mice models for tumor visualization by MRI and fluorescence imaging. The results demonstrated that a dual-targeting magnetic nanoprobe was successfully developed and applied for capturing high-purity lymphatic endothelial cells from tumor tissues, providing a starting point of clinical applications based on dual-mode imaging in cancer screening.

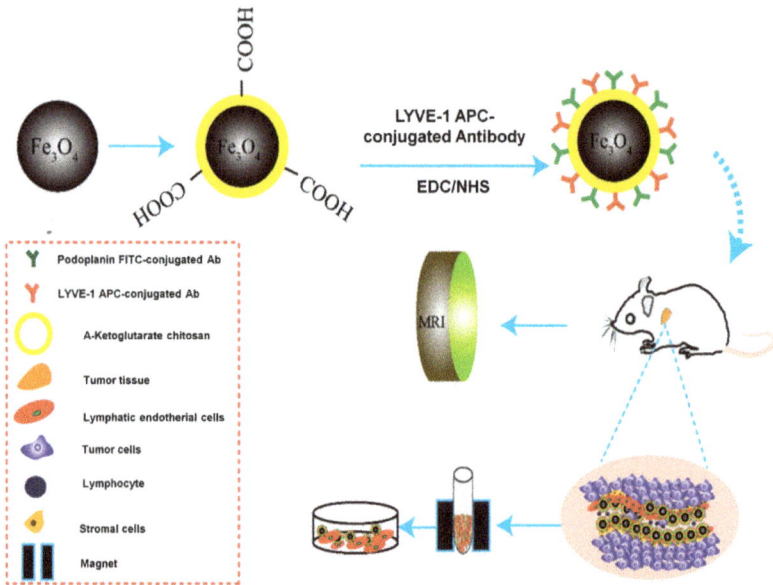

Figure 6. Schematic illustration of 2Ab/Fe$_3$O$_4$@KCTS MNPs synthesis, functionalization, and application for colorectal cancer imaging. Reproduced with permission from Springer (open access) [81].

Combining the effective features of MNPs with AuNPs some complex nanostructured materials are obtained that can be applied for cancer diagnostic and treatment by means of multiple imaging techniques and treatment strategies. These nanocomposites materials are biocompatible and can be thus further combined with other imaging and therapeutic agents (e.g., radioactive element and/or drug molecule) and biomolecules (e.g., peptide or antibody) for multimodal imaging of tumors. Therefore, a more effective treatment can be employed by the synergetic effects of combined therapy approaches [82].

Combinations between the imaging methods are also used since these dual-imaging methods may improve the accuracy of diagnosis. For instance, dual imaging of single-photon emission computed tomography (SPECT) and MRI have been applied in pancreatic and breast cancer, while MRI and optical imaging were combined for the successful diagnosis of breast cancer [3].

4.3. Cancer Treatment Using Magnetic Nanoparticles

The success in cancer treatment and the decrease in the mortality rate of patients are closely related to its diagnosis in early stages. When cancer is discovered earlier, the cure rate is greatly improved. Tumor imaging technology is used both in cancer diagnosis and treatment. Due to the high resolution and tomographic capabilities, MRI has proved to be one of the most valuable non-invasive imaging techniques. Furthermore, MNPs are the most widely researched and used contrast agents in cancer imaging. Due to the colloidal instability of MNPs, their surface modification is necessary by inducing the magnetic dipole interaction and its intrinsic surface energy. The multifunctional nanocomposite MNPs present higher potential for therapeutic and diagnostic applications [3].

MRI is related to nuclear magnetic resonance of hydrogen atoms and it usually requires the use of contrast agents for enhanced imaging. MNPs can be used as contrast agents only if they exhibit high saturation magnetization and after functionalization with compounds that increase the hydrophilicity around the Fe$_2$O$_4$ core [83].

Selective detection of cancer cells can be achieved by antibodies, thus many immunosensors have been developed for this purpose. Although, when using MNPs functionalized with antibodies specific for a type of tumor cell, the detection through the specific immunosensor can be combined with imaging through MRI and cancer treatment through hyperthermia. This strategy offers greatly improved survival rates among oncological patient's response to therapy. A first approach presents MNPs based on Fe_3O_4, having the core diameter of about 10 nm functionalized with poly-L-lysine (PLL) [83]. This complex strategy increases the stability and biocompatibility of MNPs and allows their use for combined detection, diagnosis through MRI and cancer therapy through magnetic hyperthermia. Hence, the 3D model of MNPs accumulation in tumor was also investigated for better evaluation of selectivity and in vivo toxicity.

Another MNPs-based imagistic strategy for determining the MNPs in vivo distribution is magneto-acoustic tomography. Herein, a magnetomotive force is generated by applying a short pulsed magnetic field and then using it to promote ultrasound frequencies in SPION-labelled tumor cells. After a long period of intense study and clinical trials, it can be still stated that most forms of human cancer are yet to be cured. The main reason is that this malady has many etiologies and the different types of cancer present numerous manifestations. Furthermore, multiple individuals having the same cancer respond differently to identical therapies. Moreover, the mechanisms of tumor growth and evolution still remain unsolved. Therefore, anticancer therapy is an important topic nowadays, considering the extent of this type of disease in the world. While certain types of cancer have been successfully treated, there are still many types of neoplasms that are refractory to all modern therapies.

Three major types of antineoplastic therapies are currently used, namely: surgical oncology in which the surgeon and pathologist discriminate between tumor tissue and healthy cells based on imaging techniques; chemotherapy uses antineoplastic drugs in order to eliminate cancer cells and stop their rapid multiplication; and radiation therapy exploiting the increased sensitivity to radiation of neoplastic tissue compared with normal tissue.

Surgical oncology is applied at controlling local tumor development, while chemotherapy is able to address circulating tumor cells, being thus more suitable for metastases. However, additive or synergistic and improved therapeutic effects can be obtained combining these types of therapies and minimizing the severe side-effects on healthy cells [10].

4.3.1. Drug Delivery

Targeted drug delivery is a concept that has been developed rapidly in recent years. In the case of cancers in particular, it has become one of the most popular treatment strategies since it can lead to a substantial increase in treatment efficiency and has far fewer side effects than the conventional methods used. A promising approach in this regard refers to magnetic drug delivery systems which involves the existence of a magnetic moment. Thus, various types of materials possessing magnetic properties that can be applied in magnetic targeted drug delivery are currently used as promising tools for modern therapy of several diseases, including cancers. Ideal properties for the magnetocomplexes which are to be used for targeted drug delivery must present high magnetization activity at the operational temperature. MNPs based on iron, cobalt, and nickel, are suited for this application, but the particles' dimensions and coating are of great importance. Thus, MNPs are constructed using biocompatible shells of polymers or metals, as well as nanocomposite mixtures consisting of MNPs encapsulated within porous polymers. Presence of the polymers or other coatings provides an opportunity to anchor various therapeutic drugs or DNA for targeted gene delivery [84,85].

Figure 7 is a suggestive representation of the multiple possibilities of MNPs' functionalization for application in cancer detection and treatment [85].

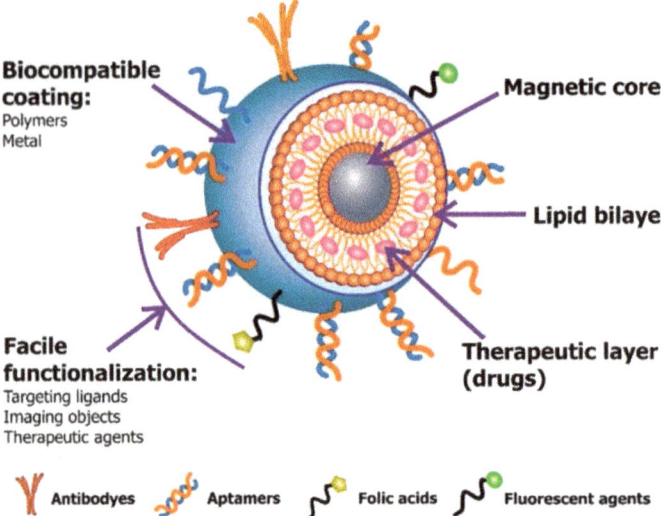

Figure 7. Schematic illustration of a multifunctional magnetic nanoparticle structure with different types of coatings, target ligands and imaging agents. Therapeutic drugs can be embedded in the coating, or conjugated on the surface. Reproduced with permission from MDPI (open access) [85].

In chemotherapy, anticancer drugs are administered through the venous circulatory system, strategy that aims at the accumulation of the drugs in the tumors, where vascularization is accentuated compared to healthy tissues. Antineoplastic drugs destroy cancer cells, while poisoning healthy tissues causing severe side effects, being one major drawbacks of chemotherapy. Thus, due to the need for more efficient approaches, an explosive development of research in the field of drug carriers, including magnetic approaches, has been extensively exploited. Furthermore, drug-delivery systems are often functionalized with biomolecular recognition sites able to specifically interact with receptors located in tumors, allowing for the selective targeted orientation of the drug carriers to cancer cells. Another very popular drug-delivery system is magnetic drug targeting which involves the use of a drug delivery vehicle with magnetism properties that can be manipulated by an EMF. Both these strategies decrease the side effects caused by antineoplastic systemic treatment [6]. Most of the MNPs used in biomedical applications are the so-called SPIONs consisting of one or multiple magnetite or maghemite cores and with biocompatible shell functionalized with various modifiers. In magnetic drug delivery a therapeutic agent is coupled to a magnetic particle, a step that is followed by their injection in the blood flow and their orientation to the target location by the aid of a magnetic field. MNPs may present small magnetic moment thus being challenging to retain it at the targets while withstanding the drag of the blood flow. To overcome this phenomenon, the magnetic field and gradient have to be extremely large, or the particles will agglomerate and cause embolism of the blood vessels. Some FePd-based magnetic nanowires were developed and used in a pilot scale in vivo experiment of targeted therapy. A magnet was designed for capture of the nanowires from the blood flow in the hind leg of a rat and no negative side effects from injection of the nanowires were found. Preliminary in vivo tests performed on animals proved that FePd nanowires were non-cytotoxic and non-immunotoxic which is an essential condition for any in vivo application and promising for future use in a clinical application [86]. Although the method was successfully applied in some modeling studies and also in animals and humans, no magnetic drug delivery applications have yet clinical use.

Commonly used chemotherapy drugs include doxorubicin (DOX), paclitaxel, cisplatin, gemcitabine, methotrexate, docetaxel, sorafenib and mitomycin C [3]. The majority of anticancer drugs present limited or no targeting capacity towards specific cancer cells. A good strategy to improve the treatment efficiency and to reduce the dose of drugs used in cancer treatment is the use of targeting-based approaches. Thus, cancer cell lines derived from liver, prostate and breast was used as a model for the implementation of a targeting-based strategy. These model cancer cells overexpress the riboflavin receptors on their cell membrane and are also sensitive to the treatment with *n*-Butylidenephthalide (BP). Fe_3O_4 MNPs were functionalized with riboflavin-50-phosphate (RFMP) through Fe-phosphate chelation and successfully used as carriers for BP to treat the model cancer cells that are also sensitive to this treatment. The results demonstrated that the as-prepared functional MNPs can be used to effectively target and inhibit the cell growth, have no toxicity toward non-targeted cells, and have the potential to be used as anti-cancer agents. More in vivo tests must be further performed in order to assess the clinical relevance of this approach [87].

Even though the concept of magnetic drug delivery was used for the first time in the 1980s [6], and the first clinical cancer therapy trials in humans using magnetic microspheres filled with 4-epidoxorubcin was reported in Germany in the 1990s (being about the treatment of advanced solid liver cancer in 14 patients) [84], the development of the domain has been achieved especially in the last 10 years after the development of stronger magnets and sophisticated magnetic probes, namely the theranostic probes that allow the combination of diagnostic and treatment. In this case, the diagnostic could be achieved through MRI or magnetic particle imaging, while the therapy could be realized by approaches such as hyperthermia, drug release or magneto-drug delivery [6].

Magnetic bioprobes are intensively explored for magnetic targeting. In this case, the uptake of drugs in drug delivery systems is usually carried out through conjugation, hydrophobic interactions or physical absorption within porous structures. as in the case of the non-magnetic ones, while the release of drugs can be accomplished by mechanical forces, varying the pH of the environment, by near-infrared (NIR) irradiation, magnetic hyperthermia or chemical reduction [6,10].

Magnetic drug targeting and delivery systems are often based on the use of an EMF from electromagnetic coils or permanent magnets. Here it was proven that the most important aspects for the effective magnetic drug delivery are the geometry of the magnet and the distance between the magnet and tumors [82,88].

Three different biopolymers, hydroxyl ethylene cellulose (HEC), nanocrystalline cellulose (NCC), and a synthetic biopolymer polyvinyl pyrrolidone (PVP) were applied for the functionalization of the surfaces of superparamagnetic Fe_3O_4 nanoparticles, these polymers being chosen based on their ionic charges which are cationic, anionic and non-ionic, respectively. The results obtained shows that the cationic polymer used in this study is more efficient for targeted delivery applications since it completely covers particle surfaces reducing their toxicity, allows better loading efficiency for anti-tumoral drugs, and does not significantly reduce magnetization of the particles in order to be driven to the targeted site under the action of an EMF [89].

The configuration that implies the use of an EMF is difficult to be applied to target areas below 5 cm under the skin, thus the concept called delivery deep inside the body was introduced. In this case a dynamic control of magnets was proposed in order to focus magnetic carriers to deep tissue targets [6]. More recently, magnetic implants seem to be a viable alternative to the use of an EMF which may cause severe problems in the case of drug delivery to some organs. A biocompatible nanodrug delivery formulation based on poly (*D, L*-lactide-co-glycolic) acid (PLGA), polyethyleneglycol (PEG) and SPIONs has been developed and evaluated for the enhanced delivery of docetaxel to breast cancer cells. The higher saturation magnetization, controllable size, satisfactory drug loading, sustained release, predominant cancer cell uptake and effective cytotoxicity make this a promising and outstanding drug delivery system for breast cancer therapy [90]. A biocompatible magnetic implant scaffold made of a magnetite/poly(lactic-co-glycolic acid) nanocomposite was reported for bone cancer, providing a more accurate cancer treatment [6]. However, more in vivo tests need to be performed before these systems could be safely applied for clinical trials.

Tumor hypoxia represents the low oxygen concentration which is generally a result of disordered vasculature that leads to distinctive hypoxic microenvironments. Traditional anticancer agents cannot penetrate into these zones, thus being ineffective in cancer treatment. As can be seen in Figure 8, MNPs loaded with drugs are guided to the tumor site under the influence of EMF as a viable magnetic drug delivery system.

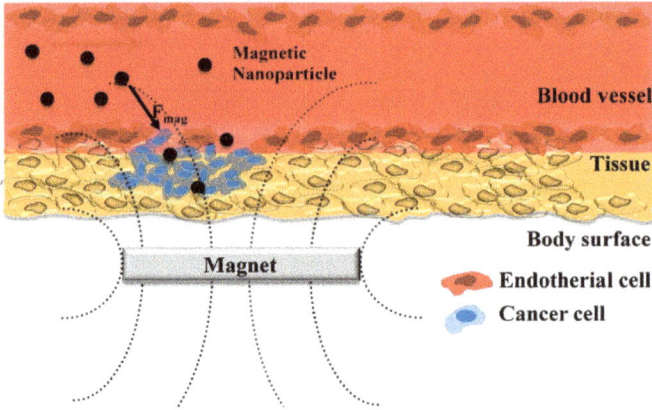

Figure 8. Schematic representation of a magnetic drug delivery system operated under the influence of external magnetic field. Reproduced with permission from Elsevier [91].

However, the development of this delivery system mandates that the MNPs behave magnetically only under the influence of EMF and are rendered inactive once the EMF is removed [84,91].

Additionally, cancer-targeted drug delivery particles still have many risks that can be overcame by using microrobots. These entities are constituted of an anti-cancer drug and MNPs to provide drug delivery to a cancer cell target lesion through electromagnetic actuation. However, viable solutions are still needed considering the inherent toxicity of MNPs that may remain in the body after the drug release. Various microrobots that can be manipulated by electromagnetic actuation (EMA) systems have been developed for various biomedical applications. These microrobots may be (i) shape morphing (changing their shape in response to external stimuli resulting in the delivery of the drug to target positions), (ii) shape-switching (using temperature or pH-responsive materials and can be manipulated by an EMA system to capture or release therapeutic drug particles), and (iii) controlled-drug releasing. Magnetic-actuated microrobots are envisaged as alternative to conventional drug therapy, but it should be noted that for biomedical applications, these devices should be made of biocompatible and biodegradable materials with no or little side-effects on humans. However, the MNPs used to magnetically drive microrobots are very small but lack a biodegrability property. Thus, it can be supposed that a part of MNPs will be excreted by human metabolism, while some MNPs will remain in the human body and affect cell metabolism, membrane integrity, cell death and proliferation, thus reducing treatment efficiency.

A novel microrobot was designed based on a gelatin/poly vinyl alcohol (PVA) based hydrogel, MNPs and polylactic-co-glycolic acid particles loaded with doxorubicin (PLGA–DOX). The targeted delivery of the drug as well as the retrieval of MNPs after drug release from the hydrogel microrobot are possible due to an integrated system based on electromagnetic actuation (EMA) and NIR spectroscopy. The targeted delivery of the hydrogel microrobot is based on the magnetic field of the EMA system. The subsequent NIR irradiation causes decomposition of the hydrogel microrobot. Only the PLGA–DOX drug particles remain in the target area for the generation of the therapeutic effect, while the MPs are recovered by the magnetic field of the EMA system (Figure 9). The hydrogel-based microrobot forms spherical microbeads and consists of gelatin/PVA hydrogel, PLGA–DOX drug particles and MNPs [92].

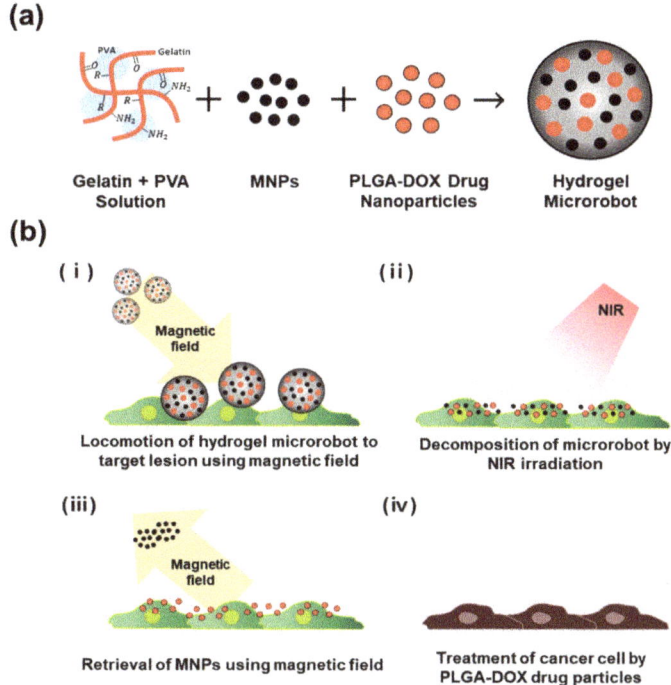

Figure 9. (a) Structure of hydrogel microrobot, consisting of gelatin/polyvinyl alcohol (PVA) hydrogel, PLGA–DOX (poly(lactic-co-glycolic acid)-doxorubicin) drug nanoparticles and MNPs (magnetic nanoparticles); **(b)** concept of the treatment process using hydrogel microrobot, where (i) hydrogel microrobot moves to a target lesion using magnetic field, (ii) hydrogel microrobot is decomposed by NIR (near-infrared) irradiation, (iii) remaining MNPs are retrieved by magnetic field, and (iv) cancer cells are treated by the remaining PLGA–DOX drug particles. Reprinted with permission from Elsevier [92].

4.3.2. Therapeutic Viruses

Another strategy in cancer treatment is based on the use of therapeutic viruses. During the last few decades, therapeutic viruses have been considered as a potential cancer therapy, adenoviruses being one of the most powerful gene-delivery systems. The protection of the virus from inactivation by cells of the immune system can be achieved after its conjugation to MNPs via electrostatic interactions. This conjugation also allows targeted transportation to specific sites, this process being known as magnetofection. Furthermore, the use of supermagnetic particles for complex formation with adenovirus particles have been also applied being promising for the potential utilization in clinical treatments [80,84]. There are still few unsolved problems relating to non-specific immune responses and low efficiency before the clinically used virus-based treatments in cancer.

4.3.3. Hyperthermia

Cancer treatment via hyperthermia is one of the most important thermo-therapeutic methods since determines the death of tumoral cells by increasing their temperature to a value between 42 and 46 °C for at least 30 minutes. Although, this method drastically reduces the negative side-effects of classical treatment, any increase of the whole body temperature genuinely promotes soft to harsh damage in healthy cells as well [80]. However, magnetic hyperthermia using MNPs brings significant advantages in comparison with other hyperthermia treatments as it is possible to adjust the proper amount of

MNPs and these can be delivered in the proper location [93]. During magnetic hyperthermia treatment, the MNPs are firstly injected directly into the tumor, followed by the application of a high-frequency alternating magnetic field, a process that causes local heating and finally thermal destruction of the tumor [83]. The strength and frequency of the magnetic field, the size and amount of MNPs are some important parameters that determine the efficiency of heat generation for successful cancer therapy [3].

Producing localized hyperthermia in cancer lesions, using MNPs, has the potential to destroy cancer cells or at least to enhance their susceptibility to radiation or chemotherapy. Several conditions are required in order to qualify MNP-based hyperthermia for clinical applications:

- the MNPs need to be functionalized for increase biocompatibility and low toxicity;
- only MNPs that are located in tumors must be heated;
- MNPs must absorb enough power to achieve cytolytic tumor temperatures without significant heating of the surrounding cells;
- these MNPs must be observable when in vivo using a non-invasive technique (MRI or fluorescence imaging) in order to prove their presence in the tumor;
- the temperature variations must be monitored in real time during the hyperthermia treatment;
- the effectiveness of the hyperthermia treatment needs to be accurately determined for optimization of all the required parameters (e.g., nanoparticle dose, administration technique, temperature, duration of the treatment);
- functionalization of the MNPs for increased selectivity when used for metastases treatment.

The activation of MNPs using an alternating magnetic field has been intensively explored recently for targeted therapeutic heating of tumors. Superparamagnetic and ferromagnetic particles, with different coatings and functionalities have been shown to be effective in tumor therapy [10,94]. There are several routes of MNPs administration in magnetic hyperthermia, the most popular being the intra-tumoral and intravenous applications. These strategies usually lead to a decrease in the efficacy of magnetic hyperthermia and also require invasive surgery, since they often determine a broad distribution of MNPs. Therefore, alternative routes for the administration of MNPs must be found. Recently, inhalable MNPs were applied in the treatment of non-small cell lung cancer. This concerns the use of MNPs functionalized with epidermal growth factor receptor and in vivo targeted use for lung cancer cells destruction through magnetic hyperthermia. Furthermore, other research led to the synthesis of some iron oxide-based MNPs functionalized with D-mannitol that can be targeted delivered by aerosol, and that were tested in vitro for human lung A549 cancer cells [80]. Although MNPs represent an area of active development for magnetically induced hyperthermia, the in vivo anti-tumor effect under low-frequency magnetic field using MNPs has not been yet demonstrated [3].

The biomineralized bacterial magnetic nanoparticles (BMPs) are another type of MNPs that have been intensively studied for possible biomedical applications, including the in vivo magnetically targeted photothermal therapy of cancer. Compared with MNPs, the BMPs have special properties such as large production, good dispersion, high crystallinity, and close-to-bulk magnetization. The BMPs were injected directly into the tumor to mice for accumulation in tumor tissues, but this was a compromise strategy before succeeding in the local accumulation after the systemic administration. A permanent magnet was used for targeting delivery with a high retention rate of BMPs in tumor tissues of mice being observed. It was also noticed that in vivo photothermal therapy with laser irradiation determined complete tumor elimination. Thus, it can be concluded that the systematically administered BMPs with magnetic targeting would be promising for biomedical and clinical applications [88].

Methoxy-PEGylated poly(amidoamine) (PAMAM) generation 3 dendrimers were synthesized and loaded with curcumin and SPIONs previously decorated with folic acid. A novel multifunctional nanoplatforms (FAmPEG-PAMAM G3-CUR@SPIONs) for the targeted thermo-chemotherapy of cancer cells was thus obtained and tested on two different cancer cell lines. It was proved that the nanocomplex could selectively bind to cancer cells and greatly enhance the targeted thermo-chemotherapy against the tumor upon alternating magnetic field excitation. Furthermore, the decoration of the nanocomplex with folate-targeting ligands modulated the response to thermo-chemotherapy by apoptosis. Future studies investigating MRI contrast enhancement performance of the nanocomplex are envisaged here [95].

4.3.4. Photodynamic Therapy

Photodynamic therapy (PDT) is an externally-activated and minimally invasive modality of cancer treatment. This strategy involves the systemic or local application of photosensitizing drugs, also called photosensitizers, followed by their photoexcitation in the tissue using light of the appropriate wavelength and power. These photosensitizers are excited in the presence of oxygen, thereby electrons from the ground state are delocalized to the excited state. This step is followed by activation with light of an appropriate wavelength, and an electron is transferred to nearby tissue, producing oxygen free radicals also known as reactive oxygen species (ROS), which cause cell damage, including for cancer. To enhance the effect of photosensitizers, the design of targeted drug delivery systems based on MNPs has become of interest. Thus, it was demonstrated that the use of MNPs determined remarkable and efficient photodynamic anticancer activity, and exhibited strong anti-cancer effects on human prostate cancer (PC-3), breast cancer (MDA-MB-231) and cervical (HeLa) cell lines [3].

As a light absorbent of low toxicity on skin and deep tissue penetration, NIR may directly kill cancer cells by photothermal therapy, which has recently become a highly controlled treatment method. In this treatment strategy, functionalized MNPs act as photothermal agents for solid tumor therapy and are used in combination with NIR. The photothermal effect of MNP clusters was initially reported for the in vitro and in vivo photothermal ablation of cancer cells. This strategy may determine an important increase in the NIR absorption and high cytotoxic effect against A549 cells [3].

Advances in nanomedicine determined the increased interest in the design and application of novel MNPs in cancer therapy. Thus, it has been more than 10 years since clinical trials were applied in order to find innovative methods for cancer imaging and therapy mainly through the activation of the immune response of the organism or by switching the magnetic field and producing localized heat effect at tumour cell's level. Based on these acquirements, MNPs are increasingly used in cancer therapy, several researches being now in the stage of in vivo or even clinical trials [96]. Furthermore, the therapeutic effects of the MNPs have recently been intensively tested by using them for drug loading and transport to the target tumor, in hyperthermal and photothermal cancer therapy.

The use of MNPs for cancer treatment have proved worthy to be considered for biomedical application and especially in nanomedicine, but precautions should still be considered as their mechanism of action in the human body is not yet elucidated. With this respect, another important issue arise in cancer treatment and is represented by the therapeutic resistance.

Due to their special properties, MNPs are also suitable for gene therapy and RNA delivery. A suggestive example in this regard is the product also called "LipoMag" consisting in nanocones of magnetite covered with cationic lipid shells that was successfully applied as a gene delivery device that can be magnetically guided [97].

Magnetic hyperthermia has been approved for clinical trials in Europe since 2007, firstly for the brain, then for prostate cancer, but the problems in this area, which restrain the use of MNPs in cancer therapy, are related to the delivery route, poor transfer efficiency of magnetic MNPs and insufficient heat at the tumor level that hinders the success of treatment [98]. Thus, intratumoral, intravenous and direct intratumoral injections are few examples of delivery strategies, all of them having both advantages and disadvantages that should be considered for clinical applications.

Combined treatment strategies in cancer are more often used. Thus, magnetic-optical hybrid nanosystems were applied for magnetic-field-guided drug delivery and dual mode PTT and PDT. The system acts as both magnetic and PTT agents for amplification of heating efficiency, and presents high accumulation of MNPs in tumors with excellent tumor regression [3]. Combined therapy between magnetic hyperthermia ionizing radiation and chemotherapy has determined a synergistic effect on several tumors and is a current reality in the practice of specialized clinics all over the world. For example, radiotherapy combined with magnetic hyperthermia was approved for clinical trials almost 20 years ago and generated good results on patients suffering with glioblastoma, while chemotherapy was combined with hyperthermia as an effective treatment of advanced pelvic cancers [96].

5. Conclusions and Perspectives

Although the research in the field of magnetic particles and their use in cancer diagnosis and treatment started several decades ago, only the recent surge of progress in nanotechnology has significantly expanded this research topic. With a wide range of biomedical applications for screening, diagnosis, monitoring and treatment of severe diseases such as cancer, MNPs are excellent candidates in meeting the healthcare needs of tomorrow.

MNPs were applied as contrast agents in imaging, but exhibit significant toxicity, thereby many restrictions have been applied in their biomedical and clinical use. Surface coating and functionalization of MNPs with different organic and inorganic layers are known to improve their features, as well as to diminish the potential toxicity for the human health.

There are several challenges associated with use of MNP-based systems for clinical applications, the most important being the in vivo behavior of MNPs. For increased efficiency of MNPs, several techniques, including reduced size and biocompatible shells of polymers or metals have been employed to improve their blood circulation and reduce the time required to reach the targeted tissues.

Despite many successful studies using MNPs as a theranostic material and even though many MNP formulations have demonstrated excellent results in small animal models, there are still many challenges to overcome when being applied in clinical trials. By improving their loading capacity, and increasing their specificity and affinity to target cancer cells, MNPs may become suitable for clinical use with integrated imaging and combined therapy with a high impact on the treatment of cancer.

The use of MNPs for drug targeted delivery is still in continuous development, and synthesis of high-performance magnetic drug delivery systems and integration of multifunctional ligands are being continuously investigated. The magnetic properties of MNPs may be exploited for specific targeting of disease biomarkers by using EMF thus offering attractive means of remotely directing therapeutic drugs specifically to a disease site, while simultaneously reducing dosage and minimizing side-effects associated with non-specific uptake of cytotoxic drugs by healthy cells.

Considerable efforts have been made in medicine related to the use of MNPs for modern and efficient therapies in cancer, but there is much more to discover until these materials can be safely used to increase life expectancy and prolong cancer patient survival. However, until the obstacles such as elimination from the body and long-term toxicity are completely overcome, their clinical applications are impossible to achieve.

Author Contributions: Conceptualization, O.H., M.T., C.C.; writing—original draft preparation, M.T., O.H., C.C.; writing—review and editing, O.H., M.T., C.C.; supervision, C.C.; project administration, C.C.; funding acquisition, C.C.

Funding: This research was funded by the Romanian National Authority for Scientific Research and Innovation, CNCS/CCCDI-UEFISCDI; grant project number PN-III-P1-1.2-PCCDI-2017-0407/ 39PCCDI/2018, within PNCDI III.

Conflicts of Interest: The authors declare no conflict of interest.

References

1. Wang, R.; Billone, P.S.; Mullett, W.M. Nanomedicine in action: An overview of cancer nanomedicine on the market and in clinical trials. *J. Nanomater.* **2013**, *2013*, 1–12. [CrossRef]
2. WHO. *Cancer*; WHO: Geneva, Switzerland, 2019.
3. Wu, M.; Huang, S. Magnetic nanoparticles in cancer diagnosis, drug delivery and treatment (Review). *Mol. Clin. Oncol.* **2017**, *7*, 738–746. [CrossRef] [PubMed]
4. Khmara, I.; Strbak, O.; Zavisova, V.; Koneracka, M.; Kubovcikova, M.; Antal, I.; Kavecansky, V.; Lucanska, D.; Dobrota, D.; Kopcansky, P. Chitosan-stabilized iron oxide nanoparticles for magnetic resonance imaging. *J. Magn. Magn. Mater.* **2019**, *474*, 319–325. [CrossRef]

5. Abu-Dief, A.M. Abdel-Mawgoud AAH. Functionalization of Magnetic Nanoparticles for Drug Delivery. *SF J. Nanochem. Nanotechnol.* **2018**, *1*, 1005.
6. Price, P.M.; Mahmoud, W.E.; Al-Ghamdi, A.A.; Bronstein, L.M. Magnetic drug delivery: Where the field is going. *Front. Chem.* **2018**, *6*, 6. [CrossRef] [PubMed]
7. Smith, M.; McKeague, M.; DeRosa, M.C. Synthesis, transfer, and characterization of core-shell gold-coated magnetic nanoparticles. *MethodsX* **2019**, *6*, 333–354. [CrossRef]
8. Rikken, R.S.M.; Nolte, R.J.M.; Maan, J.C.; van Hest, J.C.M.; Wilson, D.A.; Christianen, P.C.M. Manipulation of micro- and nanostructure motion with magnetic fields. *Soft Matter* **2014**, *10*, 1295–1308. [CrossRef]
9. Li, L.; Jiang, W.; Luo, K.; Song, H.; Lan, F.; Wu, Y.; Gu, Z. Superparamagnetic Iron Oxide Nanoparticles as MRI contrast agents for Non-invasive Stem Cell Labeling and Tracking. *Theranostics* **2013**, *3*, 595–615. [CrossRef]
10. Giustini, A.J.; Petryk, A.A.; Cassim, S.M.; Tate, J.A.; Baker, I.; Hoopes, P.J. Magnetic Nanoparticle Hyperthermia in Cancer Treatment. *Nano Life* **2010**, *01*, 17–32. [CrossRef]
11. Simeonidis, K.; Mourdikoudis, S.; Kaprara, E.; Mitrakas, M.; Polavarapu, L. Inorganic engineered nanoparticles in drinking water treatment: A critical review. *Environ. Sci. Water Res. Technol.* **2016**, *2*, 43–70. [CrossRef]
12. Baresel, C.; Schaller, V.; Jonasson, C.; Johansson, C.; Bordes, R.; Chauhan, V.; Sugunan, A.; Sommertune, J.; Welling, S. Functionalized magnetic particles for water treatment. *Heliyon* **2019**, *5*, e02325. [CrossRef] [PubMed]
13. Rabias, I.; Tsitrouli, D.; Karakosta, E.; Kehagias, T.; Diamantopoulos, G.; Fardis, M.; Stamopoulos, D.; Maris, T.G.; Falaras, P.; Zouridakis, N.; et al. Rapid magnetic heating treatment by highly charged maghemite nanoparticles on Wistar rats exocranial glioma tumors at microliter volume. *Biomicrofluidics* **2010**, *4*, 024111. [CrossRef] [PubMed]
14. Xianyu, Y.; Wang, Q.; Chen, Y. Magnetic particles-enabled biosensors for point-of-care testing. *TrAC Trends Anal. Chem.* **2018**, *106*, 213–224. [CrossRef]
15. Kralj, S.; Rojnik, M.; Kos, J.; Makovec, D. Targeting EGFR-overexpressed A431 cells with EGF-labeled silica-coated magnetic nanoparticles. *J. Nanoparticle Res.* **2013**, *15*, 1666. [CrossRef]
16. Issa, B.; Obaidat, I.M.; Albiss, B.A.; Haik, Y. Magnetic nanoparticles: Surface effects and properties related to biomedicine applications. *Int. J. Mol. Sci.* **2013**, *14*, 21266–21305. [CrossRef] [PubMed]
17. Tapeinos, C. Magnetic Nanoparticles and Their Bioapplications. In *Smart Nanoparticles for Biomedicine*; Elsevier: Amsterdam, The Netherlands, 2018; pp. 131–142. ISBN 9780128141564.
18. Liu, G.; Li, R.-W.; Chen, Y. Magnetic Nanoparticle for Biomedicine Applications. *Nanotechnol. Nanomed. Nanobiotechnol.* **2015**, *2*, 1–7. [CrossRef]
19. Jamshaid, T.; Neto, E.T.T.; Eissa, M.M.; Zine, N.; Kunita, M.H.; El-Salhi, A.E.; Elaissari, A. Magnetic particles: From preparation to lab-on-a-chip, biosensors, microsystems and microfluidics applications. *TrAC Trends Anal. Chem.* **2016**, *79*, 344–362. [CrossRef]
20. Chen, Y.T.; Kolhatkar, A.G.; Zenasni, O.; Xu, S.; Lee, T.R. Biosensing using magnetic particle detection techniques. *Sensors* **2017**, *17*, 2300. [CrossRef]
21. Revia, R.A.; Zhang, M. Magnetite nanoparticles for cancer diagnosis, treatment, and treatment monitoring: Recent advances. *Mater. Today* **2016**, *19*, 157–168. [CrossRef]
22. Rhee, I. Medical Applications of Magnetic Nanoparticles. *New Phys. Sae Mulli* **2015**, *65*, 411–431. [CrossRef]
23. Bucak, S.; Altan, C.L. Magnetic nanoparticles and cancer. In *Nanotechnology in Cancer*; Elsevier: Amsterdam, The Netherlands, 2016; pp. 105–137. ISBN 9780323390811.
24. Hajba, L.; Guttman, A. The use of magnetic nanoparticles in cancer theranostics: Toward handheld diagnostic devices. *Biotechnol. Adv.* **2016**, *34*, 354–361. [CrossRef] [PubMed]
25. Rocha-Santos, T.A.P. Sensors and biosensors based on magnetic nanoparticles. *TrAC Trends Anal. Chem.* **2014**, *62*, 28–36. [CrossRef]
26. Chen, Z.; Wu, C.; Zhang, Z.; Wu, W.; Wang, X.; Yu, Z. Synthesis, functionalization, and nanomedical applications of functional magnetic nanoparticles. *Chin. Chem. Lett.* **2018**, *29*, 1601–1608. [CrossRef]
27. Cristea, C.; Tertis, M.; Galatus, R. Magnetic nanoparticles for antibiotics detection. *Nanomaterials* **2017**, *7*, 119. [CrossRef] [PubMed]
28. Xu, J.K.; Zhang, F.F.; Sun, J.J.; Sheng, J.; Wang, F.; Sun, M. Bio and nanomaterials based on Fe_3O_4. *Molecules* **2014**, *19*, 21506–21528. [CrossRef] [PubMed]

29. Liu, C.; Zou, B.; Rondinone, A.J.; Zhang, Z.J. Reverse micelle synthesis and characterization of superparamagnetic MnFe$_2$O$_4$ spinel ferrite nanocrystallites. *J. Phys. Chem. B* **2000**, *104*, 1143–1145. [CrossRef]
30. Karade, V.C.; Dongale, T.D.; Sahoo, S.C.; Kollu, P.; Chougale, A.D.; Patil, P.S.; Patil, P.B. Effect of reaction time on structural and magnetic properties of green-synthesized magnetic nanoparticles. *J. Phys. Chem. Solids* **2018**, *120*, 161–166. [CrossRef]
31. Magdziarz, A.; Colmenares, J.C. In situ coupling of ultrasound to electro-and photo-deposition methods for materials synthesis. *Molecules* **2017**, *22*, 216. [CrossRef]
32. Abd Elrahman, A.A.; Mansour, F.R. Targeted magnetic iron oxide nanoparticles: Preparation, functionalization and biomedical application. *J. Drug Deliv. Sci. Technol.* **2019**, *52*, 702–712. [CrossRef]
33. Jahangirian, H.; Kalantari, K.; Izadiyan, Z.; Rafiee-Moghaddam, R.; Shameli, K.; Webster, T.J. A review of small molecules and drug delivery applications using gold and iron nanoparticles. *Int. J. Nanomed.* **2019**, *14*, 1633–1657. [CrossRef]
34. Mehta, R.V. Synthesis of magnetic nanoparticles and their dispersions with special reference to applications in biomedicine and biotechnology. *Mater. Sci. Eng. C* **2017**, *79*, 901–916. [CrossRef] [PubMed]
35. Kudr, J.; Haddad, Y.; Richtera, L.; Heger, Z.; Cernak, M.; Adam, V.; Zitka, O. Magnetic nanoparticles: From design and synthesis to real world applications. *Nanomaterials* **2017**, *7*, 243. [CrossRef] [PubMed]
36. Gangwar, A.; Varghese, S.S.; Meena, S.S.; Prajapat, C.L.; Gupta, N.; Prasad, N.K. Fe 3 C nanoparticles for magnetic hyperthermia application. *J. Magn. Magn. Mater.* **2019**, *481*, 251–256. [CrossRef]
37. Sun, T.; Zhang, Y.S.; Pang, B.; Hyun, D.C.; Yang, M.; Xia, Y. Engineered nanoparticles for drug delivery in cancer therapy. *Angew. Chem. Int. Ed.* **2014**, *53*, 12320–12364. [CrossRef] [PubMed]
38. Ayubi, M.; Karimi, M.; Abdpour, S.; Rostamizadeh, K.; Parsa, M.; Zamani, M.; Saedi, A. Magnetic nanoparticles decorated with PEGylated curcumin as dual targeted drug delivery: Synthesis, toxicity and biocompatibility study. *Mater. Sci. Eng. C* **2019**, *104*, 109810. [CrossRef] [PubMed]
39. Xu, Q.; Yuan, X.; Chang, J. Self-aggregates of cholic acid hydrazide-dextran conjugates as drug carriers. *J. Appl. Polym. Sci.* **2005**, *95*, 487–493. [CrossRef]
40. de Mendonça, E.S.D.T.; de Faria, A.C.B.; Dias, S.C.L.; Aragón, F.F.H.; Mantilla, J.C.; Coaquira, J.A.H.; Dias, J.A. Effects of silica coating on the magnetic properties of magnetite nanoparticles. *Surfaces Interfaces* **2019**, *14*, 34–43. [CrossRef]
41. Hosu, O.; Selvolini, G.; Cristea, C.; Marrazza, G. Electrochemical Immunosensors for Disease Detection and Diagnosis. *Curr. Med. Chem.* **2017**, *25*, 4119–4137. [CrossRef]
42. Sapsford, K.E.; Algar, W.R.; Berti, L.; Gemmill, K.B.; Casey, B.J.; Oh, E.; Stewart, M.H.; Medintz, I.L. Functionalizing nanoparticles with biological molecules: Developing chemistries that facilitate nanotechnology. *Chem. Rev.* **2013**, *113*, 1904–2074. [CrossRef]
43. Kouassi, G.K.; Irudayaraj, J. Magnetic and gold-coated magnetic nanoparticles as a DNA sensor. *Anal. Chem.* **2006**, *78*, 3234–3241. [CrossRef]
44. Wu, L.; Qu, X. Cancer biomarker detection: Recent achievements and challenges. *Chem. Soc. Rev.* **2015**, *44*, 2963–2997. [CrossRef] [PubMed]
45. Hosu, O.; Florea, A.; Cristea, C.; Sandulescu, R. Functionalized Advanced Hybrid Materials for Biosensing Applications. In *Advanced Biosensors for Health Care Applications*; Elsevier: Amsterdam, The Netherlands, 2019; pp. 171–207. ISBN 9780128157435.
46. Soloducho, J.; Cabaj, J. Electrochemical and Optical Biosensors in Medical Applications. In *Biosensors—Micro and Nanoscale Applications*; Toonika, R., Ed.; IntechOpen: London, UK, 2015; pp. 321–346. ISBN 9789537619343.
47. Hosu, O.; Selvolini, G.; Marrazza, G. Recent advances of immunosensors for detecting food allergens. *Curr. Opin. Electrochem.* **2018**, *10*, 149–156. [CrossRef]
48. Ge, S.; Sun, M.; Liu, W.; Li, S.; Wang, X.; Chu, C.; Yan, M.; Yu, J. Disposable electrochemical immunosensor based on peroxidase-like magnetic silica-graphene oxide composites for detection of cancer antigen 153. *Sens. Actuators B Chem.* **2014**, *192*, 317–326. [CrossRef]
49. Ge, S.; Liu, W.; Ge, L.; Yan, M.; Yan, J.; Huang, J.; Yu, J. In situ assembly of porous Au-paper electrode and functionalization of magnetic silica nanoparticles with HRP via click chemistry for Microcystin-LR immunoassay. *Biosens. Bioelectron.* **2013**, *49*, 111–117. [CrossRef] [PubMed]

50. Alizadeh, N.; Salimi, A.; Hallaj, R. Magnetoimmunosensor for simultaneous electrochemical detection of carcinoembryonic antigen and α-fetoprotein using multifunctionalized Au nanotags. *J. Electroanal. Chem.* **2018**, *811*, 8–15. [CrossRef]
51. Guerrero, S.; Cadano, D.; Agüí, L.; Barderas, R.; Campuzano, S.; Yáñez-Sedeño, P.; Pingarrón, J.M. Click chemistry-assisted antibodies immobilization for immunosensing of CXCL7 chemokine in serum. *J. Electroanal. Chem.* **2019**, *837*, 246–253. [CrossRef]
52. Dadfar, S.M.; Roemhild, K.; Drude, N.I.; von Stillfried, S.; Knüchel, R.; Kiessling, F.; Lammers, T. Iron oxide nanoparticles: Diagnostic, therapeutic and theranostic applications. *Adv. Drug Deliv. Rev.* **2019**, *138*, 302–325. [CrossRef]
53. Tian, L.; Qi, J.; Qian, K.; Oderinde, O.; Cai, Y.; Yao, C.; Song, W.; Wang, Y. An ultrasensitive electrochemical cytosensor based on the magnetic field assisted binanozymes synergistic catalysis of Fe3O4 nanozyme and reduced graphene oxide/molybdenum disulfide nanozyme. *Sens. Actuators B Chem.* **2018**, *260*, 676–684. [CrossRef]
54. Yang, J.; Wang, K.; Xu, H.; Yan, W.; Jin, Q.; Cui, D. Detection platforms for point-of-care testing based on colorimetric, luminescent and magnetic assays: A review. *Talanta* **2019**, *202*, 96–110. [CrossRef]
55. Xu, Q.; Liang, K.; Liu, R.Y.; Deng, L.; Zhang, M.; Shen, L.; Liu, Y.N. Highly sensitive fluorescent detection of p53 protein based on DNA functionalized Fe 3 O 4 nanoparticles. *Talanta* **2018**, *187*, 142–147. [CrossRef]
56. Hu, Y.; Li, L.; Guo, L. The sandwich-type aptasensor based on gold nanoparticles/DNA/magnetic beads for detection of cancer biomarker protein AGR2. *Sens. Actuators B Chem.* **2015**, *209*, 846–852. [CrossRef]
57. Wang, J.X.; Zhuo, Y.; Zhou, Y.; Yuan, R.; Chai, Y.Q. Electrochemiluminescence immunosensor based on multifunctional luminol-capped AuNPs@Fe$_3$O$_4$ nanocomposite for the detection of mucin-1. *Biosens. Bioelectron.* **2015**, *71*, 407–413. [CrossRef] [PubMed]
58. Li, W.; Fan, G.C.; Gao, F.; Cui, Y.; Wang, W.; Luo, X. High-activity Fe$_3$O$_4$ nanozyme as signal amplifier: A simple, low-cost but efficient strategy for ultrasensitive photoelectrochemical immunoassay. *Biosens. Bioelectron.* **2019**, *127*, 64–71. [CrossRef] [PubMed]
59. Su, D.; Teoh, C.L.; Samanta, A.; Kang, N.Y.; Park, S.J.; Chang, Y.T. The development of a highly photostable and chemically stable zwitterionic near-infrared dye for imaging applications. *Chem. Commun.* **2015**, *51*, 3989–3992. [CrossRef] [PubMed]
60. Gui, C.; Wang, K.; Li, C.; Dai, X.; Cui, D. A CCD-based reader combined with CdS quantum dot-labeled lateral flow strips for ultrasensitive quantitative detection of CagA. *Nanoscale Res. Lett.* **2014**, *9*, 57. [CrossRef]
61. Peng, J.; Guan, J.; Yao, H.; Jin, X. Magnetic colorimetric immunoassay for human interleukin-6 based on the oxidase activity of ceria spheres. *Anal. Biochem.* **2016**, *492*, 63–68. [CrossRef]
62. Domingo-Domenech, J.; Oliva, C.; Rovira, A.; Codony-Servat, J.; Bosch, M.; Filella, X.; Montagut, C.; Tapia, M.; Campás, C.; Dang, L.; et al. Interleukin 6, a nuclear factor-κB target, predicts resistance to docetaxel in hormone-independent prostate cancer and nuclear factor-κB inhibition by PS-1145 enhances docetaxel antitumor activity. *Clin. Cancer Res.* **2006**, *12*, 5578–5586. [CrossRef]
63. Lee, Y.W.; Hirani, A.A.; Kyprianou, N.; Toborek, M. Human immunodeficiency virus-1 Tat protein up-regulates interleukin-6 and interleukin-8 expression in human breast cancer cells. *Inflamm. Res.* **2005**, *54*, 380–389. [CrossRef]
64. Gao, Z.; Xu, M.; Hou, L.; Chen, G.; Tang, D. Magnetic bead-based reverse colorimetric immunoassay strategy for sensing biomolecules. *Anal. Chem.* **2013**, *85*, 6945–6952. [CrossRef]
65. Han, S.-J.; Wang, S. Magnetic Nanotechnology for Biodetection. *J. Assoc. Lab. Autom.* **2010**, *15*, 93–98. [CrossRef]
66. Serrate, D.; De Teresa, J.M.; Marquina, C.; Marzo, J.; Saurel, D.; Cardoso, F.A.; Cardoso, S.; Freitas, P.P.; Ibarra, M.R. Quantitative biomolecular sensing station based on magnetoresistive patterned arrays. *Biosens. Bioelectron.* **2012**, *35*, 206–212. [CrossRef] [PubMed]
67. Hira, S.M.; Aledealat, K.; Chen, K.S.; Field, M.; Sullivan, G.J.; Chase, P.B.; Xiong, P.; Von Molnár, S.; Strouse, G.F. Detection of target ssDNA using a microfabricated hall magnetometer with correlated optical readout. *J. Biomed. Biotechnol.* **2012**, *2012*, 1–10. [CrossRef] [PubMed]
68. Osterfeld, S.J.; Yu, H.; Gaster, R.S.; Caramuta, S.; Xu, L.; Han, S.J.; Hall, D.A.; Wilson, R.J.; Sun, S.; White, R.L.; et al. Multiplex protein assays based on real-time magnetic nanotag sensing. *Proc. Natl. Acad. Sci. USA* **2008**, *105*, 20637–20640. [CrossRef] [PubMed]

69. Xu, T.; Chi, B.; Wu, F.; Ma, S.; Zhan, S.; Yi, M.; Xu, H.; Mao, C. A sensitive label-free immunosensor for detection α-Fetoprotein in whole blood based on anticoagulating magnetic nanoparticles. *Biosens. Bioelectron.* **2017**, *95*, 87–93. [CrossRef] [PubMed]
70. Eletxigerra, U.; Martinez-Perdiguero, J.; Merino, S.; Barderas, R.; Ruiz-Valdepeñas Montiel, V.; Villalonga, R.; Pingarrón, J.M.; Campuzano, S. Estrogen receptor α determination in serum, cell lysates and breast cancer cells using an amperometric magnetoimmunosensing platform. *Sens. Bio-Sens. Res.* **2016**, *7*, 71–76. [CrossRef]
71. Lin, R.; Li, Y.; MacDonald, T.; Wu, H.; Provenzale, J.; Peng, X.; Huang, J.; Wang, L.; Wang, A.Y.; Yang, J.; et al. Improving sensitivity and specificity of capturing and detecting targeted cancer cells with anti-biofouling polymer coated magnetic iron oxide nanoparticles. *Colloids Surfaces B Biointerfaces* **2017**, *150*, 261–270. [CrossRef] [PubMed]
72. Dianping, T.; Yuan, R.; Chai, Y. Ultrasensitive Electrochemical Immunosensor for Clinical Immunoassay Using Thionine-Doped Magnetic Gold Nanospheres as Labels and Horseradish Peroxidase as Enhancer. *Anal. Chem.* **2008**, *80*, 1582–1588.
73. Tertiş, M.; Melinte, G.; Ciui, B.; Şimon, I.; Ştiufiuc, R.; Săndulescu, R.; Cristea, C. A Novel Label Free Electrochemical Magnetoimmunosensor for Human Interleukin-6 Quantification in Serum. *Electroanalysis* **2019**, *31*, 282–292. [CrossRef]
74. Taleat, Z.; Cristea, C.; Marrazza, G.; Săndulescu, R. Electrochemical Sandwich Immunoassay for the Ultrasensitive Detection of Human MUC1 Cancer Biomarker. *Int. J. Electrochem.* **2013**, *2013*, 1–6. [CrossRef]
75. Mani, V.; Chikkaveeraiah, B.V.; Patel, V.; Gutkind, J.S.; Rusling, J.F. Ultrasensitive Immunosensor for Cancer Biomarker Proteins Using Gold Nanoparticle Film Electrodes and Multienzyme-Particle Amplification. *ACS Nano* **2009**, *3*, 585–594. [CrossRef]
76. Marrazza, G.; Florea, A.; Ravalli, A.; Cristea, C.; Sa, R. An Optimized Bioassay for Mucin1 Detection in Serum. *Electroanalysis* **2015**, *27*, 1594–1601.
77. Florea, A.; Taleat, Z.; Cristea, C.; Mazloum-Ardakani, M.; Săndulescu, R. Label free MUC1 aptasensors based on electrodeposition of gold nanoparticles on screen printed electrodes. *Electrochem. Commun.* **2013**, *33*, 127–130. [CrossRef]
78. Hong, W.; Lee, S.; Cho, Y. Dual-responsive immunosensor that combines colorimetric recognition and electrochemical response for ultrasensitive detection of cancer biomarkers. *Biosens. Bioelectron.* **2016**, *86*, 920–926. [CrossRef] [PubMed]
79. Marques, R.C.B.; Costa-Rama, E.; Viswanathan, S.; Nouws, H.P.A.; Costa-García, A.; Delerue-Matos, C.; González-García, M.B. Voltammetric immunosensor for the simultaneous analysis of the breast cancer biomarkers CA 15-3 and HER2-ECD. *Sens. Actuators B Chem.* **2018**, *255*, 918–925. [CrossRef]
80. Williams, H.M. The application of magnetic nanoparticles in the treatment and monitoring of cancer and infectious diseases. *Biosci. Horizons Int. J. Student Res.* **2017**, *10*. [CrossRef]
81. Wu, S.; Liu, X.; He, J.; Wang, H.; Luo, Y.; Gong, W.; Li, Y.; Huang, Y.; Zhong, L.; Zhao, Y. A Dual Targeting Magnetic Nanoparticle for Human Cancer Detection. *Nanoscale Res. Lett.* **2019**, *14*, 228. [CrossRef]
82. Das, P.; Fatehbasharzad, P.; Colombo, M.; Fiandra, L.; Prosperi, D. Multifunctional Magnetic Gold Nanomaterials for Cancer. *Trends Biotechnol.* **2019**, *37*, 995–1010. [CrossRef]
83. Kubovcikova, M.; Koneracka, M.; Strbak, O.; Molcan, M.; Zavisova, V.; Antal, I.; Khmara, I.; Lucanska, D.; Tomco, L.; Barathova, M.; et al. Poly-L-lysine designed magnetic nanoparticles for combined hyperthermia, magnetic resonance imaging and cancer cell detection. *J. Magn. Magn. Mater.* **2019**, *475*, 316–326. [CrossRef]
84. Mody, V.V.; Cox, A.; Shah, S.; Singh, A.; Bevins, W.; Parihar, H. Magnetic nanoparticle drug delivery systems for targeting tumor. *Appl. Nanosci.* **2014**, *4*, 385–392. [CrossRef]
85. Belyanina, I.; Kolovskaya, O.; Zamay, S.; Gargaun, A.; Zamay, T.; Kichkailo, A. Targeted magnetic nanotheranostics of cancer. *Molecules* **2017**, *22*, 975. [CrossRef]
86. Pondman, K.M.; Bunt, N.D.; Maijenburg, A.W.; Van Wezel, R.J.A.; Kishore, U.; Abelmann, L.; Ten Elshof, J.E.; Ten Haken, B. Magnetic drug delivery with FePd nanowires. *J. Magn. Magn. Mater.* **2015**, *380*, 299–306. [CrossRef]
87. Wu, C.Y.; Chen, Y.C. Riboflavin immobilized Fe_3O_4 magnetic nanoparticles carried with n-butylidenephthalide as targeting-based anticancer agents. *Artif. Cells Nanomed. Biotechnol.* **2019**, *47*, 210–220. [CrossRef] [PubMed]

88. Wang, F.; Chen, C.; Chen, Y.; Wang, P.; Chen, C.; Geng, D.; Li, L.; Song, T. Magnetically targeted photothemal cancer therapy in vivo with bacterial magnetic nanoparticles. *Colloids Surfaces B Biointerfaces* **2018**, *172*, 308–314. [CrossRef] [PubMed]
89. Bekaroğlu, M.G.; Alemdar, A.; İşçi, S. Comparison of ionic polymers in the targeted drug delivery applications as the coating materials on the Fe_3O_4 nanoparticles. *Mater. Sci. Eng. C* **2019**, *103*, 109838. [CrossRef] [PubMed]
90. Panda, J.; Satapathy, B.S.; Majumder, S.; Sarkar, R.; Mukherjee, B.; Tudu, B. Engineered polymeric iron oxide nanoparticles as potential drug carrier for targeted delivery of docetaxel to breast cancer cells. *J. Magn. Magn. Mater.* **2019**, *485*, 165–173. [CrossRef]
91. Park, J.H.; Saravanakumar, G.; Kim, K.; Kwon, I.C. Targeted delivery of low molecular drugs using chitosan and its derivatives. *Adv. Drug Deliv. Rev.* **2010**, *62*, 28–41. [CrossRef] [PubMed]
92. Kim, D.i.; Lee, H.; Kwon, S.-h.; Choi, H.; Park, S. Magnetic nano-particles retrievable biodegradable hydrogel microrobot. *Sens. Actuators B Chem.* **2019**, *289*, 65–77. [CrossRef]
93. Roohi, R.; Emdad, H.; Jafarpur, K.; Mahmoudi, M.R. Determination of Magnetic Nanoparticles Injection Characteristics for Optimal Hyperthermia Treatment of an Arbitrary Cancerous Cells Distribution. *J. Test. Eval.* **2020**, *48*, 20170677. [CrossRef]
94. Alomari, M.; Jermy, B.R.; Ravinayagam, V.; Akhtar, S.; Almofty, S.A.; Rehman, S.; Bahmdan, H.; AbdulAzeez, S.; Borgio, J.F. Cisplatin-functionalized three-dimensional magnetic SBA-16 for treating breast cancer cells (MCF-7). *Artif. Cells Nanomed. Biotechnol.* **2019**, *47*, 3079–3086. [CrossRef]
95. Montazerabadi, A.; Beik, J.; Irajirad, R.; Attaran, N.; Khaledi, S.; Ghaznavi, H.; Shakeri-Zadeh, A. Folate-modified and curcumin-loaded dendritic magnetite nanocarriers for the targeted thermo-chemotherapy of cancer cells. *Artif. Cells Nanomed. Biotechnol.* **2019**, *47*, 330–340. [CrossRef]
96. Zhang, H.; Liu, X.L.; Zhang, Y.F.; Gao, F.; Li, G.L.; He, Y.; Peng, M.L.; Fan, H.M. Magnetic nanoparticles based cancer therapy: Current status and applications. *Sci. China Life Sci.* **2018**, *61*, 400–414. [CrossRef] [PubMed]
97. Namiki, Y.; Namiki, T.; Yoshida, H.; Ishii, Y.; Tsubota, A.; Koido, S.; Nariai, K.; Mitsunaga, M.; Yanagisawa, S.; Kashiwagi, H.; et al. A novel magnetic crystal–lipid nanostructure for magnetically guided in vivo gene delivery. *Nat. Nanotechnol.* **2009**, *4*, 598–606. [CrossRef] [PubMed]
98. Salunkhe, A.B.; Khot, V.M.; Pawar, S.H. Magnetic Hyperthermia with Magnetic Nanoparticles: A Status Review. *Curr. Top. Med. Chem.* **2014**, *14*, 572–594. [CrossRef] [PubMed]

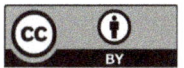

© 2019 by the authors. Licensee MDPI, Basel, Switzerland. This article is an open access article distributed under the terms and conditions of the Creative Commons Attribution (CC BY) license (http://creativecommons.org/licenses/by/4.0/).

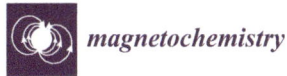

Review

The Potential Biomedical Application of NiCu Magnetic Nanoparticles

Janja Stergar [1,2,*], Irena Ban [1] and Uroš Maver [2,3,*]

1. Faculty of Chemistry and Chemical Engineering, University of Maribor, Smetanova ulica 17, SI-2000 Maribor, Slovenia; irena.ban@um.si
2. Faculty of Medicine, Institute of Biomedical Sciences, University of Maribor, Taborska ulica 8, SI-2000 Maribor, Slovenia
3. Department of Pharmacology, Faculty of Medicine, University of Maribor, Taborska ulica 8, SI-2000 Maribor, Slovenia
* Correspondence: janja.stergar@um.si (J.S.); uros.maver@um.si (U.M.); Tel.: +386-2-229-4417 (J.S.); +386-2-234-5823 (U.M.)

Received: 8 October 2019; Accepted: 15 November 2019; Published: 6 December 2019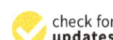

Abstract: Magnetic nanoparticles became increasingly interesting in recent years as a result of their tailorable size-dependent properties, which enable their use in a wide range of applications. One of their emerging applications is biomedicine; in particular, bimetallic nickel/copper magnetic nanoparticles (NiCu MNPs) are gaining momentum as a consequence of their unique properties that are suitable for biomedicine. These characteristics include stability in various chemical environments, proven biocompatibility with various cell types, and tunable magnetic properties that can be adjusted by changing synthesis parameters. Despite the obvious potential of NiCu MNPs for biomedical applications, the general interest in their use for this purpose is rather low. Nevertheless, the steadily increasing annual number of related papers shows that increasingly more researchers in the biomedical field are studying this interesting formulation. As with other MNPs, NiCu-based formulations were examined for their application in magnetic hyperthermia (MH) as one of their main potential uses in clinics. MH is a treatment method in which cancer tissue is selectively heated through the localization of MNPs at the target site in an alternating magnetic field (AMF). This heating destroys cancer cells only since they are less equipped to withstand temperatures above 43 °C, whereas this temperature is not critical for healthy tissue. Superparamagnetic particles (e.g., NiCu MNPs) generate heat by relaxation losses under an AMF. In addition to MH in cancer treatment, which might be their most beneficial potential use in biomedicine, the properties of NiCu MNPs can be leveraged for several other applications, such as controlled drug delivery and prolonged localization at a desired target site in the body. After a short introduction that covers the general properties of NiCu MNPs, this review explores different synthesis methods, along with their main advantages and disadvantages, potential surface modification approaches, and their potential in biomedical applications, such as MH, multimodal cancer therapy, MH implants, antibacterial activity, and dentistry.

Keywords: NiCu magnetic nanoparticles; physical and chemical methods; surface modification; biomedicine; magnetic hyperthermia; curie temperature

---

1. Introduction

Magnetic nanoparticles (MNPs) attracted much interest in the last two decades, especially in the field of biomedicine. Their appealing potential biomedical applications rely on the strategic exploitation of their (extremely) small sizes, resulting in large surface areas, which distinguish them from bulk materials [1,2]. Additionally, MNPs have various unique magnetic properties, including their superparamagnetic nature, a high magnetic susceptibility, a low Curie temperature (T_C), coercivity, and an inducible magnetic moment that allows them to be directed to a defined location or heated with an external alternating magnetic field (AMF) [3,4]. Among the properties that make MNPs ideal for biomedical applications are their biocompatibility, non-toxicity, and extensive aggregation in the desired tissue [5,6]. For their in vivo application, they must be coated by or encapsulated in a biocompatible polymer to prevent the formation of large aggregates, prevent the manipulation of their original structure, and potentially enable targeted biodegradation at the desired site in the body [7,8]. The important factors that determine the biocompatibility and toxicity of MNPs are the nature of the magnetically responsive component and the particles' final size, core composition, and coatings [9–11]. Moreover, MNPs with sizes below 100 nm are known to possess lower sedimentation rates and improved tissular diffusion [12,13].

The potential biomedical applications of MNPs require further consideration in regard to some specific properties. In addition to their composition of non-toxic and non-immunogenic materials, their sizes (and size distributions) have to be even more carefully controlled to prolong their circulation after injection in the body, as well as to allow them to pass through the capillary systems of organs and tissues to avoid vessel embolism. High magnetization is crucial for their movement in the blood so that they can be controlled using an AMF and immobilized close to the targeted pathologic tissue [2,14].

The abovementioned properties of MNPs and their ability to work at both cellular and molecular levels enabled their investigation and, in some cases, application in vitro and in vivo as part of drug delivery systems [15–17], in the targeted delivery of cytotoxic drugs [16,18,19], as active components in hyperthermia treatment [17,20,21], as contrast agents in magnetic resonance imaging (MRI) [1,22,23], as radiotherapeutics [24,25], for advanced gene delivery applications [26,27], for separation and selection [24,28], in magnetorelaxometry [29,30], as active antibacterial materials [31,32], in tissue engineering [8,33], and as part of biotherapeutics [34,35]. Figure 1 summarizes the potential applications of MNPs in biomedicine.

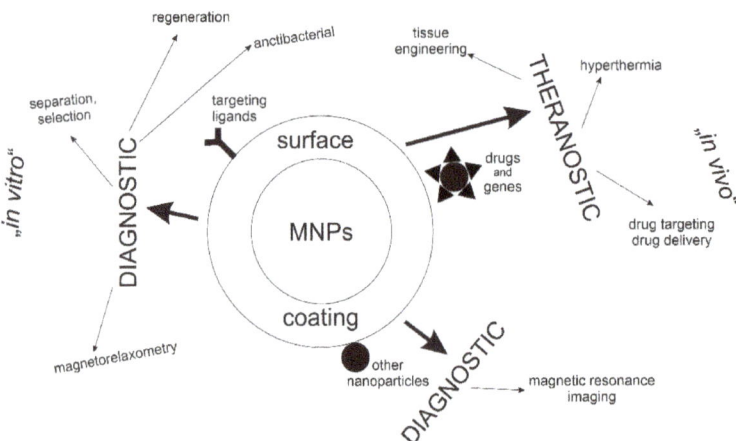

Figure 1. A schematic that illustrates the biomedical applications of magnetic nanoparticles (MNPs).

In the last decade, the authors of this paper developed several novel NiCu-based MNPs that not only exhibit all the above mentioned characteristics but also hold great promise for many different applications, which include multi-layer coatings, solar energy, and regenerative medicine, as well as in various formulations used in biomedicine [36–39]. The versatile range of potential applications, especially their applicability in biomedicine, is related to their chemical stability, proven biocompatibility with different human and animal cells, and tailorable magnetic characteristics. Their magnetic properties can be controlled using different preparation methods, ranging from mechanical milling, hydrothermal reduction reactions, and emulsion techniques, through various electrochemistry-based and sol–gel methods, to plasma evaporation [36,40–42].

Despite the obvious potential of NiCu MNPs for biomedical applications, the general interest in their use for this purpose is rather low. Nevertheless, the steadily increasing annual number of related papers shows that increasingly more researchers in the field of biomedicine are studying this interesting formulation (Figure 2).

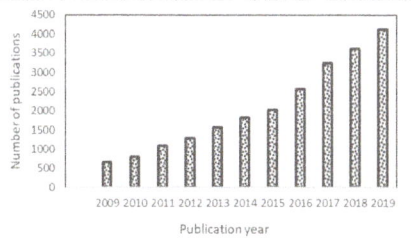
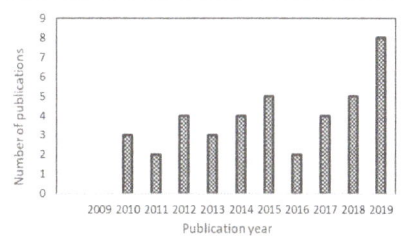

Figure 2. Research papers found using the keywords "MNPs AND biomedical applications" (left part of the figure) and "NiCu NPs AND biomedical applications" (right part of the figure). The number of papers is shown according to the year of publication. The data were obtained by searching the ScienceDirect search engine on 20 September 2019.

As is true for many other MNPs, NiCu MNPs were examined for their use in magnetic hyperthermia (MH) for the treatment of various cancers as their most interesting application type in biomedicine. For this purpose, biocompatible MNPs must be prepared. They are then applied to tumor tissues using different methods (e.g., controlled drug delivery) and subsequently heated in an AMF [38,43,44]. The heat produced through an AMF is influenced by various NP characteristics (size, shape, anisotropy, concentration in situ, and MH parameters, such as the frequency and field), which are all related (directly or indirectly) to their composition. The temperature to which the NPs are heated is defined by their Curie temperature (T_C) [39], which must be between 42 and 46 °C to maximize the selective damage to cancer cells without harming the surrounding healthy tissue [39]. This sometimes requires high frequencies, which represents an important limitation to the use of MNPs in MH [45]. For many years, most of the related research was performed on the two most well-known iron oxides (Fe_3O_4, $\gamma-Fe_2O_3$), although several other materials (e.g., Fe-doped Au NPs and $NiFe_2O_4$) were also developed and successfully employed for this purpose [39]. Furthermore, as shown in several studies, iron oxides are not without limitations, especially if adjustments to T_C play an essential role in therapeutic efficiency. Iron oxides tend to cause overheating because they have comparably higher Tc values, which can induce damage to healthy tissues in the proximity of the application site [46]. This effect does not occur with NiCu MNPs, which have a tunable T_C that is much closer to optimal therapeutic temperatures [16,36,37]. In addition to the abovementioned investigations, research studies from the last couple of years showed that NiCu MNPs have great potential in several other types of biomedical applications, such as their use in bimodal cancer treatments that combine MH and controlled drug delivery [47–49]. Nevertheless, another important factor to be considered when applying a novel formulation for MH is the overall concentration of the respective NPs at the tumor site [50,51]. Specifically, NPs with a low specific loss power (SLP) need to be more concentrated in the tumor, with the consequent disadvantages of bioaccumulation and long-term toxicity [52,53].

In Section 2, this review explores different synthesis methods, along with their main advantages and disadvantages, potential surface modification approaches, and potential in biomedical applications, such as MH, multimodal cancer therapy, MH implants, antibacterial activity, and dentistry.

2. Synthesis of Magnetic NiCu NPs

Various kinds of synthesis methods, ranging from different chemical methods to physical methods, can be used for the preparation of NiCu MNPs. Figure 3 shows a graph that reveals the most commonly used methods, along with percentages of their application for the synthesis of NiCu MNPs according to the literature (the review was performed for the years 2004–2019).

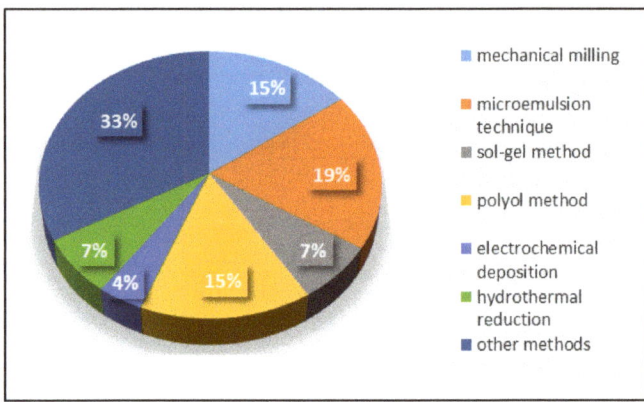

Figure 3. A comparative chart that depicts different synthesis methods of NiCu MNPs.

There are many differences between methods, especially in regard to the ability to control the particle size and the composition of the resulting particles. Furthermore, not all methods are environmentally friendly since they often rely on high temperatures and toxic chemicals (solvents and reducing compounds) and require multiple synthesis steps with low yields [54].

2.1. Mechanical Milling

Mechanical milling is a relatively simple non-equilibrium processing method in which various powdered components are mixed and milled in an inert atmosphere, resulting in the formation of NPs [55]. High-energy ball milling is widely utilized for the synthesis of various nanomaterials, nanograins, nanoalloys, nanocomposites, and nano-quasicrystalline materials. The whole process for this technique is based on the collision phenomena between the "balls" used and the powdered sample. During this process, the powdered particles in the sample are stuck between the colliding balls, which leads to particle deformation/fractionation and, hence, the formation of ultimately smaller particles in the resulting powder. The nature of these processes depends upon the mechanical behavior of the powder components, their phase equilibria, and the stress state during milling [55,56]. Figure 4 shows some examples of the mechanical milling method for the preparation of NiCu MNPs.

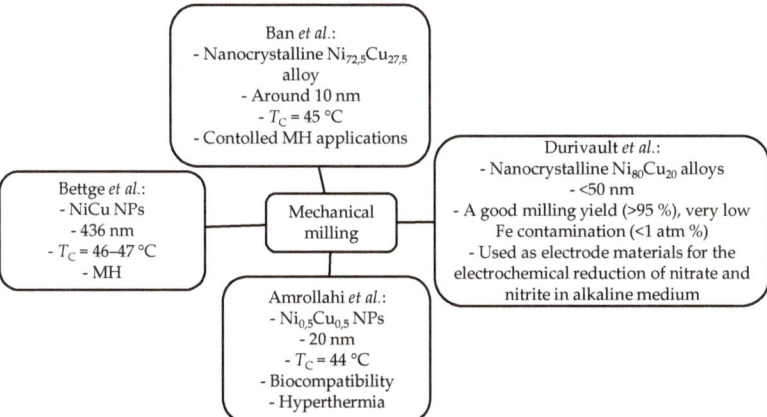

Figure 4. Mechanical milling as a method for the synthesis of NiCu MNPs MH—magnetic hyperthermia. The references to respective studies mentioned in the figure are as follows: Bettge et al. [48], Ban et al. [36], Amrollahi et al. [39], and Durivalt et al. [57].

2.2. Microemulsion Technique

In water-in-oil (W/O) microemulsion systems, fine microdroplets of the aqueous phase are trapped within assemblies of surfactant molecules (frequently in combination with a cosurfactant) dispersed in a continuous oil phase. The size of the reverse micelle is determined by the molar ratio of the water to the surfactant [3]. W/O microemulsions were shown to be an adequate, versatile, simple, and very fast procedure for preparing nanosized particles with a uniform size distribution. These are also the characteristics that could make this method useful for both in vivo and in vitro applications [2]. Figure 5 shows some examples of the microemulsion technique for the preparation of NiCu MNPs.

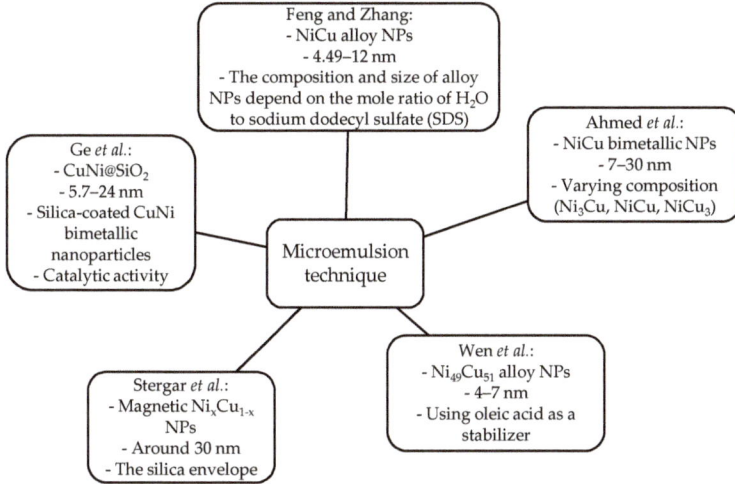

Figure 5. The microemulsion technique as a method for the synthesis of NiCu MNPs. The references to respective studies mentioned in the figure are as follows: Ge et al. [58], Feng and Zhang [42], Ahmed et al. [59], Stergar et al. [60], and Wen et al. [61].

2.3. Sol–Gel Method

The sol–gel method provides a very versatile approach to the preparation of new materials [62]. This method enables the potential control of the textural and surface properties of the resulting materials. In the sol–gel process, the final metal-oxide products are delivered after a few chemical steps: hydrolysis, condensation, and the drying process. The sol–gel method can be classified into two routes, namely, the aqueous sol–gel method and nonaqueous sol–gel method, depending on the nature of the solvent utilized [63]. Figure 6 shows some examples of the sol–gel method for the preparation of NiCu MNPs.

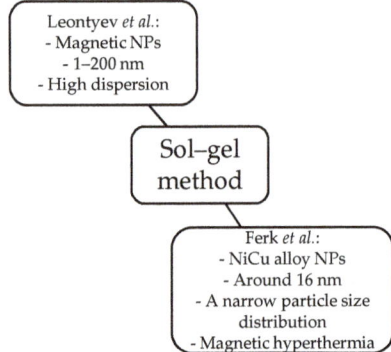

Figure 6. The sol–gel process as a method for the synthesis of NiCu MNPs. The references to respective studies mentioned in the figure are as follows: Leontyev et al. [64], and Ferk et al. [40].

2.4. Polyol Method

The polyol method involves the suspension of a metal precursor in a glycol solvent and the subsequent heating of the solution to a refluxing temperature [65]. This technique is used to synthesize metallic, oxide, and semiconductor NPs. A polyol is often used as the solvent and is combined with a reducing agent and a ligand to prevent NP agglomeration. The polyol method was shown to be very promising for the preparation of uniform NPs with a narrow size distribution for potential use in biomedical applications [65,66]. Figure 7 shows some examples of the polyol method for the preparation of NiCu MNPs.

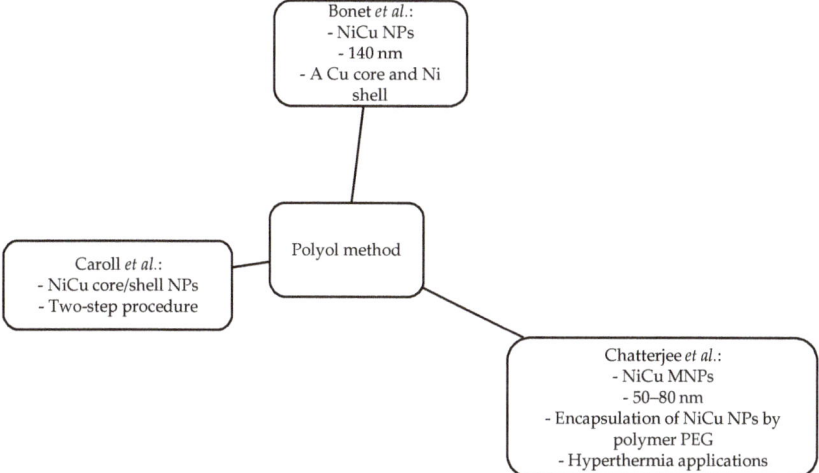

Figure 7. The polyol method as a method for the synthesis of NiCu MNPs. PEG—polyethylene glycol. The references to respective studies mentioned in the figure are as follows: Caroll et al. [67], Bonet et al. [68], and Chatterjee et al. [47].

2.5. Electrochemical Deposition

Electrodeposition of metals and alloys is of wide interest and finds application in a number of fields. The electrodeposition technique involves the use of a conducting surface, onto which metal or alloy sample coatings are deposited using electrolysis. This process is performed using an electrolyte with a strictly defined composition (bath), which can be an aqueous solution of a simple salt, complex salt, or mixture [69]. Figure 8 shows some examples of the electrochemical deposition method for the preparation of NiCu MNPs.

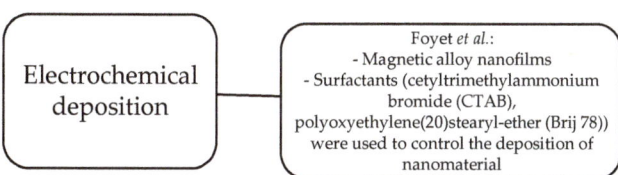

Figure 8. Electrochemical deposition as a method for the synthesis of NiCu MNPs. The reference to the mentioned study is *Foyet* et al. [70].

2.6. Hydrothermal Reduction

Hydrothermal synthesis refers to the synthesis of substances via chemical reactions in a sealed and heated solution above ambient temperature and pressure. The crystal growth is normally performed in an apparatus consisting of a steel pressure vessel called an autoclave. Hydrothermal synthesis involves water acting both as a catalyst and occasionally as a component of solid phases during synthesis at elevated temperature and pressure [71]. Figure 9 shows some examples of hydrothermal reduction for the preparation of NiCu MNPs.

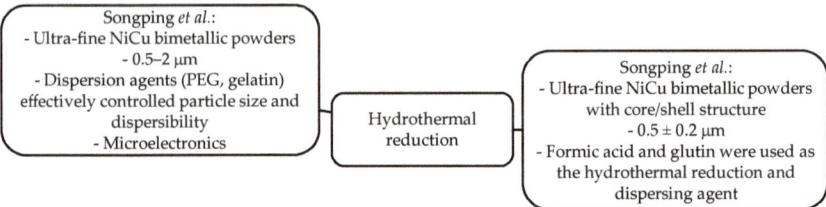

Figure 9. The hydrothermal method as a method for the synthesis of NiCu MNPs. The references to respective studies mentioned in the figure are as follows: Songping et al. [41], and Songping et al. [72].

2.7. Other Methods

MNPs can also be synthesized by other methods, such as hydrogen reduction [21,38], a combination of melting and ball milling [48], hot compressed water [54], electrical explosions [73], pulsed-spray evaporation [74], the solution combustion method [75], the sonoelectrochemical technique [76], solvothermal synthesis from metal precursors [77], and the polymeric precursor method [78]. Figure 10 summarizes some examples of other methods that were reported for the preparation of NiCu MNPs.

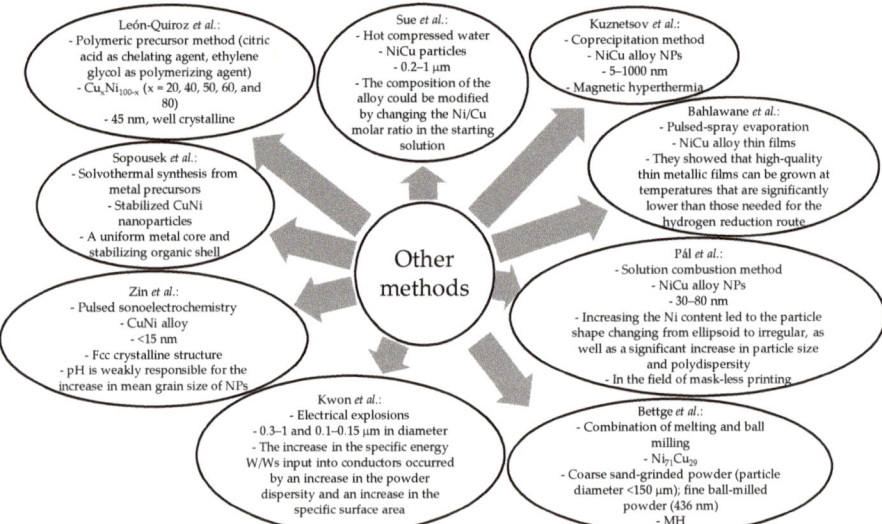

Figure 10. Other methods for the synthesis of NiCu MNPs. Fcc—face-centered cubic. The references to respective studies mentioned in the figure are as follows: León-Quiroz et al. [78], Sopousek et al. [77], Zin et al. [76], Sue et al. [54], Kuznetsov et al. [38], Bahlawane et al. [74], Pál et al. [75], Kwon et al. [73], and Bettge et al. [48].

Figure 11 shows a schematic that depicts the general outlines of the most commonly employed methods to synthesize NiCu MNPs. Furthermore, Figure 12 shows TEM or SEM micrographs of the NPs resulting from most of the mentioned synthesis methods.

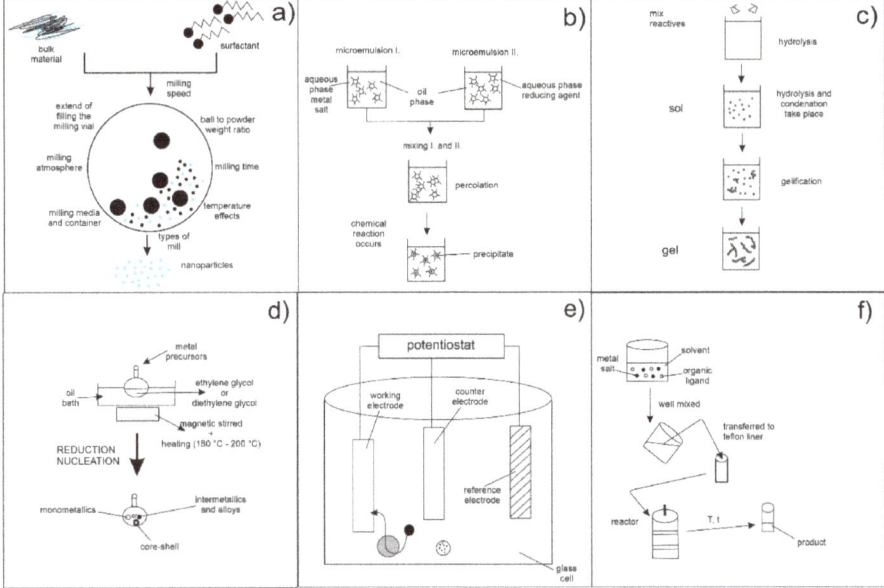

Figure 11. Schematic representation of different synthesis methods of NiCu MNPs: (**a**) mechanical milling, (**b**) microemulsion, (**c**) sol–gel, (**d**) the polyol method, (**e**) electrochemical deposition, and (**f**) hydrothermal reduction.

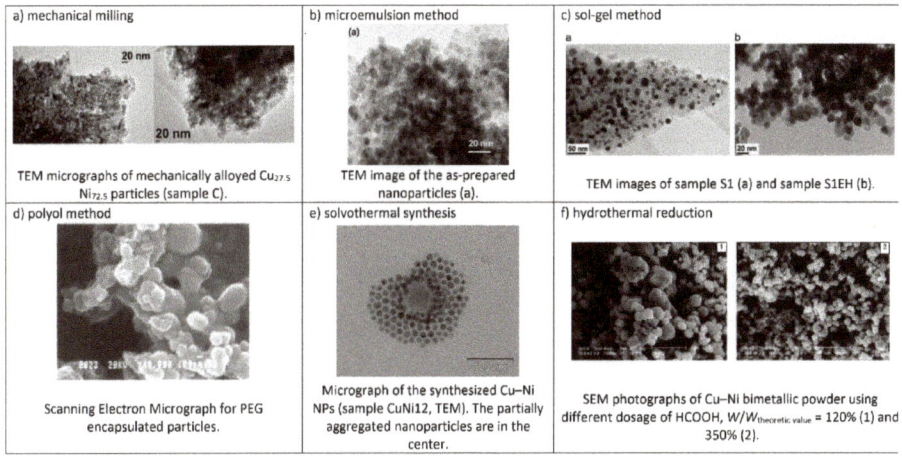

Figure 12. TEM or SEM micrographs of NiCu MNPs prepared using different synthesis methods: (**a**) mechanical milling [36], (**b**) microemulsion [79], (**c**) sol–gel [40], (**d**) the polyol method [47], (**e**) electrochemical deposition [77], and (**f**) hydrothermal reduction [41]. Permission for micrograph reuse was granted by the respective publishers.

In Table 1, we summarize the available preparation methods of different NiCu formulations and their main properties (type, size, structure) and their general usability [80]. Table 1 also compares the different NiCu MNP preparation procedures, with a focus on the general properties of the synthesized NiCu formations, their advantages and disadvantages, and their possible biomedical applications.

Table 1. Preparation methods, types of material, magnetic nanoparticle (MNP) size, advantages and disadvantages, and biomedical applications of different NiCu structures. MH—magnetic hyperthermia.

Method	Types of Material	MNP Size	Advantages	Disadvantages	Biomedical Applications	References
Mechanical milling	- Nanocrystalline Ni_xCu_{1-x} alloys - NiCu nanoparticles	10–436 nm	- A good milling yield (>95%) - Broad NP size distribution - Biocompatibility - T_C = 46–47 °C	- Fe contamination - T_C of 45 °C - Agglomeration - Agglomeration without a liquid medium	- Controlled MH applications	[36,39,48,57]
Microemulsion technique	- NiCu alloy nanoparticles	4–30 nm	- Spherical, uniform NPs - Monodispersed, spherical NPs - Crystallization behavior - Fast synthesis procedure	- A core/shell structure - Additional step (reduction)	- MH	[42,58–61]
Sol-gel method	- NiCu alloy nanoparticles	1–200 nm	- Spherical shape - Narrow NP size distribution, spherical shape	- High dispersion - The silica matrix influences magnetic behavior	- MH	[40,64]
Polyol method	- NiCu magnetic nanoparticles - NiCu core/shell nanoparticles	40–140 nm	- A uniform shape - T_C = ~77 °C - Simple procedure	- A Cu core and a Ni shell - Two-step procedure	- MH	[47,67,68]
Electrochemical deposition	- Magnetic alloy nanofilms - Ultra-fine NiCu bimetallic powders	/	- Nanostructured films	- Two peaks in the polarization curve	/	[70]
Hydrothermal technique	- Ultra-fine NiCu bimetallic powders with a core/shell structure	0.5 ± 0.2 μm	- Excellent dispersibility, a uniform size - Finest dispersibility	- Agglomeration	/	[41,72]
Other methods	- NiCu alloy nanoparticles - NiCu alloy thin films - NiCu alloy NPs	5–1000 nm	- The composition of the alloy could be controlled by changing the Ni/Cu molar ratio in the starting solution - Applying a magnetic field (44 kHz) on the liver resulted in temperature stabilization (42 °C) - Superparamagnetic behavior - Irregular shapes of NPs	- Polydispersed particles - Additional thermal treatment - Heterogeneously distributed particle size - Broad size distribution - Oxidized surface in air	- MH	[38,48,54,73–78]

3. NiCu MNP Functionalization Methods

Most MNPs require modifications to their surface for improved biocompatibility to increase the possibility of their use in biomedicine [81]. The following diverse groups of coating materials were used to modify MNP surface chemistry:

- Synthetic polymers, such as polymethylmethacrylate (PMMA), poly(lactic-*co*-glycolic acid) (PLGA), poly(vinylpyrrolidone) (PVP), polyethylene glycol (PEG), polyvinyl alcohol (PVA), and alginate [81–84];
- Natural polymers, such as dextran, starch, chitosan, pullulan, and gelatin [85–89];
- Organic surfactants, such as dodecylamine, oleic acid, oleylamine, sodium carboxymethylcellulose, and sodium oleate [90,91];
- Inorganic metals (e.g., gold and silica) are the most often used surface functionalization layers of MNPs [90,92];
- Bioactive molecules and structures, such as liposomes, lipids, ligands/receptors, and peptides [93–97].

Some of the abovementioned surface functionalization methods were employed for NiCu MNPs.

Chatterjee et al. [47] prepared PEG-functionalized NiCu MNPs using two different preparation techniques. Ultrasonication was used to prepare a stable and homogenous dispersion of NiCu MNPs in PEG as part of the first method, and an oil (a mixture of n-hexane, mineral oil, and sodium sesquioleate)/water (suspension of NiCu particles in a PEG solution) microemulsion was prepared in the second method. In the second method, ultrasonication was used to homogenize the dispersion, followed by cross-linking. TEM analysis revealed that the first approach formed more composites, while, in the second approach, the encapsulation of spherical NiCu MNPs predominated. The average sizes of the prepared NPs (and composites) were between 200 and 500 nm, and the main factor that influenced their size was the initial NP size. The encapsulated particles had a T_C in the desired range of 320–330 K, which is in the therapeutic range for MH applications. The saturation magnetization for the $Ni_{70}Cu_{30}$ composition was ~6–8 emu/g [47].

Biswas et al. [98] synthesized a NiCu nanoalloy with chain-like particles. Their preparation method was performed using two polymers: PEG and poly(4-vinylphenol) (PVPh). These materials were used to stabilize the structure of the forming nanoalloy and to control the structural features of the forming particles, respectively. Using this method, the authors obtained two types of final products, namely, NiCu–PEG and NiCu–PVPh alloy nanostructures. Simultaneously, they prepared a control NiCu alloy sample without the use of these polymers. The formed products differed in their dispersibility in organic and water-based solvents. For example, the NiCu–PEG particles could be dispersed in both water and (some) organic solvents (dioxan, xylene, acetonitrile, and ethanol). On the contrary, the NiCu–PVPh particles could be dissolved in water and in dimethylformamide (DMF). The authors used TEM analysis to assess the shapes and sizes of the prepared alloy nanostructures. For the NiCu–PEG sample, the images revealed chain-like structures that were formed from apparently spherical NPs with an average diameter of 8 ± 1.1 nm. For the other sample, NiCu–PVPh, similar nanochains were formed with a comparable average size of 7.5 ± 1.8 nm. The saturation magnetization for NiCu–PEG was 38 emu/g; it was 34 emu/g for NiCu–PVPh and 11.5 emu/g for bare CuNi. The presence of copper oxide over bare NiCu (X-ray diffraction (XRD) analysis) was probably the reason that the saturation magnetization value of bare NiCu was lower than that of the other two polymer alloy samples [98].

Araújo-Barbosa et al. [99] produced non-aggregated and monodispersed NiCu alloy NPs embedded in a chitosan matrix. A modified sol–gel method that included the use of the chitosan polymer prevented the particles from aggregating and favored the formation of particles with a narrow size distribution. The mixing step of the synthesis, which involved mixing $Ni(NO_3)_2 \times 6H_2O$ and $CuCl_2 \times 2H_2O$ with a chitosan solution, was performed at room temperature. After 20 min of stirring, they added 1 mL of glutaraldehyde and stirred for an additional 20 min. They let the dispersion rest for 1 h to allow polymerization to occur. After polymerization, they treated the precursor in vacuum at 450 °C for 1.5 h. The second heat treatment was performed in a H_2 gas atmosphere (6 mL/s) for 1.5 h at 450 °C. They prepared four samples with different compositions: $Ni_{70}Cu_{30}$, $Ni_{75}Cu_{25}$, $Ni_{81}Cu_{19}$, and $Ni_{95}Cu_5$ (all wt.%). The TEM images showed well-dispersed, non-aggregated NPs with specific morphologies. The sizes of the NPs ranged between 11 and 20 nm. Magnetic moments increased (per unit cell) with increasing Ni concentration, and the samples had a specific loss power of up to 5.86 W/g at a low field and frequency, which indicated a promising efficiency for MH [99].

Wen et al. [61] prepared NiCu MNPs by the reduction of $CuSO_4 \times 5H_2O$ and $NiCl_2 \times 6H_2O$ with KBH_4 in a positive (hexane/sodium oleate/water) system and then functionalized their surface using oleic acid directly in the formed microemulsion. The as-synthesized alloy NPs exhibited an amorphous structure and were further annealed at 923 K for 0.5 h in argon to obtain the desired crystal structure. TEM analysis of the as-synthesized NPs showed an average particle size of 4–7 nm, and the particles did not agglomerate. To prevent their agglomeration during annealing, the authors of the study coated them with oleic acid, and they used thermogravimetric analysis to show that oleic acid efficiently covered the particle surface. A weight loss between 572.2 and 651.9 K was reported as a confirmation of the presence of oleic acid in the prepared samples. According to the authors, this weight loss can be attributed to the evaporation and decomposition of oleic acid. Analysis of the magnetic properties of the synthesized MNPs revealed special soft magnetic characteristics [61].

Pramanik et al. [100] prepared NiCu NPs composed of tunable ratios of the respective metals in SiO_2 films. Initially, they formed undoped inorganic-organic hybrid solutions based on tetraethyl orthosilicate (TEOS), 3-(glycidoxypropyl) trimethoxysilane (GLYMO), n-butanol, water, methanol, HNO_3, and aluminum acetylacetonate $(Al(acac)_3)$ [100]. To perform metal ion doping, the authors prepared five different sols to achieve various Ni/Cu ratios ($Ni_{1-x}Cu_x$; $x = 0, 0.333, 0.5, 0.666, 1$). The ratio of $Ni_{1-x}Cu_x$ to SiO_2 = 20:80 was kept constant, regardless of the sol composition. The final (control) sol was undoped, and its SiO_2 content was the same as that of the other compositions. The next preparation step was the formation of silica coatings. Using the $Ni_{1-x}Cu_x$ samples, they prepared five different thin film samples and dried them in a two-step process (drying at 60 °C for 1 h, followed by drying at 90 °C for another 1 h). The as-prepared thin film samples were further heat-treated in another two-step procedure (first in air at 450 °C for 1 h and then in a 10 wt.% H_2/90 wt.% Ar atmosphere at 750 °C for 1 h). The first heat treatment step was to remove organics, and the second step was to complete the alloy formation. With the same steps, the control (undoped) NiCu coating was prepared on a polished silicon wafer. The authors then assessed the thicknesses of the prepared thin films. The average thickness was measured to be 310 ± 10 nm. Furthermore, the authors reported that the prepared film sample showed excellent adherence, as well as very good abrasion resistance [100]. From XRD diffractograms, the authors determined that a NiCu face-centered cubic (fcc) alloy was formed with an average size of 6 nm. Finally, the particle size was determined using TEM. The determined values were in agreement with those from the XRD analysis (~6.35 nm). TEM analysis further confirmed that the NiCu NPs were embedded in silica [100].

Stergar and Ferk et al. reported the preparation of NiCu MNPs using an emulsion-based approach [60] and the sol–gel process [37,40]. In both cases, the authors reported the use of silica as the stabilizing component for the prevention of MNP agglomeration. In the emulsion-based approach, they mixed the metal chlorides with hydrazine hydrate and NaOH to form a cationic water-in-oil microemulsion [101]. The silica surface protection layers (10 nm thick) were prepared from a solution of TEOS in ethanol with polyvinylpyrrolidone (PVP) as a surfactant and ultrasonication for 24 h at 60 °C. Apparently, the T_C value was not affected by the coating procedure. The magnetization of the uncoated sample was 22 emu/g, and no hysteresis or superparamagnetic behavior was observed for this sample. On the other hand, the coated particles exhibited 7 emu/g magnetization, as well as marked hysteresis. According to the obtained results, the silica-based coating effectively diminished potential agglomeration during the heat treatment while simultaneously improving the biocompatibility of the MNPs [60]. In the sol–gel process-based method, Ferk et al. also prepared NiCu MNPs, which were stabilized using silica-based functionalization [37,40]. Firstly, the authors prepared a solution of Ni and Cu salts, citric acid, and other components for the synthesis (i.e., deionized water, ethanol, and TEOS).

As in previous studies, the authors followed a multi-step drying/heating regime until the final NiCu MNP product was prepared. The process included a drying step for 72 h at room temperature and two-step calcination of the formed gel in air at 500 °C for 24 h [40] and at 800 °C for 6 h [37]. The final product was a powder mixture of Ni and Cu oxides in a silica matrix. To homogenize the product and form NiCu MNPs in silica, the authors used a H_2/Ar atmosphere. The particles exhibited a narrow particle size distribution with an average diameter of 16.6 nm. The T_C was 63 °C for $Ni_{67.5}Cu_{32.5}$, 54 °C for $Ni_{62.5}Cu_{37.5}$, and 51 °C for $Ni_{60}Cu_{40}$. In this case, the authors showed that, although silica prevented the agglomeration of the formed NiCu MNPs, it also had some negative influences on the samples. In particular, their magnetic and calorimetric properties were decreased. The as-prepared samples (in a silica matrix) were exposed to an etching solution (a mixture of NaOH/hydrazine hydrate) to obtain NiCu MNPs only. For 24 h, the samples were continuously stirred in an Ar atmosphere, after which the NiCu MNPs were collected by centrifugation [37,40].

4. Application of NiCu MNPs in Biomedicine

NiCu MNPs are still considered novel materials that can be produced through environmentally friendly methods and exhibit properties that are appropriate for biomedical use. Despite their relatively recent development, they were the subject of an increasing number of studies over the last few years (Figure 2).

As in the case of other superparamagnetic MNP investigations, most of the NiCu MNP research studies focused on MH applications [36–40,47,48,60,79,99]. In addition to the studies mentioned above, newer studies reported their potential use in bimodal cancer treatment formulations (e.g., a combination of MH and controlled drug delivery) [16], as part of medical implants [49,101], in formulations with antibacterial activity [102], and as part of dental materials [103]. The potential uses of NiCu MNPs in biomedicine are summarized in Figure 13.

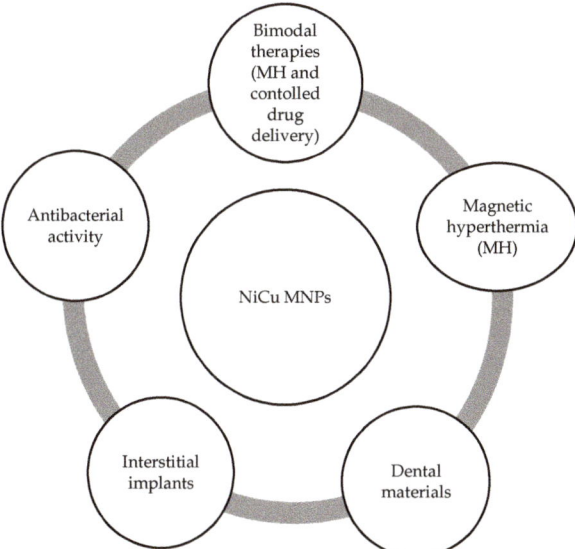

Figure 13. Potential applications of NiCu MNPs in biomedicine. The references to respective studies mentioned in the figure are as follows: Antibacterial activity [60], Bimodal therapies [17], MH [37–41,48,49,96,98,99], Interstitial implants [50,100], Dental materials [101].

Because of the steadily increasing number of research studies on NiCu-based materials for these and other types of applications, this section reviews their different uses, with an explicit focus on synthesis, functionalization, and other aspects that make them appropriate for biomedical purposes.

4.1. Magnetic Hyperthermia

MH is a promising non-invasive type of cancer therapy that makes use of MNPs that generate heat under controllable external stimuli. It uses a combination of an AMF and biocompatible MNPs with a T_C value as close as possible to 42–46 °C as heating agents. This temperature interval was proven to be ideal for destroying cancer cells with minimal harm to the healthy surrounding tissues [17]. Therefore, it is important to understand the underlying physical mechanisms via which heat is generated in small MNPs by AMFs [104]. Among the various available MNPs, NiCu MNPs with a tailorable T_C in the temperature interval 42–46 °C seem ideally suited for future effective MH formulations [36,38,39,47,48].

Bettge et al. [48] developed a new, relatively simple procedure for NiCu alloy particle synthesis that was based on the combination of ball milling and the melting of bulk materials. The resulting formulation consisted of particles with sizes below a micron that were shown to be good candidate materials for self-controlled MH treatment. The milled particles were found to be slightly above 400 nm. However, their most important finding was that the prepared formulation exhibited a T_C in the desired therapeutic range (46–47 °C), making them suitable for self-regulating MH. Using TEM analysis, the authors further determined that the particles were not uniform in shape, with some of them being spherical and the others having a flake-like appearance [48].

Chatterjee et al. [47] prepared novel NiCu NPs with a PEG surface layer using the polyol reduction technique. In addition to the other advantages of the PEG coating (e.g., decreased agglomeration, improved biocompatibility), a beneficial effect was observed on the T_C, which fell from ~77 °C to the desired ~46 °C. Furthermore, the coated NPs showed a suitable saturation magnetization of 6–8 emu/g. These findings all suggest that the prepared PEG-functionalized NPs are promising materials for use in MH [47].

Kuznetsov et al. [38] produced alloy NiCu MNPs using various methods. The authors reported that the best results were obtained by the co-precipitation of Cu and Ni salts in the presence of Na_2CO_3 at room temperature, with a consecutive reduction in a H_2 atmosphere (at 300–1000 °C). This initial particle preparation step was followed by various grinding/separation methods to achieve more uniform NP sizes, as well as a more homogenous composition. This step also enabled the control of the formulation's T_C and, thus, increased their potential for use in MH. The potential applicability of the prepared materials to cancer treatment was shown by testing this formulation on a rat liver tumor model. The results showed their effective potential use as part of magnetic fluid hyperthermia [38].

Ban et al. [36] showed the potential of a simple milling-based method to produce nanosized NiCu alloy NPs with potential application in MH. By optimizing the milling process, they were able to produce nanocrystalline $Ni_{72.5}Cu_{27.5}$ alloy NPs with an average size of 10 nm. Further, the particles exhibited a T_C in the MH suitable therapeutic range (~45 °C). The authors proved the superparamagnetic nature of the prepared NiCu NPs by showing that the hysteresis loops lacked remanent magnetization. Significant heat induction of the powdered samples indicated that they are highly promising for use in self-regulating MH [36].

Stergar et al. [101] reported another interesting synthesis approach to preparing Ni_xCu_{1-x} NPs in a water/oil (W/O) microemulsion. Although the particles were partially agglomerated (confirmed using TEM analysis), they exhibited an average size of ~30 nm. The most likely explanation for the determined T_C being very close to that of pure Ni was that the particles showed a core/shell structure. To homogenize the sample, the authors performed a heating step in a reducing atmosphere in a tube furnace at 900 °C. This led to the formation of a solid solution of Ni/Cu, which had an expected Tc value of ~65 °C according to the formulation's nominal composition. Again, a silica coating proved to be the right choice to prevent particle agglomeration without affecting the T_C value [60]. Although the developed synthesis method is very promising for the preparation of a versatile range of NiCu MNPs, the authors noted that further optimizations of the formulation are necessary to achieve a Tc in a range that is suitable for use in MH.

Ferk et al. [40] developed a sol–gel-based NiCu MNP preparation method, which yielded NPs with a narrow size distribution. The method included the reduction of Ni and Cu oxides in silica, leading to the formation of $Ni_{1-x}Cu_x$ MNPs in SiO_2. To obtain pure particles, the authors etched the silica matrix using NaOH/hydrazine hydrate. Through this processing, only $Ni_{67.5}Cu_{32.5}$ nanospheres with a narrow size distribution were retained in the sample. Thermogravimetric analysis (TGA)/single differential thermal analysis (SDTA) was used to determine a T_C value of ~65 °C for the samples [40]. This was the first study to report the successful production of superparamagnetic NiCu nanospheres with a narrow size distribution and the capability of controlling the T_C for potential application in MH [40].

Amrollahi et al. [39] used mechanical milling to produce $Ni_{0.5}Cu_{0.5}$ NPs for potential use in MH applications. The ball milling-based initial synthesis stage (30 h) was concluded with a heating step for 1 h at 500 °C. Using XRD analysis, the authors showed that only single-phase NPs were formed. The particle size and rate of agglomeration were established using TEM. The authors reported a narrow size distribution of particles with an average size of ~20 nm, although these were mostly part of larger agglomerates. Nevertheless, the potential of the prepared NPs for use in MH was proven by their measured T_C of 44 °C. To further demonstrate the suitability of these NPs for MH, the authors performed biocompatibility/cytotoxicity testing using human bone marrow stem cells (hMSCs) and proved that the formulation did not harm them [39]. A summary of various other related research studies that reported the use of NiCu MNPs in MH (including some of their most important properties) is shown in Table 2.

Table 2. Type, synthesis method, composition (w), average particle size (d_x), Curie temperature (T_C), magnetization (M_S), and specific absorption rate (SAR) of NiCu materials for MH. PEG—polyethylene glycol.

Types of Materials	Synthesis Methods	Surface Modification	w (atm. %)	d_x (nm)	T_C (°C)	M_S (emu/g)	SAR (W/g)	References
CuNi alloy NPs	Polyol reduction method —and— physical melting process	PEG	$Cu_{30}Ni_{70}$	50–80 / 300–400	43–46	45 / 6–8	/	Chatterjee et al. [47]
NiCu alloy NPs	Sol–gel method	Silica matrix	$Ni_{67.5}Cu_{32.5}$ $Ni_{62.5}Cu_{37.5}$ $Ni_{60}Cu_{40}$	15–20	51–63	3–9	0.12–0.60	Ferk et al. [37]
NiCu alloy NPs	Sol–gel method	Silica matrix	$Ni_{67.5}Cu_{32.5}$ $Ni_{70}Cu_{30}$	16	65	8	/	Ferk et al. [40]
$Cu_{1-x}Ni_x$ NPs	Cationic water-in-oil (W/O) microemulsions	Silica	$Ni_{72.5}Cu_{27.5}$ $Ni_{60}Cu_{40}$ $Ni_{70}Cu_{30}$	/	45–88	22 (uncoated) 7 (coated)	/	Stergar et al. [60]
$Ni_{1-x}Cu_x$ alloys	Modified sol–gel method	Chitosan matrix	$Ni_{75}Cu_{25}$ $Ni_{81}Cu_{19}$ $Ni_{95}Cu_5$	11–20	77–277	21–50	0.289–0.576	Araújo-Barbosa et al. [99]
CuNi NPs	Mechano-thermal method	/	$Cu_{50}Ni_{50}$	20	44	18	260.44	Amrollahi et al. [39]
CuNi alloy NPs	Co-precipitation of salts from solution followed by reduction in hydrogen and thermal treatment (sol–gel method)	NaCl matrix	25–30 atm.% of Cu	30	40–60	/	/	Kuznetsov et al. [38]
NiCu NPs	Melting and ball milling	/	$Ni_{70}Cu_{30}$ $Cu_{40}Ni_{60}$ $Cu_{30}Ni_{70}$	436	46–47	/	/	Bettge et al. [48]
Cu_xNi_{1-x} alloys	Mechanical milling	/	$Cu_{27.5}Ni_{72.5}$ $Cu_{27}Ni_{73}$ $Cu_{25}Ni_{75}$ $Cu_{20}Ni_{80}$	10–12	24–174	4.4–32.9	/	Ban et al. [36]
CuNi alloy NPs	Microemulsion method	/	$Cu_{27.5}Ni_{72.5}$	28	43	2.5–20	4.3–41.6	Stergar et al. [79]

4.2. Bimodal Cancer Therapy (A Combination of MH and Controlled Drug Delivery)

Controlled drug delivery systems have several advantages compared with traditional pharmaceutical formulations. For example, they enable drug transportation to the desired site of action in the body with minimal damage to healthy surrounding tissues. Delivery systems with these characteristics are key for drugs that exhibit a narrow therapeutic index or drugs that are directly cytotoxic to healthy cells (e.g., most antitumor drugs) [17]. Recent findings suggest that NiCu MNPs are very promising for the combination of MH and controlled drug delivery [17].

Stergar et al. [16] prepared a novel controlled drug delivery formulation composed of $Ni_{67.5}Cu_{32.5}$ MNPs in a silica matrix synthesized using the sol–gel procedure. They used the fluorescent dye rhodamine 6G to evaluate the ability of MNPs to deliver the drug to various human cells (a healthy cell line of human skin-derived fibroblasts and the cancerous cell lines HeLa and Caco-2). The progressive $Ni_{67.5}Cu_{32.5}$ MNPs were shown to be a dependable (confirmed through biocompatibility and cytotoxicity assays) and efficient delivery system (in vitro cell delivery model) to various human cell types. The obtained results indicate that the proposed formulation has a very high potential for the future development of drug delivery systems that specifically target these cells. The process explored the protection of particles during drug delivery and MH, and the results confirmed the successful application of $Ni_{67.5}Cu_{32.5}$ particles with a T_C of about 43 °C and drug accumulation in a silica protecting layer.

4.3. MH Implants

Interstitial hyperthermia using magnetic materials is known as magnetic induction hyperthermia. Soft heating or implant heating systems are excellent systems for this purpose. In these systems, the ferromagnetic material (implant) is firstly implanted in the cancer tissue, followed by the utilization of an eddy current or magnetic hysteresis loss under a high-frequency AMF to generate highly localized heating. The temperature of the cancer tissue is raised and regulated at the T_C of the implant material [105].

Paulus et al. [49] explored novel, low-T_C ferromagnetic NiCu (28 wt.% Ni) and PdCo (6.15 wt.% Pd) formulations as part of interstitial implants in prostate cancer therapy. Initially, they performed a melting step, in which both alloys were put into a carbon arc furnace. This step was followed by a heat treatment step to induce sample recrystallization (at 1000 °C). The annealed NiCu and PdCo samples were spot-welded to Cu wire connections, and the junctions were closed using a water-resistant epoxy adhesive. Potential contaminants on the sample surface were removed by polishing using a 1-µm diamond paste. The as-prepared samples proved to be more corrosion-resistant, even after longer immersion times. The authors explained this phenomenon by the formation of passivation layers on the sample surface. It was further established that the PdCo alloy outperformed the NiCu sample with regard to the corrosion stabilization time in solution. This finding was additionally backed by proving the excellent corrosion resistance of this sample in vitro. On the basis of all the findings, the authors concluded that the developed formulations are promising for the intended use, even in long-term hyperthermia applications [49].

El-Sayed et al. [101] developed a manufacturing procedure of PdNi, PdCo, and NiCu ferromagnetic thermoseeds to increase the sharpness of T_C for interstitial hyperthermia in cancer treatment. They characterized the prepared seeds by magnetic measurements as a function of temperature and magnetic field strength. The ferromagnetic thermoseeds showed a sharp decrease in ferromagnetic to paramagnetic transition temperatures at 52, 57, and 49 °C and the heat production of T_C. These seeds provided a power output at 20 °C of about 150, 200, and 75 mW/cm, as measured from the hysteresis loops. The temperature dependence of the seed power was computed from a combination of Curie and induction laws. Their computations showed a good agreement with the values calculated from the area under the hysteresis loops at an AMF with a frequency of 100 kHz and field strength of 4 kA/m. The power automatically stopped when T_C was reached, indicating that the seeds had self-limiting temperature control. This self-limitation indicates the high potential of these seeds for potential exploitation in clinics, especially for treating localized tumors [102].

4.4. Antibacterial Activity

Antibacterial activity is related to compounds that locally kill bacteria or slow their growth without being toxic to the surrounding tissue. In general, the agents can be classified as either bactericidal (agents that kill bacteria) or bacteriostatic (agents that slow bacterial growth) [106]. In the area of antibacterial agents, metal nanoparticles are of particular interest because of their high surface areas and, hence, their large number of potential active (antibacterial) sites per unit area. A distinct class of metal oxides with distinctive magnetic properties and superior biocompatibility is iron-oxide NPs [107]. Indeed, various metal NPs demonstrated broad-spectrum antibacterial properties against both Gram-positive and Gram-negative bacteria. For example, ZnO NPs were found to inhibit *Staphylococcus aureus*, and Ag NPs exhibited concentration-dependent antimicrobial activity against *Escherichia coli* and *Pseudomonas aeruginosa* [106–109]. NiCu MNPs were also previously studied for the same purpose. The example below shows their potential uses for this purpose.

Parimaladevi et al. [102] synthesized Cu, Ni, and CuNi bimetallic NPs through the solvothermal method. They added $CuSO_4$ and NaOH, $NiNO_3$ and NaOH, and $CuSO_4$ and $NiNO_3$ (1:1) to hydrazine (reducing agent) and ethylene glycol (solvent). The mixture was stirred for 15 min and transferred to an autoclave (150 °C, 5 h). The obtained precipitate was separated by centrifugation and washed repeatedly with water and ethanol. The antibacterial activity of Cu, Ni, and CuNi NPs was evaluated against Gram-positive *Staphylococcus aureus* and Gram-negative *Escherichia coli* using a standard agar well diffusion method. A standard antibacterial drug, cefixime, was used in each plate. The test results against the Gram-positive bacterium *S. aureus* showed a higher inhibition compared with the results against Gram-negative *E. coli* for all NPs. Larger zones of inhibition were recorded for CuNi NPs than the monometallic NPs; this observation is most likely the result of the unique distribution of the two different metals, enabling the simultaneous release (and activity) of two different metal ions, namely, Cu^{2+} and Ni^{2+}. The observed toxicity was similar to that of cefixime, suggesting that the CuNi NPs were utilized in abundance at sites of possible infections, such as pneumonia and strep throat. The cost-effectiveness of CuNi NPs and their lethality toward both Gram-positive and Gram-negative bacteria may lead to numerous applications, such as antibacterial coatings, paints, surfaces, and films [102].

4.5. Dental Materials

There are various applications of NPs (carbon-based nanomaterials, hydroxyapatite, iron oxide, zirconia, silica, silver, and titania) in dentistry [110]. Biocomposite materials (e.g., tiny calcium phosphate crystallites) that bear structural and chemical similarity to hydroxyapatite were shown to effectively integrate into growing human bone. This is related to the fact that hydroxyapatite is a natural nanocomposite in the body that is formed naturally by bone-derived cells. Typically, these materials are used as part of implant coatings to improve the implant's overall biocompatibility and often contribute to better wear resistance; both of these functions are important in the preparation of bone grafts. Recently, novel methods in dentistry were developed in which organically modified ceramic and its fillers are used to enhance dispersion and biocompatibility, accompanied by a simultaneous increase in the toughness of the implant. Iron-oxide nanoparticles are very useful for eradicating biofilms on dental implants. Alumina/zirconia nanocomposites are new implant materials that show better efficacy compared with ceramic materials. Zirconia-oxide nanoparticles were found to have anti-biofilm activity against certain bacteria (such as *Enterococcus faecalis*); therefore, they can be used effectively as polishing agents in dental practices [110,111]. NiCu MNPs are also emerging as potential materials for future use in dentistry. Some examples are described below.

Argueta-Figueroa et al. [103] developed various single-metal and bimetallic alloy materials based on Ni and Cu and tested their antibacterial activity. The main purpose of their study was to evaluate the formulation for use in dentistry. The bimetallic NiCu MNP formulation was prepared by chemical reduction with NaBH$_4$. Antibacterial activity was assessed against three different bacteria, namely, Gram-positive *Staphylococcus aureus*, Gram-negative *Escherichia coli*, and the more dentistry-specific pathogen *Streptococcus mutans* (Gram-positive). Using the developed preparation method for the NiCu MNPs, the authors obtained a combination of three crystal structures, namely, both metal oxides and the alloy (determined through XRD analysis). Of all the synthesis parameters, pH had one of the strongest influences on the final ratio between the metals in the samples. A narrow size distribution and an average size of around 25 nm were found. The as-prepared Cu NPs showed a bactericidal effect on all three tested bacteria, whereas the Ni NPs and the bimetallic NiCu NPs were only bacteriostatic. From the obtained results, the authors concluded that the prepared materials have great potential for future use in dentistry [103].

5. Biosafety Considerations

As is the case with all other formulations for human use, NiCu MNPs must be appropriately evaluated for their safety. This is the most important evaluation since both metal elements can have toxic effects on the human body [112]. Nevertheless, as we showed in one of our previous (in vitro) studies [16], the biocompatibility of Ni$_{67.5}$Cu$_{32.5}$ MNPs in a silica matrix should not pose a problem. For the time span of the performed study, we are also positive that no leaching of metal ions occurred, which might have negatively affected cell growth [16]. As an integral part of this review, we also present various strategies of NiCu MNP functionalization. The purpose of functionalization is often to improve the biocompatibility of the core materials with the target (human body) environment. Of the most frequently used "shells", silica is by far the most common [90,92]. Therefore, the developed MNPs have very high potential for the future development of drug delivery systems for specific applications targeting cells (and, hence, tissues). Since the core nanoalloy compositions also vary, it is also important to consider Ni/Cu ratios. For example, MNPs with the composition Cu$_{0.5}$Ni$_{0.5}$ were demonstrated to be safe for cancer treatment applications [39].

Although we understand that further studies are necessary to prove the "full" safety of NiCu MNPs for potential patients, we also acknowledge that there are already available strategies that can diminish even potential toxic effects (the bar for potential risks posed by chemotherapy agents is set relatively low) that might occur with Ni or Cu degradation products [113]. One strategy could be to take advantage of their superior magnetic properties to achieve MH with low MNP concentrations, which are non-toxic. Alternatively, as shown in Section 3, a core/shell strategy to mitigate toxicity can significantly increase the safety of the core material.

6. Conclusions

The presented review summarizes the most important aspects of the preparation of NiCu MNPs with regard to their potential use in biomedicine. This includes different possible synthesis procedures, as well as the necessary functionalization/modification steps that need to be taken to either boost their biocompatibility or prevent agglomeration, which are both factors that contribute to their improved properties for application. As can be concluded from the currently available literature, which grew for the last couple of years, NiCu MNPs could be among future formulations for use as MH formulations, drug delivery systems, or other applications. With an already proven track record of successful application (currently only in in vitro and animal models), the potential of NiCu MNPs will only grow; many research groups are now testing their suitability using various additional tissue models to determine their application as part of the abovementioned uses or even in regenerative medicine, which was not addressed above [114].

Nevertheless, NiCu MNPs do not come without hurdles. Future challenges in their development certainly include the optimization of their synthesis and functionalization, which need to be green, to yield uniform small-sized nanoparticles with a narrow size distribution that are less prone to agglomeration. Additionally, careful composition control is necessary to prepare NiCu MNPs with a

T_C in the therapeutic range to minimize potential damage to healthy tissues. By meeting all of these criteria, their potential in biomedical applications will almost be without limitations, either as part of formulations for "traditional" applications of magnetic materials (e.g., MH) or as part of novel multi-modal drug delivery systems or dentistry implants that exhibit antibacterial activity.

Funding: This research was funded by Slovenian National Agency, grant numbers P3-0036, J1-9169, and J3-1762.

Conflicts of Interest: The authors declare no conflicts of interest.

References

1. Liu, Z.; Kiessling, F.; Gätjens, J. Advanced Nanomaterials in Multimodal Imaging: Design, Functionalization, and Biomedical Applications. *J. Nanomater.* **2010**, *2010*, 15. [CrossRef]
2. Tartaj, P.; del Puerto Morales, M.; Veintemillas-Verdaguer, S.; González-Carreño, T.; Serna, C.J. The preparation of magnetic nanoparticles for applications in biomedicine. *J. Phys. D Appl. Phys.* **2003**, *36*, R182. [CrossRef]
3. Lu, A.-H.; Salabas, E.L.; Schüth, F. Magnetic Nanoparticles: Synthesis, Protection, Functionalization, and Application. *Angew. Chem. Int. Ed.* **2007**, *46*, 1222–1244. [CrossRef] [PubMed]
4. Mornet, S.; Vasseur, S.; Grasset, F.; Veverka, P.; Goglio, G.; Demourgues, A.; Portier, J.; Pollert, E.; Duguet, E. Magnetic nanoparticle design for medical applications. *Progr. Solid State Chem.* **2006**, *34*, 237–247. [CrossRef]
5. Dürr, S.; Janko, C.; Lyer, S.; Tripal, P.; Schwarz, M.; Zaloga, J.; Tietze, R.; Alexiou, C. Magnetic nanoparticles for cancer therapy. *Nanotechnol. Rev.* **2013**, *2*, 395–409. [CrossRef]
6. Ahola, S.; Salmi, J.; Johansson, L.S.; Laine, J.; Osterberg, M. Model films from native cellulose nanofibrils. Preparation, swelling, and surface interactions. *Biomacromolecules* **2008**, *9*, 1273–1282. [CrossRef]
7. Park, J.W.; Lee, G.U. Properties of mixed lipid monolayers assembled on hydrophobic surfaces through vesicle adsorption. *Langmuir* **2006**, *22*, 5057–5063. [CrossRef]
8. Gao, Y.; Liu, Y.; Xu, C. Magnetic Nanoparticles for Biomedical Applications: From Diagnosis to Treatment to Regeneration. In *Engineering in Translational Medicine*; Cai, W., Ed.; Springer: London, UK, 2014; pp. 567–583. [CrossRef]
9. Tweedle, M.F. The Chemistry of Contrast Agents in Medical Magnetic Resonance Imaging Edited by André E. Merbach and Éva Tóth (University of Lausanne). J. Wiley & Sons: Chichester, New York, Weinheim, Brisbane, Singapore, Toronto. 2001. xii + 472 pp. $160.00. ISBN: 0-471-60778-9. *J. Am. Chem. Soc.* **2002**, *124*, 884–885. [CrossRef]
10. Catherine, C.B.; Curtis, A.S.G. Functionalisation of magnetic nanoparticles for applications in biomedicine. *J. Phys. D Appl. Phys.* **2003**, *36*, R198.
11. Le Trequesser, Q.; Seznec, H.; Delville, M.-H. Functionalized nanomaterials: Their use as contrast agents in bioimaging: Mono- and multimodal approaches. *Nanotechnol. Rev.* **2013**, *2*, 125. [CrossRef]
12. Portet, D.; Denizot, B.; Rump, E.; Lejeune, J.-J.; Jallet, P. Nonpolymeric Coatings of Iron Oxide Colloids for Biological Use as Magnetic Resonance Imaging Contrast Agents. *J. Colloid Interface Sci.* **2001**, *238*, 37–42. [CrossRef] [PubMed]
13. Issa, B.; Obaidat, I.M.; Albiss, B.A.; Haik, Y. Magnetic nanoparticles: Surface effects and properties related to biomedicine applications. *Int. J. Mol. Sci.* **2013**, *14*, 21266–21305. [CrossRef] [PubMed]
14. Jordan, A.; Scholz, R.; Maier-Hauff, K.; Johannsen, M.; Wust, P.; Nadobny, J.; Schirra, H.; Schmidt, H.; Deger, S.; Loening, S.; et al. Presentation of a new magnetic field therapy system for the treatment of human solid tumors with magnetic fluid hyperthermia. *J. Magn. Magn. Mater.* **2001**, *225*, 118–126. [CrossRef]
15. Wong, J.; Prout, J.; Seifalian, A. Magnetic Nanoparticles: New Perspectives in Drug Delivery. *Curr. Pharm. Des.* **2017**, *23*, 2908–2917. [CrossRef]
16. Stergar, J.; Ban, I.; Gradišnik, L.; Maver, U. Novel drug delivery system based on NiCu nanoparticles for targeting various cells. *J. Sol-Gel Sci. Technol.* **2018**, *88*, 57–65. [CrossRef]
17. Kumar, C.S.S.R.; Mohammad, F. Magnetic nanomaterials for hyperthermia-based therapy and controlled drug delivery. *Adv. Drug Deliv. Rev.* **2011**, *63*, 789–808. [CrossRef]
18. Bernkop-Schnurch, A.; Walker, G. Multifunctional matrices for oral peptide delivery. *Crit. Rev. Ther. Drug Carr. Syst.* **2001**, *18*, 459–501. [CrossRef]
19. Chomoucka, J.; Drbohlavova, J.; Huska, D.; Adam, V.; Kizek, R.; Hubalek, J. Magnetic nanoparticles and targeted drug delivering. *Pharmacol. Res.* **2010**, *62*, 144–149. [CrossRef]

20. Salunkhe, A.B.; Khot, V.M.; Pawar, S.H. Magnetic hyperthermia with magnetic nanoparticles: A status review. *Curr. Top. Med. Chem.* **2014**, *14*, 572–594. [CrossRef]
21. Laurent, S.; Dutz, S.; Häfeli, U.O.; Mahmoudi, M. Magnetic fluid hyperthermia: Focus on superparamagnetic iron oxide nanoparticles. *Adv. Colloid Interface Sci.* **2011**, *166*, 8–23. [CrossRef]
22. Sun, C.; Lee, J.S.; Zhang, M. Magnetic nanoparticles in MR imaging and drug delivery. *Adv. Drug Deliv. Rev.* **2008**, *60*, 1252–1265. [CrossRef] [PubMed]
23. Stephen, Z.R.; Kievit, F.M.; Zhang, M. Magnetite Nanoparticles for Medical MR Imaging. *Mater. Today* **2011**, *14*, 330–338. [CrossRef]
24. Mohammed, L.; Gomaa, H.G.; Ragab, D.; Zhu, J. Magnetic nanoparticles for environmental and biomedical applications: A review. *Particuology* **2017**, *30*, 1–14. [CrossRef]
25. Hauser, A.K.; Wydra, R.J.; Stocke, N.A.; Anderson, K.W.; Hilt, J.Z. Magnetic nanoparticles and nanocomposites for remote controlled therapies. *J. Control. Release Off. J. Control. Release Soc.* **2015**, *219*, 76–94. [CrossRef]
26. McBain, S.C.; Yiu, H.H.P.; Dobson, J. Magnetic nanoparticles for gene and drug delivery. *Int. J. Nanomed.* **2008**, *3*, 169–180.
27. Majidi, S.; Sehrig, F.Z.; Samiei, M.; Milani, M.; Abbasi, E.; Dadashzadeh, K.; Akbarzadeh, A. Magnetic nanoparticles: Applications in gene delivery and gene therapy. *Artif. Cells Nanomed. Biotechnol.* **2016**, *44*, 1186–1193. [CrossRef]
28. Šafařík, I.; Šafaříková, M. Magnetic Nanoparticles and Biosciences. *Monatshefte Chem. Chem. Mon.* **2002**, *133*, 737–759. [CrossRef]
29. Ludwig, F.; Heim, E.; Mäuselein, S.; Eberbeck, D.; Schilling, M. Magnetorelaxometry of magnetic nanoparticles with fluxgate magnetometers for the analysis of biological targets. *J. Magn. Magn. Mater.* **2005**, *293*, 690–695. [CrossRef]
30. Wiekhorst, F.; Steinhoff, U.; Eberbeck, D.; Trahms, L. Magnetorelaxometry assisting biomedical applications of magnetic nanoparticles. *Pharm. Res.* **2012**, *29*, 1189–1202. [CrossRef]
31. Ismail, R.A.; Sulaiman, G.M.; Abdulrahman, S.A.; Marzoog, T.R. Antibacterial activity of magnetic iron oxide nanoparticles synthesized by laser ablation in liquid. *Mater. Sci. Eng. C* **2015**, *53*, 286–297. [CrossRef]
32. Thukkaram, M.; Sitaram, S.; Kannaiyan, S.K.; Subbiahdoss, G. Antibacterial Efficacy of Iron-Oxide Nanoparticles against Biofilms on Different Biomaterial Surfaces. *Int. J. Biomater.* **2014**, *2014*, 716080. [CrossRef] [PubMed]
33. Ito, A.; Shinkai, M.; Honda, H.; Kobayashi, T. Medical application of functionalized magnetic nanoparticles. *J. Biosci. Bioeng.* **2005**, *100*, 1–11. [CrossRef] [PubMed]
34. Mok, H.; Zhang, M. Superparamagnetic iron oxide nanoparticle-based delivery systems for biotherapeutics. *Expert Opin. Drug Deliv.* **2013**, *10*, 73–87. [CrossRef] [PubMed]
35. Williams, H.M. The application of magnetic nanoparticles in the treatment and monitoring of cancer and infectious diseases. *Biosci. Horiz. Int. J. Stud. Res.* **2017**, *10*, hzx009. [CrossRef]
36. Ban, I.; Stergar, J.; Drofenik, M.; Ferk, G.; Makovec, D. Synthesis of copper–nickel nanoparticles prepared by mechanical milling for use in magnetic hyperthermia. *J. Magn. Magn. Mater.* **2011**, *323*, 2254–2258. [CrossRef]
37. Ferk, G.; Stergar, J.; Makovec, D.; Hamler, A.; Jagličić, Z.; Drofenik, M.; Ban, I. Synthesis and characterization of Ni–Cu alloy nanoparticles with a tunable Curie temperature. *J. Alloys Compd.* **2015**, *648*, 53–58. [CrossRef]
38. Kuznetsov, A.A.; Leontiev, V.G.; Brukvin, V.A.; Vorozhtsov, G.N.; Kogan, B.Y.; Shlyakhtin, O.A.; Yunin, A.M.; Tsybin, O.I.; Kuznetsov, O.A. Local radiofrequency-induced hyperthermia using CuNi nanoparticles with therapeutically suitable Curie temperature. *J. Magn. Magn. Mater.* **2007**, *311*, 197–203. [CrossRef]
39. Amrollahi, P.; Ataie, A.; Nozari, A.; Seyedjafari, E.; Shafiee, A. Cytotoxicity Evaluation and Magnetic Characteristics of Mechano-thermally Synthesized CuNi Nanoparticles for Hyperthermia. *J. Mater. Eng. Perform.* **2015**, *24*, 1220–1225. [CrossRef]
40. Ferk, G.; Stergar, J.; Drofenik, M.; Makovec, D.; Hamler, A.; Jagličić, Z.; Ban, I. The synthesis and characterization of nickel–copper alloy nanoparticles with a narrow size distribution using sol–gel synthesis. *Mater. Lett.* **2014**, *124*, 39–42. [CrossRef]
41. Songping, W.; Jing, N.; Li, J.; Zhenou, Z. Preparation of ultra-fine copper–nickel bimetallic powders with hydrothermal–reduction method. *Mater. Chem. Phys.* **2007**, *105*, 71–75. [CrossRef]
42. Feng, J.; Zhang, C.-P. Preparation of Cu–Ni alloy nanocrystallites in water-in-oil microemulsions. *J. Colloid Interface Sci.* **2006**, *293*, 414–420. [CrossRef] [PubMed]

43. Hergt, R.; Andra, W.; d'Ambly, C.G.; Hilger, I.; Kaiser, W.A.; Richter, U.; Schmidt, H.G. Physical limits of hyperthermia using magnetite fine particles. *IEEE Trans. Magn.* **1998**, *34*, 3745–3754. [CrossRef]
44. Jordan, A.; Scholz, R.; Wust, P.; Fähling, H.; Roland, F. Magnetic fluid hyperthermia (MFH): Cancer treatment with AC magnetic field induced excitation of biocompatible superparamagnetic nanoparticles. *J. Magn. Magn. Mater.* **1999**, *201*, 413–419. [CrossRef]
45. Chang, D.; Lim, M.; Goos, J.; Qiao, R.; Ng, Y.Y.; Mansfeld, F.M.; Jackson, M.; Davis, T.P.; Kavallaris, M. Biologically Targeted Magnetic Hyperthermia: Potential and Limitations. *Front. Pharmacol.* **2018**, *9*, 831. [CrossRef]
46. Andra, W.; Nowak, H. *Magnetism in Medicine: A Handbook*, 2nd ed.; Wiley-VCH: Weinheim, Germany, 2007; 629p.
47. Chatterjee, J.; Bettge, M.; Haik, Y.; Jen Chen, C. Synthesis and characterization of polymer encapsulated Cu–Ni magnetic nanoparticles for hyperthermia applications. *J. Magn. Magn. Mater.* **2005**, *293*, 303–309. [CrossRef]
48. Bettge, M.; Chatterjee, J.; Haik, Y. Physically synthesized Ni-Cu nanoparticles for magnetic hyperthermia. *Biomagn. Res. Technol.* **2004**, *2*, 4. [CrossRef]
49. Paulus, J.A.; Parida, G.R.; Tucker, R.D.; Park, J.B. Corrosion analysis of NiCu and PdCo thermal seed alloys used as interstitial hyperthermia implants. *Biomaterials* **1997**, *18*, 1609–1614. [CrossRef]
50. Abenojar, E.C.; Wickramasinghe, S.; Bas-Concepcion, J.; Samia, A.C.S. Structural effects on the magnetic hyperthermia properties of iron oxide nanoparticles. *Prog. Nat. Sci. Mater.* **2016**, *26*, 440–448. [CrossRef]
51. Engelmann, U.M.; Roeth, A.A.; Eberbeck, D.; Buhl, E.M.; Neumann, U.P.; Schmitz-Rode, T.; Slabu, I. Combining Bulk Temperature and Nanoheating Enables Advanced Magnetic Fluid Hyperthermia Efficacy on Pancreatic Tumor Cells. *Sci. Rep.* **2018**, *8*, 13210. [CrossRef]
52. Soetaert, F.; Kandala, S.K.; Bakuzis, A.; Ivkov, R. Experimental estimation and analysis of variance of the measured loss power of magnetic nanoparticles. *Sci. Rep.* **2017**, *7*, 6661. [CrossRef]
53. Allia, P.; Barrera, G.; Tiberto, P. Nonharmonic Driving Fields for Enhancement of Nanoparticle Heating Efficiency in Magnetic Hyperthermia. *Phys. Rev. Appl.* **2019**, *12*, 034041. [CrossRef]
54. Sue, K.; Tanaka, S.; Hiaki, T. Synthesis of Ni–Cu Particles by Hydrogen Reduction in Hot-compressed Water. *Chem. Lett.* **2006**, *35*, 50–51. [CrossRef]
55. Wang, L.-L.; Jiang, J.-S. Preparation of α-Fe_2O_3 nanoparticles by high-energy ball milling. *Phys. B Condens. Matter* **2007**, *390*, 23–27. [CrossRef]
56. Ali, M.E.; Ullah, M.; Maamor, A.; Hamid, S.B.A. Surfactant Assisted Ball Milling: A Simple Top down Approach for the Synthesis of Controlled Structure Nanoparticle. *Adv. Mater. Res.* **2014**, *832*, 356–361. [CrossRef]
57. Durivault, L.; Brylev, O.; Reyter, D.; Sarrazin, M.; Bélanger, D.; Roué, L. Cu–Ni materials prepared by mechanical milling: Their properties and electrocatalytic activity towards nitrate reduction in alkaline medium. *J. Alloys Compd.* **2007**, *432*, 323–332. [CrossRef]
58. Ge, Y.; Gao, T.; Wang, C.; Shah, Z.H.; Lu, R.; Zhang, S. Highly efficient silica coated CuNi bimetallic nanocatalyst from reverse microemulsion. *J. Colloid Interface Sci.* **2017**, *491*, 123–132. [CrossRef]
59. Ahmed, J.; Ramanujachary, K.V.; Lofland, S.E.; Furiato, A.; Gupta, G.; Shivaprasad, S.M.; Ganguli, A.K. Bimetallic Cu–Ni nanoparticles of varying composition ($CuNi_3$, CuNi, Cu_3Ni). *Colloids Surf. A Physicochem. Eng. Asp.* **2008**, *331*, 206–212. [CrossRef]
60. Stergar, J.; Ban, I.; Drofenik, M.; Ferk, G.; Makovec, D. *Synthesis and Characterization of Silica-Coated $Cu_{1-x}Ni_x$ Nanoparticles*; Institute of Electrical and Electronics Engineers: New York, NY, USA, 2012; p. 4.
61. Wen, M.; Liu, Q.-Y.; Wang, Y.-F.; Zhu, Y.-Z.; Wu, Q.-S. Positive microemulsion synthesis and magnetic property of amorphous multicomponent Co-, Ni- and Cu-based alloy nanoparticles. *Colloids Surf. A Physicochem. Eng. Asp.* **2008**, *318*, 238–244. [CrossRef]
62. Wang, X.L.; Ben Ahmed, N.; Alvarez, G.S.; Tuttolomondo, M.V.; Helary, C.; Desimone, M.F.; Coradin, T. Sol-gel Encapsulation of Biomolecules and Cells for Medicinal Applications. *Curr. Top. Med. Chem.* **2015**, *15*, 223–244. [CrossRef]
63. Brinker, C.J.; Scherer, G.W. *Sol-Gel Science: The Physics and Chemistry of Sol-Gel Processing*; Academic Press: Boston, MA, USA, 1990.
64. Leontyev, V. Magnetic properties of Ni and Ni–Cu nanoparticles. *Phys. Status Solidi (b)* **2013**, *250*, 103–107. [CrossRef]

65. Hachani, R.; Lowdell, M.; Birchall, M.; Hervault, A.; Mertz, D.; Begin-Colin, S.; Thanh, N.T. Polyol synthesis, functionalisation, and biocompatibility studies of superparamagnetic iron oxide nanoparticles as potential MRI contrast agents. *Nanoscale* **2016**, *8*, 3278–3287. [CrossRef] [PubMed]
66. Songvorawit, N.; Tuitemwong, K.; Tuitemwong, P. Single Step Synthesis of Amino-Functionalized Magnetic Nanoparticles with Polyol Technique at Low Temperature. *ISRN Nanotechnol.* **2011**, *2011*, 6. [CrossRef]
67. Carroll, K.J.; Calvin, S.; Ekiert, T.F.; Unruh, K.M.; Carpenter, E.E. Selective Nucleation and Growth of Cu and Ni Core/Shell Nanoparticles. *Chem. Mater.* **2010**, *22*, 2175–2177. [CrossRef]
68. Bonet, F.; Grugeon, S.; Dupont, L.; Urbina, R.H.; Guéry, C.; Tarascon, J.M. Synthesis and characterization of bimetallic Ni–Cu particles. *J. Solid State Chem.* **2003**, *172*, 111–115. [CrossRef]
69. Jayakrishnan, D.S. 5—Electrodeposition: The versatile technique for nanomaterials. In *Corrosion Protection and Control Using Nanomaterials*; Saji, V.S., Cook, R., Eds.; Woodhead Publishing: Sawston, UK, 2012; pp. 86–125. [CrossRef]
70. Foyet, A.; Hauser, A.; Schäfer, W. Double template electrochemical deposition and characterization of NiCo and NiCu alloys nanoparticles and nanofilms. *J. Solid State Electrochem.* **2007**, *12*, 47–55. [CrossRef]
71. Feng, S.H.; Li, G.H. Chapter 4—Hydrothermal and Solvothermal Syntheses. In *Modern Inorganic Synthetic Chemistry*, 2nd ed.; Xu, R., Xu, Y., Eds.; Elsevier: Amsterdam, The Netherlands, 2017; pp. 73–104. [CrossRef]
72. Songping, W.; Li, J.; Jing, N.; Zhenou, Z.; Song, L. Preparation of ultra fine copper–nickel bimetallic powders for conductive thick film. *Intermetallics* **2007**, *15*, 1316–1321. [CrossRef]
73. Kwon, Y.S.; An, V.V.; Ilyin, A.P.; Tikhonov, D.V. Properties of powders produced by electrical explosions of copper–nickel alloy wires. *Mater. Lett.* **2007**, *61*, 3247–3250. [CrossRef]
74. Bahlawane, N.; Premkumar, P.A.; Tian, Z.; Hong, X.; Qi, F.; Kohse-Höinghaus, K. Nickel and Nickel-Based Nanoalloy Thin Films from Alcohol-Assisted Chemical Vapor Deposition. *Chem. Mater.* **2010**, *22*, 92–100. [CrossRef]
75. Pál, E.; Kun, R.; Schulze, C.; Zöllmer, V.; Lehmhus, D.; Bäumer, M.; Busse, M. Composition-dependent sintering behaviour of chemically synthesised CuNi nanoparticles and their application in aerosol printing for preparation of conductive microstructures. *Colloid Polym. Sci.* **2012**, *290*, 941–952. [CrossRef]
76. Zin, V.; Brunelli, K.; Dabalà, M. Characterization of Cu–Ni alloy electrodeposition and synthesis of nanoparticles by pulsed sonoelectrochemistry. *Mater. Chem. Phys.* **2014**, *144*, 272–279. [CrossRef]
77. Sopousek, J.; Vrestal, J.; Pinkas, J.; Broz, P.; Bursik, J.; Styskalik, A.; Skoda, D.; Zobac, O.; Lee, J. Cu–Ni nanoalloy phase diagram—Prediction and experiment. *Calphad* **2014**, *45*, 33–39. [CrossRef]
78. de León-Quiroz, E.L.; Puente-Urbina, B.A.; Vázquez-Obregón, D.; García-Cerda, L.A. Preparation and structural characterization of CuNi nanoalloys obtained by polymeric precursor method. *Mater. Lett.* **2013**, *91*, 67–70. [CrossRef]
79. Stergar, J.; Ferk, G.; Ban, I.; Drofenik, M.; Hamler, A.; Jagodič, M.; Makovec, D. The synthesis and characterization of copper–nickel alloy nanoparticles with a therapeutic Curie point using the microemulsion method. *J. Alloys Compd.* **2013**, *576*, 220–226. [CrossRef]
80. Ban, I.; Stergar, J.; Maver, U. NiCu magnetic nanoparticles: Review of synthesis methods, surface functionalization approaches, and biomedical applications. *Nanotechnol. Rev.* **2018**, *7*, 187. [CrossRef]
81. Hao, R.; Xing, R.; Xu, Z.; Hou, Y.; Gao, S.; Sun, S. Synthesis, Functionalization, and Biomedical Applications of Multifunctional Magnetic Nanoparticles. *Adv. Mater.* **2010**, *22*, 2729–2742. [CrossRef]
82. An, L.; Li, Z.; Wang, Y.; Yang, B. Synthesis of Fe_3O_4/PMMA Nanocomposite Particles by Surface-Initiated ATRP and Characterization. *Chem. J. Chin. Univ.* **2006**, *27*, 1372–1375.
83. Morales, M.A.; Finotelli, P.; Coaquira, J.A.H.; Rocha-Leão, M.H.; Diaz-Aguila, C.; Baggio-Saitovitch, E.; Rossi, A.M. In situ synthesis and magnetic studies of iron oxide nanoparticles in calcium-alginate matrix for biomedical applications. *Mater. Sci. Eng. C* **2008**, *28*, 253–257. [CrossRef]
84. Yallapu, M.M.; Foy, S.P.; Jain, T.K.; Labhasetwar, V. PEG-functionalized magnetic nanoparticles for drug delivery and magnetic resonance imaging applications. *Pharmaceut. Res.* **2010**, *27*, 2283–2295. [CrossRef]
85. Kim, D.K.; Mikhaylova, M.; Wang, F.H.; Kehr, J.; Bjelke, B.; Zhang, Y.; Tsakalakos, T.; Muhammed, M. Starch-Coated Superparamagnetic Nanoparticles as MR Contrast Agents. *Chem. Mater.* **2003**, *15*, 4343–4351. [CrossRef]
86. Li, G.-Y.; Jiang, Y.-R.; Huang, K.-L.; Ding, P.; Yao, L.-L. Kinetics of adsorption of Saccharomyces cerevisiae mandelated dehydrogenase on magnetic Fe3O4–chitosan nanoparticles. *Colloids Surf. A Physicochem. Eng. Asp.* **2008**, *320*, 11–18. [CrossRef]

87. Saranya, D.; Rajan, R.; Suganthan, V.; Murugeswari, A.; Raj, N.A.N. Synthesis and Characterization of Pullulan Acetate Coated Magnetic Nanoparticle for Hyperthermic Therapy. *Procedia Mater. Sci.* **2015**, *10*, 2–9. [CrossRef]
88. Berry, C.C.; Wells, S.; Charles, S.; Curtis, A.S. Dextran and albumin derivatised iron oxide nanoparticles: Influence on fibroblasts in vitro. *Biomaterials* **2003**, *24*, 4551–4557. [CrossRef]
89. Gaihre, B.; Aryal, S.; Khil, M.S.; Kim, H.Y. Encapsulation of Fe_3O_4 in gelatin nanoparticles: Effect of different parameters on size and stability of the colloidal dispersion. *J. Microencapsul.* **2008**, *25*, 21–30. [CrossRef] [PubMed]
90. Gupta, A.K.; Gupta, M. Synthesis and surface engineering of iron oxide nanoparticles for biomedical applications. *Biomaterials* **2005**, *26*, 3995–4021. [CrossRef] [PubMed]
91. Shete, P.B.; Patil, R.M.; Tiwale, B.M.; Pawar, S.H. Water dispersible oleic acid-coated Fe3O4 nanoparticles for biomedical applications. *J. Magn. Magn. Mater.* **2015**, *377*, 406–410. [CrossRef]
92. Silva, S.M.; Tavallaie, R.; Sandiford, L.; Tilley, R.D.; Gooding, J.J. Gold coated magnetic nanoparticles: From preparation to surface modification for analytical and biomedical applications. *Chem. Commun.* **2016**, *52*, 7528–7540. [CrossRef]
93. Martínez-González, R.; Estelrich, J.; Busquets, M.A. Liposomes Loaded with Hydrophobic Iron Oxide Nanoparticles: Suitable T_2 Contrast Agents for MRI. *Int. J. Mol. Sci.* **2016**, *17*, 1209. [CrossRef]
94. Liang, J.; Zhang, X.; Miao, Y.; Li, J.; Gan, Y. Lipid-coated iron oxide nanoparticles for dual-modal imaging of hepatocellular carcinoma. *Int. J. Nanomed.* **2017**, *12*, 2033–2044. [CrossRef]
95. Huang, H.-C.; Chang, P.-Y.; Chang, K.; Chen, C.-Y.; Lin, C.-W.; Chen, J.-H.; Mou, C.-Y.; Chang, Z.-F.; Chang, F.-H. Formulation of novel lipid-coated magnetic nanoparticles as the probe for in vivo imaging. *J. Biomed. Sci.* **2009**, *16*, 86. [CrossRef]
96. Hauser, A.K.; Anderson, K.W.; Hilt, J.Z. Peptide conjugated magnetic nanoparticles for magnetically mediated energy delivery to lung cancer cells. *Nanomedicine* **2016**, *11*, 1769–1785. [CrossRef]
97. Scarberry, K.E.; Dickerson, E.B.; McDonald, J.F.; Zhang, Z.J. Magnetic Nanoparticle–Peptide Conjugates for in Vitro and in Vivo Targeting and Extraction of Cancer Cells. *J. Am. Chem. Soc.* **2008**, *130*, 10258–10262. [CrossRef] [PubMed]
98. Biswas, M.; Saha, A.; Dule, M.; Mandal, T.K. Polymer-Assisted Chain-like Organization of CuNi Alloy Nanoparticles: Solvent-Adoptable Pseudohomogeneous Catalysts for Alkyne–Azide Click Reactions with Magnetic Recyclability. *J. Phys. Chem. C* **2014**, *118*, 22156–22165. [CrossRef]
99. Araújo-Barbosa, S.; Morales, M.A. Nanoparticles of $Ni_{1-x}Cu_x$ alloys for enhanced heating in magnetic hyperthermia. *J. Alloys Compd.* **2019**, *787*, 935–943. [CrossRef]
100. Pramanik, S.; Pal, S.; Bysakh, S.; De, G. Cu_xNi_{1-x} alloy nanoparticles embedded SiO_2 films: Synthesis and structure. *J. Nanopart. Res.* **2010**, *13*, 321–329. [CrossRef]
101. El-Sayed, A.H.; Aly, A.A.; Ei-Sayed, N.I.; Mekawy, M.M.; Ei-Gendy, A.A. Calculation of heating power generated from ferromagnetic thermal seed (PdCo-PdNi-CuNi) alloys used as interstitial hyperthermia implants. *J. Mater. Sci. Mater. Med.* **2007**, *18*, 523–528. [CrossRef]
102. Parimaladevi, R.; Parvathi, V.P.; Lakshmi, S.S.; Umadevi, M. Synergistic effects of copper and nickel bimetallic nanoparticles for enhanced bacterial inhibition. *Mater. Lett.* **2018**, *211*, 82–86. [CrossRef]
103. Argueta-Figueroa, L.; Morales-Luckie, R.A.; Scougall-Vilchis, R.J.; Olea-Mejía, O.F. Synthesis, characterization and antibacterial activity of copper, nickel and bimetallic Cu–Ni nanoparticles for potential use in dental materials. *Progr. Nat. Sci. Mater. Int.* **2014**, *24*, 321–328. [CrossRef]
104. Pankhurst, Q.A.; Connolly, J.; Jones, S.K.; Dobson, J. Applications of magnetic nanoparticles in biomedicine. *J. Phys. D Appl. Phys.* **2003**, *36*, R167. [CrossRef]
105. Shimizu, T.; Matsui, M. New magnetic implant material for interstitial hyperthermia. *Sci. Technol. Adv. Mat.* **2003**, *4*, 469–473. [CrossRef]
106. Arokiyaraj, S.; Saravanan, M.; Udaya Prakash, N.K.; Valan Arasu, M.; Vijayakumar, B.; Vincent, S. Enhanced antibacterial activity of iron oxide magnetic nanoparticles treated with *Argemone mexicana* L. leaf extract: An in vitro study. *Mater. Res. Bull.* **2013**, *48*, 3323–3327. [CrossRef]
107. Prabhu, Y.T.; Rao, K.V.; Kumari, B.S.; Kumar, V.S.S.; Pavani, T. Synthesis of Fe_3O_4 nanoparticles and its antibacterial application. *Int. Nano Lett.* **2015**, *5*, 85–92. [CrossRef]
108. Wang, L.; Hu, C.; Shao, L. The antimicrobial activity of nanoparticles: Present situation and prospects for the future. *Int. J. Nanomed.* **2017**, *12*, 1227–1249. [CrossRef] [PubMed]

109. Ramalingam, B.; Parandhaman, T.; Das, S.K. Antibacterial Effects of Biosynthesized Silver Nanoparticles on Surface Ultrastructure and Nanomechanical Properties of Gram-Negative Bacteria viz. Escherichia coli and Pseudomonas aeruginosa. *ACS Appl. Mater. Interfaces* **2016**, *8*, 4963–4976. [CrossRef] [PubMed]
110. Priyadarsini, S.; Mukherjee, S.; Mishra, M. Nanoparticles used in dentistry: A review. *J. Oral Biol. Craniofac. Res.* **2018**, *8*, 58–67. [CrossRef]
111. Besinis, A.; De Peralta, T.; Tredwin, C.J.; Handy, R.D. Review of Nanomaterials in Dentistry: Interactions with the Oral Microenvironment, Clinical Applications, Hazards, and Benefits. *ACS Nano* **2015**, *9*, 2255–2289. [CrossRef]
112. Minocha, S.; Mumper, R.J. Effect of carbon coating on the physico-chemical properties and toxicity of copper and nickel nanoparticles. *Small* **2012**, *8*, 3289–3299. [CrossRef]
113. Shih, K.; Tang, Y. Prolonged toxicity characteristic leaching procedure for nickel and copper aluminates. *J. Environ. Monit. JEM* **2011**, *13*, 829–835. [CrossRef]
114. Milojević, M.; Gradišnik, L.; Stergar, J.; Klemen, M.S.; Stožer, A.; Vesenjak, M.; Dobnik Dubrovski, P.; Maver, T.; Mohan, T.; Kleinschek, K.S.; et al. Development of multifunctional 3D printed bioscaffolds from polysaccharides and NiCu nanoparticles and their application. *Appl. Surf. Sci.* **2019**, *488*, 836–852. [CrossRef]

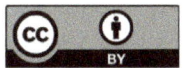

© 2019 by the authors. Licensee MDPI, Basel, Switzerland. This article is an open access article distributed under the terms and conditions of the Creative Commons Attribution (CC BY) license (http://creativecommons.org/licenses/by/4.0/).

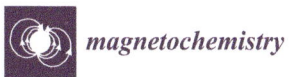

Review

Iron Oxide Labeling and Tracking of Extracellular Vesicles

Yuko Tada and Phillip C. Yang *

School of Medicine, Department of Medicine, Division of Cardiovascular Medicine and Cardiovascular Institute, Stanford University, 269 Campus Drive, CCSR 3115C, Stanford, CA 94305, USA; ytada@stanford.edu
* Correspondence: phillip@stanford.edu, Tel.: +1-650-498-8008

Received: 30 September 2019; Accepted: 5 November 2019; Published: 7 November 2019

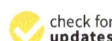

Abstract: Extracellular vesicles (EVs) are essential tools for conveying biological information and modulating functions of recipient cells. Implantation of isolated or modulated EVs can be innovative therapeutics for various diseases. Furthermore, EVs could be a biocompatible drug delivery vehicle to carry both endogenous and exogenous biologics. Tracking EVs should play essential roles in understanding the functions of EVs and advancing EV therapeutics. EVs have the characteristic structures consisting of the lipid bilayer and specific membrane proteins, through which they can be labeled efficiently. EVs can be labeled either directly using probes or indirectly by transfection of reporter genes. Optical imaging (fluorescent imaging and bioluminescent imaging), single-photon emission computed tomography (SPECT)/positron emission tomography (PET), and magnetic resonance imaging (MRI) are currently used for imaging EVs. Labeling EVs with superparamagnetic iron oxide (SPIO) nanoparticles for MRI tracking is a promising method that can be translated into clinic. SPIO can be internalized by most of the cell types and then released as SPIO containing EVs, which can be visualized on T2*-weighted imaging. However, this method has limitations in real-time imaging because of the life cycle of SPIO after EV degradation. Further studies will be needed to validate SPIO labeling by other imaging modalities in preclinical studies. The emerging technologies of labeling and imaging EVs with SPIO in comparison with other imaging modalities are reviewed in this paper.

Keywords: extracellular vesicles; superparamagnetic iron oxide nanoparticles; magnetic resonance imaging (MRI)

---

1. Introduction

Extracellular vesicles (EVs), which represent microvesicle and exosome secretomes, are produced by most of the cell types under physiological and pathological conditions, playing essential roles in intercellular communications. EVs secreted from cells migrate through interstitial fluid or systemic circulation and transfer their cargos consisting of nucleic acids, proteins, lipids, and mitochondrial fractions to their recipient cells [1–3]. mRNAs from EVs can be translated in the recipient cells and miRNA from EVs can modulate gene expression and biological functions [4]. For instance, cardiomyocytes exchange EVs with cardiac fibroblasts and endothelial cells inside the interstitium. Myocardial function is modified by those interstitial cell-derived EVs in adaptive responses both in beneficial or harmful ways. miR-21* (the passenger strand miRNA), transferred from fibroblast-derived EVs stimulates myocardial hypertrophy [5]. Endothelial cell-derived exosomes increase miR-146a expression level in cardiomyocytes, leading to impaired metabolic activity and contractile dysfunction [6]. EV therapy could modulate and enhance the innate repair capacities. The usefulness of EVs in tissue repair or regeneration have been suggested by many researchers. EVs from bone marrow stem cells modified the functions of endothelial cells and cardiomyocytes to improve cardiac function with enhanced angiogenesis [7]. Mesenchymal stem cell (MSC)-derived EVs reduced myocardial infarct size following the ischemia reperfusion in animal models [8,9].

Due to their unique characteristics including nano-scale size, biogenesis potential, endogenous lipid bilayer membrane, signal transduction system, and effectors of various biological information, EVs can be useful in numerous ways in diagnostic and therapeutic roles. Furthermore, EV therapy could have distinctive advantages compared to stem cell therapy. They are potentially less toxic and less likely to suffer immune rejections. The dose could be optimized to achieve higher concentration of effectors. Finally, EVs have wider delivery options since EVs have intrinsic capacities to cross tissue and cellular barriers. With higher biocompatibility and less toxicity, EVs may replace artificial lipid nanoparticles in the future as drug delivery vehicles to deliver exogenous and endogenous therapeutic cargos. Due to these potentials of EVs, monitoring the distribution and fate of secreted or implanted EVs in vitro or in vivo is one of the essential strategies in understanding their functions and advancing the EV-mediated diagnostics or therapeutics. Appropriate biodistribution of EVs is key to their efficacy and safety.

Among the existing labeling and tracking technologies including optical imaging, nuclear imaging and magnetic resonance imaging (MRI), labeling with superparamagnetic iron oxide (SPIO) nanoparticles for MRI tracking is a promising method. SPIO are the magnetic nanoparticles, which are clinically used as MRI contrast agents to detect cancers, inflammation, vascular flows, or tissue perfusion [10–12]. In regenerative medicine, stem cells have been successfully labeled with SPIO and tracked after implantation [13–15]. Finally, the technology of labeling and tracking EVs with SPIO is currently under development.

Here, we review the emerging technologies of labeling and imaging EV with SPIO and compare them with other imaging modalities.

2. Extracellular Vesicles

2.1. Microvesicles and Exosomes

Exosomes and microvesicles are two of the major components of EVs, which differ in their size, biogenesis potential, and secretion pathways [16,17]. Exosomes are smaller vesicles (40–150 nm) and technically indicate the vesicles passing through 220-nm pore filters or recovered by high-speed ultracentrifugation. Exosomes are formed in the multivesicular bodies (MVB) and released by the fusion of plasma membrane. In the beginning of this process, cells generate early endosomes by endocytosis. During the maturation to late endosomes, some endosomes shed intraluminal vesicles (ILV) within themselves to become MVBs. MVBs migrate to the cell membrane and fuse with the membrane and release exosomes [18]. By contrast, microvesicles are bigger vesicles compared to exosomes (150–1000 nm) and released from the plasma membrane by budding. However, it is difficult to separate them completely. EVs are released both under physiological and pathological conditions. For instance, adult cardiomyocytes are known to release various sized EVs [19]. Nano-scale EVs can be visualized by electron microscopy (Figure 1). Although cardiomyocytes release EVs under physiological conditions, cellular stresses caused by hypoxia/reoxygenation or reactive oxygen species enhance EV release and modify the protein profile of EVs [4].

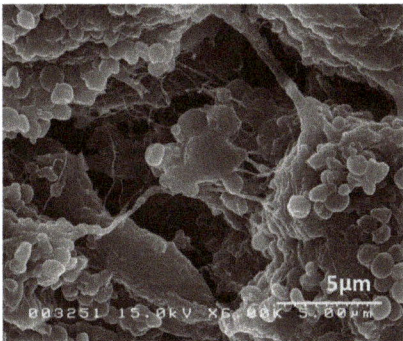

Figure 1. Scanning electron microscopy images of extracellular vesicles (EVs) released from cardiomyocytes. Cardiac tissues from a healthy mouse were collected and prepared (primary fixation with 2.5% glutaraldehyde, secondary fixation with osmium tetroxide, dehydration, mounting, and ion sputter coating). The sample was observed by scanning electron microscope (Hitachi S-4500). [Unpublished data].

2.2. The Structural Properties of EVs

The lipid or protein components of EV membranes determine their biodistribution and uptake by recipient cells [20]. EVs have the lipid bilayer membrane consisting of proteins and lipids with abundant lipid rafts, which are important structures in labeling them with imaging probes. In spite of the similarity to the plasma membrane, EV membranes contain some specific surface lipid components designated for ligand-receptor pairing and resultant cellular uptake of EVs [21]. EVs are enriched with anionic phospholipid phosphatidylserine (PS), which is recognized by macrophages [22–24]. The integrin composition of the membrane renders the affinity with certain tissues [25]. EV surface protein glycosylation affects biodistribution of EVs [26]. EV internalization is caused by several mechanisms such as lipid raft-, clathrin-, and caveolae-dependent endocytosis, micropinocytosis, and phagocytosis [20,27]. The routes of EV uptake could also be affected by EV type or conditions of the extracellular space (acidic/basic, hypoxic, extracellular matrix components). It is likely cells and EVs have some systems that can let EVs escape from the degrading pathways after being taken up by cells [28]. Unmodified EVs suffer from rapid clearance and low accumulation in target tissues and cells. Similar to liposomes, intravenously administered EVs are delivered to the reticuloendothelial system mainly the liver and spleen and are rapidly cleared from circulation via, in part, the macrophage-dependent pathway [29,30].

Exosomes contain common biomarkers such as Alix, tumor susceptibility gene 101 (Tsg101), Annexin XI, and tetraspanins (CD9, CD81, and CD63) [31]. Several proteins such as actinin-4 and mitofilin are more favorably expressed in large or medium-sized EVs [32]. Exosomes and microvesicles share some surface biomarker proteins, including MHC, flotillin, heat-shock proteins, and tetraspanins CD63 and CD9 [32]. On the other hand, vesicular proteins vary from one cell type to the other [33]. The cellular origin of EVs influence surface protein profile including integrin subunits, tetraspanins, and fibronectin [20]. Proteomic analysis revealed that the EVs secreted from adult cardiomyocytes uniquely include cytosolic, sarcomeric, and mitochondrial proteins, such as myomesin, myosin-binding protein C, VCP, tropomyosin, and α-crystallin [34]. The unique protein profiles define different targeting characteristics of EVs.

3. Labeling and Imaging of EVs

3.1. Imaging Modalities of EV Labeling and Tracking

While no ideal imaging technology has been developed for in vivo EV labeling and tracking, rigorous research for EV imaging has been performed utilizing optical imaging (fluorescence imaging (FLI) and bioluminescence imaging (BLI)), single-photon emission computed tomography (SPECT)/positron emission tomography (PET), and magnetic resonance imaging (MRI). Many kinds of probes or vectors for labeling EVs are available on the market. Each method has its strength and weakness related to the spatial or temporal resolution, sensitivity, specificity, clinical availability, safety, and complexity of the technique. In EV labeling, it is fundamental not to disturb the integrity of the EV membranes in order to maintain their morphology and physiological functions.

The methods for labeling are largely categorized into direct labeling and indirect labeling. In the direct labeling, probes are directly bound to the target (EV) surface or transported inside the cells or EVs via physiological mechanisms. After cells are directly labeled, labeled EVs are created inside the cells and released. One of the advantages of the direct labeling method is that it is simple and relatively physiological without need for any gene modification. In general, the critical problem with direct labeling is that signals may persist longer than the actual lifetime of EVs in the body because of the aggregation or re-binding of the probes by other cells or substrates. By contrast, in indirect labeling, reporter genes such as luciferase or fluorescence binding proteins are transfected with donor cells, followed by the expression of the reporter genes or fluorescence tagged EV membrane proteins. The indirect labeling method could evaluate the in vivo lifetime of EVs and transfer of EV components to the recipient cells more accurately and be suitable for real-time monitoring [35].

3.2. FLI, BLI, and PET/SPECT

FLI has been widely used for labeling EVs. Fluorescent proteins or organic dyes emit signals under excitation with an external light source, which are detected by an in vivo imaging system. Small lipophilic fluorophores are used to label isolated EVs due to its affinity to lipids on the membrane and produce a strong and stable fluorescence signal. PKH67 (Ex. 490 nm/Em. 502 nm), PKH26 (Ex.551 nm/Em. 565 nm), and $DiOC_{18}$ (7) (DiR) (Ex.750 nm/Em.780 nm) are representative lipophilic carbocyanine dyes used for EV labeling [36–38]. DiR is a Near-infrared (NIR) dye, which is advantageous for in vivo applications due to the high signal to noise ratio (SNR), minimal autofluorescence, and enhanced tissue penetration [39]. However, several drawbacks of the lipophilic dyes are known that make them unideal probes for EV labeling and in vivo tracking. Binding of lipophilic dye is not EV membrane specific. Due to their relatively long in vivo half-life of 5 to >100 days, after degradation of EVs, the dyes remain intact and bind to other lipid components non-specifically in the extracellular space or the recipient cells [40]. The dyes could also promote EV aggregation [41]. As a result, in vivo signal from these lipid dyes yield inaccurate information regarding the fates of EVs compared to signals obtained by BLI [35].

The membrane-targeted indirect labeling methods are also used for FLI. Fluorescent proteins such as green fluorescent protein (GFP) or red fluorescent protein (RFP) fused with membrane protein markers are transfected to donor cells. Cells transfected with CD63-GFP plasmid express GFP-tagged EV membrane anchoring protein [42]. Lai et al. reported a method to fuse fluorescent proteins with a palmitoylation signal of EV membrane [43]. By fusing fluorescent proteins (enhanced GFP or tandem dimer Tomato) with a consensus palmitoylation sequence, these reporters are expressed on the whole cell membrane. This is followed by labeling of EVs of variable sizes on their membranes. Notably, the fused protein was expressed mostly on the inner membrane of EVs, which could avoid potential disturbance to EV surface function. Using this EV labeling technique, they visualized bidirectional cell-cell translocation of EVs. In addition, the implantation of the labeled thymoma cells enabled visualization of EV release from the tumors in vivo, revealing that the tumor releases more EVs in the peripheral regions, accompanying infiltration of immune cells compared to the tumor core area of the highest tumor cell density [43].

BLI is a powerful in vivo optical imaging tool. In BLI, luciferases, most commonly *Photinus pyralis* luciferase (firefly; Fluc), *Renilla reniformis* luciferase (sea pansy; Tluc), and *Gaussia princeps* luciferase (marine copepod; Gluc) are used as reporters. Luciferases emit bioluminescence via oxidation of their respective substrate with either ATP and Mg (Fluc-D-luciferin), or oxygen alone (Rluc and

Gluc-coelenterazine), when the enzyme is expressed in vivo as a molecular reporter [44]. Gluc emit over 1000-fold stronger bioluminescence compared to Rluc and Fluc [45]. Reporter luciferase genes need to be inserted into the genome of the donor cells. BLI has high SNR since the mammalian tissues have little intrinsic bioluminescence. Lai et al. developed a method that transfects donor cells with lentivirus vectors encoding Gluc combined with transmembrane domain [35,46]. EVs that share lipid bilayer components with a cellular membrane then express transmembrane domain bound Gluc. This method has an excellent temporal resolution and enables tracking of the accurate fate of EVs in vivo. Decreased Gluc signal indicates decreased availability of external EVs and internal degradation of Gluc transcripts. EVs accumulated in the kidneys, liver, lungs, and spleen. Intravenously administered EVs have a half-life of < 30 min in most tissues and are cleared from the body by 6 h post injection [35].

The application of BLI and FLI is limited to the small animals because of the limited signal penetration (only several centimeters) [44]. It could give valuable information in preclinical research. The obtained signals are semi-quantitative as signal strength strongly depends on the tissue depth and has limited sensitivity to signals from deep tissues. Another limitation is that the expression level of reporter proteins restricts the fluorescence or bioluminescence signals.

PET/SPECT label substrates with high-energy gamma-emitting radiotracers. They are widely used as clinical imaging tools. PET and SPECT are very sensitive techniques and are extensively used for in vivo tracking of nanomaterials. They rely on detection of high-energy gamma rays, which have no penetration limits. The high energy of emitted photons minimize the attenuation and scattering effects, enabling the accurate quantification of signals in the whole body. PET achieves better sensitivity and spatial resolution compared to SPECT. Although tracers with different half-life and decay profiles are used, short half-life of the radioactive tracers might limit long-term tracking [47]. However, it might not be a problem in EV tracking because of their short lifetime in vivo. Both direct and indirect labeling with 99mTc or [^{125}I] NaI tracers are used to image EVs on SPECT [48,49]. Direct radiolabeling was performed for in vivo real time EV tracking on PET using the commercial [^{124}I] NaI probe (half-life >4 days) to form a covalent bond to tyrosine of EV membrane protein [26].

3.3. SPIO and MRI

Compared to the optical imaging or SPECT/PET, MRI has the most exquisite spatial resolution although the sensitivity of MRI is relatively low. MRI without accompanying any radiation exposure is superior to nuclear labeling in terms of safety. The labeling methods developed for MRI can be compatible with clinical application. It can be also combined with simultaneous anatomical assessment, functional evaluation and tissue characterization. This capability enables precise localization of EVs and assessment of their specific regional effects in the different areas of tissue injury to correlate EV engraftment with therapeutic efficacy. The strength and weakness of EV labeling using MRI are summarized in Table 1.

Table 1. Pros and cons of superparamagnetic iron oxide (SPIO) labeling.

Pros	Cons
Clinical translation is easy	False positive signals
Excellent spatial resolution	Low sensitivity
No gene modification required	Real time observation is difficult
No interference with surface membrane	Quantification might not be accurate
No radiation	Whole body scan is not easy
Simultaneous assessment of anatomy/function/ tissue characterics is possible	Potential interference with cellular/vesicular function

Superparamagnetic iron oxide nanoparticles (SPIO) are magnetic nanoparticles most commonly used for visualizing cells on MRI. It could be applied for EVs in a similar manner. SPIO nanoparticles are attractive probes for EV labeling because of their small size and biocompatibility. SPIO enable detection of labeled objects in the tissues longitudinally. The superparamagnetic core of SPIO produces local field homogeneity, which enhances transverse relaxation (=T2* relaxation effect) and produces negative contrast [50]. Large susceptibility effects of SPIO make the signal void much larger than the particle size, enhancing detectability. Negative contrast in the tissues containing SPIO can be detected on a T2*-weighted gradient echo sequence consisting of long TR/TE and low flip angle [51]. In general, quantification of SPIO accumulation from signal loss on MRI is difficult [52]. T2* mapping can be useful for quantifying accumulation of SPIO, which is created by several gradient echo sequences at different TEs to calculate T2* decrease on the T2* decay curve [14].

SPIO consists of the functional core, coating, and surface properties. Those properties determine the efficiency of cellular uptake, distribution, metabolism, and potential toxicity. The functional core producing the superparamagnetic property is a single-domain iron oxide molecule (<10 nm diameter in general) containing Fe_3O_4 (magnetite), gamma-Fe_2O_3 (maghemite), or alpha-Fe_2O_3 (hematite) [53]. SPIO are coated with biocompatible polymers such as dextran and carboxydextran, which can prevent aggregations, structural changes and degradation [54,55]. SPIO are classified into standard SPIO (SSPIO, >50 nm), ultra-small SPIO (USPIO, 10–50 nm), and very-small SPIO (VSPIO, <10 nm) based on their hydrodynamic diameters [56]. The larger magnetic susceptibility of SSPIO yields larger R2 relaxation and higher T2-shortening effects compared to the effects caused by USPIO [57]. However, the size of USPIO is more suitable for labeling nano-scale EVs (Figure 2). SPIO are clinically used as MRI contrast agents for evaluating blood volume fraction, perfusion, and cancer metastasis [10–12]. Unfortunately, manufacturers of most of them were discontinued because of the safety reasons or infrequent use (Table 2). Currently, ferumoxytol is the only clinically available USPIO. Ferumoxytol is approved by FDA for iron replacement therapy for renal anemia patients. However, it has been also used off-label as an MRI contrast agent [58]. Clinical compatibility of labeling agents is critical in applying EV labeling in humans. Therefore, labeling with ferumoxytol is an attractive method and several groups have reported the method to label cells with ferumoxytol [59,60].

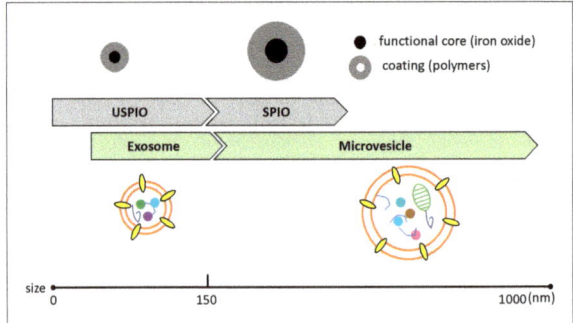

Figure 2. Comparison of size between ultra-small SPIO (USPIO) and SPIO (upper), and exosome and microvesicles (lower). [Unpublished figure].

Table 2. Clinical SPIO (cited from [61]).

Generic Name	Brand Name	Classification	Coating	Diameter (nm)	Status
Ferumoxide	Feridex/Endorem	SSPIO	dextran	120-180	discontinued
Ferumoxtran-10	Combidex/Sinerem	USPIO	dextran	15-30	discontinued
Ferucarbotran	Resovist/Cliavist	SSPIO	carboxydextran	60	discontinued
Ferucarbotran	Supravist	USPIO	carboxydextran	21	discontinued
Feruglose	Clariscan	USPIO	pegylated starch	20	discontinued
Ferumoxytol	Feraheme	USPIO	carboxymethyl dextran	30	FDA approved

3.4. EV Labeling with SPIO

SPIO can label cells directly. Subsequently, labeled EVs are created inside the cells and released. In this method, donor cells are incubated with the culture medium containing SPIO. Most of the cell types except for phagocytes such as neutrophils and macrophages do not have the capacity of phagocytizing particles. Therefore, iron-oxide nanoparticles are prepared with facilitators such as poly-L-Lysine, protamine, or some transfection reagents, which facilitate cellular uptake of SPIO [62]. These cationic compounds facilitate interaction of SPIO with the negatively charged cell membrane and subsequent endosomal uptake mainly by Clathrin-mediated endocytosis [27]. Most cell types without phagocytizing capacity can be labeled by this method. Donor cells which incorporate SPIO then release vesicles containing SPIO. USPIO taken up by human bone marrow derived MSC (hBM-MSCs) were found to traffic to the intracellular vesicles expressing EV markers such as CD9, CD63, and CD81, which indicated that the intracellular localization of internalized SPIOs is actively regulated and the deposited SPIO are ready to be released from cells [63]. The SPIO internalization can be confirmed by electron microscopy (Figure 3). Accumulation of SPIO labeled EVs in the tissue is detected on T2*-weighted MRI (Figure 3). Busato et al. labeled exosomes isolated from adipose stem cells with commercial USPIO by this cell labeling method. They injected isolated labeled exosomes in the hindlimb and detected them on MRI [64,65]. They labeled cells with 200 µgFe/mL of USPIO and found 0.634 µg of iron was contained per 100 µg of exosomes. Injection of 5 µg of exosomes produced sufficient signals to detect on MRI. Histologically, Prussian Blue staining confirms the existence of SPIO in the tissue (Figure 3). The amount of SPIO internalization depends on the incubation time (cell and SPIO) and the iron concentration [64]. EV iron content is significantly correlated with intracellular iron content. Therefore, a strategy should be made to label donor cells with the highest SPIO concentration possible [65]. T2* negative contrast depends on the concentration of loaded SPIO in the vesicles and the number of labeled exosomes.

The labeled EVs had the similar capacity of being taken up by cells in vitro [63]. This direct SPIO labeling method is likely to maintain the morphology and the physiological characteristics of the EVs intact. The major limitation of SPIO-labeling is the persistence of in vivo signal after EV degradation. Signals from EVs labeled with SPIO cannot be distinguished from signals originating from other cells taking up SPIO after EV degradation. In the past report, significant MRI signal was derived from SPIO-containing macrophages 3 weeks after transplantation of SPIO-labeled cells despite only a few viable transplanted cells remaining in the tissue [66].

Another representative method to label EV with SPIO is the direct vesicle labeling via electroporation. Hu et al. labeled melanoma exosomes with USPIO (SPION5, 4.5 nm in diameter) by electroporation. Labeled melanoma exosomes were injected into the foot pad and their migration into the ipsilateral local lymph node was detected 48 h post injection by T2* mapping [67]. The potential disadvantage of electroporation method is that this could damage the membrane as the strong electric field by electroporation causes pore formation in the EV membrane to let iron oxide particles be inside [68].

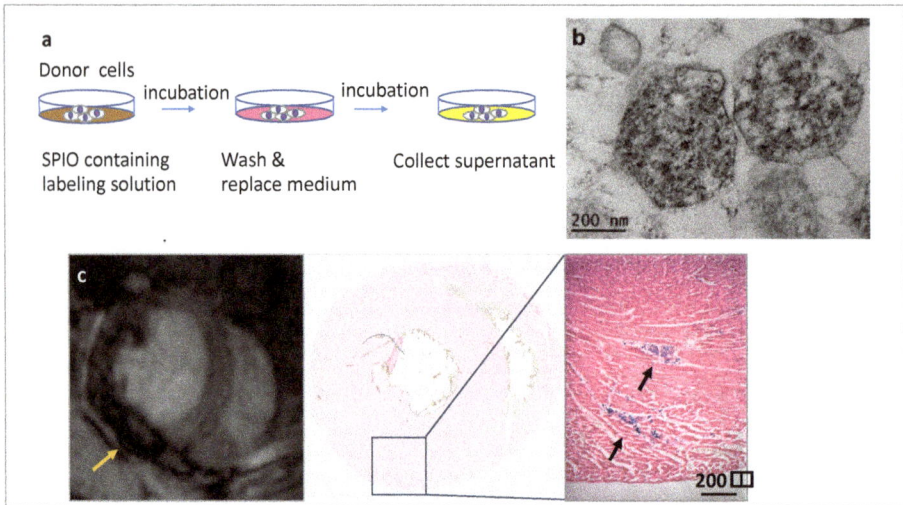

Figure 3. (a) The diagram of the method of labeling with SPIO. (b) Transmission electron microscopy of labeled extracellular vesicles (EVs). SPIO are detected as black particles inside the vesicles. (c) In vivo magnetic resonance imaging (MRI) detection of SPIO labeled EVs injected in the mouse heart (left). The image was acquired with a GE 3.0T Signa scanner. Prussian blue staining of the slice from the excised heart (middle) proved the iron oxide particles stained blue in the myocardium (right: high magnification). [Unpublished data].

3.5. Effects of Labeling on the Functions of EVs

SPIO generally has low toxicity to cells. However, some in vitro experiments suggested the possibility that iron oxide or the facilitators could cause cellular stress (mitochondrial dysfunction and reactive oxygen species generation), alterations in gene expression and cell differentiation, decreased cell proliferation, and promotion of pro-inflammatory environment, depending on their concentrations [69]. Cellular/vesicular iron concentration could interfere with cell viability and production of EVs. Therefore, the optimization of iron concentration, incubation time, cell viability, and MRI image contrast are the crucial points [65]. Further research will be required to clarify the effect of SPIO on EVs.

4. Summary and Outlook

Technology to image EVs are developing rapidly and more and more labeling probes are becoming available. They are useful for visualizing intercellular EV translocations and biodistribution of implanted EVs in preclinical small animal models. It is important to select the appropriate labeling method and imaging modality based on the purpose. Labeling of EVs with SPIO for MRI detection is clinically compatible and especially useful when specific organs are targeted. It has limitations in real-time monitoring and whole-body imaging. EV labeling using SPIO has just started and further studies are needed in the future to establish the method and its usefulness. The SPIO signal on MRI needs to be verified by precise histological evaluation and comparison with signals obtained from in vivo real-time monitoring using BLI, FLI, or SPECT/PET.

Advancement of the EV imaging technology could strongly help understand the functions and kinetics of EVs, and which in turn, help advance imaging techniques. Further studies are necessary, focusing on labeling of various kinds of EVs with different origins and targets, gaining more stable and stronger signals, utilizing completely biocompatible methods with high safety, improving the detection and quantification method, and enabling accurate real-time monitoring.

EV labeling and tracking will give us valuable information when we try to apply them as drug delivery systems. However, current technologies rely on the labeling of the external EVs and it is quite challenging to visualize the biodistributions of internal EVs. A more comprehensive approach is required to truly understand the roles of EVs.

Author Contributions: Y.T.; writing—original draft preparation, P.C.Y.; writing—review and editing.

Funding: NIH UM1 (P.Y.): NIH K24 (P.Y.).

Conflicts of Interest: The authors declare no conflict of interest.

References

1. Kourembanas, S. Exosomes: Vehicles of intercellular signaling, biomarkers, and vectors of cell therapy. *Annu. Rev. Physiol.* **2015**, *77*, 13–27. [CrossRef]
2. Torralba, D.; Baixauli, F.; Sánchez-Madrid, F. Mitochondria Know No Boundaries: Mechanisms and Functions of Intercellular Mitochondrial Transfer. *Front. Cell Dev. Biol.* **2016**, *4*, 107. [CrossRef]
3. Coly, P.M.; Boulanger, C.M. Extracellular Mitochondria and Vesicles. *Circ. Res.* **2019**, *125*, 53–54. [CrossRef] [PubMed]
4. Cervio, E.; Barile, L.; Moccetti, T.; Vassalli, G. Exosomes for Intramyocardial Intercellular Communication. *Stem Cells Int.* **2015**, *2015*, 482171. [CrossRef] [PubMed]
5. Bang, C.; Batkai, S.; Dangwal, S.; Gupta, S.K.; Foinquinos, A.; Holzmann, A.; Just, A.; Remke, J.; Zimmer, K.; Zeug, A.; et al. Cardiac fibroblast-derived microRNA passenger strand-enriched exosomes mediate cardiomyocyte hypertrophy. *J. Clin. Investig.* **2014**, *124*, 2136–2146. [CrossRef] [PubMed]
6. Halkein, J.; Tabruyn, S.P.; Ricke-Hoch, M.; Haghikia, A.; Nguyen, N.Q.; Scherr, M.; Castermans, K.; Malvaux, L.; Lambert, V.; Thiry, M.; et al. MicroRNA-146a is a therapeutic target and biomarker for peripartum cardiomyopathy. *J. Clin. Investig.* **2013**, *123*, 2143–2154. [CrossRef] [PubMed]
7. Sahoo, S.; Klychko, E.; Thorne, T.; Misener, S.; Schultz, K.M.; Millay, M.; Ito, A.; Liu, T.; Kamide, C.; Agrawal, H.; et al. Exosomes from human CD34(+) stem cells mediate their proangiogenic paracrine activity. *Circ. Res.* **2011**, *109*, 724–728. [CrossRef] [PubMed]
8. Timmers, L.; Lim, S.K.; Arslan, F.; Armstrong, J.S.; Hoefer, I.E.; Doevendans, P.A.; Piek, J.J.; El Oakley, R.M.; Choo, A.; Lee, C.N.; et al. Reduction of myocardial infarct size by human mesenchymal stem cell conditioned medium. *Stem Cell Res.* **2007**, *1*, 129–137. [CrossRef] [PubMed]
9. Arslan, F.; Lai, R.C.; Smeets, M.B.; Akeroyd, L.; Choo, A.; Aguor, E.N.; Timmers, L.; van Rijen, H.V.; Doevendans, P.A.; Pasterkamp, G.; et al. Mesenchymal stem cell-derived exosomes increase ATP levels, decrease oxidative stress and activate PI3K/Akt pathway to enhance myocardial viability and prevent adverse remodeling after myocardial ischemia/reperfusion injury. *Stem Cell Res.* **2013**, *10*, 301–312. [CrossRef]
10. Finn, J.P.; Nguyen, K.L.; Han, F.; Zhou, Z.; Salusky, I.; Ayad, I.; Hu, P. Cardiovascular MRI with ferumoxytol. *Clin. Radiol.* **2016**, *71*, 796–806. [CrossRef]
11. Rivera-Rivera, L.A.; Schubert, T.; Johnson, K.M. Measurements of cerebral blood volume using quantitative susceptibility mapping, R. *NMR Biomed.* **2019**, e4175. [CrossRef] [PubMed]
12. Toth, G.B.; Varallyay, C.G.; Horvath, A.; Bashir, M.R.; Choyke, P.L.; Daldrup-Link, H.E.; Dosa, E.; Finn, J.P.; Gahramanov, S.; Harisinghani, M.; et al. Current and potential imaging applications of ferumoxytol for magnetic resonance imaging. *Kidney Int.* **2017**, *92*, 47–66. [CrossRef] [PubMed]
13. Huang, Z.; Li, C.; Yang, S.; Xu, J.; Shen, Y.; Xie, X.; Dai, Y.; Lu, H.; Gong, H.; Sun, A.; et al. Magnetic resonance hypointensive signal primarily originates from extracellular iron particles in the long-term tracking of mesenchymal stem cells transplanted in the infarcted myocardium. *Int. J. Nanomed.* **2015**, *10*, 1679–1690. [CrossRef]
14. Bos, C.; Delmas, Y.; Desmoulière, A.; Solanilla, A.; Hauger, O.; Grosset, C.; Dubus, I.; Ivanovic, Z.; Rosenbaum, J.; Charbord, P.; et al. In vivo MR imaging of intravascularly injected magnetically labeled mesenchymal stem cells in rat kidney and liver. *Radiology* **2004**, *233*, 781–789. [CrossRef]
15. Mathiasen, A.B.; Hansen, L.; Friis, T.; Thomsen, C.; Bhakoo, K.; Kastrup, J. Optimal labeling dose, labeling time, and magnetic resonance imaging detection limits of ultrasmall superparamagnetic iron-oxide nanoparticle labeled mesenchymal stromal cells. *Stem Cells Int.* **2013**, *2013*, 353105. [CrossRef]

16. Zaborowski, M.P.; Balaj, L.; Breakefield, X.O.; Lai, C.P. Extracellular Vesicles: Composition, Biological Relevance, and Methods of Study. *Bioscience* **2015**, *65*, 783–797. [CrossRef]
17. Van Niel, G.; D'Angelo, G.; Raposo, G. Shedding light on the cell biology of extracellular vesicles. *Nat. Rev. Mol. Cell Biol.* **2018**, *19*, 213–228. [CrossRef]
18. Colombo, M.; Raposo, G.; Théry, C. Biogenesis, secretion, and intercellular interactions of exosomes and other extracellular vesicles. *Annu. Rev. Cell Dev. Biol.* **2014**, *30*, 255–289. [CrossRef]
19. Gupta, S.; Knowlton, A.A. HSP60 trafficking in adult cardiac myocytes: Role of the exosomal pathway. *Am. J. Physiol. Heart Circ. Physiol.* **2007**, *292*, H3052–H3056. [CrossRef]
20. Murphy, D.E.; de Jong, O.G.; Brouwer, M.; Wood, M.J.; Lavieu, G.; Schiffelers, R.M.; Vader, P. Extracellular vesicle-based therapeutics: Natural versus engineered targeting and trafficking. *Exp. Mol. Med.* **2019**, *51*, 32. [CrossRef]
21. Théry, C.; Ostrowski, M.; Segura, E. Membrane vesicles as conveyors of immune responses. *Nat. Rev. Immunol.* **2009**, *9*, 581–593. [CrossRef] [PubMed]
22. Matsumoto, A.; Takahashi, Y.; Nishikawa, M.; Sano, K.; Morishita, M.; Charoenviriyakul, C.; Saji, H.; Takakura, Y. Role of Phosphatidylserine-Derived Negative Surface Charges in the Recognition and Uptake of Intravenously Injected B16BL6-Derived Exosomes by Macrophages. *J. Pharm. Sci.* **2017**, *106*, 168–175. [CrossRef] [PubMed]
23. Zwaal, R.F.; Bevers, E.M.; Comfurius, P.; Rosing, J.; Tilly, R.H.; Verhallen, P.F. Loss of membrane phospholipid asymmetry during activation of blood platelets and sickled red cells; mechanisms and physiological significance. *Mol. Cell Biochem.* **1989**, *91*, 23–31. [CrossRef] [PubMed]
24. Miyanishi, M.; Tada, K.; Koike, M.; Uchiyama, Y.; Kitamura, T.; Nagata, S. Identification of Tim4 as a phosphatidylserine receptor. *Nature* **2007**, *450*, 435–439. [CrossRef] [PubMed]
25. Hoshino, A.; Costa-Silva, B.; Shen, T.L.; Rodrigues, G.; Hashimoto, A.; Tesic Mark, M.; Molina, H.; Kohsaka, S.; Di Giannatale, A.; Ceder, S.; et al. Tumour exosome integrins determine organotropic metastasis. *Nature* **2015**, *527*, 329–335. [CrossRef]
26. Royo, F.; Cossío, U.; Ruiz de Angulo, A.; Llop, J.; Falcon-Perez, J.M. Modification of the glycosylation of extracellular vesicles alters their biodistribution in mice. *Nanoscale* **2019**, *11*, 1531–1537. [CrossRef]
27. Hillaireau, H.; Couvreur, P. Nanocarriers' entry into the cell: Relevance to drug delivery. *Cell Mol. Life Sci.* **2009**, *66*, 2873–2896. [CrossRef]
28. Izquierdo-Useros, N.; Naranjo-Gómez, M.; Archer, J.; Hatch, S.C.; Erkizia, I.; Blanco, J.; Borràs, F.E.; Puertas, M.C.; Connor, J.H.; Fernández-Figueras, M.T.; et al. Capture and transfer of HIV-1 particles by mature dendritic cells converges with the exosome-dissemination pathway. *Blood* **2009**, *113*, 2732–2741. [CrossRef]
29. Charoenviriyakul, C.; Takahashi, Y.; Morishita, M.; Matsumoto, A.; Nishikawa, M.; Takakura, Y. Cell type-specific and common characteristics of exosomes derived from mouse cell lines: Yield, physicochemical properties, and pharmacokinetics. *Eur. J. Pharm. Sci.* **2017**, *96*, 316–322. [CrossRef]
30. Abra, R.M.; Hunt, C.A. Liposome disposition in vivo. III. Dose and vesicle-size effects. *Biochim. Biophys. Acta* **1981**, *666*, 493–503. [CrossRef]
31. Lötvall, J.; Hill, A.F.; Hochberg, F.; Buzás, E.I.; Di Vizio, D.; Gardiner, C.; Gho, Y.S.; Kurochkin, I.V.; Mathivanan, S.; Quesenberry, P.; et al. Minimal experimental requirements for definition of extracellular vesicles and their functions: A position statement from the International Society for Extracellular Vesicles. *J. Extracell. Vesicles* **2014**, *3*, 26913. [CrossRef] [PubMed]
32. Kowal, J.; Arras, G.; Colombo, M.; Jouve, M.; Morath, J.P.; Primdal-Bengtson, B.; Dingli, F.; Loew, D.; Tkach, M.; Théry, C. Proteomic comparison defines novel markers to characterize heterogeneous populations of extracellular vesicle subtypes. *Proc. Natl. Acad. Sci. USA* **2016**, *113*, E968–E977. [CrossRef] [PubMed]
33. Dickhout, A.; Koenen, R.R. Extracellular Vesicles as Biomarkers in Cardiovascular Disease; Chances and Risks. *Front. Cardiovasc. Med.* **2018**, *5*, 113. [CrossRef] [PubMed]
34. Malik, Z.A.; Kott, K.S.; Poe, A.J.; Kuo, T.; Chen, L.; Ferrara, K.W.; Knowlton, A.A. Cardiac myocyte exosomes: Stability, HSP60, and proteomics. *Am. J. Physiol. Heart Circ. Physiol.* **2013**, *304*, H954–H965. [CrossRef] [PubMed]
35. Lai, C.P.; Mardini, O.; Ericsson, M.; Prabhakar, S.; Maguire, C.; Chen, J.W.; Tannous, B.A.; Breakefield, X.O. Dynamic biodistribution of extracellular vesicles in vivo using a multimodal imaging reporter. *ACS Nano* **2014**, *8*, 483–494. [CrossRef]

36. Liu, H.; Gao, W.; Yuan, J.; Wu, C.; Yao, K.; Zhang, L.; Ma, L.; Zhu, J.; Zou, Y.; Ge, J. Exosomes derived from dendritic cells improve cardiac function via activation of CD4 (+) T lymphocytes after myocardial infarction. *J. Mol. Cell Cardiol.* **2016**, *91*, 123–133. [CrossRef]
37. Usman, W.M.; Pham, T.C.; Kwok, Y.Y.; Vu, L.T.; Ma, V.; Peng, B.; Chan, Y.S.; Wei, L.; Chin, S.M.; Azad, A.; et al. Efficient RNA drug delivery using red blood cell extracellular vesicles. *Nat. Commun.* **2018**, *9*, 2359. [CrossRef]
38. Wiklander, O.P.; Nordin, J.Z.; O'Loughlin, A.; Gustafsson, Y.; Corso, G.; Mäger, I.; Vader, P.; Lee, Y.; Sork, H.; Seow, Y.; et al. Extracellular vesicle in vivo biodistribution is determined by cell source, route of administration and targeting. *J. Extracell. Vesicles* **2015**, *4*, 26316. [CrossRef]
39. Di Rocco, G.; Baldari, S.; Toietta, G. Towards Therapeutic Delivery of Extracellular Vesicles: Strategies for. *Stem Cells Int.* **2016**, *2016*, 5029619. [CrossRef]
40. Rieck, B. Unexpected durability of PKH 26 staining on rat adipocytes. *Cell Biol. Int.* **2003**, *27*, 445–447. [CrossRef]
41. Pužar Dominkuš, P.; Stenovec, M.; Sitar, S.; Lasič, E.; Zorec, R.; Plemenitaš, A.; Žagar, E.; Kreft, M.; Lenassi, M. PKH26 labeling of extracellular vesicles: Characterization and cellular internalization of contaminating PKH26 nanoparticles. *Biochim. Biophys. Acta Biomembr.* **2018**, *1860*, 1350–1361. [CrossRef]
42. Suetsugu, A.; Honma, K.; Saji, S.; Moriwaki, H.; Ochiya, T.; Hoffman, R.M. Imaging exosome transfer from breast cancer cells to stroma at metastatic sites in orthotopic nude-mouse models. *Adv. Drug Deliv. Rev.* **2013**, *65*, 383–390. [CrossRef]
43. Lai, C.P.; Kim, E.Y.; Badr, C.E.; Weissleder, R.; Mempel, T.R.; Tannous, B.A.; Breakefield, X.O. Visualization and tracking of tumour extracellular vesicle delivery and RNA translation using multiplexed reporters. *Nat. Commun.* **2015**, *6*, 7029. [CrossRef]
44. Sadikot, R.T.; Blackwell, T.S. Bioluminescence imaging. *Proc. Am. Thorac. Soc.* **2005**, *2*, 537–540. [CrossRef]
45. Badr, C.E.; Tannous, B.A. Bioluminescence imaging: Progress and applications. *Trends Biotechnol.* **2011**, *29*, 624–633. [CrossRef]
46. Lai, C.P.; Tannous, B.A.; Breakefield, X.O. Noninvasive in vivo monitoring of extracellular vesicles. *Methods Mol. Biol.* **2014**, *1098*, 249–258. [CrossRef]
47. Velly, H.; Bouix, M.; Passot, S.; Penicaud, C.; Beinsteiner, H.; Ghorbal, S.; Lieben, P.; Fonseca, F. Cyclopropanation of unsaturated fatty acids and membrane rigidification improve the freeze-drying resistance of Lactococcus lactis subsp. lactis TOMSC161. *Appl. Microbiol. Biotechnol.* **2015**, *99*, 907–918. [CrossRef]
48. Varga, Z.; Gyurkó, I.; Pálóczi, K.; Buzás, E.I.; Horváth, I.; Hegedűs, N.; Máthé, D.; Szigeti, K. Radiolabeling of Extracellular Vesicles with (99m)Tc for Quantitative In Vivo Imaging Studies. *Cancer Biother. Radiopharm.* **2016**, *31*, 168–173. [CrossRef]
49. Morishita, M.; Takahashi, Y.; Nishikawa, M.; Sano, K.; Kato, K.; Yamashita, T.; Imai, T.; Saji, H.; Takakura, Y. Quantitative analysis of tissue distribution of the B16BL6-derived exosomes using a streptavidin-lactadherin fusion protein and iodine-125-labeled biotin derivative after intravenous injection in mice. *J. Pharm. Sci.* **2015**, *104*, 705–713. [CrossRef]
50. Ghugre, N.R.; Coates, T.D.; Nelson, M.D.; Wood, J.C. Mechanisms of tissue-iron relaxivity: Nuclear magnetic resonance studies of human liver biopsy specimens. *Magn. Reson. Med.* **2005**, *54*, 1185–1193. [CrossRef]
51. Nitz, W.R.; Reimer, P. Contrast mechanisms in MR imaging. *Eur. Radiol.* **1999**, *9*, 1032–1046. [CrossRef] [PubMed]
52. Li, Z.; Suzuki, Y.; Huang, M.; Cao, F.; Xie, X.; Connolly, A.J.; Yang, P.C.; Wu, J.C. Comparison of reporter gene and iron particle labeling for tracking fate of human embryonic stem cells and differentiated endothelial cells in living subjects. *Stem Cells* **2008**, *26*, 864–873. [CrossRef] [PubMed]
53. Thorek, D.L.; Chen, A.K.; Czupryna, J.; Tsourkas, A. Superparamagnetic iron oxide nanoparticle probes for molecular imaging. *Ann. Biomed. Eng.* **2006**, *34*, 23–38. [CrossRef]
54. Moraes, L.; Vasconcelos-dos-Santos, A.; Santana, F.C.; Godoy, M.A.; Rosado-de-Castro, P.H.; Jasmin; Azevedo-Pereira, R.L.; Cintra, W.M.; Gasparetto, E.L.; Santiago, M.F.; et al. Neuroprotective effects and magnetic resonance imaging of mesenchymal stem cells labeled with SPION in a rat model of Huntington's disease. *Stem Cell Res.* **2012**, *9*, 143–155. [CrossRef]

55. Bull, E.; Madani, S.Y.; Sheth, R.; Seifalian, A.; Green, M.; Seifalian, A.M. Stem cell tracking using iron oxide nanoparticles. *Int. J. Nanomed.* **2014**, *9*, 1641–1653. [CrossRef]
56. Thorek, D.L.; Tsourkas, A. Size, charge and concentration dependent uptake of iron oxide particles by non-phagocytic cells. *Biomaterials* **2008**, *29*, 3583–3590. [CrossRef]
57. Metz, S.; Bonaterra, G.; Rudelius, M.; Settles, M.; Rummeny, E.J.; Daldrup-Link, H.E. Capacity of human monocytes to phagocytose approved iron oxide MR contrast agents in vitro. *Eur. Radiol.* **2004**, *14*, 1851–1858. [CrossRef]
58. Vasanawala, S.S.; Nguyen, K.L.; Hope, M.D.; Bridges, M.D.; Hope, T.A.; Reeder, S.B.; Bashir, M.R. Safety and technique of ferumoxytol administration for MRI. *Magn. Reson. Med.* **2016**, *75*, 2107–2111. [CrossRef]
59. Thu, M.S.; Bryant, L.H.; Coppola, T.; Jordan, E.K.; Budde, M.D.; Lewis, B.K.; Chaudhry, A.; Ren, J.; Varma, N.R.; Arbab, A.S.; et al. Self-assembling nanocomplexes by combining ferumoxytol, heparin and protamine for cell tracking by magnetic resonance imaging. *Nat. Med.* **2012**, *18*, 463–467. [CrossRef]
60. Castaneda, R.T.; Khurana, A.; Khan, R.; Daldrup-Link, H.E. Labeling stem cells with ferumoxytol, an FDA-approved iron oxide nanoparticle. *J. Vis. Exp.* **2011**, e3482. [CrossRef]
61. Jung, J.-H.; Tada, Y.; Yang, P.C. Novel MRI Contrast from Magnetotactic Bacteria to Evaluate In Vivo Stem Cell Engraftment. In *Biological, Physical and Technical Basics of Cell Engineering*; Springer: Singapore, 2018; pp. 365–380.
62. Suzuki, Y.; Zhang, S.; Kundu, P.; Yeung, A.C.; Robbins, R.C.; Yang, P.C. In vitro comparison of the biological effects of three transfection methods for magnetically labeling mouse embryonic stem cells with ferumoxides. *Magn. Reson. Med.* **2007**, *57*, 1173–1179. [CrossRef]
63. Dabrowska, S.; Del Fattore, A.; Karnas, E.; Frontczak-Baniewicz, M.; Kozlowska, H.; Muraca, M.; Janowski, M.; Lukomska, B. Imaging of extracellular vesicles derived from human bone marrow mesenchymal stem cells using fluorescent and magnetic labels. *Int. J. Nanomed.* **2018**, *13*, 1653–1664. [CrossRef]
64. Busato, A.; Bonafede, R.; Bontempi, P.; Scambi, I.; Schiaffino, L.; Benati, D.; Malatesta, M.; Sbarbati, A.; Marzola, P.; Mariotti, R. Magnetic resonance imaging of ultrasmall superparamagnetic iron oxide-labeled exosomes from stem cells: A new method to obtain labeled exosomes. *Int. J. Nanomed.* **2016**, *11*, 2481–2490. [CrossRef]
65. Busato, A.; Bonafede, R.; Bontempi, P.; Scambi, I.; Schiaffino, L.; Benati, D.; Malatesta, M.; Sbarbati, A.; Marzola, P.; Mariotti, R. Labeling and Magnetic Resonance Imaging of Exosomes Isolated from Adipose Stem Cells. *Curr. Protoc. Cell Biol.* **2017**, *75*, 3.44.1–3.44.15. [CrossRef]
66. Terrovitis, J.; Stuber, M.; Youssef, A.; Preece, S.; Leppo, M.; Kizana, E.; Schär, M.; Gerstenblith, G.; Weiss, R.G.; Marbán, E.; et al. Magnetic resonance imaging overestimates ferumoxide-labeled stem cell survival after transplantation in the heart. *Circulation* **2008**, *117*, 1555–1562. [CrossRef]
67. Hu, L.; Wickline, S.A.; Hood, J.L. Magnetic resonance imaging of melanoma exosomes in lymph nodes. *Magn. Reson. Med.* **2015**, *74*, 266–271. [CrossRef]
68. Johnsen, K.B.; Gudbergsson, J.M.; Skov, M.N.; Christiansen, G.; Gurevich, L.; Moos, T.; Duroux, M. Evaluation of electroporation-induced adverse effects on adipose-derived stem cell exosomes. *Cytotechnology* **2016**, *68*, 2125–2138. [CrossRef]
69. Jasmin; Torres, A.L.; Nunes, H.M.; Passipieri, J.A.; Jelicks, L.A.; Gasparetto, E.L.; Spray, D.C.; Campos de Carvalho, A.C.; Mendez-Otero, R. Optimized labeling of bone marrow mesenchymal cells with superparamagnetic iron oxide nanoparticles and in vivo visualization by magnetic resonance imaging. *J. Nanobiotechnol.* **2011**, *9*, 4. [CrossRef]

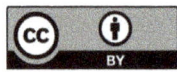

© 2019 by the authors. Licensee MDPI, Basel, Switzerland. This article is an open access article distributed under the terms and conditions of the Creative Commons Attribution (CC BY) license (http://creativecommons.org/licenses/by/4.0/).

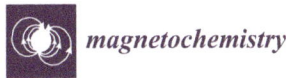

Review

Magnetic Particle Bioconjugates: A Versatile Sensor Approach

Sadagopan Krishnan [1,*,†] and K. Yugender Goud [2,†]

1. Department of Chemistry, Oklahoma State University, Stillwater, OK 74078, USA
2. Department of Chemistry, National Institute of Technology Warangal, Telangana 506004, India; yugenderkotagiri@gmail.com
* Correspondence: gopan.krishnan@okstate.edu
† Equal contribution.

Received: 16 October 2019; Accepted: 14 November 2019; Published: 19 November 2019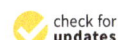

Abstract: Nanomaterial biosensors have revolutionized the entire scientific, technology, biomedical, materials science, and engineering fields. Among all nanomaterials, magnetic nanoparticles, microparticles, and beads are unique in offering facile conjugation of biorecognition probes for selective capturing of any desired analytes from complex real sample matrices (e.g., biofluids such as whole blood, serum, urine and saliva, tissues, food, and environmental samples). In addition, rapid separation of the particle-captured analytes by the simple use of a magnet for subsequent detection on a sensor unit makes the magnetic particle sensor approach very attractive. The easy magnetic isolation feature of target analytes is not possible with other inorganic particles, both metallic (e.g., gold) and non-metallic (e.g., silica), which require difficult centrifugation and separation steps. Magnetic particle biosensors have thus enabled ultra-low detection with ultra-high sensitivity that has traditionally been achieved only by radioactive assays and other tedious optical sources. Moreover, when traditional approaches failed to selectively detect low-concentration analytes in complex matrices (e.g., colorimetric, electrochemistry, and optical methods), magnetic particle-incorporated sensing strategies enabled sample concentration into a defined microvolume of large surface area particles for a straightforward detection. The objective of this article is to highlight the ever-growing applications of magnetic materials for the detection of analytes present in various real sample matrices. The central idea of this paper was to show the versatility and advantages of using magnetic particles for a variety of sample matrices and analyte types and the adaptability of different transducers with the magnetic particle approaches.

Keywords: magnetic particles; sensor; biomarkers; cells/cancer cells; food analytes; pathogens; pharmaceuticals; real sample matrices; optical; electrochemical; surface sensitive methods

1. Introduction

Most chemical and biological detection labels are limited to one transducer type or, sometimes, a few at best. In contrast, nanomaterials are not limited to a particular type of transducer, and they can be employed to a wide range of transducers. Moreover, nanomaterials can be used as labels for signal amplification and detection in sensors and assays. Because of these astonishing properties, nanomaterial sensors can be used with various detection methods (e.g., sensors based on optical, electrical, electrochemical, mass, mechanical, luminescent, and other physical properties). Thus, the unusual versatility of nanomaterial sensors supersedes traditional approaches and enables the analysis of complex sample matrices [1,2]. The magnetic separability of nanomaterials allows selective capturing of desired target analytes from complex real sample matrices through the analyte-specific probes. The bioconjugation is made feasible through viable chemical functionalization of magnetic materials to link desired molecular probes for analyte detection in sensors. Chemical and bio sensors constitute one common theme of involving magnetic particle applications [1,3–9], and other equally important areas include biomedical imaging [10–17], food science [18–20], drug delivery [21–23], disease treatment [24,25], nanomedicine [26], diagnostics [27–32], catalysis [33–40], separation and purification [41,42], health [43], and environmental applications [44–47]. Thus, a plethora of studies have been reviewed for the unusually broad research fields in which magnetic materials play crucial roles. In addition to several characteristics such as optical, electrochemical, and catalytic properties of magnetic particles, their biocompatibility and tunable chemical functionalities and geometries (i.e., size and shape) pave the way for their in vivo applications. A literature search by the authors conveys that the research progress, number of publications, and reviews on magnetic particles and their applications in a vast range of topics have gained never-ceasing attention. This article specifically focused on magnetic particle (both nano and micro) and magnetic bead-based biosensors for the detection of biomarkers (for the most part) and other classes of analytes.

Xianyu et al. [4] recently reviewed the advances in magnetic particle-based biosensors for point-of-care testing and mechanisms of assaying biomarkers. They additionally outlined the milestones that limit the realization of real-world applications of certain magnetic materials. They emphasized the need to synthesize high-quality magnetic particles with control over their size distribution and magnetization and the need of portable and miniaturized magnetic signal readout systems. Farka et al. [48] recently published a very informative and comprehensive review of nanomaterials, including magnetic materials for immunochemical biosensors and assays. They discussed several types of transducers (e.g., optical, electrochemical, surface-sensitive methods, and transistors) and covered a range of target analytes including proteins, small molecules, cancer cells, toxic substances, and pathogens.

With regard to the specific needs of successfully utilizing magnetic materials for ultra-low analyte detection with high sensitivity, several strategies are being explored. Magnetic preconcentration of desired analytes, (basically, capturing low concentrations of target analytes from real samples onto a large surface area of magnetic particles; as a result, the analyte molecules are concentrated in small geometric areas to enable sensitive detection) to minimize the effect of interference from coexisting irrelevant molecules in sample matrices, has been explored. In addition, the use of an external magnetic field to selectively attract desired target analytes attached to magnetic conjugates onto the sensor surface is another strategy. Furthermore, sensitive detection and imaging of magnetically tagged analytes (or their complexes with biorecognition molecules) in solutions have also been explored in sensors [48]. Another review discussed the transduction mechanisms and applications of complementary metal-oxide-semiconductor biosensor designs based on magnetic and other particles for in vitro diagnosis [49].

In a typical heterogeneous biosensor design, the analyte molecules in the magnetic conjugates diffuse to the sensor surface to generate signals. In contrast, magnetic particle sensors in which the analytes are detected in the whole solution volume of the sample as a homogeneous sensing approach have also been developed [50]. Sample preparation steps are shown to be reduced in the homogeneous sensor assay, and the combined diffusion of analyte molecules and capture probes is shown to reduce the total assay time compared with a heterogeneous assay. In this article, we will mainly focus on the heterogeneous sensor systems that are shown to offer high sensitivity, reduced nonspecific or false positive signals, ultra-low detection limits, and tunability to attain a wide dynamic range of detection.

In addition to the synthesis and sensor application of iron oxide-based magnetic particles, considerable focus has been also placed on making hybrid magnetic materials (e.g., core/shell, bimetallic, and alloys) and composites with other materials (e.g., polymers, graphene, chitosan, and carbon nanostructures) to obtain a multifactorial advantage from a single end material [51–56]. We also present here several examples on core/shell and nanocomposite magnetic materials. This article is not a comprehensive review of magnetic nanoparticles or biosensors.

2. Rationale for the Selection of Transducer

On deciding the type of sensor signal transducers, major factors, such as the molecular properties of the analytes, detection limits required, and the design of suitable biorecognition process for selective detection, are considered. For a redox-active analyte or reagents that can offer redox-active products, electrochemical methods are suitable and offer sensitive detection (e.g., amperometric, potentiometric, and impedance sensors) (Table 1). When the analyte concentration is large enough (e.g., micromolar to millimolar range) and can be selectively visualized by the naked eye by a color reaction, the colorimetric detection is advantageous. For ultra-low detection limits, fluorescence, luminescence, and surface-sensitive optical methods (e.g., surface-enhanced Raman scattering and surface plasmon resonance) have been developed using magnetic nanomaterials (Table 2). Thus, each transducer has its significance depending on the target analyte nature and the associated extractable molecular properties in the sensor design.

Molecular Recognition Probes

Antibodies and aptamers for proteins and small molecules, complementary nucleotides for deoxyribonucleic acid (DNA) and ribonucleic acid (RNA) hybridization, enzymes for specific substrates by either direct or indirect catalytic conversions, receptors for ligands, and non-enzymatic molecular probes (e.g., molecularly imprinted polymers) for analytes are commonly used approaches in magnetic biosensors. For example, a magnetic force-aided electrochemical sensor was developed using sandwich biorecognitions from an aptamer and antibody combination for the detection of thrombin in serum samples [57]. Similarly, a magnetic field-induced self-assembly of Fe_3O_4(magnetite)@polyaniline nanoparticles incorporated with a molecularly imprinted polymer biorecognition element-delivered electrochemical sensing of creatinine in human plasma and urine samples [58]. Electrochemical glucose biosensing by glucose oxidase, on an electrode consisting of gold nanoparticles/bovine serum albumin/Fe_3O_4 nanocomposite [59], is an example for enzymatic biorecognition event (Figure 1-I–III).

An antibody biorecognition probe immobilized on a magnetic ($CoFe_2O_4$) metal–organic framework (MOF)@Au tetrapods (AuTPs) surface, with toluidine blue as the surface-enhanced Raman spectroscopy (SERS) tag, was used for detection of N-terminal pro-brain natriuretic peptides [54]. This strategy offered a large dynamic range with ultra-low detection limits. Effective magnetic bead-based separation and highly selective aptamer recognition of G-quadruplex formation of the anterior gradient homolog 2 (AGR2) protein, cancer biomarker, offered picomolar detection limits. This system also utilized gold nanoparticles. The detection was based on UV–vis spectrometry [60]. Another antibody-conjugated magnetic-bead sensor detected chloramphenicol antibiotic based on a competitive surface-enhanced Raman scattering method [61] (Figure 2-I,II).

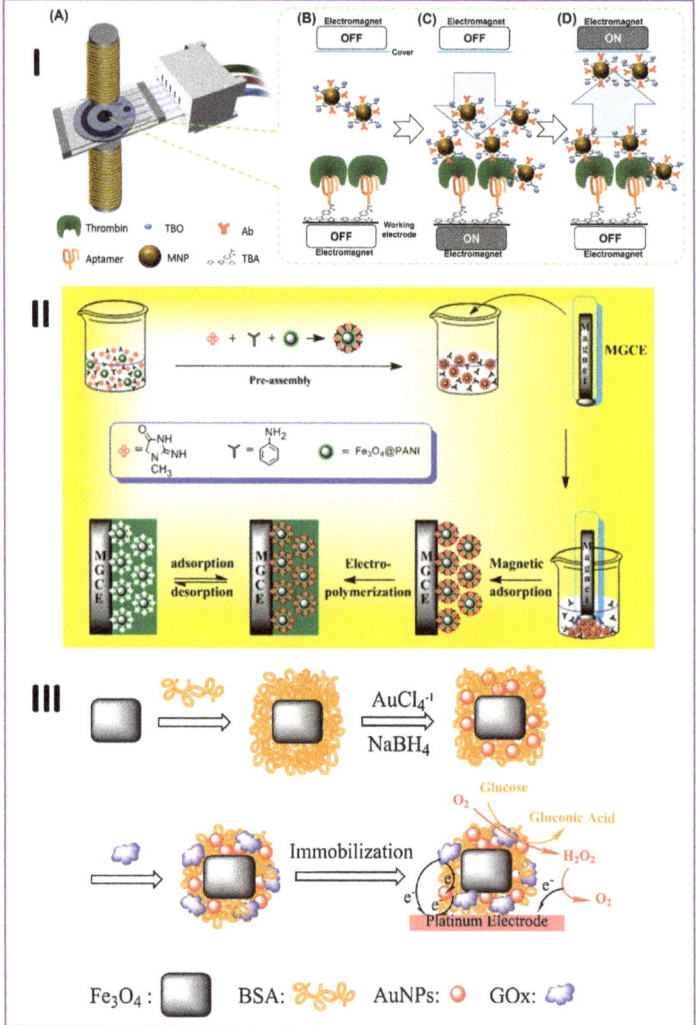

Figure 1. (**I**) (**A**) Sensing system composed of an electrochemical sensor, a pair of electromagnets, and a sample chamber. (**B–D**) The process of magnetic force-assisted electrochemical sandwich assays (MESA) is illustrated: (**B**) the sample loading step to mix the sample solution and the magnetic nanoparticle (MNP) bioconjugates with antibody and toluidine blue O (MNP@Ab-TBO); (**C**) the reaction step to form sandwich complexes on the electrode surface; and (**D**) the removal step to remove unbound MNP@Ab-TBO from the electrode surface. Reproduced with permission from Reference [57]. Copyright 2018 Elsevier. (**II**) Schematic representation of the preparation of the molecularly imprinted electrochemical sensor (MIES) for detection of creatinine. Reproduced with permission from Reference [58]. Copyright 2014 Elsevier. (**III**) Schematic illustration of the preparation of a GOx/AuNPs/BSA/Fe$_3$O$_4$/Pt electrode. Reproduced with permission from Reference [59]. Copyright 2016 Elsevier. Abbreviations: TBA - 2,2′:5′,5″-terthiophene-3′-p-benzoic acid; MGCE - magnetic glassy carbon electrode; Fe$_3$O$_4$@PANI - magnetite@polyaniline; BSA - bovine serum albumin; AuNPs - gold nanoparticles; GOx - glucose oxidase.

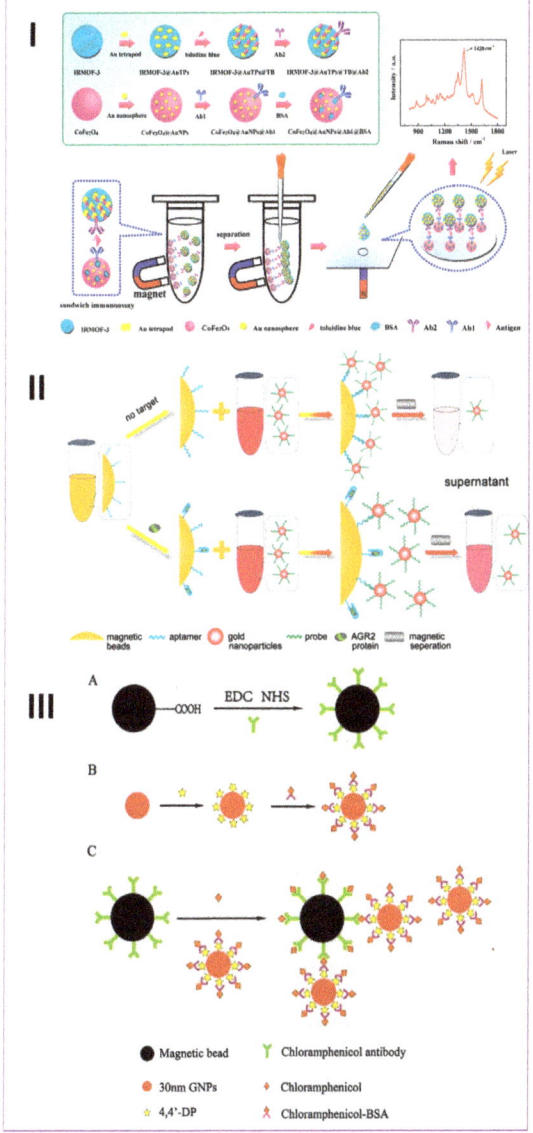

Figure 2. (**I**) Schematic representation of the surface-enhanced Raman spectroscopy (SERS)-based sandwich immunosensor for the detection of N-terminal pro-brain natriuretic peptides (NT-proBNPs). Reproduced with permission from Reference [54]. (**II**) Schematic representation of anterior gradient homolog 2 (AGR2) protein detection procedure. Reproduced with permission from Reference [60]. Copyright 2015 Elsevier. (**III**) (**A**) Preparation of MNPs modified with chloramphenicol antibody. (**B**) Preparation of SERS tags. (**C**) SERS-based magnetic immunosensor for chloramphenicol. Reproduced with permission from Reference [61]. Copyright 2016 Elsevier. Abbreviations: IRMOF- amino-functionalized metal–organic framework; AuTPs - gold tetrapods; AuNPs - gold nanoparticles; TB - toluidine blue; GNPs - gold nanoparticles; 4,4'-DP - 4,4'-dipyridyl; EDC - 1-Ethyl-3-(3-dimethylaminopropyl)carbodiimide; NHS - N-Hydroxysuccinimide.

Magnetic particle sensors for detection of various classes of analytes in a variety of complex sample matrices. In the subsequent sections, we extend our discussion to selective classes of analytes and various sample matrices, biorecognition materials, and transducers that best addressed the sensor purpose and analytical performance.

3. Biomarkers

Biomarkers indicate normal versus abnormal conditions based on the levels of their concentrations in organs, tissues, and circulating body fluids. Hence, sensors that allow selective and required sensitive detection of the biomarkers are significant in diagnosis and treatment. We present here a few examples of biomarker sensors based on magnetic materials which use various transducers. Recently, Gooding et al. [62] devised a novel microRNA detection probe consisting of a DNA sequence attached to gold-coated magnetic nanoparticles. By electrically reconfiguring the nanoparticle probe, they achieved electrochemical (square wave voltammetry) detection of microRNA in whole blood samples over a wide concentration range from attomolar to nanomolar. Such ultrasensitive magnetic nanoparticle tools are significant for clinical diagnostics.

Similarly, magnetic nanoparticle-based voltammetric and electrochemical mass sensors recently enabled the detection of ultra-low clinically relevant picomolar serum insulin concentrations (Figure 3A(a,b),B) [63,64]. In the electrochemical mass sensor, magnetic isolation of insulin from a serum sample reduced the interference from the sample matrix and non-specific background signals which was quantitatively estimated by comparing the background signals for magnetically treated serum control response with that of a solution-based bulk serum control response (Figure 3A-b) [63]. Furthermore, enriching the surface –COOH groups of pyrenyl-carbon nanostructures by combined covalent and non-covalent carboxylation improved the sensitivity of serum insulin immunosensing compared to only a carboxylated nanotube-based sensor (Figure 3C) [65]. Another quartz crystal microbalance (QCM) mass sensor method has been reported for detection of thrombin (in diluted serum or fibrinogen-precipitated plasma samples) by a magnetic microbead polymeric material and detection on an aptamer-immobilized QCM crystal based on oscillation frequency decrease [66]. Translating the quantitative knowledge derived from a single-sample QCM analysis sensor into a relatively better throughput surface plasmon imaging gold array enabled magnetic nanoparticle captured serum insulin (50% serum in buffer) detection at picomolar concentrations (Figure 3D) [67]. Advancements in microfluidic designs enabled on-line protein capturing by magnetic beads and ultrasensitive electrochemical detection of interleukin cancer biomarkers (IL-6 and IL-8) in undiluted calf serum [68]. In addition to electrochemical detection, surface plasmon spectroscopy that offers detection with binding insights [69] has been successfully developed with a polyamidoamine (PAMAM)-magnetic nanoparticle quantum dot modification on a gold array for a dual imaging-based detection of blood insulin and glycated hemoglobin (20 time diluted whole blood samples in buffer) (Figure 3E) [70]. Subsequently, fluorescence imaging of the sensor array allowed an independent validation of the method. Table 1 presents various magnetic nanoparticles based electrochemical sensors for the detection of a wide range of analytes. Cyclic, square-wave, and differential voltammetry, and amperometric techniques have been widely used as electrochemical transducers. Moreover, the analytes ranged from small molecules such as glucose, bisphenol A, and ciprofloxacin antibiotics to various protein biomarkers, pesticides, and illicit drugs. The analyte recognition elements include enzymes, aptamers, antibodies, and molecularly imprinted polymers. The wide variety of sample matrices covered were blood, serum, plasma, urine, milk, juice, meat samples, and water (Table 1).

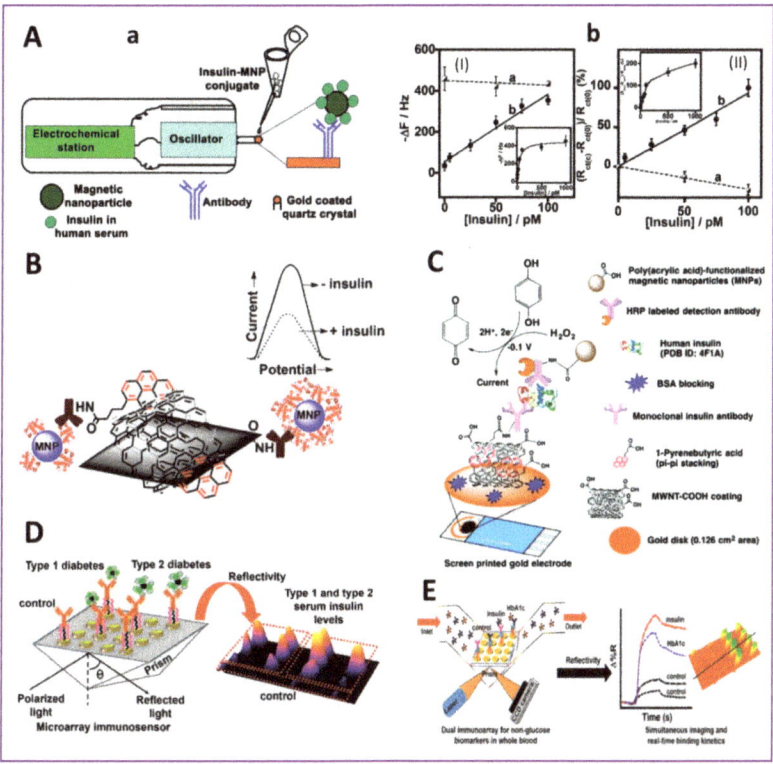

Figure 3. (**A**) An electrochemical mass sensor for clinically relevant detection of insulin in human serum conjugated to magnetic nanoparticles and captured onto antibody immobilized gold-coated quartz resonators was reported in this study: (**a**) Schematic of the electrochemical quartz crystal microbalance (eQCM) sensor and (**b**) sensor responses (QCM and Faradaic impedance) showing the significant reduction of non-specific signals for control serum due to the magnetic nanoparticle capturing of insulin and detection upon binding onto the surface antibody sensor, enabling picomolar detection limits. This is not possible by doing the assay from a solution form of the serum insulin sample due to the inability of ultra-low picomolar signals to overcome the large background signal response of the un-spiked serum solution control. Reproduced with permission from Reference [63]. Copyright 2014 Royal Society of Chemistry. (**B**) This report presented the first serum insulin voltammetric immunosensor for diagnosis of type-1 and type-2 diabetic disorders based on fasting serum insulin levels. The sensor was composed of multiwalled carbon nanotube-pyrenebutyric acid frameworks on edge plane pyrolytic graphite electrodes to which anti-insulin antibody was covalently attached. Magnetically captured insulin from 50% serum in buffer was detected upon binding onto the surface insulin-antibody sensor. Reproduced with permission from Reference [64]. Copyright 2015 American Chemical Society. (**C**) Schematic of a combined covalent and noncovalent carboxylation of carbon nanotubes for sensitivity enhancement of clinical immunosensors (demonstrated here with serum insulin). Reproduced with permission from Reference [65]. Copyright 2016 Royal Society of Chemistry. (**D**) Schematic of a magnetic optical microarray imager for diagnosing type of diabetes in clinical fasting blood serum samples based on picomolar insulin concentrations. Reproduced with permission from Reference [67]. Copyright 2016 American Chemical Society. (**E**) Schematic of a magnetite-quantum dot immunoarray for plasmon-coupled fluorescence imaging of blood insulin and glycated hemoglobin. Reproduced with permission from Reference [70]. Copyright 2017 American Chemical Society.

Table 1. Magnetic nanoparticle (MNP)-based electrochemical sensors for the detection of various analytes.

S. No.	Application	Transduction Method	Recognition Element	Analyte	Interface	Real Sample	Range	LOD	Reference
1	Medical	Voltammetry	Molecularly Imprinted Polymers (MIPs)	Hemoglobin	GCE[1]/Fe$_3$O$_4$@SiO$_2$/MMIP	Blood	0.005–0.1 mg mL^{-1}	0.001 mg mL^{-1}	[71]
2	Environmental	Differential Pulse Voltammetry (DPV)	MIP	Bisphenol A	SPCE[2]/AuNPs/ CBNPs[5]/Fe$_3$O$_4$/MMIP[3]	Mineral water	0.07–10 μM	8.8 nM	[72]
3	Medical	DPV	Chemical	Ciprofloxacin	CPE/Fe$_3$O$_4$/CMNPs	Serum, Urine	0.05–75 μM L^{-1}	0.01 μM L^{-1}	[73]
4	Food Clinical	DPV	MIP	N-Acyl-homoserine -lactones	MGCE[5]/Fe$_3$O$_4$@SiO$_2$-MIP		2.5×10^{-9}–1.0×10^{-7} mol L^{-1}	8×10^{-10} mol L^{-1}	[74]
5	Food	DPV	MIP	Kanamycin	CE[4]/MWCNTs/Fe$_3$O$_4$/PMMA	Milk, Chicken, Pig	1×10^{-10}–1.0×10^{-6} mol L^{-1}	2.3×10^{-11} mol L^{-1}	[75]
6	Food	Cyclic Voltammetry (CV)	Enzyme	Peroxide	Pt/MRGO[6]/chi/HRP	Orange juice	20–1000 μM 48.08 μA μM^{-1}·cm^{-2}	2 μM	[76]
7	Security	DPV		Morphine	CPE/CHT[7]/Fe$_3$O$_4$	Serum, Urine	10–2000 nM	3 nM	[77]
8	Food	DPV		Quercetin and Tryptophan	CPE/Fe$_3$O$_4$@NiO core/shell nanoparticles	Human breast milk, cow milk, and honey	0.08–60 μM 0.1–120 μM	2.18 nM 14.23 nM	[78]
9	Medical	DPV	Antibody (Ab)	Prostate specific antigen (PSA)	Ab$_2$/MB[8]/ Au@Fe$_3$O$_4$@COF/GCE	Serum	0.0001–10 ng mL^{-1}	30 fg mL^{-1}	[79]
10	Medical	Amperometry	Enzyme	Glucose	GOx[14]/AuNPs/BSA/Fe$_3$O$_4$/PtE	-	0.25–7.0 mM	3.54 μM	[59]
11	Medical	DPV		Ractopamine	MSPE/RGO/Fe$_3$O$_4$	Pork meat	0.05–100 μM	13 nM	[80]
12	Medical	Amperometry	Aptamer-Antibody	Thrombin	pTBA/Apt/thrombin/ MNP@Ab-TBO[9]/SPCE	Serum	1–500 nM	0.49	[57]
13	Security	Square Wave Voltammetry (SWV)		Organo-phosphates	Fe$_3$O$_4$@ZrO$_2$/MCCE	-	7.60×10^{-8}–9.12×10^{-5} M	1.52×10^{-8} M	[81]
14	Medical	DPV	MIP	Creatinine	MCCE/Fe$_3$O$_4$@PANI[10] NPs/MIP	Plasma, Urine	0.02–1 μM L^{-1}	0.35 nM L^{-1}	[58]
15	Medical	DPV		Progesterone	Fe$_3$O$_4$@GQD[11]/ f-MWCNTs[12]/GCE	Serum	0.01–3.0 μM	2.18 nM	[82]
16	Medical	Amperometry		PSA, Prostate specific membrane antigen (PSMA) Cancer biomarker	Fe$_3$O$_4$@GO/Ab/PSMA		61 fg mL^{-1}–3.9 pg mL^{-1} 9.8 fg mL^{-1}–10 pg mL^{-1}	15 fg mL^{-1} 4.8 fg mL^{-1}	[83]
17	Medical	DPV		PSA, PSMA, IL6, Platelet factor 4 (PF4)	MNP/HRP[13]-Ab		0.05–2 pg mL^{-1}		[84]

GCE[1]: Glassy carbon electrode; SPCE[2]: screen-printed carbon electrode; MMIPs[3]: magnetic molecularly imprinted polymers; CE[4]: carbon electrode; CBNPs[4]: carbon black nanoparticles; MGCE[5]: magnetic glassy carbon electrode; MRGO[6]: magnetic reduced graphene oxide; CHT[7]: chitosan; MB[8]: methylene blue; TBO[9]: toluidine blue O; PANI[10]: polyaniline; GQD[11]: graphene quantum dots; MWCNTs[12]: multiwalled carbon nanotubes; HRP[13]: horseradish peroxidase; GOx: glucose oxidase.

A nanocomposite that consists of glucose oxidase with reduced graphene oxide and magnetic nanoparticles on a magnetic sticker attached to a screen-printed electrode was shown to offer micromolar glucose amperometric detection in simple aqueous solutions [55]. An antibody conjugation to a magnetic nitrogen-doped graphene-modified gold electrode was used for voltammetric detection of amyloid-beta peptide 1–42 (Aβ42), a biomarker of Alzheimer's disease, in solution [85]. However, the applicability of such sensors for practical sample matrices of biofluids would be more significant.

A recently reported magnetic-focus-lateral flow-colorimetric biosensor offered a million-fold improvement in sensitivity over the conventional lateral flow systems toward detection of the valosin-containing protein of relevance to cervical cancer [53] (Figure 4A(a,b)). The sensor applicability for protein mixtures extracted from the tissue of cervical cancer patients was successfully demonstrated. Spectral correlation interferometry, capable of picometer resolution of measured thickness changes of a layer of molecules or nanoparticles, was designed for sensitive detection of prostate-specific antigen by a magnetic nanoparticle-bioprobe amplification strategy [86] (Figure 4B). Another study utilized anodic stripping voltammetry for sensitive DNA detection on a magnetic porous pseudo-carbon paste electrode [87].

A magnetic bead-based colorimetric biosensor allowed for detection of two inflammatory salivary biomarkers, human neutrophil elastase and cathepsin-G, in solution and spiked saliva samples. The sensor utilized proteolytic activity-induced color changes with biomarker concentration. The sensor was validated with patients' saliva analysis [88]. Magnetic particles possess peroxidase-like enzymatic activity. This property has been extensively used in both electrochemical and optical sensors for analyte detection. An illustration would be the enzymatic colorimetric glucose sensors based on magnetic particles that exploited the peroxidase-like activity of these particles [89]. In this report, glucose oxidase was covalently attached to carboxylated magnetic beads (1 µm size) for spectrophotometric detection of glucose in solutions or that spiked in plasma samples using o-phenylenediamine dihydrochloride reagent.

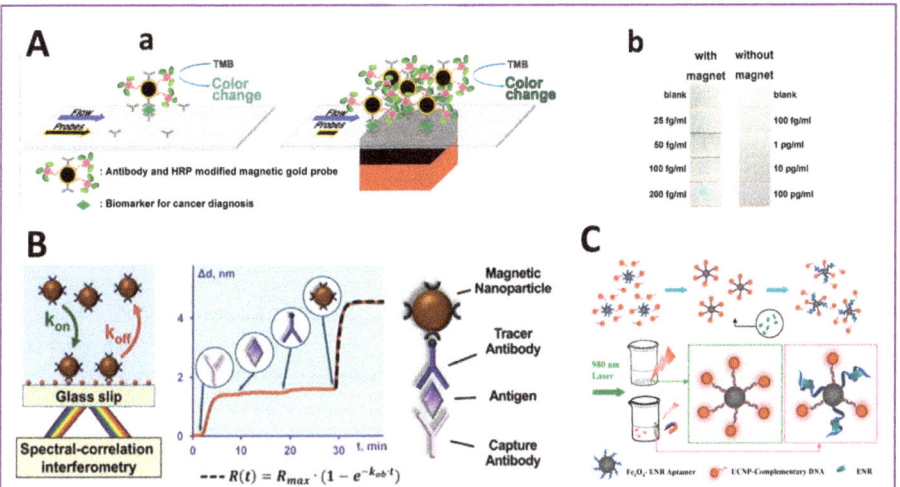

Figure 4. (**A**) (**a**) Schematic depicting the effect of magnetic focus lateral flow biosensor. Without the magnet, the magnetic probe-labeled targets move along with the sample flow on the lateral flow strip, resulting in a low capture efficiency (left). With magnet, the probe-labeled targets are focused at the signal generation zone due to the magnetic focus thus increasing the capture efficiency of labeled targets (right). (**b**) Comparison of the detection results with and without magnet. Reproduced with permission from Reference [53]. Copyright 2019 American Chemical Society. (**B**) Sandwich immunoassay for t-PSA: on the left—sensograms demonstrating all assay steps in absence of t-PSA (lower blue curve)

and in the presence of 1 µg/ml t-PSA (upper red curve); on the right—scheme of sandwich assay: 1—capture antibody, 2—antigen, 3—biotinylated tracer antibody, 4—magnetic nanoparticle coated by streptavidin. Reproduced with permission from Reference [86]. Copyright 2016 Elsevier. (**C**) Schematic diagram of upconversion nanoparticles (UCNPs) luminescence-based aptasensor for the selective detection of ENR. Reproduced with permission from Reference [90]. Copyright 2016 Elsevier. Abbreviations: TMB - Tetramethyl benzidine; HRP - Horseradish peroxidase; UCNPs - Upconversion nanoparticles; ENR – Enrofloxacin.

An enzymatic biosensor composed of poly(dopamine)-modified magnetic nanoparticles, covalently attached with a PAMAM dendrimer (ethylenediamine core polyamidoamine G-4; fourth-generation) and additionally incorporated with platinum nanoparticles, was used for amperometric detection of micromolar xanthine in fish samples [91]. Similarly, magnetic nanocomposite materials with carbon nanostructures (e.g., graphene and nanotubes) have been devised for sensitive electrochemical enzymatic glucose detection in spiked urine samples [92] and progesterone in human serum samples and pharmaceutical products [82] with good recoveries. Magnetic susceptibility measurements combined with a optomagnetic method was developed for detection of C-reactive protein in serum from the agglutination of magnetic nanoparticles conjugated with the protein antibody [93]. A chemiluminescent biosensor combining magnetic beads with platinum nanoparticles for thyroid-stimulating hormone detection in serum has been devised [94].

Protein A/G-functionalized 2 µm magnetic beads successfully isolated glutamic acid decarboxylase-65 autoantibody from 10% serum and enabled sensitive (picomolar) detection on the glutamic acid decarboxylase-65 immobilized carboxylated graphene surface [95] (Figure 5A(a,b)). In this report, the correlation of picomolar affinities between surface plasmon resonance and electrochemical immunosensors was demonstrated. Furthermore, multiplex biosensing of a panel of biomarkers allows reliable and rapid quantification of several analytes in complex clinical matrices. A new surface plasmon-imaging array based on core/shell Fe_3O_4@Au nanoparticles enabled combined detection of two interleukin proteins and two microRNAs in a diluted serum (Figure 5B) [96]. The gold shell can facilitate the enhancement of the plasmon signals and the magnetic core for easy separation and magnetic isolation of desired target analytes present in complex sample matrices. Moreover, the core/shell material exhibited higher plasmonic signals than the individual nanoparticle components of similar hydrodynamic sizes [96]. Such multifunctional magnetic materials and composites offer several distinct properties but centralized into a single component to enable designing ultra-sensitive sensors [59,97–101]. A multiplex sensor featuring magnetic nanoparticle–antibody conjugates for detection of ovarian cancer biomarkers, CA-125, β-2M, and ApoA1, has been reported [102]. Fluorescence spectroscopy and surface plasmon resonance analysis were utilized. Thus, emerging directions of magnetic particle biosensor designs [103] are pushing the limits of applications to increasingly complex real samples and multianalyte biosensing. One other example of a biocatalytic real-sample system is the design of magnetic nanoparticle-based liver microsomal biofilms (subcellular liver fractions containing drug-metabolizing cytochrome P450 enzymes with their reductase) for reduced-nicotinamide adenine dinucleotide phosphate (NADPH)-free direct electrochemical drug biosensing and stereoselective metabolite production [104] (Figure 5C).

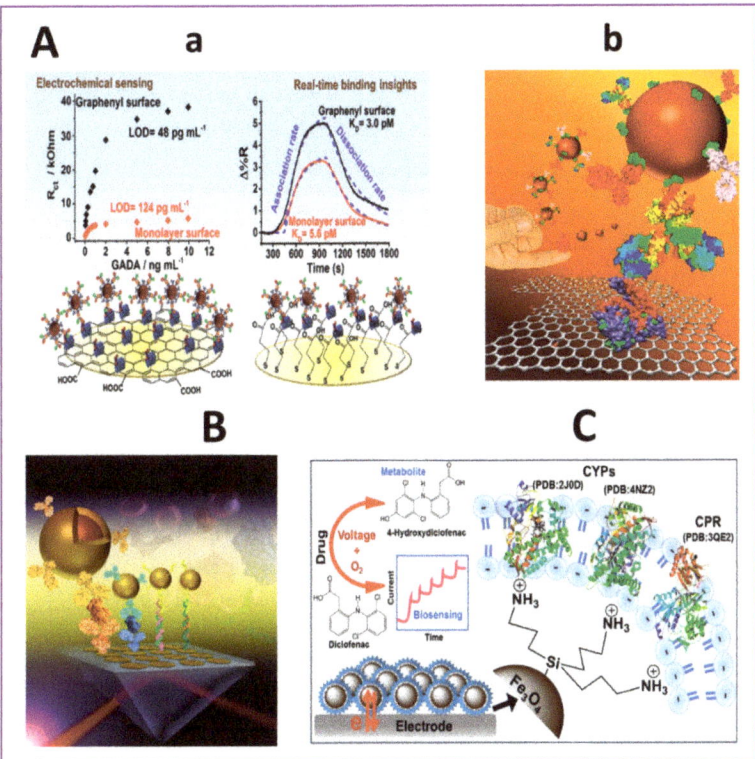

Figure 5. (**A**) (**a**) Electrochemical and surface plasmon correlation of serum autoantibody immunosensors with binding insights. In this report, a comparative account of carboxylated graphenyl and mercapto-monolayer surfaces was made for the detection of serum glutamic acid decarboxylase-65 autoantibody (GADA), a biomarker of type 1 diabetes and (**b**) schematic representation. Reproduced with permission from Reference [95]. Copyright 2018 American Chemical Society. (**B**) Schematic representation of a multiplexed surface plasmon imaging of serum biomolecules. In this report, Fe_3O_4@Au core/shell nanoparticles carrying analyte-specific second biorecognition element (the first one was immobilized on the sensor surface) were used for signal amplification purpose and presented with plasmonic simulation insights. Reproduced with permission from Reference [96]. Copyright 2019 Elsevier. (**C**) Schematic of a biocatalytic system constructed by electrostatically immobilizing drug-metabolizing human liver microsomes (HLMs, negatively charged due to the phospholipids) onto positively charged amine-functionalized magnetic nanoparticles (100 nm hydrodynamic diameter). This report presented electrochemical biosensing of cytochrome P450 (CYP)-specific drug candidates and electrocatalyzing drug conversion into metabolites with electron mediation in the biofilm by cytochrome P450-reductase (CPR). Reproduced with permission from Reference [104]. Copyright 2018 Elsevier.

Katz et al. [105] reported a novel magnetic field-activated binary deoxyribozyme sensor for fluorescent detection of a specific messenger RNA that is a cancer biomarker. The sensor functioned well when internalized in live MCF-7 breast cancer cells and activated by a magnetic field. The sensor utilized two types of magnetic bead bioconjugates that carried different components of a multicomponent deoxyribozyme sensor. The sensor function was activated only in the presence of a specific target messenger RNA and upon an applied magnetic field thus adding control over the selectivity [106]. Pang et al. [107] designed a DNA probe Fe_3O_4@Ag magnetic nanoparticle biosensor for capturing microRNA from cancer cells and detection at ultra-low concentrations (0.3 fM). In this study, surface-enhanced Raman scattering with a duplex-specific nuclease signal amplification strategy was used. Application for point-of-care clinical diagnostics of microRNA has been envisioned. Discussed above are a range of illustrative examples of bioanalytes, and, in the subsequent sections, we highlight magnetic particle sensors developed for other analyte classes.

4. Food Analytes, Pathogens, and Pharmaceuticals

In addition to the important detection advantages of the magnetic particle sensor approaches for a range of diagnostically useful biomarkers and small molecules, the broader applicability for food, pathogens, and pharmaceuticals are illustrated in this section. Food and pharmaceuticals represent two essential components for sustaining life and health. Biosensors play important roles in the detection of foodborne pathogens and the development of valuable therapeutic molecules. Andreescu et al. [108], in the year 2015, published an excellent review of the design and development of nanoparticle-based (including magnetic) sensors for food safety assessment. They covered both colorimetric and electrochemical detection of chemical and biological contaminants (e.g., pesticides, heavy metals, bacterial pathogens, and natural toxins). Therefore, we provide some representative recent reports specifically on magnetic material sensors for food contaminants, pathogens, and pharmaceuticals.

An impedimetric electrochemical aptasensor allowed rapid and sensitive detection of *Escherichia coli* [109]. The sensor system contained biotinylated polyclonal antibodies bound strongly to streptavidin-modified magnetic nanoparticles for selective separation of target bacteria from the sample in a coaxial capillary designed with high-gradient magnetic fields. For measuring impedance signals with the bacteria concentration, urease-catalyzed hydrolysis of urea into ammonium ions and carbonate ions in the capillary was used. A disposable amperometric sensor based on core/shell $Fe_3O_4@SiO_2$ superparamagnetic nanoparticles conjugated with specific bioreceptors for selective detection and quantification of *Brettanomyces bruxellensis* (Brett) and total yeast content in wine has been developed (Figure 6) [110]. Maghemite nanoparticles (Fe_2O_3) have been identified to be an efficient and reliable material for removal of citrinin, a nephrotoxic mycotoxin, from food samples [111]. Table 2 presents various magnetic nanoparticles based optical sensors for detection of a wide range of analytes. Colorimetric, luminescence, surface plasmon resonance (SPR), and other surface-sensitive techniques are illustrated as representative transducers. Aptamers, peptides, antibodies, and MIPs are presented as recognition elements. The analytes ranged from proteins, hormones, peptides, miRNA, and bacteria to small molecules (Table 2).

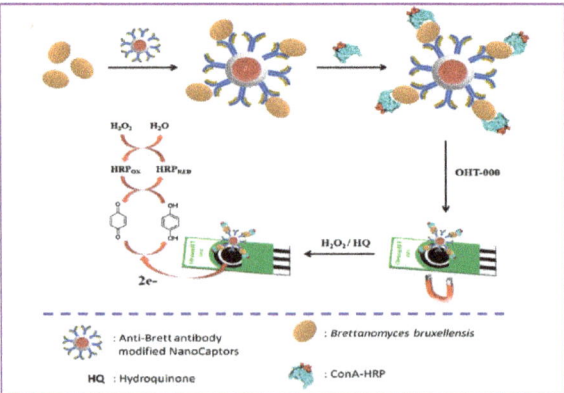

Figure 6. Schematic display of the steps involved in the preparation and performance of the biosensor for Brett (Ab-B sensor). Reproduced with permission from Reference [110]. Copyright 2019 Elsevier. Abbreviations: ConA - Concanavalin A.

Table 2. Magnetic nanoparticle (MNP)-based optical sensors for the detection of various analytes.

S.No.	Transduction Method	Recognition Element	Analyte	Assay	Range	LOD	Reference
1	Ultraviolet-Visible (UV-Vis)	Aptamer	Cancer biomarker AGR2[1]	Au NPs/DNA/MBs	10–1280 pM	6.6 pM	[60]
2	Surface Plasmon Resonance (SPR)	Aptamer	Thrombin	Fe_3O_4@Au NPs/Apt	0.1–100 nM	0.1 nM	[112]
3	Colorimetric	Ab	Listeria	MNB-MAb-Listeria-PAb-AuNP-urease	1.1×10^2–1.1×10^6 CFU mL^{-1}	102 CFU mL^{-1}	[113]
4	Colorimetric	Peptide	E. coli.	MNP[2]/Peptide/AuNPs/SAM	30–300 CFU mL^{-1}	12 CFU mL^{-1}	[114]
5	Photonic crystal	Ab	soluble transferrin receptor	fAb-IONs[3]	0.01–0.2 µg mL^{-1}	-	[115]
6	Surface Enhanced Raman Spectroscopy (SERS)	Ab	chloramphenicol	AuNPs/MNPs/Ab	0–10 ng mL^{-1}	1 pg mL^{-1}	[61]
7	Chemiluminescence	MIP	Lysozyme	ILs[3]-Fe_3O_4@DA/GO[6]/β-CD[4]	1.0×10^{-9}–8.0×10^{-8} mg mL^{-1}	3.0×10^{-10} mg mL^{-1}	[116]
8	Chemiluminescence	Enzyme-Ab	Thyroid stimulant hormone	Pt NPs/HRP-Ab/magnetic beads	0.013–12 mU L^{-1}	0.005 mU L^{-1}	[94]
9	SERS		MiRNA let-7b (cancer cells)	Fe_3O_4@Ag NPs	0–1000 pM	0.3 fM	[107]
10	SERS	Ab	Ovarian cancer Multiplexed (CA-125, β2-M and ApoA1)	MNPs/Abs		0.26 U mL^{-1}, 0.55 ng mL^{-1}, and 7.7 ng mL^{-1}	[102]
11	SERS	Ab	N-Terminal pro-brain natriuretic peptide (heart failure)	$CoFe_2O_4$@AuNPs/MOFs	1 fg mL^{-1}–1 ng mL^{-1}	0.75 fg mL^{-1}	[54]
12	SERS		Carcinoembryonic antigen	MBA-labeled NiFe@Au NPs	0–1 ng mL^{-1}	0.1 pM	[56]
13	SERS			Fe_3O_4@Au Core/shell nanoparticles			[96]

AGR2[1]: anterior gradient homolog 2; MNP[2]: magnetic nanoparticles; IONs[3]: iron oxide nanoparticles; ILs[3]: ionic liquids; β-CD[4]: β-cyclodextrins[5]; GO[6]: graphene oxide.

Aptamer-functionalized magnetite (Fe_3O_4) conjugated upconversion nanoparticles were constructed to quantify trace enrofloxacin (a fluoroquinolone antibiotic) in fish samples; hybridization reaction-based luminescent intensity decreased when the analyte concentration was used as the signal transduction output [90] (Figure 4C). The "upconversion" terminology is related to the property of high-energy photon emission by a shorter wavelength excitation source of lower energy such as near-infrared photons. Other representative magnetic nanoparticle sensors for separation and/or detection include colorimetric tetracycline detection [117], chloramphenicol [61], lysozyme (an antimicrobial enzyme) [116], aflatoxins [118] (a review covering electrochemical, optical, and mass-sensitive biosensors), *Listeria monocytogenes* (a Gram-positive bacterium) [119], *Staphylococcus aureus* (a Gram-positive bacterium) [120], *Salmonella enteritidis* (a Gram-negative bacterium) [121], impedimetric hepatitis B virus DNA [122], and *Vibrio cholerae* DNA detection [123,124].

5. Environment

Environmental biosensors play significant roles in human safety and protecting the planet from devastations. Nanotechnology as a whole has contributed to the development of modern real-time environmental sensors (e.g., pollution monitoring, agriculture, renewable energy, water, and aviation) [47,125,126]. Herein, we illustrate literature reports on magnetic particle-based environmental biosensor system for organophosphorus pesticides, which are known to be toxic agricultural wastes despite their widespread use. Co-immobilization of carboxylic acid group-modified magnetic nanoparticles and acetylcholinesterase enzyme onto an electropolymerized surface of 4,7-di(furan-2-yl)benzo[c][1,2,5]-thiadiazole allowed sensitive micromolar detection of paraoxon and trichlorfon used as model organophosphates [127]. Amperometric current signals were used as the transduction method. Good reproducibility, long-term stability over 10 days, and applicability of the sensor for analysis in real tap water samples were demonstrated. Another acetylcholinesterase-magnetic particle electrochemical biosensor operated in flow injection analysis also delivered sensitive detection of organophosphate insecticides [128].

Summary/Prospects

The versatile nature of magnetic materials for applications with a range of transduction and biorecognition principles is detailed. Moreover, magnetic sensor designs for the detection of a broad range of analytes present in various complex real sample matrices of relevance to disease diagnosis, health, food, agriculture, energy, and environment are highlighted. Future directions in the field are aimed at synthesizing new multifunctional magnetic materials that offer simplicity and rapid detection platforms from the prior methods and quantitative insights into size and shape distributions as well as chemical and surface functionality aspects of magnetic materials. Moreover, efficient strategies for oriented and other modes of immobilization of bioprobes, their quantitative characterizations, activity, bioconjugation and catalytic efficiency, need of reproducibility, and long-term stability of sensor designs are being addressed. Emerging magnetic particle biosensor designs with multifunctional and multiplex features are discussed. Improvements on the scientific rigor of methodologies and approaches developed and standardization of protocols for reliable end applications are some of the currently emphasized benchmarks for successful magnetic particle sensor designs.

Author Contributions: S.K. and K.Y.G. contributed equally in the preparation of this review article.

Funding: This research received no external funding.

Conflicts of Interest: The authors declare no conflicts of interest.

References

1. Hasanzadeh, M.; Shadjou, N.; de la Guardia, M. Iron and iron-oxide magnetic nanoparticles as signal-amplification elements in electrochemical biosensing. *TrAC Trends Anal. Chem.* **2015**, *72*, 1–9. [CrossRef]
2. Kudr, J.; Haddad, Y.; Richtera, L.; Heger, Z.; Cernak, M.; Adam, V.; Zitka, O. Magnetic nanoparticles: From design and synthesis to real world applications. *Nanomaterials* **2017**, *7*, 243. [CrossRef] [PubMed]
3. Jamshaid, T.; Neto, E.T.T.; Eissa, M.M.; Zine, N.; Kunita, M.H.; El-Salhi, A.E.; Elaissari, A. Magnetic particles: From preparation to lab-on-a-chip, biosensors, microsystems and microfluidics applications. *TrAC Trends Anal. Chem.* **2016**, *79*, 344–362. [CrossRef]
4. Xianyu, Y.; Wang, Q.; Chen, Y. Magnetic particles-enabled biosensors for point-of-care testing. *TrAC Trends Anal. Chem.* **2018**, *106*, 213–224. [CrossRef]
5. Giouroudi, I.; Kokkinis, G. Recent advances in magnetic microfluidic biosensors. *Nanomaterials* **2017**, *7*, 171. [CrossRef]
6. Ravalli, A.; Marrazza, G. Gold and magnetic nanoparticles-based electrochemical biosensors for cancer biomarker determination. *J. Nanosci. Nanotechnol.* **2015**, *15*, 3307–3319. [CrossRef]
7. Lan, L.; Yao, Y.; Ping, J.; Ying, Y. Recent advances in nanomaterial-based biosensors for antibiotics detection. *Biosens. Bioelectron.* **2017**, *91*, 504–514. [CrossRef]
8. Kurbanoglu, S.; Ozkan, S.A.; Merkoçi, A. Nanomaterials-based enzyme electrochemical biosensors operating through inhibition for biosensing applications. *Biosens. Bioelectron.* **2017**, *89*, 886–898. [CrossRef]
9. Yoo, S.M.; Lee, S.Y. Optical biosensors for the detection of pathogenic microorganisms. *Trends Biotechnol.* **2016**, *34*, 7–25. [CrossRef]
10. Yu, E.Y.; Bishop, M.; Zheng, B.; Ferguson, R.M.; Khandhar, A.P.; Kemp, S.J.; Krishnan, K.M.; Goodwill, P.W.; Conolly, S.M. Magnetic particle imaging: A novel in vivo imaging platform for cancer detection. *Nano Lett.* **2017**, *17*, 1648–1654. [CrossRef]
11. Salamon, J.; Hofmann, M.; Jung, C.; Kaul, M.G.; Werner, F.; Them, K.; Reimer, R.; Nielsen, P.; Vom Scheidt, A.; Adam, G.; et al. Magnetic particle/magnetic resonance imaging: In-vitro MPI-guided real time catheter tracking and 4D angioplasty using a road map and blood pool tracer approach. *PLoS ONE* **2016**, *11*, e0156899. [CrossRef] [PubMed]
12. Arami, H.; Teeman, E.; Troksa, A.; Bradshaw, H.; Saatchi, K.; Tomitaka, A.; Gambhir, S.S.; Häfeli, U.O.; Liggitt, D.; Krishnan, K.M. Tomographic magnetic particle imaging of cancer targeted nanoparticles. *Nanoscale* **2017**, *9*, 18723–18730. [CrossRef] [PubMed]
13. Shen, Z.; Wu, A.; Chen, X. Iron oxide nanoparticle based contrast agents for magnetic resonance imaging. *Mol. Pharm.* **2017**, *14*, 1352–1364. [CrossRef] [PubMed]
14. Knopp, T.; Hofmann, M. Online reconstruction of 3D magnetic particle imaging data. *Phys. Med. Biol.* **2016**, *61*, N257–N267. [CrossRef]
15. Arami, H.; Khandhar, A.P.; Tomitaka, A.; Yu, E.; Goodwill, P.W.; Conolly, S.M.; Krishnan, K.M. In vivo multimodal magnetic particle imaging (MPI) with tailored magneto/optical contrast agents. *Biomaterials* **2015**, *52*, 251–261. [CrossRef]
16. Teeman, E.; Shasha, C.; Evans, J.E.; Krishnan, K.M. Intracellular dynamics of superparamagnetic iron oxide nanoparticles for magnetic particle imaging. *Nanoscale* **2019**, *11*, 7771–7780. [CrossRef]
17. Möddel, M.; Knopp, T.; Werner, R.; Weller, D.; Salamon, J.M. *Toward Employing the Full Potential of Magnetic Particle Imaging: Exploring Visualization Techniques and Clinical Use Cases for Real-Time 3D Vascular Imaging*; SPIE-Intl Soc Optical Eng: Washington, DC, USA, 2019; p. 65.
18. Vasilescu, C.; Todea, A.; Nan, A.; Circu, M.; Turcu, R.; Benea, I.C.; Peter, F. Enzymatic synthesis of short-chain flavor esters from natural sources using tailored magnetic biocatalysts. *Food Chem.* **2019**, *296*, 1–8. [CrossRef]
19. Zeng, Y.; Zhu, Z.; Du, D.; Lin, Y. Nanomaterial-based electrochemical biosensors for food safety. *J. Electroanal. Chem.* **2016**, *781*, 147–154. [CrossRef]
20. Rotariu, L.; Lagarde, F.; Jaffrezic-Renault, N.; Bala, C. Electrochemical biosensors for fast detection of food contaminants—Trends and perspective. *TrAC Trends Anal. Chem.* **2016**, *79*, 80–87. [CrossRef]
21. Pon-On, W.; Tithito, T.; Maneeprakorn, W.; Phenrat, T.; Tang, I.M. Investigation of magnetic silica with thermoresponsive chitosan coating for drug controlled release and magnetic hyperthermia application. *Mater. Sci. Eng. C* **2019**, *97*, 23–30. [CrossRef]

22. Zahn, D.; Weidner, A.; Saatchi, K.; Häfeli, U.O.; Dutz, S. Biodegradable magnetic microspheres for drug targeting, temperature controlled drug release, and hyperthermia. *Curr. Dir. Biomed. Eng.* **2019**, *5*, 161–164. [CrossRef]
23. Chandra, S.; Noronha, G.; Dietrich, S.; Lang, H.; Bahadur, D. Dendrimer-magnetic nanoparticles as multiple stimuli responsive and enzymatic drug delivery vehicle. *J. Magn. Magn. Mater.* **2015**, *380*, 7–12. [CrossRef]
24. Legge, C.J.; Colley, H.E.; Lawson, M.A.; Rawlings, A.E. Targeted magnetic nanoparticle hyperthermia for the treatment of oral cancer. *J. Oral Pathol. Med.* **2019**. [CrossRef] [PubMed]
25. Yao, X.; Niu, X.; Ma, K.; Huang, P.; Grothe, J.; Kaskel, S.; Zhu, Y. Graphene quantum dots-capped magnetic mesoporous Silica nanoparticles as a multifunctional platform for controlled drug delivery, magnetic hyperthermia, and photothermal therapy. *Small* **2017**, *13*, 1602225. [CrossRef]
26. Alcantara, D.; Lopez, S.; García-Martin, M.L.; Pozo, D. Iron oxide nanoparticles as magnetic relaxation switching (MRSw) sensors: Current applications in nanomedicine. *Nanomed. Nanotechnol. Biol. Med.* **2016**, *12*, 1253–1262. [CrossRef]
27. Lam, T.; Devadhasan, J.P.; Howse, R.; Kim, J. A chemically patterned microfluidic paper-based analytical device (C-µPAD) for point-of-care diagnostics. *Sci. Rep.* **2017**, *7*, 1188. [CrossRef]
28. Dhavalikar, R.; Bohórquez, A.C.; Rinaldi, C. Image-guided thermal therapy using magnetic particle imaging and magnetic fluid hyperthermia. In *Nanomaterials for Magnetic and Optical Hyperthermia Applications*; Elsevier: Amsterdam, The Netherlands, 2019; pp. 265–286.
29. Chałupniak, A.; Morales-Narváez, E.; Merkoçi, A. Micro and nanomotors in diagnostics. *Adv. Drug Deliv. Rev.* **2015**, *95*, 104–116. [CrossRef]
30. Zhang, Y.; Nguyen, N.T. Magnetic digital microfluidics—A review. *Lab Chip* **2017**, *17*, 994–1008. [CrossRef]
31. Kim, K.; Guo, J.; Liang, Z.; Fan, D. Artificial micro/nanomachines for bioapplications: Biochemical delivery and diagnostic sensing. *Adv. Funct. Mater.* **2018**, *28*. [CrossRef]
32. Ferhan, A.R.; Jackman, J.A.; Park, J.H.; Cho, N.J. Nanoplasmonic sensors for detecting circulating cancer biomarkers. *Adv. Drug Deliv. Rev.* **2018**, *125*, 48–77. [CrossRef]
33. Liu, B.; Zhang, Z. Catalytic conversion of biomass into chemicals and fuels over magnetic catalysts. *ACS Catal.* **2016**, *6*, 326–338. [CrossRef]
34. Vaghari, H.; Jafarizadeh-Malmiri, H.; Mohammadlou, M.; Berenjian, A.; Anarjan, N.; Jafari, N.; Nasiri, S. Application of magnetic nanoparticles in smart enzyme immobilization. *Biotechnol. Lett.* **2016**, *38*, 223–233. [CrossRef] [PubMed]
35. Meffre, A.; Mehdaoui, B.; Connord, V.; Carrey, J.; Fazzini, P.F.; Lachaize, S.; Respaud, M.; Chaudret, B. Complex nano-objects displaying both magnetic and catalytic properties: A proof of concept for magnetically induced heterogeneous catalysis. *Nano Lett.* **2015**, *15*, 3241–3248. [CrossRef] [PubMed]
36. Ye, Z.; Li, C.; Skillen, N.; Xu, Y.; McCabe, H.; Kelly, J.; Robertson, P.; Bell, S.E.J. A one-pot method for building colloidal nanoparticles into bulk dry powders with nanoscale magnetic, plasmonic and catalytic functionalities. *Appl. Mater. Today* **2019**, *15*, 398–404. [CrossRef]
37. Premaratne, G.; Nerimetla, R.; Matlock, R.; Sunday, L.; Hikkaduwa Koralege, R.S.; Ramsey, J.D.; Krishnan, S. Stability, scalability, and reusability of a volume efficient biocatalytic system constructed on magnetic nanoparticles. *Catal. Sci. Technol.* **2016**, *6*, 2361–2369. [CrossRef]
38. Krishnan, S.; Walgama, C. Electrocatalytic features of a heme protein attached to polymer-functionalized magnetic nanoparticles. *Anal. Chem.* **2013**, *85*, 11420–11426. [CrossRef]
39. Jiang, W.; Dong, L.; Li, H.; Jia, H.; Zhu, L.; Zhu, W.; Li, H. Magnetic supported ionic liquid catalysts with tunable pore volume for enhanced deep oxidative desulfurization. *J. Mol. Liq.* **2019**, *274*, 293–299. [CrossRef]
40. Kluender, E.J.; Hedrick, J.L.; Brown, K.A.; Rao, R.; Meckes, B.; Du, J.S.; Moreau, L.M.; Maruyama, B.; Mirkin, C.A. Catalyst discovery through megalibraries of nanomaterials. *Proc. Natl. Acad. Sci. USA* **2019**, *116*, 40–45. [CrossRef]
41. Wang, Y.; Chen, Q.; Gan, C.; Yan, B.; Han, Y.; Lin, J. A review on magnetophoretic immunoseparation. *J. Nanosci. Nanotechnol.* **2016**, *16*, 2152–2163. [CrossRef]
42. Wu, J.; Wei, X.; Gan, J.; Huang, L.; Shen, T.; Lou, J.; Liu, B.; Zhang, J.X.J.; Qian, K. Multifunctional magnetic particles for combined circulating tumor cells isolation and cellular metabolism detection. *Adv. Funct. Mater.* **2016**, *26*, 4016–4025. [CrossRef]

43. Arduini, F.; Micheli, L.; Moscone, D.; Palleschi, G.; Piermarini, S.; Ricci, F.; Volpe, G. Electrochemical biosensors based on nanomodified screen-printed electrodes: Recent applications in clinical analysis. *TrAC Trends Anal. Chem.* **2016**, *79*, 114–126. [CrossRef]
44. Rufus, A.; Sreeju, N.; Philip, D. Size tunable biosynthesis and luminescence quenching of nanostructured hematite (α-Fe2O3) for catalytic degradation of organic pollutants. *J. Phys. Chem. Solids* **2019**, *124*, 221–234. [CrossRef]
45. Zhou, Y.; Tang, L.; Zeng, G.; Zhang, C.; Zhang, Y.; Xie, X. Current progress in biosensors for heavy metal ions based on DNAzymes/DNA molecules functionalized nanostructures: A review. *Sens. Actuators B Chem.* **2016**, *223*, 280–294. [CrossRef]
46. Reverté, L.; Prieto-Simón, B.; Campàs, M. New advances in electrochemical biosensors for the detection of toxins: Nanomaterials, magnetic beads and microfluidics systems. A review. *Anal. Chim. Acta* **2016**, *908*, 8–21. [CrossRef] [PubMed]
47. Giraldo, J.P.; Wu, H.; Newkirk, G.M.; Kruss, S. Nanobiotechnology approaches for engineering smart plant sensors. *Nat. Nanotechnol.* **2019**, *14*, 541–553. [CrossRef]
48. Farka, Z.; Juřík, T.; Kovář, D.; Trnková, L.; Skládal, P. Nanoparticle-based immunochemical biosensors and assays: Recent advances and challenges. *Chem. Rev.* **2017**, *117*, 9973–10042. [CrossRef]
49. Lei, K.M.; Mak, P.I.; Law, M.K.; Martins, R.P. CMOS biosensors for: In vitro diagnosis-transducing mechanisms and applications. *Lab Chip* **2016**, *16*, 3664–3681. [CrossRef]
50. Schrittwieser, S.; Pelaz, B.; Parak, W.J.; Lentijo-Mozo, S.; Soulantica, K.; Dieckhoff, J.; Ludwig, F.; Guenther, A.; Tschöpe, A.; Schotter, J. Homogeneous biosensing based on magnetic particle labels. *Sensors* **2016**, *16*, 828. [CrossRef]
51. Schelhas, L.T.; Banholzer, M.J.; Mirkin, C.A.; Tolbert, S.H. Magnetic confinement and coupling in narrow-diameter Au-Ni nanowires. *J. Magn. Magn. Mater.* **2015**, *379*, 239–243. [CrossRef]
52. Moraes Silva, S.; Tavallaie, R.; Sandiford, L.; Tilley, R.D.; Gooding, J.J. Gold coated magnetic nanoparticles: From preparation to surface modification for analytical and biomedical applications. *Chem. Commun.* **2016**, *52*, 7528–7540. [CrossRef]
53. Ren, W.; Mohammed, S.I.; Wereley, S.; Irudayaraj, J. Magnetic focus lateral flow sensor for detection of cervical cancer biomarkers. *Anal. Chem.* **2019**, *91*, 2876–2884. [CrossRef] [PubMed]
54. He, Y.; Wang, Y.; Yang, X.; Xie, S.; Yuan, R.; Chai, Y. Metal organic frameworks combining CoFe 2 O 4 magnetic nanoparticles as highly efficient SERS sensing platform for ultrasensitive detection of N-terminal pro-brain natriuretic peptide. *ACS Appl. Mater. Interfaces* **2016**, *8*, 7683–7690. [CrossRef] [PubMed]
55. Pakapongpan, S.; Poo-arporn, R.P. Self-assembly of glucose oxidase on reduced graphene oxide-magnetic nanoparticles nanocomposite-based direct electrochemistry for reagentless glucose biosensor. *Mater. Sci. Eng. C* **2017**, *76*, 398–405. [CrossRef] [PubMed]
56. Li, J.; Skeete, Z.; Shan, S.; Yan, S.; Kurzatkowska, K.; Zhao, W.; Ngo, Q.M.; Holubovska, P.; Luo, J.; Hepel, M.; et al. Surface enhanced raman scattering detection of cancer biomarkers with bifunctional nanocomposite probes. *Anal. Chem.* **2015**, *87*, 10698–10702. [CrossRef] [PubMed]
57. Chung, S.; Moon, J.M.; Choi, J.; Hwang, H.; Shim, Y.B. Magnetic force assisted electrochemical sensor for the detection of thrombin with aptamer-antibody sandwich formation. *Biosens. Bioelectron.* **2018**, *117*, 480–486. [CrossRef]
58. Wen, T.; Zhu, W.; Xue, C.; Wu, J.; Han, Q.; Wang, X.; Zhou, X.; Jiang, H. Novel electrochemical sensing platform based on magnetic field-induced self-assembly of Fe3O4@Polyaniline nanoparticles for clinical detection of creatinine. *Biosens. Bioelectron.* **2014**, *56*, 180–185. [CrossRef]
59. He, C.; Xie, M.; Hong, F.; Chai, X.; Mi, H.; Zhou, X.; Fan, L.; Zhang, Q.; Ngai, T.; Liu, J. A highly sensitive glucose biosensor based on gold nanoparticles/bovine serum albumin/Fe_3O_4 biocomposite nanoparticles. *Electrochim. Acta* **2016**, *222*, 1709–1715. [CrossRef]
60. Hu, Y.; Li, L.; Guo, L. The sandwich-type aptasensor based on gold nanoparticles/DNA/magnetic beads for detection of cancer biomarker protein AGR2. *Sens. Actuators B Chem.* **2015**, *209*, 846–852. [CrossRef]
61. Yang, K.; Hu, Y.; Dong, N. A novel biosensor based on competitive SERS immunoassay and magnetic separation for accurate and sensitive detection of chloramphenicol. *Biosens. Bioelectron.* **2016**, *80*, 373–377. [CrossRef]

62. Tavallaie, R.; McCarroll, J.; Le Grand, M.; Ariotti, N.; Schuhmann, W.; Bakker, E.; Tilley, R.D.; Hibbert, D.B.; Kavallaris, M.; Gooding, J.J. Nucleic acid hybridization on an electrically reconfigurable network of gold-coated magnetic nanoparticles enables microRNA detection in blood. *Nat. Nanotechnol.* **2018**, *13*, 1066–1071. [CrossRef]
63. Singh, V.; Krishnan, S. An electrochemical mass sensor for diagnosing diabetes in human serum. *Analyst* **2014**, *139*, 724–728. [CrossRef] [PubMed]
64. Singh, V.; Krishnan, S. Voltammetric immunosensor assembled on carbon-pyrenyl nanostructures for clinical diagnosis of type of diabetes. *Anal. Chem.* **2015**, *87*, 2648–2654. [CrossRef] [PubMed]
65. Niroula, J.; Premaratne, G.; Ali Shojaee, S.; Lucca, D.A.; Krishnan, S. Combined covalent and noncovalent carboxylation of carbon nanotubes for sensitivity enhancement of clinical immunosensors. *Chem. Commun.* **2016**, *52*, 13039–13042. [CrossRef] [PubMed]
66. Bayramoglu, G.; Ozalp, C.; Oztekin, M.; Guler, U.; Salih, B.; Arica, M.Y. Design of an aptamer-based magnetic adsorbent and biosensor systems for selective and sensitive separation and detection of thrombin. *Talanta* **2019**, *191*, 59–66. [CrossRef] [PubMed]
67. Singh, V.; Rodenbaugh, C.; Krishnan, S. Magnetic optical microarray imager for diagnosing type of diabetes in clinical blood serum samples. *ACS Sens.* **2016**, *1*, 437–443. [CrossRef] [PubMed]
68. Otieno, B.A.; Krause, C.E.; Latus, A.; Chikkaveeraiah, B.V.; Faria, R.C.; Rusling, J.F. On-line protein capture on magnetic beads for ultrasensitive microfluidic immunoassays of cancer biomarkers. *Biosens. Bioelectron.* **2014**, *53*, 268–274. [CrossRef] [PubMed]
69. Walgama, C.; Al Mubarak, Z.H.; Zhang, B.; Akinwale, M.; Pathiranage, A.; Deng, J.; Berlin, K.D.; Benbrook, D.M.; Krishnan, S. Label-free real-time microarray imaging of cancer protein-protein interactions and their inhibition by small molecules. *Anal. Chem.* **2016**, *88*, 3130–3135. [CrossRef]
70. Singh, V.; Nerimetla, R.; Yang, M.; Krishnan, S. Magnetite-quantum dot immunoarray for plasmon-coupled-fluorescence imaging of blood insulin and glycated hemoglobin. *ACS Sens.* **2017**, *2*, 909–915. [CrossRef]
71. Sun, B.; Ni, X.; Cao, Y.; Cao, G. Electrochemical sensor based on magnetic molecularly imprinted nanoparticles modified magnetic electrode for determination of Hb. *Biosens. Bioelectron.* **2017**, *91*, 354–358. [CrossRef]
72. Ben Messaoud, N.; Ait Lahcen, A.; Dridi, C.; Amine, A. Ultrasound assisted magnetic imprinted polymer combined sensor based on carbon black and gold nanoparticles for selective and sensitive electrochemical detection of Bisphenol A. *Sens. Actuators B Chem.* **2018**, *276*, 304–312. [CrossRef]
73. Dehdashtian, S.; Gholivand, M.B.; Shamsipur, M.; Azadbakht, A.; Karimi, Z. Fabrication of a highly sensitive and selective electrochemical sensor based on chitosan-coated Fe_3O_4 magnetic nanoparticle for determination of antibiotic ciprofloxacin and its application in biological samples. *Can. J. Chem.* **2016**, *94*, 803–811. [CrossRef]
74. Jiang, H.; Jiang, D.; Shao, J.; Sun, X. Magnetic molecularly imprinted polymer nanoparticles based electrochemical sensor for the measurement of Gram-negative bacterial quorum signaling molecules (N-acyl-homoserine-lactones). *Biosens. Bioelectron.* **2016**, *75*, 411–419. [CrossRef] [PubMed]
75. Long, F.; Zhang, Z.; Yang, Z.; Zeng, J.; Jiang, Y. Imprinted electrochemical sensor based on magnetic multi-walled carbon nanotube for sensitive determination of kanamycin. *J. Electroanal. Chem.* **2015**, *755*, 7–14. [CrossRef]
76. Waifalkar, P.P.; Chougale, A.D.; Kollu, P.; Patil, P.S.; Patil, P.B. Magnetic nanoparticle decorated graphene based electrochemical nanobiosensor for H_2O_2 sensing using HRP. *Colloids Surf. B Biointerfaces* **2018**, *167*, 425–431. [CrossRef] [PubMed]
77. Dehdashtian, S.; Gholivand, M.B.; Shamsipur, M.; Kariminia, S. Construction of a sensitive and selective sensor for morphine using chitosan coated Fe_3O_4 magnetic nanoparticle as a modifier. *Mater. Sci. Eng. C* **2016**, *58*, 53–59. [CrossRef] [PubMed]
78. Tajyani, S.; Babaei, A. A new sensing platform based on magnetic Fe_3O_4@NiO core/shell nanoparticles modified carbon paste electrode for simultaneous voltammetric determination of Quercetin and Tryptophan. *J. Electroanal. Chem.* **2018**, *808*, 50–58. [CrossRef]
79. Liang, H.; Xu, H.; Zhao, Y.; Zheng, J.; Zhao, H.; Li, G.; Li, C.-P. Ultrasensitive electrochemical sensor for prostate specific antigen detection with a phosphorene platform and magnetic covalent organic framework signal amplifier. *Biosens. Bioelectron.* **2019**, *144*, 111691. [CrossRef]

80. Poo-arporn, Y.; Pakapongpan, S.; Chanlek, N.; Poo-arporn, R.P. The development of disposable electrochemical sensor based on Fe_3O_4-doped reduced graphene oxide modified magnetic screen-printed electrode for ractopamine determination in pork sample. *Sens. Actuators B Chem.* **2019**, *284*, 164–171. [CrossRef]
81. Li, N.N.; Kang, T.F.; Zhang, J.J.; Lu, L.P.; Cheng, S.Y. Fe_3O_4@ZrO_2 magnetic nanoparticles as a new electrode material for sensitive determination of organophosphorus agents. *Anal. Methods* **2015**, *7*, 5053–5059. [CrossRef]
82. Arvand, M.; Hemmati, S. Magnetic nanoparticles embedded with graphene quantum dots and multiwalled carbon nanotubes as a sensing platform for electrochemical detection of progesterone. *Sens. Actuators B Chem.* **2017**, *238*, 346–356. [CrossRef]
83. Sharafeldin, M.; Bishop, G.W.; Bhakta, S.; El-Sawy, A.; Suib, S.L.; Rusling, J.F. Fe_3O_4 nanoparticles on graphene oxide sheets for isolation and ultrasensitive amperometric detection of cancer biomarker proteins. *Biosens. Bioelectron.* **2017**, *91*, 359–366. [CrossRef] [PubMed]
84. Tang, C.K.; Vaze, A.; Shen, M.; Rusling, J.F. High-throughput electrochemical microfluidic immunoarray for multiplexed detection of cancer biomarker proteins. *ACS Sens.* **2016**, *1*, 1036–1043. [CrossRef] [PubMed]
85. Li, S.S.; Lin, C.W.; Wei, K.C.; Huang, C.Y.; Hsu, P.H.; Liu, H.L.; Lu, Y.J.; Lin, S.C.; Yang, H.W.; Ma, C.C.M. Non-invasive screening for early Alzheimer's disease diagnosis by a sensitively immunomagnetic biosensor. *Sci. Rep.* **2016**, *6*, 25155. [CrossRef] [PubMed]
86. Orlov, A.V.; Nikitin, M.P.; Bragina, V.A.; Znoyko, S.L.; Zaikina, M.N.; Ksenevich, T.I.; Gorshkov, B.G.; Nikitin, P.I. A new real-time method for investigation of affinity properties and binding kinetics of magnetic nanoparticles. *J. Magn. Magn. Mater.* **2015**, *380*, 231–235. [CrossRef]
87. Xu, L.; Xie, S.; Du, J.; He, N. Porous magnetic pseudo-carbon paste electrode electrochemical biosensor for DNA detection. *J. Nanosci. Nanotechnol.* **2017**, *17*, 238–243. [CrossRef] [PubMed]
88. Wignarajah, S.; Suaifan, G.A.R.Y.; Bizzarro, S.; Bikker, F.J.; Kaman, W.E.; Zourob, M. Colorimetric assay for the detection of typical biomarkers for periodontitis using a magnetic nanoparticle biosensor. *Anal. Chem.* **2015**, *87*, 12161–12168. [CrossRef]
89. Martinkova, P.; Opatrilova, R.; Kruzliak, P.; Styriak, I.; Pohanka, M. Colorimetric glucose assay based on magnetic particles having pseudo-peroxidase activity and immobilized glucose oxidase. *Mol. Biotechnol.* **2016**, *58*, 373–380. [CrossRef]
90. Liu, X.; Su, L.; Zhu, L.; Gao, X.; Wang, Y.; Bai, F.; Tang, Y.; Li, J. Hybrid material for enrofloxacin sensing based on aptamer-functionalized magnetic nanoparticle conjugated with upconversion nanoprobes. *Sens. Actuators B Chem.* **2016**, *233*, 394–401. [CrossRef]
91. Borisova, B.; Sánchez, A.; Jiménez-Falcao, S.; Martín, M.; Salazar, P.; Parrado, C.; Pingarrón, J.M.; Villalonga, R. Reduced graphene oxide-carboxymethylcellulose layered with platinum nanoparticles/PAMAM dendrimer/magnetic nanoparticles hybrids. Application to the preparation of enzyme electrochemical biosensors. *Sens. Actuators B Chem.* **2016**, *232*, 84–90. [CrossRef]
92. Baghayeri, M.; Veisi, H.; Ghanei-Motlagh, M. Amperometric glucose biosensor based on immobilization of glucose oxidase on a magnetic glassy carbon electrode modified with a novel magnetic nanocomposite. *Sens. Actuators B Chem.* **2017**, *249*, 321–330. [CrossRef]
93. Fock, J.; Parmvi, M.; Strömberg, M.; Svedlindh, P.; Donolato, M.; Hansen, M.F. Comparison of optomagnetic and AC susceptibility readouts in a magnetic nanoparticle agglutination assay for detection of C-reactive protein. *Biosens. Bioelectron.* **2017**, *88*, 94–100. [CrossRef] [PubMed]
94. Choi, G.; Kim, E.; Park, E.; Lee, J.H. A cost-effective chemiluminescent biosensor capable of early diagnosing cancer using a combination of magnetic beads and platinum nanoparticles. *Talanta* **2017**, *162*, 38–45. [CrossRef] [PubMed]
95. Premaratne, G.; Niroula, J.; Patel, M.K.; Zhong, W.; Suib, S.L.; Kaan Kalkan, A.; Krishnan, S. Electrochemical and surface-plasmon correlation of a serum-autoantibody immunoassay with binding insights: Graphenyl surface versus mercapto-monolayer surface. *Anal. Chem.* **2018**, *90*, 12456–12463. [CrossRef] [PubMed]
96. Premaratne, G.; Dharmaratne, A.C.; Al Mubarak, Z.H.; Mohammadparast, F.; Andiappan, M.; Krishnan, S. Multiplexed surface plasmon imaging of serum biomolecules: Fe_3O_4@Au Core/shell nanoparticles with plasmonic simulation insights. *Sens. Actuators B Chem.* **2019**, *299*, 126956. [CrossRef]

97. Sanaeifar, N.; Rabiee, M.; Abdolrahim, M.; Tahriri, M.; Vashaee, D.; Tayebi, L. A novel electrochemical biosensor based on Fe3O4 nanoparticles-polyvinyl alcohol composite for sensitive detection of glucose. *Anal. Biochem.* **2017**, *519*, 19–26. [CrossRef]

98. Zhang, C.; Si, S.; Yang, Z. A highly selective photoelectrochemical biosensor for uric acid based on core-shell Fe_3O_4@C nanoparticle and molecularly imprinted TiO_2. *Biosens. Bioelectron.* **2015**, *65*, 115–120. [CrossRef]

99. Rouhi, M.; Mansour Lakouraj, M.; Baghayeri, M.; Hasantabar, V. Novel conductive magnetic nanocomposite based on poly (indole-co-thiophene) as a hemoglobin diagnostic biosensor: Synthesis, characterization and physical properties. *Int. J. Polym. Mater. Polym. Biomater.* **2017**, *66*, 12–19. [CrossRef]

100. Zhang, W.; Li, X.; Zou, R.; Wu, H.; Shi, H.; Yu, S.; Liu, Y. Multifunctional glucose biosensors from Fe_3O_4 nanoparticles modified chitosan/graphene nanocomposites. *Sci. Rep.* **2015**, *5*, 11129. [CrossRef]

101. Yuan, Y.H.; Wu, Y.D.; Chi, B.Z.; Wen, S.H.; Liang, R.P.; Qiu, J.D. Simultaneously electrochemical detection of microRNAs based on multifunctional magnetic nanoparticles probe coupling with hybridization chain reaction. *Biosens. Bioelectron.* **2017**, *97*, 325–331. [CrossRef]

102. Pal, M.K.; Rashid, M.; Bisht, M. Multiplexed magnetic nanoparticle-antibody conjugates (MNPs-ABS) based prognostic detection of ovarian cancer biomarkers, CA-125, β-2M and ApoA1 using fluorescence spectroscopy with comparison of surface plasmon resonance (SPR) analysis. *Biosens. Bioelectron.* **2015**, *73*, 146–152. [CrossRef]

103. Ahmed, A.; Hassan, I.; Mosa, I.M.; Elsanadidy, E.; Sharafeldin, M.; Rusling, J.F.; Ren, S. An ultra-shapeable, smart sensing platform based on a multimodal ferrofluid-infused surface. *Adv. Mater.* **2019**, *31*, 1807201. [CrossRef] [PubMed]

104. Nerimetla, R.; Premaratne, G.; Liu, H.; Krishnan, S. Improved electrocatalytic metabolite production and drug biosensing by human liver microsomes immobilized on amine-functionalized magnetic nanoparticles. *Electrochim. Acta* **2018**, *280*, 101–107. [CrossRef]

105. Bakshi, S.F.; Guz, N.; Zakharchenko, A.; Deng, H.; Tumanov, A.V.; Woodworth, C.D.; Minko, S.; Kolpashchikov, D.M.; Katz, E. Magnetic field-activated sensing of mRNA in living cells. *J. Am. Chem. Soc.* **2017**, *139*, 12117–12120. [CrossRef] [PubMed]

106. Bakshi, S.; Zakharchenko, A.; Minko, S.; Kolpashchikov, D.; Katz, E. Towards nanomaterials for cancer theranostics: A system of DNA-modified magnetic nanoparticles for detection and suppression of RNA marker in cancer cells. *Magnetochemistry* **2019**, *5*, 24. [CrossRef]

107. Pang, Y.; Wang, C.; Wang, J.; Sun, Z.; Xiao, R.; Wang, S. Fe_3O_4@Ag magnetic nanoparticles for microRNA capture and duplex-specific nuclease signal amplification based SERS detection in cancer cells. *Biosens. Bioelectron.* **2016**, *79*, 574–580. [CrossRef]

108. Bülbül, G.; Hayat, A.; Andreescu, S. Portable nanoparticle-based sensors for food safety assessment. *Sensors* **2015**, *15*, 30736–30758. [CrossRef]

109. Wang, L.; Huang, F.; Cai, G.; Yao, L.; Zhang, H.; Lin, J. An electrochemical aptasensor using coaxial capillary with magnetic nanoparticle, urease catalysis and PCB electrode for rapid and sensitive detection of escherichia coli O157:H7. *Nanotheranostics* **2017**, *1*, 403. [CrossRef]

110. Villalonga, M.L.; Borisova, B.; Arenas, C.B.; Villalonga, A.; Arévalo-Villena, M.; Sánchez, A.; Pingarrón, J.M.; Briones-Pérez, A.; Villalonga, R. Disposable electrochemical biosensors for Brettanomyces bruxellensis and total yeast content in wine based on core-shell magnetic nanoparticles. *Sens. Actuators B Chem.* **2019**, *279*, 15–21. [CrossRef]

111. Magro, M.; Moritz, D.E.; Bonaiuto, E.; Baratella, D.; Terzo, M.; Jakubec, P.; Malina, O.; Čépe, K.; De Aragao, G.M.F.; Zboril, R.; et al. Citrinin mycotoxin recognition and removal by naked magnetic nanoparticles. *Food Chem.* **2016**, *203*, 505–512. [CrossRef]

112. Chen, H.; Qi, F.; Zhou, H.; Jia, S.; Gao, Y.; Koh, K.; Yin, Y. Fe_3O_4@Au nanoparticles as a means of signal enhancement in surface plasmon resonance spectroscopy for thrombin detection. *Sens. Actuators B Chem.* **2015**, *212*, 505–511. [CrossRef]

113. Chen, Q.; Huang, F.; Cai, G.; Wang, M.; Lin, J. An optical biosensor using immunomagnetic separation, urease catalysis and pH indication for rapid and sensitive detection of Listeria monocytogenes. *Sens. Actuators B Chem.* **2018**, *258*, 447–453. [CrossRef]

114. Suaifan, G.A.R.Y.; Alhogail, S.; Zourob, M. Paper-based magnetic nanoparticle-peptide probe for rapid and quantitative colorimetric detection of Escherichia coli O157:H7. *Biosens. Bioelectron.* **2017**, *92*, 702–708. [CrossRef] [PubMed]

115. Peterson, R.D.; Chen, W.; Cunningham, B.T.; Andrade, J.E. Enhanced sandwich immunoassay using antibody-functionalized magnetic iron-oxide nanoparticles for extraction and detection of soluble transferrin receptor on a photonic crystal biosensor. *Biosens. Bioelectron.* **2015**, *74*, 815–822. [CrossRef] [PubMed]
116. Duan, H.; Wang, X.; Wang, Y.; Sun, Y.; Li, J.; Luo, C. An ultrasensitive lysozyme chemiluminescence biosensor based on surface molecular imprinting using ionic liquid modified magnetic graphene oxide/β-cyclodextrin as supporting material. *Anal. Chim. Acta* **2016**, *918*, 89–96. [CrossRef] [PubMed]
117. Wang, Y.; Sun, Y.; Dai, H.; Ni, P.; Jiang, S.; Lu, W.; Li, Z.; Li, Z. A colorimetric biosensor using Fe_3O_4 nanoparticles for highly sensitive and selective detection of tetracyclines. *Sens. Actuators B Chem.* **2016**, *236*, 621–626. [CrossRef]
118. Wang, X.; Niessner, R.; Tang, D.; Knopp, D. Nanoparticle-based immunosensors and immunoassays for aflatoxins. *Anal. Chim. Acta* **2016**, *912*, 10–23. [CrossRef] [PubMed]
119. Wang, D.; Chen, Q.; Huo, H.; Bai, S.; Cai, G.; Lai, W.; Lin, J. Efficient separation and quantitative detection of Listeria monocytogenes based on screen-printed interdigitated electrode, urease and magnetic nanoparticles. *Food Control* **2017**, *73*, 555–561. [CrossRef]
120. Suaifan, G.A.R.Y.; Alhogail, S.; Zourob, M. Rapid and low-cost biosensor for the detection of Staphylococcus aureus. *Biosens. Bioelectron.* **2017**, *90*, 230–237. [CrossRef]
121. Liu, X.; Hu, Y.; Zheng, S.; Liu, Y.; He, Z.; Luo, F. Surface plasmon resonance immunosensor for fast, highly sensitive, and in situ detection of the magnetic nanoparticles-enriched Salmonella enteritidis. *Sens. Actuators B Chem.* **2016**, *230*, 191–198. [CrossRef]
122. Mashhadizadeh, M.H.; Talemi, R.P. Synergistic effect of magnetite and gold nanoparticles onto the response of a label-free impedimetric hepatitis B virus DNA biosensor. *Mater. Sci. Eng. C* **2016**, *59*, 773–781. [CrossRef]
123. Low, K.F.; Rijiravanich, P.; Singh, K.K.B.; Surareungchai, W.; Yean, C.Y. An electrochemical genosensing assay based on magnetic beads and gold nanoparticle-loaded latex microspheres for vibrio cholerae detection. *J. Biomed. Nanotechnol.* **2015**, *11*, 702–710. [CrossRef] [PubMed]
124. Narmani, A.; Kamali, M.; Amini, B.; Kooshki, H.; Amini, A.; Hasani, L. Highly sensitive and accurate detection of Vibrio cholera O1 OmpW gene by fluorescence DNA biosensor based on gold and magnetic nanoparticles. *Process Biochem.* **2018**, *65*, 46–54. [CrossRef]
125. Antonacci, A.; Arduini, F.; Moscone, D.; Palleschi, G.; Scognamiglio, V. Nanostructured (Bio)sensors for smart agriculture. *TrAC Trends Anal. Chem.* **2018**, *98*, 95–103. [CrossRef]
126. Abegaz, B.W.; Datta, T.; Mahajan, S.M. Sensor technologies for the energy-water nexus—A review. *Appl. Energy* **2018**, *210*, 451–466. [CrossRef]
127. Dzudzevic Cancar, H.; Soylemez, S.; Akpinar, Y.; Kesik, M.; Göker, S.; Gunbas, G.; Volkan, M.; Toppare, L. A novel Acetylcholinesterase biosensor: Core-shell magnetic nanoparticles incorporating a conjugated polymer for the detection of organophosphorus pesticides. *ACS Appl. Mater. Interfaces* **2016**, *8*, 8058–8067. [CrossRef]
128. Dominguez, R.B.; Alonso, G.A.; Muñoz, R.; Hayat, A.; Marty, J.L. Design of a novel magnetic particles based electrochemical biosensor for organophosphate insecticide detection in flow injection analysis. *Sens. Actuators B Chem.* **2015**, *208*, 491–496. [CrossRef]

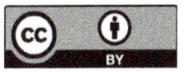 © 2019 by the authors. Licensee MDPI, Basel, Switzerland. This article is an open access article distributed under the terms and conditions of the Creative Commons Attribution (CC BY) license (http://creativecommons.org/licenses/by/4.0/).

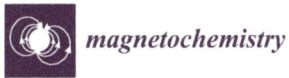

Review

Optical-Based (Bio) Sensing Systems Using Magnetic Nanoparticles

Recep Üzek [1], Esma Sari [2] and Arben Merkoçi [3,4,*]

1. Department of Chemistry, Faculty of Science, Hacettepe University, Ankara 06800, Turkey; ruzek@hacettepe.edu.tr
2. Vocational School of Health Services, Medical Laboratory Techniques, Yüksek İhtisas University, Ankara 06800, Turkey; esma.sari@hotmail.com
3. Catalan Institute of Nanoscience and Nanotechnology (ICN2), CSIC and BIS, Bellaterra, 08193 Barcelona, Spain
4. Catalan Institution for Research and Advanced Studies (ICREA), Pg. Lluís Companys 23, 08010 Barcelona, Spain
* Correspondence: arben.merkoci@icn2.cat; Tel.: +34-937374604

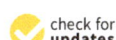

Received: 23 September 2019; Accepted: 22 October 2019; Published: 25 October 2019

Abstract: In recent years, various reports related to sensing application research have suggested that combining the synergistic impacts of optical, electrical or magnetic properties in a single technique can lead to a new multitasking platform. Owing to their unique features of the magnetic moment, biocompatibility, ease of surface modification, chemical stability, high surface area, high mass transference, magnetic nanoparticles have found a wide range of applications in various fields, especially in sensing systems. The present review is comprehensive information about magnetic nanoparticles utilized in the optical sensing platform, broadly categorized into four types: surface plasmon resonance (SPR), surface-enhanced Raman spectroscopy (SERS), fluorescence spectroscopy and near-infrared spectroscopy and imaging (NIRS) that are commonly used in various (bio) analytical applications. The review also includes some conclusions on the state of the art in this field and future aspects.

Keywords: optical sensor; magnetic nanoparticle; imaging; surface plasmon resonance; surface-enhanced Raman spectroscopy; fluorescence spectroscopy; near infrared spectroscopy

---

1. Introduction

In recent years, great interest has been shown in the field of nanotechnology in general and particularly its applications in the manufacturing of novel materials with added magnetic, electrical, optical, and biological properties for various areas. Among these nanomaterials with added properties, magnetic nanoparticles (MNPs) are quite interesting given their unique physico-chemical structure. The plethora of applications has been described for MNPs that are directly associated with modulation of the chemical structure, size distribution, and magnetic moment [1,2]. In addition, MNPs were found to possess a number of intrinsic properties such as biocompatibility, low toxicity, ease of surface modification, chemical stability, high surface area, high mass transference besides others [3]. Although all kind of MNPs, like other nanoparticles, can be used in different ways, size, and surface have a severe impact on the application area. For example, MNPs over 28 nm are ferrimagnetic and commonly used for magnetic separation and for electronic instruments as ferrofluids. MNPs below 28 nm, on the other side, are super-paramagnetic and are generally preferred for biomedical applications [4].

MNPs are generally divided, regarding their chemical structure, into metal oxides, pure metals, and magnetic nanocomposites. This distinct class of MNPs and application areas are depicted in

Figure 1. Metal oxides are most commonly used for biomedical applications, such as cell labeling and imaging [5–8], diagnostic and therapeutic agents [9]. Among metal oxides, iron oxides are commonly used since they have better biocompatibility [10]. In contrast to metal oxides, pure metals as a class of MNPs have limited application areas due to their chemical instability [11] and large size distributions [12]. Although rarely reported, the use of pure metal nanoparticles is generally found in electronic devices such as ultra-high-density magnetic storage devices [13–15]. In other respects, the use of magnetic nanocomposites, particularly in a sensor, biosensor and detection systems, has become increasingly common in recent years [16–19]. Disadvantages of MNPs, such as their tendency to aggregate to reduce surface energies, and oxidation in air, are among the major obstacles to the spread of their more frequent use in the applications [20]. Therefore, from the application point of view, researchers have proposed a new approach to the development of new materials by coating polymer, silica or other materials over MNPs, so-called magnetic nanocomposites [21–23].

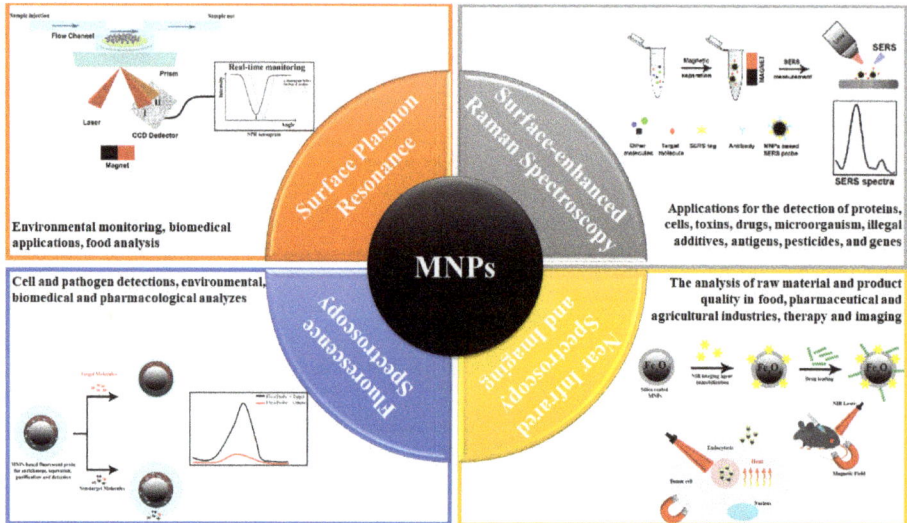

Figure 1. The main applications of optical-based (bio) sensing systems using magnetic nanoparticles (MNPs) in biomedical and environmental fields.

In practice, the feasible features of MNPs are not only affected by their structure but also by their fabrication techniques and surrounding environments [4,24,25]. MNPs can be prepared in the following three routes to suit the final desired application. The majority of these methods are based on the chemical methods or "bottom-up" synthesis procedures, which include co-precipitation, high-temperature thermal decomposition and/or reduction, sol-gel synthesis, flow-injection synthesis, oxidation method, electrochemical method, aerosol/vapor-phase method, supercritical fluid method, and synthesis using nanoreactors [5,25]. Chemical synthesis is controllable for almost all the processing conditions, and indeed, there has been a report indicating that this may be one reason for the "popularity" of chemical techniques for synthesis [26]. Alternatively, MNPs can be formed via physical methods through a simple non-chemical "top-down" dispersion technique, e.g., gas-phase deposition and electron-beam lithography [5,25,27]. Traditionally, physical methods have been the less preferred synthesis techniques for MNPs given an inability to control the size of particles down to the nanometer scale using these methods [27]. On the other hand, bio-reduction in the so-called microorganism approach, which has allowed large quantities of production, ensures the high yield, good reproducibility, and stability, as well as low cost [5,27]. In optical-based (bio)sensing systems, multifunctional composites such as Fe_3O_4@Ag, Fe_3O_4@Au, etc., are mainly prepared by two methods: core-shell structure (1) and immobilization on the core (2) [28,29]. In both methods, magnetic nanoparticles are first coated with silica shells to increase the stability of the magnetic nanoparticles and to facilitate their modification. In the first of these directions, Ag or Au is reduced by using chemical compounds such as NaBH$_4$, citric acid, etc. on the surface of the magnetic core. In the second method, gold or silver nanoparticles are prepared in different forms such as spherical, cubes or nanorods and then immobilized to the surface of the magnetic core by physical or chemical methods. In physical immobilization, it is usually carried out by modification of the magnetic core with polymers such as oleic acid, etc., and then bonded to the magnetic surface by the secondary interactions. In chemical immobilization, the surface of magnetic and Au or Ag nanoparticles are first modified with functional groups such as carboxyl or amine, and then the chemical immobilization is performed by modification method such as 1-Ethyl-3-(3-dimethylaminopropyl) carbodiimide/N-hydroxysuccinimide (EDC/NHS) coupling, etc.

After synthesis of MNPs, the common analytical techniques used for the characterization of MNPs are: ultraviolet (UV)–visible spectrophotometry, dynamic light scattering (DLS), scanning electron microscopy (SEM), transmission electron microscopy (TEM), Fourier transform infrared spectroscopy (FTIR), atomic force microscopy (AFM), powder X-ray diffraction (XRD), X-ray fluorescence (XRF) and energy-dispersive spectroscopy (EDS) [30,31].

There is no doubt that the extensive literature that can be associated with the term of biosensor shows that the related field of research is very attractive. In the first approach, a biosensor can be simply defined as a device that intimately combines a biological sensing element with a transducer [32]. In an efficient biosensor design, it is essential to convert the biological interaction to a signal which is transduced by physical, chemical, optical, thermal or electrochemical actions, into observable information and analyzed quantitatively [33]. Even though electrical and electrochemical platforms are the most advanced and used biosensor platforms, these systems have drawbacks owing to the extra reduction/oxidizing agent being involved [34]. While the biosensor can be built in a comparable manner based on optical and electrochemical transducers, it obviously demonstrates distinct working features [32]. Optical biosensors play a prominent role in sensing applications because they have distinct advantages: for example, high-precision detection and label-free design [34]. Optical biosensors also offer the possibility of immune electromagnetic interference, capable of remote sensing, and can perform multiplex detection within a single device [35]. The next generation of sensing equipment for daily use is optical biosensor platforms, based on absorbance, photoluminescence and surface plasmon resonance (SPR) [34]. In addition, coupling the synergistic effects of the optical properties and magnetic properties in a single method may offer new multitasking platforms for (bio)sensing, biolabeling/imaging, cell sorting/separation, and photothermal therapy [36].

In this comprehensive review, we will discuss optical biosensing systems based on the use of MNPs. Under this category, there exist a number of optical-sensing methods by using MNPs, including SPR, surface-enhanced Raman spectroscopy (SERS), fluorescence spectroscopy and near-infrared spectroscopy and imaging (NIRS).

2. Surface Plasmon Resonance (SPR)

Surface plasmon resonance (SPR) is a complex physical phenomenon occurring on an electrically conductive noble metal layer at the interface between two media (i.e. high refractive indices of sensor's glass surface and low refractive indices of buffer) when p-polarized light under conditions of total internal reflection [37,38]. Interest in the SPR effect started with an explanation as the energy of photons absorbed by the free electrons of the metallic layer reduced the amplitude of the incident light that comes with a certain angle. Despite the SPR effect being successfully explained in 1968, SPR as a method of determination in the field of biosensor was first mentioned in 1983 by Wijaya et al. Although fluorescence or absorbance based optical methods have been used since earlier times, SPR as surface-based optical method has been developed very rapidly and has attracted considerable interest in biosensing platform [38]. Investigation of biomolecular interactions with SPR is considered an exceedingly powerful analysis method due to SPR's remarkable properties as an analytical tool such as its label-free nature, real-time, highly precise, a short time and simplicity. Despite the usefulness of SPR, the conventional SPR methods are mainly hampered by the detection of low concentration, low molecular weight biomolecules due to trivial changes of the refractive index in the binding process. Several approaches to overcome this challenge have been offered by researchers based on the use of nanoparticles [39,40]. Until now, decorating SPR surfaces with MNPs seems to be the most widely attested. Especially the application of MNPs in SPR sensing has attracted great focus owing to advantages which are (1) capture of the target molecules from the complex sample and (2) high refractive index and high molecular weight of MNPs to recruit the SPR signal [41,42]. Due to the aforementioned desired properties of MNPs, these compounds are widely used for environmental monitoring, biomedical applications, food analysis, etc. [43–46]. The principle of the SPR system with MNPs was illustrated in Figure 2 [47].

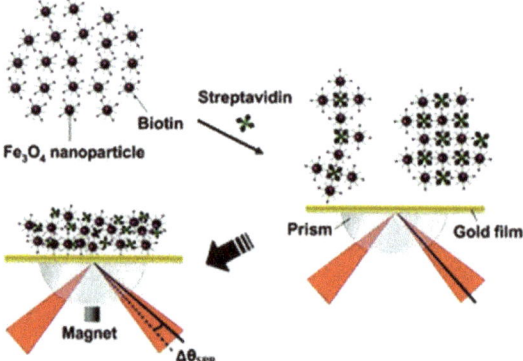

Figure 2. Amplification of the surface plasmon resonance (SPR) response signal with MNPs [47]. Reproduced with permission of the Royal Society of Chemistry.

In 2018, Sun and co-workers reported the SPR biosensor based on hollow gold nanospheres and improved sandwich assay with magnetic nanoparticles to detect rabbit IgG. While the reduced graphene layer (rGO) was covered with Ag nanoparticles to obtain SPR surface, Fe_3O_4 MNPs were utilized to capture the analyte of interest easily from the medium. In order to bind the antibody to the surface without modification and avoid agglomeration of nanoparticles, polydopamine (PDA) was used. These researchers showed that the detection of rabbit IgG by gold nanostructures resulted in the 132 times lower concentration when compared with a conventional SPR biosensor. The changes in the SPR signal caused by the magneto-sandwich immunoassay were further compared with the signal of hollow gold nanospheres. Their investigation showed that the 8 times higher enhancement in the SPR signal was related to the magneto-sandwich immunoassay [48]. In another study, aptamer immobilized SPR-based biosensors were developed by utilizing core-shell AuNPs and MNPs (MNPs) as the plasmonic coupling partners for the detection of thrombin as a model analyte. Aptamer immobilized AuNPs-MNPs conjugate-based SPR biosensors exhibited a considerable response to the thrombin with the limits of detection (LOD) of 0.6 nM. As compared to the SPR signal shift with a control group that is based on SPR signal without AuNPs-MNPs conjugate, AuNPs-MNPs conjugate based SPR angle shift was enlarged for 5 times at the 100 nM concentration [49]. A summary of the different applications of the MNPs by combining the synergistic effects of the SPR is summarized in Table 1.

Table 1. Examples of the application of MNPs in SPR system.

Magnetic Part	SPR System	Applications	Advantages	[R]
Active layer consisting of Fe_3O_4 + Polyethylene glycol (PEG4000)	Silver-coated prism-coupled SPR System	Plant DNA	Target analyte could not be detected without using a magnetic part.	[50]
Polydopamine-Ag capped Fe_3O_4 NPs reduced with graphene oxide	Gold film of SPR chip was electromagnetically coupled with hollow gold nanoparticles	Rabbit IgG	Detection limit 132 times lower than conventional SPR and 8 times lower than immunosandwich assay.	[48]
Gold capped Fe_3O_4 nanoparticles (GMNPs)	Conventional SPR system with gold chip	Thrombin	SPR angle shift is enlarged for 5 times comparing with that of control group without GMNPs	[49]
MNPs conjugated with antibody	Conventional SPR system with gold chip	Pathogenic Bacteria	MNPs offer a sensing enhancement of 4 orders of magnitude.	[51]
Magneto plasmonic nanoparticles (core shell gold capped MNPs)	Conventional SPR system	Antigen (Tuberculosis marker protein)	Implementation of magneto-plasmonic NPs outcomes in 30-fold extension of the SPR signal at the limit of detection.	[52]
Nanohybrids containing Fe_3O_4 NPs and hollow gold sphere nanoparticles.	SPR chip coated with carboxyl functionalized graphene oxide sheet.	Human IgG	Detection limit is approximately 260-fold lower than that acquired with sandwich assay by routine SPR biosensors.	[53]
Polydopamine-wrapped magnetic multi-walled carbon nanotubes	Capture antibody-immobilized SPR-sensing film modified by hollow gold nanoparticles and polydopamine	Protein (Human cardiac troponin I, CTnI)	Minimum detectable SPR response for the concentration of target molecule is 1000 times lower than that achieved by the traditional SPR immunoassay.	[54]
Magnetic fluid photonic crystal (i.e. kind of colloid compassed of MNPs dispersed in carrier liquid)	Kretschmann configuration (prism coupling) SPR system.	—	The excellent benefit of elevated sensitivity is with the combination of magnetic fluid photonic crystal and SPR.	[55]
Aptamer-immobilized Fe_3O_4 nanoparticles with organic clusters	Kretschmann configuration (prism coupling) SPR system.	Protein (prion disease associated isoform, PrP^{Sc})	The SPR scheme involves magnetic NPs-organic clusters that allow for a 215-fold rise in the immediate SPR signal.	[46]
Streptavidin-coated MNPs	Grating-coupled SPR (GC-SPR) with wavelength interrogation.	Lipid (Extracellular vesicles, EVs)	Target could not be detected with the direct SPR detection platform at such low concentrations.	[56]
Fe-C core shell–aptamer conjugation	Prism-coupling SPR system	Protein (prion disease associated isoform, PrP^{Sc})	The detection sensitivity of PrP^{Sc} has been improved by about 10 times relative to the direct format of SPR detection.	[57]
Antibody-functionalized MNPs	Antibody-immobilized SPR immunoassay	Hormone (Estradiol)	The MNPs showed outstanding ability to amplify the SPR signal.	[45]
PEG4000 functionalized Fe_3O_4 MNPs	SPR set up device in Kretschmann configuration and He/Ne laser beam.	Microalgae	Microalgae population has been successfully monitored with the proposed system.	[58]
MNPs antibody conjugates	Conventional SPR spectroscopy	Cancer Biomarkers	To differentiate ovarian cancer, this multiplexed scheme accomplished sensitivity and specificity of up to 94% and 98%, respectively.	[59]

3. Surface-Enhanced Raman Spectroscopy (SERS)

Surface-enhanced Raman scattering (SERS) based on the enhancement of molecular Raman scattering by surface plasmons after the interaction between light and nanostructures is a surface-sensitive technique that is used for the detection of target with high molecular sensitivity and specificity at ultra-trace concentrations, including single molecules and provides more details on the chemical structure and conformation of target molecule [60]. The enhancement of the Raman signal is explained by two mechanisms: chemical enhancement arising from the charge transfer between the nanostructures and the adsorbed target and electromagnetic enhancement stemming from the electromagnetic field effect of the adsorbed target by stimulating the surface plasmons of nanostructures [61,62]. Since the enhancement of molecular Raman scattering mainly occurred by electromagnetic enhancement, novel nanostructures have been developed to achieve high enhancement factors by changing the plasmonic properties. The surface plasmons of nanostructures can be changed with the physical and chemical properties of nanostructures such as shape, size, type, and composition, etc. thus directly affecting the sensitivity and selectivity of SERS [63]. Because of their higher enhancement factors and the accessibility of plasmonic resonances in the visible and NIR areas, the plasmonic nanostructures (PNS) based on Au and Ag are most often preferred to produce SERS substrate [64]. Because of their higher enhancement factors and the accessibility of plasmonic resonances in the visible and NIR areas, the plasmonic nanostructures based on Au and Ag are most often preferred to produce SERS substrates. The SERS substrates have been successfully manufactured for the detection of targets such as biomolecules, cells, microorganisms, environmental pollutants, etc.

Although SERS has many important advantages, there are still needs for improvement of the reproducibility and stability of SERS substrates and the analysis of biological fluids and real environmental samples. These improvements can be achieved using MNPs or magnetic nanocomposites because of their unique properties such as strong superparamagnetic property, low toxicity, biocompatibility, easy preparation, and high adsorption ability. As outlined in Table 2, MNPs in SERS analysis have been used for the detection of proteins [65–68], cells [69–71], toxins [72], drugs [73,74], microorganisms [75–78], illegal additives [79,80], antigens [81,82], pesticides [83], and genes [84,85].

Table 2. Selected examples of surface-enhanced Raman spectroscopy (SERS) sensors based on MNPs.

Type of PNS	Size of PNS, nm	Forms of MNPs	Size of MNPs, nm	Reporter [1]	Analyte	Detection limit	[R]
Au NPs	15	γ-Fe$_2$O$_3$ covered with silica shell and polymer shell	64	DTNB	Tau protein	25 fM	[65]
Au NPs	20	γ-Fe$_2$O$_3$ MNPs covered with silica and Au shell	160	DTNB	Telomerase activity	1 cell/mL	[67]
Triangular Ag nanoprisms	40	γ-Fe$_2$O$_3$ MNPs MNPs	21	MBA	Tumor cells	1 cell/mL	[69]
Au NPs	20	γ-Fe$_2$O$_3$ covered with silica shell	25	MBA	Microcystin-LR	2.0 pg/mL	[72]
Au NPs	20	Fe$_3$O$_4$ magnetic microspheres covered with SiO$_2$ shell and Au nanoparticles	500	Cyanine	Sildenafil citrate	10 nM	[74]
Au NPs	31	γ-Fe$_2$O$_3$ encapsulated with polymer	330	MBA and DSNB	*S. typhimurium*	10 cells/mL	[77]
Au NPs	30	γ-Fe$_2$O$_3$ MNPs	500	DP	Chloramphenicol	1.0 pg/mL	[79]
Ag NPs	20	Fe$_3$O$_4$ MNPs covered with GO and Ag NPs	500	-	Chloramphenicol	0.1 nM	[80]
Au NPs	60	ParaMNPs	200	IR-792 and NB	West Nile virus Antigen and Rift Valley fever virus Antigen	5 fg/mL	[81]
Au NPs	30	γ-Fe$_2$O$_3$ MNPs	500	DP	PSA antigen	5 pg/mL	[82]
Ag/SiO$_2$ core-shell NPs	35	γ-Fe$_2$O$_3$ MNPs covered with silica shell	50	Rhodamine B	DNA	5 µM	[84]
Ag shell	30	γ-Fe$_2$O$_3$ MNPs covered with Ag shell	300	Cyanine	miRNA	0.3 fM	[85]
Ag shell	8	γ-Fe$_2$O$_3$ MNPs covered with Ag shell	300	PATP	Thiram	1.0 nM	[86]
Au@Ag core-shell NPs	32	γ-Fe$_2$O$_3$ MNPs covered with polymer shell	36	MBT	Kanamycin	2 pg/mL	[87]
Ni@Au and Ni@Ag NPs	212 and 222	Ni MNPs	89	rhodamine 6G	rhodamine 6G	1 mM	[88]
Au Shell	35	γ-Fe$_2$O$_3$ MNPs covered with Au shell	50	-	Microcystin-LR	3 fM	[89]
Au Shell	15	Fe$_3$O$_4$ MNPs covered with Au shell	17-30	pthiocresol	Pthiocresol	4.5 pM	[90]
Au nanocubes and nanospheres	51	DNA modified Fe$_3$O$_4$ magnetic beads	1000	Cyanine	DNA	1 pM	[91]
Silver layers on reporter-coated AuNPs	60	Protein G modified Fe$_3$O$_4$ magnetic beads	1000	MBA, DTNB, and TFMBA	Cytokines	4.5 pg mL	[92]

[1] DTNB: 5,5'-dithiobis(2-dinitrobenzoic acid); DP: 4,4'-dipyridyl; MBA: 4-Mercaptobenzoic acid; NB: Infrared-792(IR-792) and Nile blue; PATB: p-aminothiophenol.

As mentioned above, gold (Au) nanostructures in the manufacture of SERS substrates are one of the most widely used metallic nanostructures for the plasmonic substrate. As an example, Zengin et al. [65] applied a sandwich assay for the ultrasensitive detection of tau protein by using monoclonal anti-tau immobilized hybrid MNPs as a probe and polyclonal anti-tau functionalized Au nanoparticles as SERS tags. Firstly, MNPs (γ-Fe$_2$O$_3$) were coated with silica for easy modification and then the hybrid structure was coated with polymer shell by Reversible Addition–Fragmentation chain Transfer (RAFT) polymerization. After the modification of the polymer shell, the monoclonal anti-tau was immobilized on the surface of the hybrid MNPs to obtain the capture probe. Gold nanoparticles were synthesized by citrate reduction with a diameter of 15 ± 8 nm and then, the gold nanoparticles were first modified with a layer of Raman reporter, 5,5-dithiobis(2-dinitrobenzoic acid) (DTNB) to obtain the homogeneous sandwich assay. Finally, their surfaces were functionalized with polyclonal anti-tau to prepare SERS tags. In this study, the MNPs used in sandwich assay provided easy and rapid detection of the tau protein with a detection limit of 25 fM. As another example, Yang et al. [79] performed a similar approach for the detection of chloramphenicol (CAP) by using magnetic separation. For the preparation of SERS tags, gold nanoparticles were first modified with 4,4'-dipyridyl (DP) as SERS reporter and then functionalized with chloramphenicol-bovine serum albumin (BSA) conjugate. CAP antibody was immobilized on the surface of carboxyl-functionalized magnetic beads (average diameter 500 nm) by EDC/NHS coupling reaction for magnetically and selectively separation of CAP. The limit of detection was obtained as 1.0 pg/mL for CAP in aqueous solution and also this SERS immunosensor system based on MNPs was applied to detect CAP in real samples and CAP was detected in the CAP concentration range of 0–5x10^5 pg/mL. The selectivity experiment and real sample analysis indicate that this immunosensor is fast, sensitive and specific for the detection of CAP in the aqueous solution. As an example of toxin analysis, He et al. [72] developed an aptasensor based on SERS with MNPs for the detection of microcystin-LR (MC-LR) (Figure 3). After the synthesis of Au nanoparticles, its surface was modified with SERS reporter, MBA and then functionalized with MC-LR aptamer as SERS probe. MNPs were first covered with silica for easy immobilization of biomolecule and then the complementary DNA to MC-LR aptamer was immobilized on the surfaces of MNPs by biotin/avidin affinity as a capture probe. The developed aptasensor based on magnetic SERS was successfully applied to the selective and specific detection of MC-LR in tap water with the limit of detection, 2.0 pg/mL. As another approach, Yang et al. [81] developed an aptasensor based on magnetic SERS for the detection of prostate-specific antigen (PSA). PSA-aptamer was immobilized on the surface of the magnetic nanoparticle by EDC/NHS coupling reaction for the specific separation of PSA in the matrix. Au NPs were functionalized with DNA of PSA-complementary as a signal probe. The sandwich assay was applied for detection of PSA and LOD was obtained as 5.0 pg/mL and 25 pg/mL in aqueous solution and human serum, respectively. In another study for the detection of antigens, Neng et al. [82] performed the multiplex detection of antigens by using two sets of a spectrally distinct reporter for the preparation of the SERS probe. For the preparation of the SERS probe, the Raman reporter dyes Infrared-792 (IR-792) and Nile blue (NB) were bound separately on the surface of Au NPs and IR-792-coated Au NPs were modified with anti-E IgG and the NB-coated Au NPs were functionalized with anti-N IgG for specific recognition of each target antigen. For capture probe, paramagnetic nanoparticles were first coated with silica and then functionalized with anti-E and anti-N IgG. Briefly, the following procedure was applied for the assay: the antigens were first separated magnetically with the capture probe and then mixed with the antigen modified Au NPs. In the developed SERS sensor, LOD was around 5 fg/mL for both antigens. This study demonstrated the suitability of magnetic particles in SERS for the multiple detection of targets. In a study to examine the performance of SERS based on MNPs in the detection of microorganisms, polymeric MNPs were synthesized as a capture probe and Au NPs were modified with SERS reporter and specific antibody for the detection of *S. typhimurium* in the food product [77]. MBA (4-mercapto benzoic acid) and 5,5'-dithiobis(succinimidyl-2-nitrobenzoate) (DSNB) were used as SERS reporter. After the application of sandwich assay for the detection of microorganism, the limit of detection (LOD) of MBA and DSNB was obtained as 100 cells/mL, and 10 cells/mL, respectively, in a spiked food product. The enhanced sensitivity of DSNB as a SERS reporter is due to its molecular characteristics that provide higher Raman scattering. In this study, higher reproducibility is obtained as it provides better solubility in water by coating the magnetic cores with polymer film.

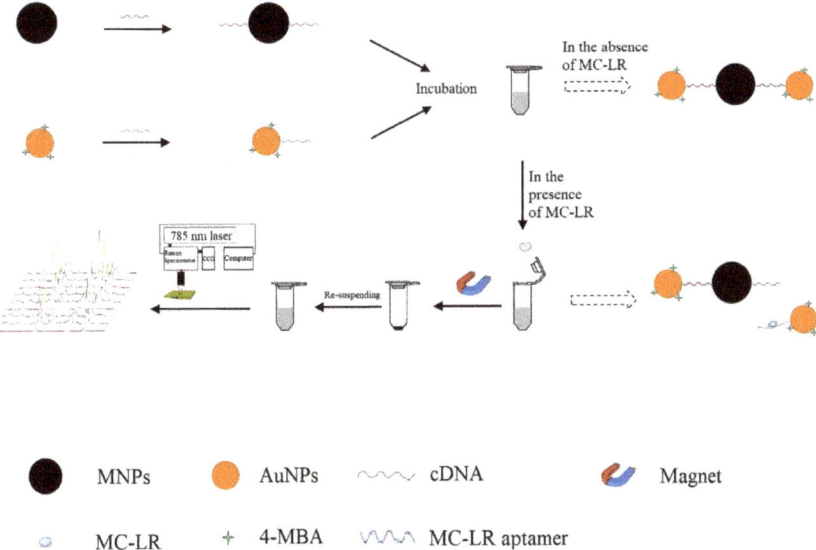

Figure 3. Illustration of the principle for the analysis of microcystin-LR (MC-LR) based on the SERS-based aptasensor. Reprinted [72] © 2019, with permission from Elsevier.

In SERS substrate, the other widely used nanostructures are silver nanostructures to create plasmonic surfaces. As an example, Liang et al. [84] developed a DNA hybridization assay based on magnetic SERS for DNA sequences related to HIV. In this strategy, Ag/SiO$_2$ core-shell nanoparticle-modified with Raman tags (Rhodamine B) were prepared as SERS probe and MNPs covered with silica shell were functionalized with oligonucleotides related HIV as capture probe. The hybridization reaction was performed between these probes. After the magnetical separation of DNA related to HIV from 3 µM solution, the DNA was successfully detected via the SERS probe. In another approach for the detection of genes, Pang et al. [85] developed a SERS sensor based on functionalized Fe$_3$O$_4$@Ag magnetic nanoparticle for the detection of microRNA (miRNA) in total RNA extract from cancer cells. In this application, unlike the others, MNPs were not only functionalized with the capture agent but also functionalized with the SERS signal reporter. This study has demonstrated the advantage of MNPs which are used to concentrate, capture and purify the target gene with the detection limit of 0.3 fM by using a single hybrid nanostructure. Furthermore, a similar strategy has been applied to the detection of microorganisms [76]. In another example, a seed-mediated strategy was applied to obtain an Ag shell on the surface of MNPs after the SiO$_2$ coating to use the detection of pesticide thiram [86] and the limit of detection was achieved as 1.0 nM for thiram.

The SERS applications of plasmonic nanostructures in different shapes are becoming quite attractive because of increasing the enhancement factor of SERS. As an example, Ruan et al. [69] developed SERS sensor based on triangular silver nanoprisms (AgNPR) and superparamagnetic iron oxide nanoparticles with a function of capture, enrichment, detection, and release for the tumor cells analysis. Firstly, AgNPR was modified with MBA and functionalized with rBSA (i.e., reductive bovine serum albumin) and FA (i.e., folic acid) generating the SERS probe. Then, MNPs were also modified with rBSA and FA generating the capture probe to be used for the capturing, enriching and detecting of cancer cells from blood samples. The LOD was obtained as 1 cell/mL and the results demonstrate that nanoprisms have stronger electromagnetic enhancement compared to nanospheres due to their asymmetric shape. In another example of the SERS applications of plasmonic nanostructures in different shapes, the dual-mode nanoprobes based on SERS and fluorescence detection were developed by using Raman reporter-tagged Au@Ag core–shell nanorods and quantum dots onto the silica nanospheres for IgG detection as mentioned Figure 4 [66]. In this study, LOD was obtained as 0.1 pg/mL by applying a sandwich assay.

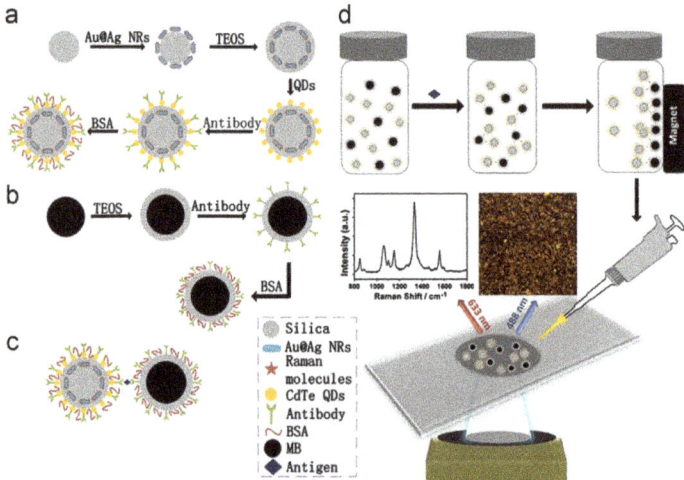

Figure 4. (a) Synthesis and surface functionalization procedure of the dual mode nanoprobe; (b) the synthesis and surface modification procedure of the magnetic beads (MBs); (c) illustration of the structure of the sandwich type nanocomplex formed during the immuno-reaction. For simplicity, only a single nanoprobe, antigen, and MB particle is drawn in the picture; (d) the aqueous phase immunoassay protocol. Reprinted [66] © 2013, with permission from Elsevier.

Zong et al. [67] developed a dual-mode sensor system based on colorimetry and magnetic SERS for the detection of telomerase. Au NPs were functionalized with DTNB and telomeric repeat complementary oligonucleotide to produce a bifunctional reporting tag in SERS and colorimetry. MNPs were first coated with silica and Au shell and then modified with telomerase substrate oligonucleotide as capture prob. The coating of Au shell provides easy modification and colorimetric detection via color change after the capturing. LODs of SERS and colorimetry were obtained as 1 tumor cell/mL and 10 tumor cells/mL, respectively.

As a consequence, MNPs are generally used in two different approaches in SERS applications. In the first one, it is designed as a capture probe for enrichment, purification and separation, and then the detection process by interacting with SERS tag based on the sandwich assay. In the other approach, the magnetic core is modified with SERS reporters such as BMA, DTNB, DP, etc. and plasmonic nanostructures such as Au or Ag shell and used directly as a capture probe and SERS probe. The approaches have advantages in itself as well as the approach being determined according to the analysis to be performed.

4. Fluorescence Spectroscopy

Various investigations have been conducted to address the impacts of the dual signal strategy to ameliorate the detection performance of the sensing system [93,94]. Different techniques that merge with MNPs have been used to serve as an all-in-one sensing system [95,96]. Among these techniques, signal amplification labels relying on the enzyme or DNA labeling, dye labeling, and fluorophore labeling have exhibited great promise thanks to the synchronous properties [94,97,98]. Among numerous composite materials, the magneto-fluorescent nanocomposites have a great potential application due to their merits such as optical activity (biolabeling and bioimaging of fluorescent particles) and magnetic field guide opportunity [99–102]. Fluorometric assays have many advantages for biological applications such as higher sensitivity caused by their robust chemical and optical properties. Apart from their intrinsic properties, fluorescent particles have been frequently used for a sensing platform due to their outstanding advantages such as rapid, sensitive and low cost [103–105]. However, there are still some challenges such as an inevitable false signal caused by non-specific adsorption in real samples. Thus, the magnetization of particles was utilized to capture and separated target agents from complex matrices to avoid false signals [106–108]. Furthermore, MNPs can be adopted to utilize as contrast agents for magnetic resonance imaging (MRI) [100,109,110]. Magneto-fluorometric methods for sensing of numerous materials such as heavy metals [111,112], toxins [113], drugs [114,115], pesticide [116], biological materials i.e. DNA [117,118], cell [119,120], bacteria [121], etc. have been investigated. A summary of the different applications of fluorescence-based MNPs is given in Table 3.

Table 3. Some examples of fluorescence-based MNPs sensors.

Types of NPs	Capture probe	Size nm	Signal Probe	Size nm	Method	Target	LOD	[R]
MNPs@CuNCs	Folate receptor functionalized MNPs	300	Fluorescent copper nanoclusters	20	Sandwich assay	Streptavidin and biotin	0.47 nM and 3.1 nM	[93]
MNPs@FMs	Monoclonal antibodies (MAbs) immobilized Fe_3O_4 MNPs	150	PAbs functionalized fluorescent microspheres (FMs)	150	Microfluidic biosensor- smartphone based fluorescent microscopic system	Salmonella typhimurium	58 CFU/mL	[122]
MNPs@SiO$_2$@BSA@Au-Myo-SNP@RhX	Fe_3O_4 MNPs@SiO2@BSA@Au@antibody	292	SNP@RhX@antibody conjugates	85	Sandwich assay	myoglobin	0.28 ng/mL	[123]
MNPs-aptamer/TRFLNPs-cDNA	Fe_3O_4 MNPs functionalized with ZEN aptamers	55	$NaYF_4$: Ce/Tb modified complementary DNA (TRFLNPs-cDNA)	34	Sandwich assay	Zearalenone (ZEN)	0.21 pg/mL	[124]
MNPs@ssDNA-FAM	Fe_3O_4 MNPs functionalized with ssDNA	50	carboxyfluorescein (FAM)	-	Sandwich assay	Total mercury (Hg)	0.49 nM	[125]
Aptamer-conjugated FMNPs	Specific aptamer modified fluorescent magnetic nanoparticles (FMNPs)	100	-	-	Smartphone-based detection	Staphylococcus aureus	10 CFU/mL	[126]
CoFe$_2$O$_4$@dopamine@HSA@PDI-4NH$_2$	CoFe$_2$O$_4$@dopamine@HSA@PDI-4NH$_2$	190	PDI-4NH$_2$ (Perylene diimide) carboxyfluorescein	-	Fluorescence imaging	Cell imaging	-	[127]
Fe$_3$O$_4$@aptamer 1@ IFN-γ@aptamer-FAM@dsDNA	Fe$_3$O$_4$-aptamer 1/ IFN-γ/ aptamer	100-300	modified aptamer and dsDNA (FAM@dsDNA)	-	Aptamer/protein/aptamerpolymer supersandwich fluorescence sensor	Interferon gamma (IFN-γ)	0.175 fM	[128]
Fe$_3$O$_4$@SiO$_2$-NH$_2$-morin	Fe$_3$O$_4$@SiO$_2$-NH$_2$	78	Morin	-	Fluorescence titrations	Cu^{2+}	7.5 nM	[129]
Fe$_3$O$_4$@SiO$_2$@Au MNPs	Fe$_3$O$_4$@SiO$_2$@Au MNPs	11	BSA-Au NCs	-	H2O2 quenching	glucose	3.0 μM	[130]
MNP-2nd DNA probe-target DNA-1st DNA probe-GNP-barcode DNA	Second target specific DNA probe modified Fe$_3$O$_4$ MNPs	45	First target-specific DNA probe 1 (1pDNA) and bio-barcode DNA coated Au NPs (GNP)	23	Sandwich assay	Exotoxin A gene sequence	1.2 ng/mL	[131]
MNPs-PEI-ssDNA	MNPs-PEI-ssDNA	78	dye-labeled DNA	-	Sandwich assay	lipopolysaccharide	35 ng/mL	[132]

MNPs@CuNCs: Magnetic nanoparticles-fluorescent copper nanoclusters; Rhodamine Red-X: RhX; SNP: Silica nanoparticle.

Liu et al. synthesized magnetic-fluorescent nanoparticles that were able to separate DNA. These research findings have indicated that the adsorption capacity was increased by using this approach. These nanoparticles also allowed to perform an experiment with only a small amount of nanocomposite except the necessity of radioactive probe [98].

According to the work of Cao et al., MNPs and highly fluorescent copper nanoclusters were prepared respectively by following approaches, streptavidin immobilization onto the surface afterward of the co-precipitation method and polymerization by using poly(T) as a template. The primary benefits of this research are that the dual-signal obtained from the supernatant and the re-dispersed precipitate confirmed each other and be integrated in order to result in a solid and quantitative detection [93].

In the case of Kim et al. research, dye-doped silica nanoparticles as fluorescent tagging and MNPs as a concentrating agent were utilized. The nanoparticles mentioned were used for the determination of enrofloxacin by combining with laser-induced fluorescence microscopy. The proposed technique has greatly improved the detection limit when it's compared with conventional methods such as ELISA [133].

A publication by Zarei-Ghobadi et al. has reported the fabrication of a genosensor for detection of target DNA based on the photoluminescence quenching of fluorescent dots in presence of Fe_3O_4 MNPs. The described nano(bio)sensor highlights the utilization of MNPs coated by the gold layer which enabled higher surface area as a quencher of fluorescent carbon dots. Also, the proposed sensor system was introduced as a good candidate for biosensing applications due to their advantages such as ease-synthesis, high biocompatibility, cost-effectivity and strong adsorption ability [134].

Another example of fluorescence shell tagging on MNPs was used to distinguish three cancer cell lines with different expression levels. A significant advantage in this study consists of the dual-mode nanoprobe which can be employed not only in the fluorescence measurements but also magnetic resonance-based cancer cell targeting [94].

Wang's group developed a bio-nanocomposite that has two parts i.e. superparamagnetic Fe_3O_4 nanoclusters as core and fluorescent dye molecule covalently doped onto silica layers to use an imaging and a photothermal therapy agent. In this contribution, bio-nanocomposite obtained were successfully applied in the specific photothermal therapy of colorectal cancer cells with high stability and reproducibility advantages [107]

Another genomagnetic separation based on fluorescence assay was offered by Liu et al. for the detection of mercury in the canned fish sample. The proposed system was successfully applied for monitoring of trace amounts of mercury even after reused for 6 cycling times [125].

Niazi et al. were also developed a novel magneto fluorescent nanosphere by combining aptamer functionalized Fe_3O_4 and $NaYF_4$:Ce/Tb fluorescence nanoparticles for the detection of mycotoxin called zearalenone. Time-resolved fluorescence (TRFL) nanoparticles were labeled with complementary DNA to obtain the signal probe while amine-functionalized MNPs were labeled with zearalenone (ZEN) aptamer to obtain the capture probe. This novel bio-nanocomposite exhibits distinctive features such as stable, specific, convenient and rapid measurements. The schematic protocol for this magneto-fluorescent assay is shown in Figure 5 [124].

Fluorescent chemosensor assay was performed for the detection of target molecules which was based on internal charge transfer. Briefly, in the presence of target molecules interaction between magneto-fluorescent particles and Cu^{2+} that causes quenching due to the coordination with sensing platform was decreased distinctly because of the decomplexation result with an increase in the fluorescence intensity. The developed chemosensor in this study was successfully used for the monitoring of glutathione oxidized as a template molecule [135].

Another approach to use MNPs in combination with fluorescent structures has been proposed by Wang et al. Major novelty in this research was reported as utilizing not only fluorescent DNA nanotag but also enriched MNPs with DNA for the first time. Among various advantages, such as low non-specific adsorption, ultra-high sensitivity, easy preparation i.e., the proposed technique offers significant promise due to allowing the detection of even a single protein, in that case, human IgG [136].

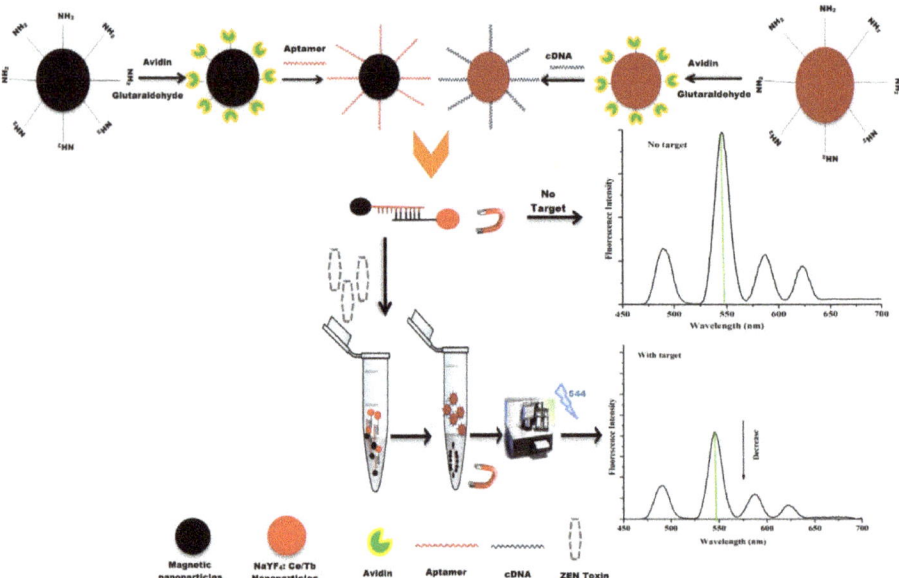

Figure 5. The detection principle based on MNPs as capture probe and fluorescent nanoparticles as a signal probe [124].

Wang and Jiang investigated solvothermal synthesizes of CePO$_4$:Tb, Gd hollow nanospheres which showed significant properties such as peroxidase mimetic activity and magnetic-fluorescent abilities into one nano-entity. The aforementioned properties made the prepared composite nanomaterials as potential applications in biocatalysis and bioimaging [110].

Other promising research was reported localized magnetic field distributions in a microchannel by using nickel powder [137]. They have captured the red fluorescent MNPs with the proposed platform [138–140]. Results have shown a great potential application in chemistry, biology, biomedicine and tissue engineering.

5. Near Infrared Spectroscopy (NIRS) and Imaging

Near-infrared spectroscopy (NIRS) based on the measurement of absorption of electromagnetic radiation, including wavelengths of 750 to 2500 nm is a type of vibration spectroscopy. The absorption bands originate mostly from the vibrations of molecular bonds such as C-H, O-H, C-O, and N-H within the structure [141]. The Spectra consisting of absorption bands allows the quantitative and qualitative analysis of the molecule being analyzed. However, the NIR radiation can easily penetrate into the body and also NIR radiation is scattered less than UV or visible radiation. Hence, the information based on imaging from the inner body can be obtained by analyzing its spectrum of NIRS [142]. Besides these features, NIRS has important advantages such as being fast and simple, and requiring little sample amount without pre-treatment. There are many applications for the analysis of raw material and product quality in food, pharmaceutical and agricultural industries [141,143,144]. Some applications are summarized in Table 4. In recent years, the new generation NIRS devices developed as functional near-infrared spectroscopy (fNIRS) have been also used for the diagnosis especially in biomedical applications such as neuroimaging, sugar blood, etc.

Table 4. Some applications of near-infrared spectroscopy (NIRS) sensors based on MNPs.

Types of NPs*	Size, nm	MNPs form	NIR agent	Target	Methods	Advantages	[R]
CMNPs	45	Fe_3O_4	Cy5.5	Tumor cells	Specific cancer-targeting and magnetic resonance/near-infrared(MR/NIR) imaging	Dual imaging, excellent structural stability with biocompatible and biodegradable	[145]
Fe_3O_4@PPy-PEG	89	Fe_3O_4	Polypyrrole (PPy)	Tumor cells	Photothermal therapy, magnetic targeting	Combination of combined the Fenton reaction and photothermal and magnet-guided cancer therapy	[146]
MFG-SiNc$_4$	40	Magnetic graphene	SiNc$_4$ and fluorescein	Tumor cells	Photodynamic/photothermal therapeutic	Time and cost effective treatments with a minimal therapy dose	[147]
DOX-Fe_3O_4@PAAP	170	Fe_3O_4	Hydrophobic Fe_3O_4	Doxorubicin (DOX)	In situ drug release and combined photothermal-chemotherapy	Fast and effective thermosensitive drug delivery	[148]
CdHgTe@DMF	100	Magnetic layered double hydroxide	Quantum dots of CdHgTe	Tumor cells	Drug delivery, optical bioimaging and magnetic targeted therapy	Slow-release curative effect and good cell imaging	[149]
Fe_3O_4-Aurods-Fe_3O_4 nanodumbbells	70	Fe_3O_4	Au Nanorods (Aurods)	Multiple pathogens	Detection, magnetic separation, and photokilling of multiple pathogens	Tunable nanoprobes for multiplex detection	[36]

* CMNPs: PSI-g-C12-PEG-folate cross-linked magnetic nanoparticles; MFG-SiNc$_4$: magnetic and fluorescent graphene (MFG) functionalized with SiNc$_4$; PAAP: poly (acrylamide-co-aniline)-g-PEG; DMF: dextran-magnetic layered double hydroxide-fluorouracil; PEG: Polyethylene glycol.

MNPs are widely used in NIRS due to their superior properties as targeting and MRI agent to improve the resolution and therapy by the development of dual-mode imaging and therapy systems. As an example, Zhou et al. [150] developed the multimodal theranostic platform by using the Fe_3O_4 magnetic nanoparticle as an MRI contrast agent and Indocyanine Green (IR820) as an NIR imaging agent. Firstly, Fe_3O_4-chitosan quaternary ammonium salt (CSQ-Fe) conjugate was synthesized to increase the stability and biocompatible of MNPs. Then, CSQ-Fe modified with IR820 and fluorescein isothiocyanate (FITC), separately. IR-CSQ-Fe and FITC-CSQ-Fe have similar size distribution and zeta potential and also their behavior in cellular uptake is quite comparable. Therefore, FITC-CSQ-Fe was used to determine the cellular uptake of IR820-CSQ-Fe. As a result, cell viability, long-time stability, MRI imaging, and photodynamic therapy tests indicate that IR-CSQ-Fe can be used as MRI and contrast agent for cancer diagnosis and detection. In another study, Zhou et al. [151] synthesized the Fe_3O_4 MNPs modified with NIR dye for sentinel lymph node mapping via the dual-mode imaging probe including MRI and NIR imaging. These conjugates performed better than small conventional dyes. Yang et al. [145] prepared biodegradable and biocompatible polymer-modified MNPs and functionalized with NIR dye Cy5.5 for specific cancer targeting and dual-mode imaging in vivo. Firstly, poly(succinimide) (PSI)-g-C$_{12}$-PEG-folate was synthesized to improve biodegradable and biocompatible characteristics and then modified with Fe_3O_4 MNPs and NIR dye Cy5.5 for dual imaging. Consequently, MNPs were coated with a polymer and this hybrid material has an efficient NIR signal, high MRI sensitivity, an active targeting function, and good structural stability. Wu et al. [146] developed a new strategy for cancer imaging and therapy based on a combination of Fe_3O_4 MNPs and polypyrole (PPy) in vivo Fenton reaction as illustrated in Figure 6. Fe_3O_4 magnetic core used for targeting the tumor site by applying the magnetic field was coated with PPy shell as near-infrared (NIR) light absorber for converting into heat for the photothermal ablation of tumors (PTT) and then modified functionalized with polyethylene glycol. Moreover, PPy coating not only provided PTT but also prevented $Fe^{2+/3+}$ release from Fe_3O_4 MNPs. This approach indicated the first time that the releasing of iron ions from Fe_3O_4 in acidic medium and the Fenton reaction were enhanced by the photothermal effect. As a result, this hybrid nanoparticle obtained the combination of Fenton reaction and PPy as photothermal therapy provided efficient tumor damage without the effecting of normal organs. In another study, Huang et al. [152] synthesized chlorin e6 (Ce6) as a photosensitizer coated on the surface of Fe_3O_4 MNPs for gastric cancer imaging and therapy. As in other NIRS applications, MNPs have been used as targeting and MRI agents in this application and final multifunctional nanocarriers exhibited good water solubility and less cytotoxicity and good biocompatibility with high photodynamic efficiency. As a consequence, the synthesized multifunctional nanocarriers performed targeting PDT and dual-mode NIR fluorescence imaging and MRI of gastric cancer tissue in vivo. In another similar study, graphene oxide was modified with ferrocene for targeting and functionalized with fluorescein for NIR fluorescence imaging [147]. After these modifications, the surface of nanoparticles was modified with silicon 2,3-naphthalocyanine bis (trihexylsilyloxide)(SiNc$_4$) as a photosensitizer. SiN$_{C4}$ was an ability to use in the photodynamic (PDT) and photothermal (PTT) therapies. This theranostic nanocarrier was used for cost and time-effective treatments with dual-mode imaging and phototherapy of cancer cells by a single light source. Cho et al. [153] designed the injectable nanocarrier based on hydrogel and collagen for drug delivery, phototherapy, and imaging. In this study, the high drug-loading capacity of hydrogel was utilized.

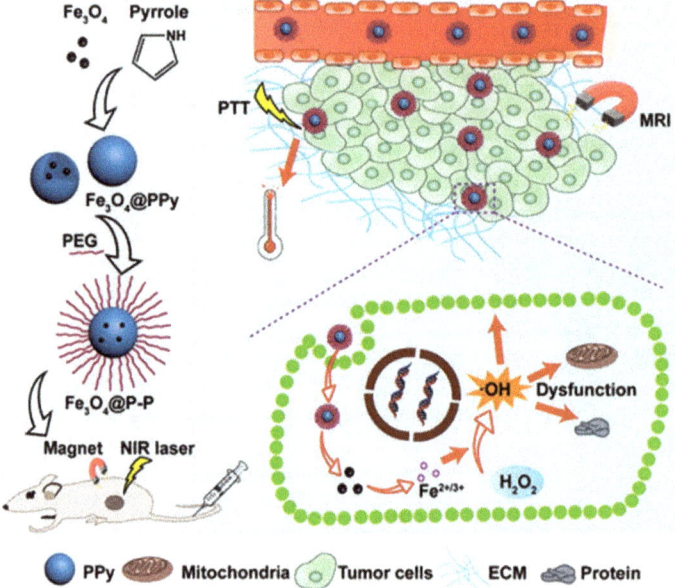

Figure 6. Schematic illustration of the synthetic route of Fe3O4@P−P NPs and the proposed synergistic antitumor mechanism of Fe3O4@P−P NPs. Reprinted with permission from [146]. Copyright American Chemical Society, 2018.

In addition to cell imaging and phototherapy, magnetic nanoparticle-mediated NIRS was used for pathogen detection. As an example, Wang and Irudayaraj [36] developed multifunctional nanoparticles based on gold nanorods and Fe$_3$O$_4$ MNPs for the simultaneous detection of multiple pathogens in a single sample, based on plasmon absorbance, magnetic separation, and thermal ablation. In this study, the plasmonic properties of gold nanorods were an ability to undertake multiple detections and MNPs were used for targeting, imaging and photothermal therapy.

Due to their small size and motility with the potential of the biomedical applications, microrobots have recently attracted attention. In vivo studies are especially prominent for the diagnosis and treatment of disease. In a study, Lee et al. [154] developed a thermosensitive hydrogel-based soft microrobot for targeting and drug delivery by applying NIR stimuli. The microrobot was mainly fabricated with alginate and NIPAM hydrogel for the thermosensitivity and drug loading and Fe$_3$O$_4$ MNPs were encapsulated into perfluoroalkoxy (PFA) tube for the targeting with a magnetic field. For drug release, a therapeutic drug, doxorubicin (DOX), was loaded into the microrobot. In this study, the drug delivery with the microrobot was performed efficiently in cancer cell treatment through in vitro Hep3B cell testing by NIR and electromagnetic actuation systems.

In conclusion, MNPs have been effectively used to develop multifunctional dual imaging and targeting systems for the purpose of drug release, targeting, thermal therapy, and imaging in NIRS applications.

6. Conclusions and Future Challenges

In recent years, MNPs have attracted much attention because of their unique properties such as biocompatibility, low toxicity, chemical stability, high surface area, easy synthesis, and modification, etc. to develop the multifunctional nanoparticle-based optical-sensing systems. Studies in this field generally consist of two main steps: (1) easy pre-modification process to improve low toxicity, solubility, and stability; (2) a second modification step with a specific recognition agent for targeting, imaging, diagnosis, separation, purification, and treatment. The most important disadvantage of MNPs is the aggregation and this problem can be overcome by the first modification such as silica or polymer coating, etc. The main disadvantage of optical sensors is the low sensitivity and selectivity of complex matrices such as body fluids, environmental samples, etc. and this problem is largely overcome by using the MNPs with a magnetic field. Moreover, the synthesis and characterization of MNPs need to be improved in (bio) sensing devices. In the future, optical sensors tend to miniaturization, implantability or wearability with high measuring accuracy for the multiple detections in (bio) sensing applications. Therefore, MNPs need to be adapted to such modifications for the integration of this field.

Author Contributions: Conceptualization, writing—review and editing R.Ü., E.S., A.M.; funding acquisition, A.M.

Funding: The ICN2 is funded by the CERCA Programme / Generalitat de Catalunya. The ICN2 is supported by the Severo Ochoa program of the Spanish Ministry of Economy, Industry and Competitiveness (MINECO, grant No. SEV-2017-0706). Financial support was obtained under MINECO project MAT2017-87202-P.

Conflicts of Interest: The authors declare no conflict of interest.

References

1. Koh, I.; Josephson, L. Magnetic nanoparticle sensors. *Sensors (Basel)* **2009**, *9*, 8130–8145. [CrossRef]
2. Nikiforov, V.N.; Filinova, E.Y. Biomedical Applications of Magnetic Nanoparticles. In *Magnetic Nanoparticles*; Gubin, S.P., Ed.; Wiley-VCH Verlag GmbH & Co. KGaA: Weinheim, Germany, 2009; pp. 393–444.
3. Mou, X.; Ali, Z.; Li, S.; He, N. Applications of Magnetic Nanoparticles in Targeted Drug Delivery System. *J. Nanosci. Nanotechnol.* **2015**, *15*, 54–62. [CrossRef]
4. Bao, Y.; Wen, T.; Samia, A.C.; Khandhar, A.; Krishnan, K.M. Magnetic Nanoparticles: Material Engineering and Emerging Applications in Lithography and Biomedicine. *J. Mater. Sci.* **2016**, *51*, 513–553. [CrossRef]
5. Rocha-Santos, T.A.P. Sensors and biosensors based on magnetic nanoparticles. *Trends Anal. Chem.* **2014**, *62*, 28–36. [CrossRef]
6. Colombo, M.; Carregal-Romero, S.; Casula, M.F.; Gutierrez, L.; Morales, M.P.; Bohm, I.B.; Heverhagen, J.T.; Prosperi, D.; Parak, W.J. Biological applications of magnetic nanoparticles. *Chem. Soc. Rev.* **2012**, *41*, 4306–4334. [CrossRef] [PubMed]
7. Mejías, R.; Pérez-Yagüe, S.; Roca, A.G.; Pérez, N.; Villanueva, Á.; Cañete, M.; Mañes, S.; Ruiz-Cabello, J.; Benito, M.; Labarta, A. Liver and brain imaging through dimercaptosuccinic acid-coated iron oxide nanoparticles. *Nanomedicine* **2010**, *5*, 397–408. [CrossRef] [PubMed]
8. Anbarasu, M.; Anandan, M.; Chinnasamy, E.; Gopinath, V.; Balamurugan, K. Synthesis and characterization of polyethylene glycol (PEG) coated Fe3O4 nanoparticles by chemical co-precipitation method for biomedical applications. *Spectrochim. Acta A Mol. Biomol. Spectrosc.* **2015**, *135*, 536–539. [CrossRef] [PubMed]
9. Figuerola, A.; Di Corato, R.; Manna, L.; Pellegrino, T. From iron oxide nanoparticles towards advanced iron-based inorganic materials designed for biomedical applications. *Pharmacol. Res.* **2010**, *62*, 126–143. [CrossRef] [PubMed]
10. Li, X.; Wei, J.; Aifantis, K.E.; Fan, Y.; Feng, Q.; Cui, F.Z.; Watari, F. Current investigations into magnetic nanoparticles for biomedical applications. *J. Biomed. Mater. Res. A* **2016**, *104*, 1285–1296. [CrossRef]

11. Chen, Q.; Rondinone, A.J.; Chakoumakos, B.C.; Zhang, Z.J. Synthesis of superparamagnetic MgFe2O4 nanoparticles by coprecipitation. *J. Magn. Magn. Mater.* **1999**, *194*, 1–7. [CrossRef]
12. Puntes, V.F.; Krishnan, K.M.; Alivisatos, A.P. Colloidal nanocrystal shape and size control: The case of cobalt. *Science* **2001**, *291*, 2115–2117. [CrossRef] [PubMed]
13. Weller, D.; Moser, A. Thermal effect limits in ultrahigh-density magnetic recording. *IEEE Trans. Magn.* **1999**, *35*, 4423–4439. [CrossRef]
14. Andres, R.P.; Bein, T.; Dorogi, M.; Feng, S.; Henderson, J.I.; Kubiak, C.P.; Mahoney, W.; Osifchin, R.G.; Reifenberger, R. "Coulomb Staircase" at Room Temperature in a Self-Assembled Molecular Nanostructure. *Science* **1996**, *272*, 1323–1325. [CrossRef] [PubMed]
15. Sun, S.; Murray, C.B.; Weller, D.; Folks, L.; Moser, A. Monodisperse FePt nanoparticles and ferromagnetic FePt nanocrystal superlattices. *Science* **2000**, *287*, 1989–1992. [CrossRef] [PubMed]
16. Chen, X.J.; Zhu, J.W.; Chen, Z.X.; Xu, C.B.; Wang, Y.; Yao, C. A novel bienzyme glucose biosensor based on three-layer Au-Fe3O4@SiO2 magnetic nanocomposite. *Sens. Actuators B Chem.* **2011**, *159*, 220–228. [CrossRef]
17. Baghayeri, M.; Nazarzadeh Zare, E.; Mansour Lakouraj, M. A simple hydrogen peroxide biosensor based on a novel electro-magnetic poly (p-phenylenediamine) @ Fe3O4 nanocomposite. *Biosens. Bioelectron.* **2014**, *55*, 259–265. [CrossRef]
18. Baghayeri, M.; Veisi, H.; Ghanei-Motlagh, M. Amperometric glucose biosensor based on immobilization of glucose oxidase on a magnetic glassy carbon electrode modified with a novel magnetic nanocomposite. *Sens. Actuators B Chem.* **2017**, *249*, 321–330. [CrossRef]
19. Zhao, Y.; Zhang, W.; Lin, Y.; Du, D. The vital function of Fe3O4@Au nanocomposites for hydrolase biosensor design and its application in detection of methyl parathion. *Nanoscale* **2013**, *5*, 1121–1126. [CrossRef]
20. Liu, J.; Qiao, S.Z.; Hu, Q.H.; Lu, G.Q. Magnetic nanocomposites with mesoporous structures: Synthesis and applications. *Small* **2011**, *7*, 425–443. [CrossRef]
21. Corma, A. From microporous to mesoporous molecular sieve materials and their use in catalysis. *Chem. Rev.* **1997**, *97*, 2373–2419. [CrossRef]
22. Lu, A.H.; Schuth, F. Nanocasting: A versatile strategy for creating nanostructured porous materials. *Adv. Mater.* **2006**, *18*, 1793–1805. [CrossRef]
23. Ying, J.Y.; Mehnert, C.P.; Wong, M.S. Synthesis and applications of supramolecular-templated mesoporous materials. *Angew. Chem. Int. Ed.* **1999**, *38*, 56–77. [CrossRef]
24. Kudr, J.; Haddad, Y.; Richtera, L.; Heger, Z.; Cernak, M.; Adam, V.; Zitka, O. Magnetic Nanoparticles: From Design and Synthesis to Real World Applications. *Nanomaterials (Basel)* **2017**, *7*, 243. [CrossRef] [PubMed]
25. Leena, M.; Gomaa, H.; Ragab, D.; Zhu, J. Magnetic nanoparticles for environmental and biomedical applications. *Particuology* **2017**, *30*, 1–14.
26. Willard, M.A.; Kurihara, L.K.; Carpenter, E.E.; Calvin, S.; Harris, V.G. Chemically prepared magnetic nanoparticles. *Int. Mater. Rev.* **2004**, *49*, 125–170. [CrossRef]
27. Reddy, L.H.; Arias, J.L.; Nicolas, J.; Couvreur, P. Magnetic nanoparticles: design and characterization, toxicity and biocompatibility, pharmaceutical and biomedical applications. *Chem. Rev.* **2012**, *112*, 5818–5878. [CrossRef]
28. Kango, S.; Kalia, S.; Celli, A.; Njuguna, J.; Habibi, Y.; Kumar, R. Surface modification of inorganic nanoparticles for development of organic–inorganic nanocomposites—A review. *Prog. Polymer Sci.* **2013**, *38*, 1232–1261. [CrossRef]
29. Mahmoudi, M.; Sant, S.; Wang, B.; Laurent, S.; Sen, T. Superparamagnetic iron oxide nanoparticles (SPIONs): development, surface modification and applications in chemotherapy. *Adv. Drug Deliv. Rev.* **2011**, *63*, 24–46. [CrossRef]
30. da Silva, B.F.; Pérez, S.; Gardinalli, P.; Singhal, R.; Mozeto, A.A.; Barceló, D. Analytical chemistry of metallic nanoparticles in natural environments. *Trends Anal. Chem.* **2011**, *30*, 528–540. [CrossRef]
31. Madkour, L.H. Biogenic–biosynthesis metallic nanoparticles (MNPs) for pharmacological, biomedical and environmental nanobiotechnological applications. *Chron. Pharm. Sci. J.* **2018**, *2*, 384–444.
32. Coulet, P.R. What is a Biosensor. In *Biosensor Principles and Applications*; Coulet, P.R., Blum, L.J., Eds.; CRC Press: New York, NY, USA, 1991; pp. 1–8.
33. Suvarnaphaet, P.; Pechprasarn, S. Graphene-Based Materials for Biosensors: A Review. *Sensors (Basel)* **2017**, *17*, 2161. [CrossRef] [PubMed]

34. Tereshchenko, A.; Bechelany, M.; Viter, R.; Khranovskyy, V.; Smyntyna, V.; Starodub, N.; Yakimova, R. Optical biosensors based on ZnO nanostructures: advantages and perspectives. A review. *Sens. Actuators B Chem.* **2016**, *229*, 664–677. [CrossRef]
35. Fan, X.; White, I.M.; Shopova, S.I.; Zhu, H.; Suter, J.D.; Sun, Y. Sensitive optical biosensors for unlabeled targets: a review. *Anal. Chim. Acta* **2008**, *620*, 8–26. [CrossRef] [PubMed]
36. Wang, C.; Irudayaraj, J. Multifunctional magnetic-optical nanoparticle probes for simultaneous detection, separation, and thermal ablation of multiple pathogens. *Small* **2010**, *6*, 283–289. [CrossRef]
37. Englebienne, P.; Van Hoonacker, A.; Verhas, M. Surface plasmon resonance: principles, methods and applications in biomedical sciences. *Spectrosc. Int. J.* **2003**, *17*, 255–273. [CrossRef]
38. Tudos, A.J.; Schasfoort, R.B.M. Introduction to Surface Plasmon Resonance. In *Handbook of Surface Plasmon Resonance*; Royal Society of Chemistry: London, UK, 2008; pp. 1–14. [CrossRef]
39. Van Der Merwe, P.A. Surface plasmon resonance. In *Protein-Ligand Interactions: Hydrodynamics Calorimetry*; Oxford University Press: Oxford, UK, 2001; Volume 1, pp. 137–170.
40. Olaru, A.; Bala, C.; Jaffrezic-Renault, N.; Aboul-Enein, H.Y. Surface plasmon resonance (SPR) biosensors in pharmaceutical analysis. *Crit. Rev. Anal. Chem.* **2015**, *45*, 97–105. [CrossRef]
41. Nguyen, H.H.; Park, J.; Kang, S.; Kim, M. Surface plasmon resonance: A versatile technique for biosensor applications. *Sensors (Basel)* **2015**, *15*, 10481–10510. [CrossRef]
42. Yang, D.; Ma, J.; Peng, M.; Zhang, Q.; Luo, Y.; Hui, W.; Jin, T.; Cui, Y. Building nanoSPR biosensor systems based on gold magnetic composite nanoparticles. *J. Nanosci. Nanotechnol.* **2013**, *13*, 5485–5492. [CrossRef]
43. Liu, X.; Li, L.; Liu, Y.Q.; Shi, X.B.; Li, W.J.; Yang, Y.; Mao, L.G. Ultrasensitive detection of deltamethrin by immune magnetic nanoparticles separation coupled with surface plasmon resonance sensor. *Biosens. Bioelectron.* **2014**, *59*, 328–334. [CrossRef]
44. Lee, J.R.; Bechstein, D.J.; Ooi, C.C.; Patel, A.; Gaster, R.S.; Ng, E.; Gonzalez, L.C.; Wang, S.X. Magneto-nanosensor platform for probing low-affinity protein-protein interactions and identification of a low-affinity PD-L1/PD-L2 interaction. *Nat. Commun.* **2016**, *7*, 12220. [CrossRef]
45. Jia, Y.T.; Peng, Y.; Bai, J.L.; Zhang, X.H.; Cui, Y.G.; Ning, B.A.; Cui, J.S.; Gao, Z.X. Magnetic nanoparticle enhanced surface plasmon resonance sensor for estradiol analysis. *Sens. Actuators B Chem.* **2018**, *254*, 629–635. [CrossRef]
46. Lou, Z.; Han, H.; Zhou, M.; Wan, J.; Sun, Q.; Zhou, X.; Gu, N. Fabrication of Magnetic Conjugation Clusters via Intermolecular Assembling for Ultrasensitive Surface Plasmon Resonance (SPR) Detection in a Wide Range of Concentrations. *Anal. Chem.* **2017**, *89*, 13472–13479. [CrossRef] [PubMed]
47. Lee, K.S.; Lee, M.; Byun, K.M.; Lee, I.S. Surface plasmon resonance biosensing based on target-responsive mobility switch of magnetic nanoparticles under magnetic fields. *J. Mater. Chem.* **2011**, *21*, 5156–5162. [CrossRef]
48. Li, S.; Wu, Q.; Ma, P.; Zhang, Y.; Song, D.; Wang, X.; Sun, Y. A sensitive SPR biosensor based on hollow gold nanospheres and improved sandwich assay with PDA-Ag@Fe3O4/rGO. *Talanta* **2018**, *180*, 156–161. [CrossRef] [PubMed]
49. Chen, H.X.; Qi, F.J.; Zhou, H.; Jia, S.S.; Gao, Y.M.; Koh, K.; Yin, Y.M. Fe3O4@Au nanoparticles as a means of signal enhancement in surface plasmon resonance spectroscopy for thrombin detection. *Sens. Actuators B Chem.* **2015**, *212*, 505–511. [CrossRef]
50. Ekariyani, N.Y.; Wardani, D.P.; Suharyadi, E.; Daryono, B.S.; Abraha, K. The use of Fe3O4 magnetic nanoparticles as the active layer to detect plant's DNA with surface plasmon resonance (SPR) based biosensor. In Proceedings of the 1st International Conference on Science and Technology, Yogyakarta, Indonesia, 11–13 November 2015; p. 150016.
51. Liu, X.; Hu, Y.X.; Zheng, S.; Liu, Y.; He, Z.; Luo, F. Surface plasmon resonance immunosensor for fast, highly sensitive, and in situ detection of the magnetic nanoparticles-enriched Salmonella enteritidis. *Sens. Actuators B Chem.* **2016**, *230*, 191–198. [CrossRef]
52. Zou, F.; Wang, X.X.; Qi, F.J.; Kohn, K.; Lee, J.; Zhou, H.J.; Chen, H.X. Magneto-plamonic nanoparticles enhanced surface plasmon resonance TB sensor based on recombinant gold binding antibody. *Sens. Actuators B Chem.* **2017**, *250*, 356–363. [CrossRef]
53. Wu, Q.; Sun, Y.; Zhang, D.; Li, S.; Wang, X.; Song, D. Magnetic field-assisted SPR biosensor based on carboxyl-functionalized graphene oxide sensing film and Fe3O4-hollow gold nanohybrids probe. *Biosens. Bioelectron.* **2016**, *86*, 95–101. [CrossRef]

54. Wu, Q.; Sun, Y.; Zhang, D.; Li, S.; Zhang, Y.; Ma, P.; Yu, Y.; Wang, X.; Song, D. Ultrasensitive magnetic field-assisted surface plasmon resonance immunoassay for human cardiac troponin I. *Biosens. Bioelectron.* **2017**, *96*, 288–293. [CrossRef]
55. Ying, Y.; Zhao, Y.; Lv, R.-Q.; Hu, H.-F. Magnetic field measurement using surface plasmon resonance sensing technology combined with magnetic fluid photonic crystal. *IEEE Trans. Instrum. Meas.* **2015**, *65*, 170–176. [CrossRef]
56. Reiner, A.T.; Ferrer, N.G.; Venugopalan, P.; Lai, R.C.; Lim, S.K.; Dostalek, J. Magnetic nanoparticle-enhanced surface plasmon resonance biosensor for extracellular vesicle analysis. *Analyst* **2017**, *142*, 3913–3921. [CrossRef] [PubMed]
57. Yuan, C.; Lou, Z.; Wang, W.; Yang, L.; Li, Y. Synthesis of Fe(3)C@C from Pyrolysis of Fe(3)O(4)-Lignin Clusters and Its Application for Quick and Sensitive Detection of PrP(Sc) through a Sandwich SPR Detection Assay. *Int. J. Mol. Sci.* **2019**, *20*, 741. [CrossRef] [PubMed]
58. Nurrohman, D.; Oktivina, M.; Suharyadi, E.; Suyono, E.; Abraha, K. Monitoring Microalgae Population Growth by using Fe3O4 Nanoparticles-based Surface Plasmon Resonance (SPR) Biosensor. In Proceedings of the IOP Conference Series: Materials Science and Engineering, Universitas Negeri Malang, Malang, Indonesia, 27–28 September 2016; p. 012077.
59. Pal, M.K.; Rashid, M.; Bisht, M. Multiplexed magnetic nanoparticle-antibody conjugates (MNPs-ABS) based prognostic detection of ovarian cancer biomarkers, CA-125, β-2M and ApoA1 using fluorescence spectroscopy with comparison of surface plasmon resonance (SPR) analysis. *Biosens. Bioelectron.* **2015**, *73*, 146–152. [CrossRef] [PubMed]
60. Campion, A.; Kambhampati, P. Surface-enhanced Raman scattering. *Chem. Soc. Rev.* **1998**, *27*, 241–250. [CrossRef]
61. Stiles, P.L.; Dieringer, J.A.; Shah, N.C.; Van Duyne, R.P. Surface-enhanced Raman spectroscopy. *Annu. Rev. Anal. Chem. (Palo Alto Calif.)* **2008**, *1*, 601–626. [CrossRef]
62. Sharma, B.; Frontiera, R.R.; Henry, A.I.; Ringe, E.; Van Duyne, R.P. SERS: Materials, applications, and the future. *Mater. Today* **2012**, *15*, 16–25. [CrossRef]
63. Pilot, R.; Signorini, R.; Durante, C.; Orian, L.; Bhamidipati, M.; Fabris, L. A Review on Surface-Enhanced Raman Scattering. *Biosensors (Basel)* **2019**, *9*, 57. [CrossRef]
64. Fan, M.; Andrade, G.F.; Brolo, A.G. A review on the fabrication of substrates for surface enhanced Raman spectroscopy and their applications in analytical chemistry. *Anal. Chim. Acta* **2011**, *693*, 7–25. [CrossRef]
65. Zengin, A.; Tamer, U.; Caykara, T. A SERS-based sandwich assay for ultrasensitive and selective detection of Alzheimer's tau protein. *Biomacromolecules* **2013**, *14*, 3001–3009. [CrossRef]
66. Zong, S.; Wang, Z.; Zhang, R.; Wang, C.; Xu, S.; Cui, Y. A multiplex and straightforward aqueous phase immunoassay protocol through the combination of SERS-fluorescence dual mode nanoprobes and magnetic nanobeads. *Biosens. Bioelectron.* **2013**, *41*, 745–751. [CrossRef]
67. Zong, S.; Wang, Z.; Chen, H.; Hu, G.; Liu, M.; Chen, P.; Cui, Y. Colorimetry and SERS dual-mode detection of telomerase activity: combining rapid screening with high sensitivity. *Nanoscale* **2014**, *6*, 1808–1816. [CrossRef] [PubMed]
68. Mo, A.H.; Landon, P.B.; Gomez, K.S.; Kang, H.; Lee, J.; Zhang, C.; Janetanakit, W.; Sant, V.; Lu, T.; Colburn, D.A.; et al. Magnetically-responsive silica-gold nanobowls for targeted delivery and SERS-based sensing. *Nanoscale* **2016**, *8*, 11840–11850. [CrossRef] [PubMed]
69. Ruan, H.M.; Wu, X.X.; Yang, C.C.; Li, Z.H.; Xia, Y.Z.; Xue, T.; Shen, Z.Y.; Wu, A.G. A Supersensitive CTC Analysis System Based on Triangular Silver Nanoprisms and SPION with Function of Capture, Enrichment, Detection, and Release. *ACS Biomater. Sci. Eng.* **2018**, *4*, 1073–1082. [CrossRef]
70. Kim, H.M.; Kim, D.M.; Jeong, C.; Park, S.Y.; Cha, M.G.; Ha, Y.; Jang, D.; Kyeong, S.; Pham, X.H.; Hahm, E.; et al. Assembly of Plasmonic and Magnetic Nanoparticles with Fluorescent Silica Shell Layer for Tri-functional SERS-Magnetic-Fluorescence Probes and Its Bioapplications. *Sci. Rep.* **2018**, *8*, 13938. [CrossRef]
71. Chen, L.; Hong, W.; Guo, Z.; Sa, Y.; Wang, X.; Jung, Y.M.; Zhao, B. Magnetic assistance highly sensitive protein assay based on surface-enhanced resonance Raman scattering. *J. Colloid Interface Sci.* **2012**, *368*, 282–286. [CrossRef]
72. He, D.; Wu, Z.; Cui, B.; Jin, Z. A novel SERS-based aptasensor for ultrasensitive sensing of microcystin-LR. *Food Chem.* **2019**, *278*, 197–202. [CrossRef]

73. Hwang, H.; Kim, S.H.; Yang, S.M. Microfluidic fabrication of SERS-active microspheres for molecular detection. *Lab Chip* **2011**, *11*, 87–92. [CrossRef]
74. Yu, S.; Liu, Z.; Wang, W.; Jin, L.; Xu, W.; Wu, Y. Disperse magnetic solid phase microextraction and surface enhanced Raman scattering (Dis-MSPME-SERS) for the rapid detection of trace illegally chemicals. *Talanta* **2018**, *178*, 498–506. [CrossRef]
75. Hardiansyah, A.; Chen, A.-Y.; Liao, H.-L.; Yang, M.-C.; Liu, T.-Y.; Chan, T.-Y.; Tsou, H.-M.; Kuo, C.-Y.; Wang, J.-K.; Wang, Y.-L. Core-shell of FePt@SiO2-Au magnetic nanoparticles for rapid SERS detection. *Nanoscale Res. Lett.* **2015**, *10*, 412. [CrossRef]
76. Wang, C.; Gu, B.; Liu, Q.; Pang, Y.; Xiao, R.; Wang, S. Combined use of vancomycin-modified Ag-coated magnetic nanoparticles and secondary enhanced nanoparticles for rapid surface-enhanced Raman scattering detection of bacteria. *Int. J. Nanomed.* **2018**, *13*, 1159–1178. [CrossRef]
77. Chattopadhyay, S.; Sabharwal, P.K.; Jain, S.; Kaur, A.; Singh, H. Functionalized polymeric magnetic nanoparticle assisted SERS immunosensor for the sensitive detection of S. typhimurium. *Anal. Chim. Acta* **2019**, *1067*, 98–106. [CrossRef] [PubMed]
78. Kim, K.; Choi, J.Y.; Lee, H.B.; Shin, K.S. Silanization of Ag-deposited magnetite particles: an efficient route to fabricate magnetic nanoparticle-based Raman barcode materials. *ACS Appl. Mater. Interfaces* **2010**, *2*, 1872–1878. [CrossRef]
79. Yang, K.; Hu, Y.; Dong, N. A novel biosensor based on competitive SERS immunoassay and magnetic separation for accurate and sensitive detection of chloramphenicol. *Biosens. Bioelectron.* **2016**, *80*, 373–377. [CrossRef] [PubMed]
80. Yu, S.; Liu, Z.; Li, H.; Zhang, J.; Yuan, X.X.; Jia, X.; Wu, Y. Combination of a graphene SERS substrate and magnetic solid phase micro-extraction used for the rapid detection of trace illegal additives. *Analyst* **2018**, *143*, 883–890. [CrossRef]
81. Yang, K.; Hu, Y.; Dong, N.; Zhu, G.; Zhu, T.; Jiang, N. A novel SERS-based magnetic aptasensor for prostate specific antigen assay with high sensitivity. *Biosens. Bioelectron.* **2017**, *94*, 286–291. [CrossRef]
82. Neng, J.; Harpster, M.H.; Wilson, W.C.; Johnson, P.A. Surface-enhanced Raman scattering (SERS) detection of multiple viral antigens using magnetic capture of SERS-active nanoparticles. *Biosens. Bioelectron.* **2013**, *41*, 316–321. [CrossRef]
83. Alula, M.T.; Lemmens, P.; Bo, L.; Wulferding, D.; Yang, J.; Spende, H. Preparation of silver nanoparticles coated ZnO/Fe3O4 composites using chemical reduction method for sensitive detection of uric acid via surface-enhanced Raman spectroscopy. *Anal. Chim. Acta* **2019**, *1073*, 62–71. [CrossRef]
84. Liang, Y.; Gong, J.L.; Huang, Y.; Zheng, Y.; Jiang, J.H.; Shen, G.L.; Yu, R.Q. Biocompatible core-shell nanoparticle-based surface-enhanced Raman scattering probes for detection of DNA related to HIV gene using silica-coated magnetic nanoparticles as separation tools. *Talanta* **2007**, *72*, 443–449. [CrossRef]
85. Pang, Y.F.; Wang, C.W.; Wang, J.; Sun, Z.W.; Xiao, R.; Wang, S.Q. Fe3O4@Ag magnetic nanoparticles for microRNA capture and duplex-specific nuclease signal amplification based SERS detection in cancer cells. *Biosens. Bioelectron.* **2016**, *79*, 574–580. [CrossRef]
86. Song, J.; Chen, Z.P.; Jin, J.W.; Chen, Y.; Yu, R.Q. Quantitative surface-enhanced Raman spectroscopy based on the combination of magnetic nanoparticles with an advanced chemometric model. *Chemom. Intell. Lab. Syst.* **2014**, *135*, 31–36. [CrossRef]
87. Zengin, A.; Tamer, U.; Caykara, T. Extremely sensitive sandwich assay of kanamycin using surface-enhanced Raman scattering of 2-mercaptobenzothiazole labeled gold@silver nanoparticles. *Anal. Chim. Acta* **2014**, *817*, 33–41. [CrossRef] [PubMed]
88. Hou, X.M.; Zhang, X.L.; Chen, S.T.; Kang, H.Z.; Tan, W.H. Facile synthesis of Ni/Au, Ni/Ag hybrid magnetic nanoparticles: New active substrates for surface enhanced Raman scattering. *Colloids Surf. A Physicochem. Eng. Asp.* **2012**, *403*, 148–154. [CrossRef]
89. Hassanain, W.A.; Izake, E.L.; Schmidt, M.S.; Ayoko, G.A. Gold nanomaterials for the selective capturing and SERS diagnosis of toxins in aqueous and biological fluids. *Biosens. Bioelectron.* **2017**, *91*, 664–672. [CrossRef] [PubMed]
90. Qu, H.; Lai, Y.; Niu, D.; Sun, S. Surface-enhanced Raman scattering from magneto-metal nanoparticle assemblies. *Anal. Chim. Acta* **2013**, *763*, 38–42. [CrossRef] [PubMed]

91. Kim, M.; Ko, S.M.; Chungyeon, L.; Son, J.; Kim, J.; Kim, J.-M.; Nam, J.-M. Hierarchic Interfacial Nanocube Assembly for Sensitive, Selective and Quantitative DNA Detection with Surface-Enhanced Raman Scattering. *Anal. Chem.* **2019**. [CrossRef]
92. Li, D.; Jiang, L.; Piper, J.A.; Maksymov, I.S.; Greentree, A.D.; Wang, E.; Wang, Y. Sensitive and Multiplexed SERS Nanotags for the Detection of Cytokines Secreted by Lymphoma. *ACS Sens.* **2019**, *4*, 2507–2514. [CrossRef]
93. Cao, J.; Wang, W.; Bo, B.; Mao, X.; Wang, K.; Zhu, X. A dual-signal strategy for the solid detection of both small molecules and proteins based on magnetic separation and highly fluorescent copper nanoclusters. *Biosens. Bioelectron.* **2017**, *90*, 534–541. [CrossRef]
94. Qin, J.; Li, K.; Peng, C.; Li, X.; Lin, J.; Ye, K.; Yang, X.; Xie, Q.; Shen, Z.; Jin, Y.; et al. MRI of iron oxide nanoparticle-labeled ADSCs in a model of hindlimb ischemia. *Biomaterials* **2013**, *34*, 4914–4925. [CrossRef]
95. Mahmoudi, M.; Shokrgozar, M.A. Multifunctional stable fluorescent magnetic nanoparticles. *Chem. Commun. (Camb.)* **2012**, *48*, 3957–3959. [CrossRef]
96. Ebrahiminezhad, A.; Ghasemi, Y.; Rasoul-Amini, S.; Barar, J.; Davaran, S. Preparation of novel magnetic fluorescent nanoparticles using amino acids. *Colloids Surf. B Biointerfaces* **2013**, *102*, 534–539. [CrossRef]
97. Lee, H.U.; Jung, D.U.; Lee, J.H.; Song, Y.S.; Park, C.; Kim, S.W. Detection of glyphosate by quantitative analysis of fluorescence and single DNA using DNA-labeled fluorescent magnetic core-shell nanoparticles. *Sens. Actuators B Chem.* **2013**, *177*, 879–886. [CrossRef]
98. Liu, C.H.; Sahoo, S.L.; Tsao, M.H. Acridine orange coated magnetic nanoparticles for nucleus labeling and DNA adsorption. *Colloids Surf. B Biointerfaces* **2014**, *115*, 150–156. [CrossRef] [PubMed]
99. Chen, O.; Riedemann, L.; Etoc, F.; Herrmann, H.; Coppey, M.; Barch, M.; Farrar, C.T.; Zhao, J.; Bruns, O.T.; Wei, H.; et al. Magneto-fluorescent core-shell supernanoparticles. *Nat. Commun.* **2014**, *5*, 5093. [CrossRef] [PubMed]
100. Wei, Z.; Wu, Y.; Zhao, Y.; Mi, L.; Wang, J.; Wang, J.; Zhao, J.; Wang, L.; Liu, A.; Li, Y.; et al. Multifunctional nanoprobe for cancer cell targeting and simultaneous fluorescence/magnetic resonance imaging. *Anal. Chim. Acta* **2016**, *938*, 156–164. [CrossRef]
101. Ruan, J.; Ji, J.; Song, H.; Qian, Q.; Wang, K.; Wang, C.; Cui, D. Fluorescent magnetic nanoparticle-labeled mesenchymal stem cells for targeted imaging and hyperthermia therapy of in vivo gastric cancer. *Nanoscale Res. Lett.* **2012**, *7*, 309. [CrossRef]
102. Icten, O.; Kose, D.A.; Matissek, S.J.; Misurelli, J.A.; Elsawa, S.F.; Hosmane, N.S.; Zumreoglu-Karan, B. Gadolinium borate and iron oxide bioconjugates: Nanocomposites of next generation with multifunctional applications. *Mater. Sci. Eng. C* **2018**, *92*, 317–328. [CrossRef]
103. Syed, M.A. Advances in nanodiagnostic techniques for microbial agents. *Biosens. Bioelectron.* **2014**, *51*, 391–400. [CrossRef]
104. Bhaisare, M.L.; Gedda, G.; Khan, M.S.; Wu, H.F. Fluorimetric detection of pathogenic bacteria using magnetic carbon dots. *Anal. Chim. Acta* **2016**, *920*, 63–71. [CrossRef]
105. Wu, Z.; Xu, E.; Chughtai, M.F.J.; Jin, Z.; Irudayaraj, J. Highly sensitive fluorescence sensing of zearalenone using a novel aptasensor based on upconverting nanoparticles. *Food Chem.* **2017**, *230*, 673–680. [CrossRef]
106. Clemente, C.S.; Ribeiro, V.G.P.; Sousa, J.E.A.; Maia, F.J.N.; Barreto, A.C.H.; Andrade, N.F.; Denardin, J.C.; Mele, G.; Carbone, L.; Mazzetto, S.E.; et al. Porphyrin synthesized from cashew nut shell liquid as part of a novel superparamagnetic fluorescence nanosystem. *J. Nanopart. Res.* **2013**, *15*, 1739. [CrossRef]
107. Wang, F.; Xu, L.; Zhang, Y.; Petrenko, V.A.; Liu, A. An efficient strategy to synthesize a multifunctional ferroferric oxide core@ dye/SiO 2@ Au shell nanocomposite and its targeted tumor theranostics. *J. Mater. Chem. B* **2017**, *5*, 8209–8218. [CrossRef]
108. Myklatun, A.; Cappetta, M.; Winklhofer, M.; Ntziachristos, V.; Westmeyer, G.G. Microfluidic sorting of intrinsically magnetic cells under visual control. *Sci. Rep.* **2017**, *7*, 6942. [CrossRef]
109. Yin, M.; Li, Z.; Liu, Z.; Ren, J.; Yang, X.; Qu, X. Photosensitizer-incorporated G-quadruplex DNA-functionalized magnetofluorescent nanoparticles for targeted magnetic resonance/fluorescence multimodal imaging and subsequent photodynamic therapy of cancer. *Chem. Commun. (Camb.)* **2012**, *48*, 6556–6558. [CrossRef] [PubMed]
110. Wang, W.; Jiang, X.; Chen, K. CePO 4: Tb, Gd hollow nanospheres as peroxidase mimic and magnetic–fluorescent imaging agent. *Chem. Commun.* **2012**, *48*, 6839–6841. [CrossRef] [PubMed]

111. Zheng, J.; Nie, Y.; Hu, Y.; Li, J.; Li, Y.; Jiang, Y.; Yang, R. Time-resolved fluorescent detection of Hg 2+ in a complex environment by conjugating magnetic nanoparticles with a triple-helix molecular switch. *Chem. Commun.* **2013**, *49*, 6915–6917. [CrossRef]
112. Xu, Y.H.; Zhou, Y.; Li, R.X. Simultaneous fluorescence response and adsorption of functionalized Fe3O4@SiO2 nanoparticles to Cd2+, Zn2+ and Cu2+. *Colloids Surf. A Physicochem. Eng. Asp.* **2014**, *459*, 240–246. [CrossRef]
113. Chen, Q.; Hu, W.; Sun, C.; Li, H.; Ouyang, Q. Synthesis of improved upconversion nanoparticles as ultrasensitive fluorescence probe for mycotoxins. *Anal. Chim. Acta* **2016**, *938*, 137–145. [CrossRef]
114. Liu, Z.; Koczera, P.; Doleschel, D.; Kiessling, F.; Gatjens, J. Versatile synthetic strategies for PBCA-based hybrid fluorescent microbubbles and their potential theranostic applications to cell labelling and imaging. *Chem. Commun. (Camb.)* **2012**, *48*, 5142–5144. [CrossRef]
115. Chang, L.; Chen, S.; Jin, P.; Li, X. Synthesis of multifunctional fluorescent magnetic graphene oxide hybrid materials. *J. Colloid Interface Sci.* **2012**, *388*, 9–14. [CrossRef]
116. Hua, X.; You, H.; Luo, P.; Tao, Z.; Chen, H.; Liu, F.; Wang, M. Upconversion fluorescence immunoassay for imidaclothiz by magnetic nanoparticle separation. *Anal. Bioanal. Chem.* **2017**, *409*, 6885–6892. [CrossRef]
117. Jin, M.; Liu, X.; van den Berg, A.; Zhou, G.; Shui, L. Ultrasensitive DNA detection based on two-step quantitative amplification on magnetic nanoparticles. *Nanotechnology* **2016**, *27*, 335102. [CrossRef] [PubMed]
118. Li, N.; Gao, Z.F.; Kang, B.H.; Li, N.B.; Luo, H.Q. Sensitive mutant DNA biomarker detection based on magnetic nanoparticles and nicking endonuclease assisted fluorescence signal amplification. *RSC Adv.* **2015**, *5*, 20020–20024. [CrossRef]
119. Quarta, A.; Bernareggi, D.; Benigni, F.; Luison, E.; Nano, G.; Nitti, S.; Cesta, M.C.; Di Ciccio, L.; Canevari, S.; Pellegrino, T.; et al. Targeting FR-expressing cells in ovarian cancer with Fab-functionalized nanoparticles: a full study to provide the proof of principle from in vitro to in vivo. *Nanoscale* **2015**, *7*, 2336–2351. [CrossRef] [PubMed]
120. Portnoy, E.; Polyak, B.; Inbar, D.; Kenan, G.; Rai, A.; Wehrli, S.L.; Roberts, T.P.; Bishara, A.; Mann, A.; Shmuel, M.; et al. Tracking inflammation in the epileptic rat brain by bi-functional fluorescent and magnetic nanoparticles. *Nanomedicine* **2016**, *12*, 1335–1345. [CrossRef]
121. Wan, Y.; Sun, Y.; Qi, P.; Wang, P.; Zhang, D. Quaternized magnetic nanoparticles-fluorescent polymer system for detection and identification of bacteria. *Biosens. Bioelectron.* **2014**, *55*, 289–293. [CrossRef]
122. Wang, S.; Zheng, L.; Cai, G.; Liu, N.; Liao, M.; Li, Y.; Zhang, X.; Lin, J. A microfluidic biosensor for online and sensitive detection of Salmonella typhimurium using fluorescence labeling and smartphone video processing. *Biosens. Bioelectron.* **2019**, *140*, 111333. [CrossRef]
123. Wang, Y.; Sun, H.; Li, R.; Ke, P.; Zhu, H.; Guo, H.; Liu, M.; Sun, H. An immunomagnetic separation based fluorescence immunoassay for rapid myoglobin quantification in human blood. *Anal. Methods* **2016**, *8*, 7324–7330. [CrossRef]
124. Niazi, S.; Wang, X.; Pasha, I.; Khan, I.M.; Zhao, S.; Shoaib, M.; Wu, S.; Wang, Z. A novel bioassay based on aptamer-functionalized magnetic nanoparticle for the detection of zearalenone using time resolved-fluorescence NaYF4: Ce/Tb nanoparticles as signal probe. *Talanta* **2018**, *186*, 97–103. [CrossRef]
125. Shen, T.; Yue, Q.; Jiang, X.; Wang, L.; Xu, S.; Li, H.; Gu, X.; Zhang, S.; Liu, J. A reusable and sensitive biosensor for total mercury in canned fish based on fluorescence polarization. *Talanta* **2013**, *117*, 81–86. [CrossRef]
126. Shrivastava, S.; Lee, W.-I.; Lee, N.-E. Culture-free, highly sensitive, quantitative detection of bacteria from minimally processed samples using fluorescence imaging by smartphone. *Biosens. Bioelectron.* **2018**, *109*, 90–97. [CrossRef]
127. Yao, Q.; Zheng, Y.; Cheng, W.; Chen, M.; Shen, J.; Yin, M. Difunctional fluorescent HSA modified CoFe 2 O 4 magnetic nanoparticles for cell imaging. *J. Mater. Chem. B* **2016**, *4*, 6344–6349. [CrossRef]
128. Wen, D.; Liu, Q.; Cui, Y.; Kong, J.; Yang, H.; Liu, Q. DNA based click polymerization for ultrasensitive IFN-γ fluorescent detection. *Sens. Actuators B Chem.* **2018**, *276*, 279–287. [CrossRef]
129. De La Rosa-Romo, L.M.; Oropeza-Guzmán, M.T.; Olivas-Sarabia, A.; Pina-Luis, G. Flavone functionalized magnetic nanoparticles: A new fluorescent sensor for Cu2+ ions with nanomolar detection limit. *Sens. Actuators B Chem.* **2016**, *233*, 459–468. [CrossRef]
130. Luo, S.; Liu, Y.; Rao, H.; Wang, Y.; Wang, X. Fluorescence and magnetic nanocomposite Fe3O4@ SiO2@ Au MNPs as peroxidase mimetics for glucose detection. *Anal. Biochem.* **2017**, *538*, 26–33. [CrossRef] [PubMed]

131. Amini, B.; Kamali, M.; Salouti, M.; Yaghmaei, P. Fluorescence bio-barcode DNA assay based on gold and magnetic nanoparticles for detection of Exotoxin A gene sequence. *Biosens. Bioelectron.* **2017**, *92*, 679–686. [CrossRef]
132. Ma, L.; Sun, N.; Meng, Y.; Tu, C.; Cao, X.; Wei, Y.; Chu, L.; Diao, A. Harnessing the affinity of magnetic nanoparticles toward dye-labeled DNA and developing it as an universal aptasensor revealed by lipopolysaccharide detection. *Anal. Chim. Acta* **2018**, *1036*, 107–114. [CrossRef]
133. Kim, S.; Ko, J.; Lim, H.B. Application of magnetic and core-shell nanoparticles to determine enrofloxacin and its metabolite using laser induced fluorescence microscope. *Anal. Chim. Acta* **2013**, *771*, 37–41. [CrossRef]
134. Zarei-Ghobadi, M.; Mozhgani, S.H.; Dashtestani, F.; Yadegari, A.; Hakimian, F.; Norouzi, M.; Ghourchian, H. A genosensor for detection of HTLV-I based on photoluminescence quenching of fluorescent carbon dots in presence of iron magnetic nanoparticle-capped Au. *Sci. Rep.* **2018**, *8*, 15593. [CrossRef]
135. Ma, Y.; Zheng, B.; Zhao, Y.; Yuan, H.; Cai, Y.; Du, J.; Xiao, D. A sensitive and selective chemosensor for GSSG detection based on the recovered fluorescence of NDPA-Fe(3)O(4)@SiO(2)-Cu(II) nanomaterial. *Biosens. Bioelectron.* **2013**, *48*, 138–144. [CrossRef]
136. Xue, Q.; Wang, L.; Jiang, W. A versatile platform for highly sensitive detection of protein: DNA enriching magnetic nanoparticles based rolling circle amplification immunoassay. *Chem. Commun. (Camb.)* **2012**, *48*, 3930–3932. [CrossRef]
137. Yu, X.; Wen, C.Y.; Zhang, Z.L.; Pang, D.W. Control of magnetic field distribution by using nickel powder@PDMS pillars in microchannels. *RSC Adv.* **2014**, *4*, 17660–17666. [CrossRef]
138. Song, E.Q.; Hu, J.; Wen, C.Y.; Tian, Z.Q.; Yu, X.; Zhang, Z.L.; Shi, Y.B.; Pang, D.W. Fluorescent-magnetic-biotargeting multifunctional nanobioprobes for detecting and isolating multiple types of tumor cells. *ACS Nano* **2011**, *5*, 761–770. [CrossRef] [PubMed]
139. Xie, H.Y.; Xie, M.; Zhang, Z.L.; Long, Y.M.; Liu, X.; Tang, M.L.; Pang, D.W.; Tan, Z.; Dickinson, C.; Zhou, W. Wheat germ agglutinin-modified trifunctional nanospheres for cell recognition. *Bioconjug. Chem.* **2007**, *18*, 1749–1755. [CrossRef] [PubMed]
140. Xie, H.Y.; Zuo, C.; Liu, Y.; Zhang, Z.L.; Pang, D.W.; Li, X.L.; Gong, J.P.; Dickinson, C.; Zhou, W. Cell-targeting multifunctional nanospheres with both fluorescence and magnetism. *Small* **2005**, *1*, 506–509. [CrossRef]
141. Reich, G. Near-infrared spectroscopy and imaging: basic principles and pharmaceutical applications. *Adv. Drug Deliv. Rev.* **2005**, *57*, 1109–1143. [CrossRef]
142. Sakudo, A. Near-infrared spectroscopy for medical applications: Current status and future perspectives. *Clin. Chim. Acta* **2016**, *455*, 181–188. [CrossRef]
143. Roggo, Y.; Chalus, P.; Maurer, L.; Lema-Martinez, C.; Edmond, A.; Jent, N. A review of near infrared spectroscopy and chemometrics in pharmaceutical technologies. *J. Pharm. Biomed. Anal.* **2007**, *44*, 683–700. [CrossRef]
144. Büning-Pfaue, H. Analysis of water in food by near infrared spectroscopy. *Food Chem.* **2003**, *82*, 107–115. [CrossRef]
145. Yang, H.M.; Park, C.W.; Park, S.; Kim, J.D. Cross-linked magnetic nanoparticles with a biocompatible amide bond for cancer-targeted dual optical/magnetic resonance imaging. *Colloids Surf. B Biointerfaces* **2018**, *161*, 183–191. [CrossRef]
146. Wu, H.; Cheng, K.; He, Y.; Li, Z.; Su, H.; Zhang, X.; Sun, Y.; Shi, W.; Ge, D. Fe3O4-based multifunctional nanospheres for amplified magnetic targeting photothermal therapy and Fenton reaction. *ACS Biomater. Sci. Eng.* **2018**, *5*, 1045–1056. [CrossRef]
147. Gollavelli, G.; Ling, Y.C. Magnetic and fluorescent graphene for dual modal imaging and single light induced photothermal and photodynamic therapy of cancer cells. *Biomaterials* **2014**, *35*, 4499–4507. [CrossRef] [PubMed]
148. Wu, L.; Zong, L.; Ni, H.; Liu, X.; Wen, W.; Feng, L.; Cao, J.; Qi, X.; Ge, Y.; Shen, S. Magnetic thermosensitive micelles with upper critical solution temperature for NIR triggered drug release. *Biomater. Sci.* **2019**, *7*, 2134–2143. [CrossRef] [PubMed]
149. Jin, X.; Zhang, M.; Gou, G.; Ren, J. Synthesis and Cell Imaging of a Near-Infrared Fluorescent Magnetic "CdHgTe–Dextran-Magnetic Layered Double Hydroxide–Fluorouracil" Composite. *J. Pharm. Sci.* **2016**, *105*, 1751–1761. [CrossRef] [PubMed]

150. Zhou, H.; Hou, X.; Liu, Y.; Zhao, T.; Shang, Q.; Tang, J.; Liu, J.; Wang, Y.; Wu, Q.; Luo, Z.; et al. Superstable Magnetic Nanoparticles in Conjugation with Near-Infrared Dye as a Multimodal Theranostic Platform. *ACS Appl. Mater. Interfaces* **2016**, *8*, 4424–4433. [CrossRef]
151. Zhou, Z.; Chen, H.; Lipowska, M.; Wang, L.; Yu, Q.; Yang, X.; Tiwari, D.; Yang, L.; Mao, H. A dual-modal magnetic nanoparticle probe for preoperative and intraoperative mapping of sentinel lymph nodes by magnetic resonance and near infrared fluorescence imaging. *J. Biomater. Appl.* **2013**, *28*, 100–111. [CrossRef]
152. Huang, P.; Li, Z.; Lin, J.; Yang, D.; Gao, G.; Xu, C.; Bao, L.; Zhang, C.; Wang, K.; Song, H.; et al. Photosensitizer-conjugated magnetic nanoparticles for in vivo simultaneous magnetofluorescent imaging and targeting therapy. *Biomaterials* **2011**, *32*, 3447–3458. [CrossRef]
153. Cho, S.H.; Kim, A.; Shin, W.; Heo, M.B.; Noh, H.J.; Hong, K.S.; Cho, J.H.; Lim, Y.T. Photothermal-modulated drug delivery and magnetic relaxation based on collagen/poly(gamma-glutamic acid) hydrogel. *Int. J. Nanomedicine* **2017**, *12*, 2607–2620. [CrossRef]
154. Lee, H.; Choi, H.; Lee, M.; Park, S. Preliminary study on alginate/NIPAM hydrogel-based soft microrobot for controlled drug delivery using electromagnetic actuation and near-infrared stimulus. *Biomed. Microdevices* **2018**, *20*, 103. [CrossRef]

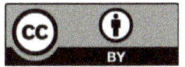

© 2019 by the authors. Licensee MDPI, Basel, Switzerland. This article is an open access article distributed under the terms and conditions of the Creative Commons Attribution (CC BY) license (http://creativecommons.org/licenses/by/4.0/).

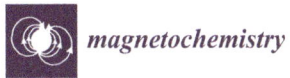

Review

Magnetic Particles-Based Analytical Platforms for Food Safety Monitoring

Reem Khan [1], Abdur Rehman [1], Akhtar Hayat [2,*] and Silvana Andreescu [1,*]

1. Department of Chemistry and Biomolecular Science, Clarkson University, Potsdam, New York, NY 13699, USA; rekhan@clarkson.edun.edu (R.K.); rehmana@clarkson.edu (A.R.)
2. Interdisciplinary Research Centre in Biomedical Materials (IRCBM), COMSATS University Islamabad (CUI), Lahore Campus, Lahore 54000, Pakistan
* Correspondence: akhtarhayat@cuilahore.edu.pk (A.H.); eandrees@clarkson.edu (S.A.); Tel.: +1-315-268-2394 (S.A.); Fax: +1-315-268-6610 (S.A.)

Received: 29 September 2019; Accepted: 14 November 2019; Published: 18 November 2019

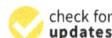

Abstract: Magnetic nanoparticles (MNPs) have attracted growing interest as versatile materials for the development of analytical detection and separation platforms for food safety monitoring. This review discusses recent advances in the synthesis, functionalization and applications of MNPs in bioanalysis. A special emphasis is given to the use of MNPs as an immobilization support for biomolecules and as a target capture and pre-concentration to increase selectivity and sensitivity of analytical platforms for the monitoring of food contaminants. General principles and examples of MNP-based platforms for separation, amplification and detection of analytes of interest in food, including organic and inorganic constituents are discussed.

Keywords: magnetic nanoparticles; surface functionalization; immobilization support; separation probe; analytical platform; food safety

---

1. Introduction

Nanotechnology provides a broad range of opportunities for designing nanomaterials with unique physicochemical characteristics offering new and unique capabilities for designing analytical platforms for detection, separation and tracking of food constituents. Magnetic nanoparticles (MNPs) with sizes ranging from 10–100 nm consisting of magnetic elements such as iron, manganese, chromium, gadolinium, cobalt, nickel, and their alloys have found a broad range of applications in sensors, diagnostics, biomedical devices and in the food sector [1]. The reduction of material dimensions form macro to nanoscale changes their optical, electrical and magnetic characteristics. MNPs of sizes typically below 30 nm exhibit superparamagnetic properties with zero coercivity and hysteresis. The application of an external magnetic field causes magnetization of MNPs. When MNPs are functionalized with specific biorecognition molecules, for example, antibodies (Ab), application of a magnetic field enables facile separation and pre-concentration of target analytes from complex matrices such as food. Therefore, the MNPs' location and motion can be controlled by an externally applied magnetic field and visualized by using magnetic resonance imaging (MRI). The toxicity and biocompatibility of MNPs is dependent on the nature, particle size, coating and the core material of the magnetically responsive component (Fe, Mg, Mn, Ni, Co).

The most commonly employed MNPs are iron oxides such as magnetite (Fe_3O_4) and its oxidized form, maghemite (γ-Fe_2O_3). These particles have been explored for biomedical and food applications owing to their biocompatibility, non-immunogenic and non-toxic characteristics and the ability to prepare them in small particle sizes [2]. Ferrous oxide NPs are the only United States Fodo and Drug Administration (US FDA) approved MNPs that retain zero magnetism after removal of an external magnetic field [1]. MNPs based on other materials, such as cobalt and nickel, despite a high magnetism have received little interest due to their toxicity and tendency to rapidly oxidize at the surface [3]. The magnetic behavior of individual NPs arise from their narrow, finite-size and surface effects, which all affect their properties [4]. MNPs can be used in bare form, surface coated or functionalized with molecular recognition sites for specific binding to enable applications in bio-separation, biosensing, information storage, catalysis and diagnostic imaging [1]. The physicochemical characteristics of NPs depend on the size, surface area, effective sedimentation rate and dispersity [1,5].

In the food sector, MNPs can be used as colorants and sources of bioavailable iron. MNPs modified with immunorecognition reagents have been used to improve detection of food borne pathogens [6]. MNPs are commonly used in magnetic solid-phase extraction for the recovery of analytes in the preparation of biological, environmental and food samples [7]. The use of MNPs can simplify the extraction process and increase sensitivity of measurements by providing selective isolation and enrichment of analytes using an external magnetic field. In this article, we discuss the synthesis, structure, properties and applications of MNPs in the development of analytical assays and sensors for food monitoring and highlight the advantages and limitations of MNPs for sample pre-treatment and pre-concentration in the food sector. Several examples of magneto-switchable devices with controlled sensing and actuation properties are provided.

2. Synthesis of MNPs

Various forms and sizes of MNPs are available and can be purchased from several companies or they can be prepared using established procedures [8–10]. Methods to synthesize MNPs (iron oxide, metal, metal alloys, magnetic composite materials) include biomineralization, physical and chemical methods [11–13]. Biomineralization involves the use of living organisms to prepare magnetic particles. MNPs fabricated by biomineralization are prepared as natural magnetosomes (nanosized magnetic iron oxide crystals coated with protein) involving magnetotactic bacteria. Magnetosomes of 20 to 45 nm have been synthesized in laboratory under simulated environment of bacterial anaerobic habitat. There is significant research focusing on the development of chemical methods which emulate the biomineralization process to synthesize MNPs [14–16].

Physical methods for MNPs synthesis can be either "top down" or "bottom up" procedures. Top down methods employ the size reduction of coarse macroscopic magnetic materials to the nanometer range by milling. The main limitation of this method is the difficulty to control the particle size and shape [15]. Bottom up techniques rely on condensation of NPs from their liquid or gaseous phase. An example if the laser evaporation technique employed for the synthesis of MNPs in which coarse particles of metal oxides are temperature treated to evaporate the solvent, followed by condensation and nucleation resulting in synthesis of 20–50 nm particles [15,17,18].

Wet chemical methods for the preparation of MNPs can be distinguished as (a) high-temperature thermal decomposition and/or reduction, (b) co-precipitation and (c) template synthesis in the interior of micelles [1]. Other methods are template-directed and can involve micro emulsion, thermal decomposition, solvo-thermal, solid state, spray pyrolysis, self-assembly, lithography, sono-chemical, microwave assisted, carbon arc techniques or glycothermal synthesis, among others [19,20]. The most common chemical method employed for MNPs synthesis involve co-precipitation and nucleation of particles from ions in solution. During the co-precipitation process, a super saturation stage followed by a burst nucleation occurs with formation of nuclei which gradually grow in size and cause the monodisperse particles to diffuse from solution into solute. The co-precipitation principle to achieve monodisperse particles is represented by the La Mer-Dinegar model [18] of homogeneous precipitation shown in Figure 1. In general, the co-precipitation method requires low temperatures and metal salts and the properties of MNPs can be tailored by controlling the reaction pH, temperature, stirring speed and metal ion concentration.

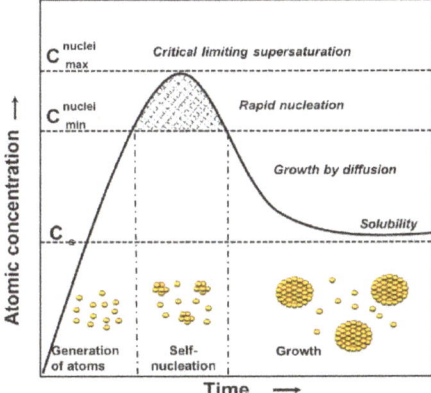

Figure 1. Mechanism of La Mer's nucleation condition. Reprinted with permission from Reference [18] Copyrights 1950, American Chemical Society.

MNPs synthesis can also be achieved by thermal decomposition of the chemical structure of organometallic compounds at elevated temperatures by cleavage of chemical bonds. This method is mostly employed for organometallic compounds (acetyl acetonates) in organic solvents (benzyl ether, carbonyls and Ethylene diamine) with surface active agent such as oleic acid, oleyl amine, polyvinyl pyrrolidone (PVP), cetyltrimethyl ammonium bromide (CTAB) and hexadecyl amine. Morphology and size of MNPs can be controlled by varying the precursor composition (Figure 2) [21]. The thermal decomposition method is used to synthesize MNPs with good crystallinity, controlled morphology and size distribution (4–45 nm) [22,23]. For example thermal decomposition of FeCup$_3$ (Cup: *N*-nitroso phenyl hydroxyl amine) at elevated temperatures of 250 °C–300 °C allowed fabrication of maghemite nanocrystals with a size range of 3–9 nm. The method can also be used to synthesize MNPs of transition metals (Co, Ni and Fe) [24]. To obtain the 3D MNPs, hot solutions of metal precursor and surfactant is mixed with a reducing agent. The morphology of the MNPs shown in Figure 2 was controlled by controlling the decomposition time. A shorter duration of (2–4 h) resulted in spherical particles while longer decomposition time (10–12 h) resulted in cubic MNPs [21,24].

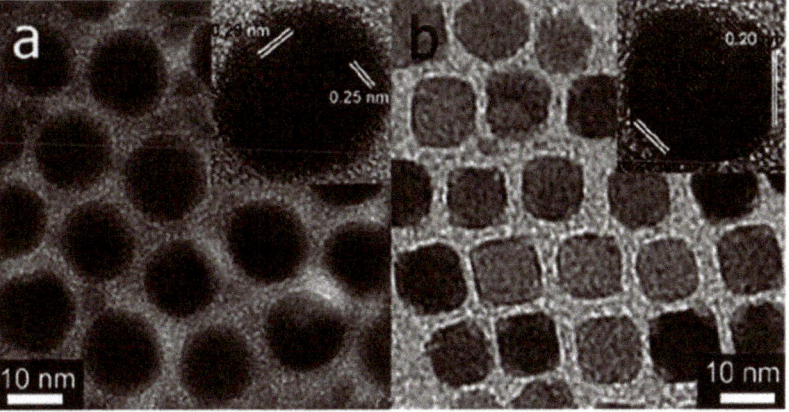

Figure 2. Ttransmission electron microscopy (HR TEM) images of monodisperse (**a**) nanosphere, (**b**) nanocubes by thermal decomposition method. Reprinted with permission from reference [21] Copyrights 2008, American Chemical Society.

Excellent control of particle size and shape can be achieved by hydrothermal synthesis. This procedure involves the synthesis of MNPs at high vapor pressure and high boiling point. During this reaction, phase separation occurs at the solid-liquid interface resulting in monodisperse Fe_3O_4 and MFe_2O_4 nanocrystals [25]. This synthesis method has been used to fabricate a variety of metal, rare earth, fluorescent, polymeric and magnetic metallic nanocrystals at different reaction conditions [26–28]. High MNPs yield with short reaction times was achieved by microwave radiation. Wang et al. [6] reported the synthesis of a highly crystalline cubical spinel $M_{II}Fe_2O_4$ (M = Co, Mn, Ni) structure by exposing the precursors to microwave radiation for 10 min. The fabrication of magnetite (Fe_3O_4) and hematite (α-Fe_2O_3) particle by microwave radiation involved the use of $FeCl_3$, polyethylene glycol and $N_2H_4 \cdot H_2O$ precursors. The final condition of Fe_3O_4 was controlled by controlling the quantity of $N_2H_4 \cdot H_2O$ [6]. Another method to prepare MNPs involves a multistep template assisted fabrication which requires the use of a base template tailed by subsequent deposition of a magnetic material. MNPs nuclei grow at the hole and defects of the template resulting in MNPs of a morphology tailored to the template. The physical properties (size, morphology) of MNPs can be controlled by the selection of a base template of desired properties. This technique allows fabricating MNPs of complex structure (nanotubes, nanorods, nanocubes, hexagonal and octahedrons) with controlled size and morphology [29].

3. Surface Modification of MNPs

To enhance solubility, stability and biocompatibility and achieve target specificity, MNPs are generally modified with surface ligands. MNPs which are hydrophobic in nature can be functionalized by ligand exchange [25,27] or encapsulated within a phospholipid bilayer to make them hydrophilic [6,28]. Other methods involve encapsulation within materials that have affinity for the iron oxide core such as gold [30,31], SiO_2 [31,32] or carbon [33] which enhances their surface properties while maintaining the magnetic functions for applications [19].

Modification of super paramagnetic NPs (Fe_2O_3, 13.5 nm in diameter) with lactoferrin or ceruloplasmin protein enabled stabilization of MNPs at room temperature and prevented non-specific adsorption. To achieve target specificity through the attachment of antibodies commercial tosylated polystyrene MNPs (Fe_2O_3) were coated with a gold layer. Other methods involve coating with polymers, silica [34] or organic layers [17]. MNPs modified by charged layers facilitated adsorption of biomolecules by electrostatic interactions. Matsunaga et al. [35] devised a technique for electrostatic-based DNA extraction in which negatively charged DNA is extracted by electrostatic interaction of positively charged NH_2-MNPs. MNPs coated with a dense amino layer using an aminosilane reagent, 3-[2-2-aminoethy(amino)-ethylamino-propyetrimethoxysilane] in toluene solution enabled fabrication of NH_2-functionalizaed MNPs. [35]. Polyamidoamine dendrimer remodified [36] and aminosilane-coated MNPs [37] were also used in adsorption-based DNA extraction techniques. For such applications, the MNPs surface was chemically modified with carboxyl and amino groups that were further used to covalently immobilize biomolecules. In addition to surface stabilizers, the coatings can include fluorescent labels [38] such that the particles can be manipulated through the use of an external magnetic field and simultaneously visualizing their position through fluorescence methods. Surface modification can also be achieved through physical means via encapsulation and sorption [39]. Various natural (gelatin, dextran, starch chitosan) and synthetic polymers (PVA, PEG, PMMA, PLA, PANI etc.) have been used to functionalize the surface of MNPs to prevent the agglomeration and enhance the selectivity for specific target. [39].

4. Applications of MNPs in Bioanalysis

4.1. Enzyme Immobilization Support

Owing to their biocomptability and magnetic properties, MNPs have various applications in the food industry as enzyme immbolization support and separator for protein purification. Modification of the MNPs with bioactive molecules tipically involves surface modification with hydroxyl -OH, carboxyl –COOH and amino –NH$_2$ functional groups [40]. Most food applications invloves catalytic enzymes such as, that is, carbohydrase, protease, lipase, lysozymes and oxidoreductase. Free enzymes are unstable to changes in pH, temperature and ionic solutions and are difficult to recycle if they are used in solution. Their stability and reuseability can be improved by immobilization [41] on various supports throug organic and inorganic linkers [42–45]. MNPsprovide a large surface area with a high enzyme loading capability. Enzyme immobilized on MNPs offers lower diffusion coefficient in solution [46]. Immobilized enzyme @ MNPs can be collected with ease and at low cost from enzyme complex mixture with the aid of external magnetic field [47,48].

Enymes immobilization on MNPs can be carried out by physical adsorption and covalent bonding. Covalent bonding provides strong enzyme adherence to MNPs surface but limits the enzyme activity, as this immobilization involves strong covalent interaction between the surface of MNPs and the functional groups of the enzymes [49]. The physical adsorption method is based on simple enzyme adhesion through weak ionic, H-bonding and van der Waals forces between the surface-modified MNPs and enzymes. Physically-immobilized enzymes on MNPs are more succeptable to changes in temperature, pH and ionic strength [49]. Immobilization though (strept)avidin–biotin affinity bonds can also be used for protein immoblization (Figure 3). The high specificity and binding affinity ($K_d \approx 10^{-15}$ M) of (strept)avidin and biotin makes this approach appealing for protein immobilization applications [50].

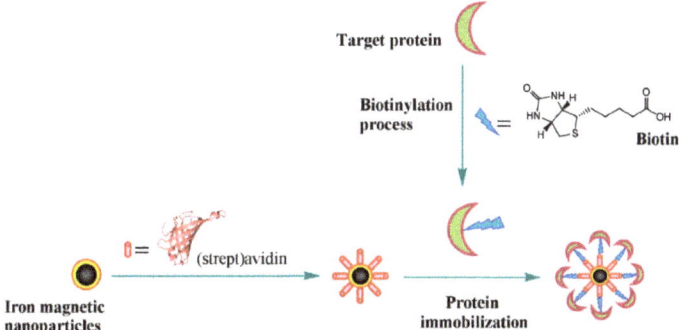

Figure 3. The (strept) avidin–biotin method for protein immobilization onto iron magnetic nanoparticles. Reproduced with permission from Reference [50], MDPI, [2014].

In order to enable protein binding on MNPs, the particles are first functionalized with amino or carboxyl functional groups. An example is the use of organic (lauric acid $C_{12}H_{24}O_2$) and inorganic (silicone dioxide SiO_2) materials. Covalent cross-linking involves coupling agents (e.g., glutaraldehyde) which provide the aldehyde group for covalent interaction between MNPs and enzymes. Enzymes immobilized via covalent bonding are more stable than those immobilized by physical adsorption [51,52]. However, covalent bonding can cause conformational changes and possible alteration of the enzyme active site reducing the activity of the immobilized enzyme. It was reported that when the concentration of the coupling agent was <0.4% the effect on the recovered enzyme activity is minimal. However greater concentrations (>4%) were found to reduce the enzyme activity due to confrmational changes induced by the interaction with the coupling agent for example, (glutraldehyde) [53,54]. Huang et al. [55] reported a simple method for the immobilization of lipase enzyme via direct bounding to MNPs by using 1-ethyl-3-(3-dimethylaminopropyl) carbodiimide hydrochloride (EDC), which enhanced its specific activity. It was reported that the specific activity of immobilized lipase was enhanced up to 1.41 times than the free form [55]. In a similar way, Liu et al. [56] immobilized lipase on lauric acid stabilized-MNPs by using EDC as a coupling agent; the specific activity of the immobilized lipase was 1.8 times higher than that of the free enzyme. A number of studies concluded that enzymes activity can be enhanced by immobilization on functionalized MNPs [56].

4.2. MNPs as Pre-Concentration and Capture Probe

Sample preparation is a critical step in almost all analytical procedures and directly influences the accuracy of measurements. Inappropriate sample preparation can cause contamination, loss of analyte, erroneous compositional data and so forth, particularly in environmental, biological or food samples in which the analytes are present in trace or ultra-trace levels or when samples are complex. Therefore, isolation or pre-concentration of analyte before analysis is a necessary step for achieving accurate qualitative and quantitative analysis. Isolation of an analyte from the primary matrix is meant to reduce the effect of interfering species but the conventional separation methods are high cost, time consuming and involve laborious procedures.

Separation of analytes from food samples can be achieved by solid phase extraction (SPE) that provides rapid enrichment of the analyte using an economical and simple procedure. MNPs represent an alternative approach and can be used to concentrate and then magnetically separate a large amount of analytes by virtue of their large surface area and magnetic properties [57]. Integration of MNPs in conventional SPE was the basis for the development of an advanced, automated and time saving extraction technique [58]. In this combined use, called magnetic-dispersive solid phase extraction (M-DSPE), the MNPs served as a sorbent in SPE. Contrary to conventional SPE where the sorbent is always packed into cartridges, the M-DSPE utilize MNPs that are directly placed into the sample which after extraction are isolated by applying an external magnetic field. Such magnetic isolation of MNPs after analyte adsorption eliminates post centrifugation or filtration processes. The analyte-sorbent interaction mainly depends on the surface chemistry of the MNPs and the tailoring of their properties to selectively interact with the analyte of interest. In general, the interaction between the sorbent and the analyte are polarity-based, ionic, van der Waals, hydrophobicity based, dipole-dipole, pi-pi and dipole induced dipole type interactions. Due to irreversibility, chemical bonding is usually avoided in MSPE. After the extraction step, the analyte is eluted from the surface of the magnetic sorbent by using a suitable solvent and thus the sorbent is regenerated and can be reused (Figure 4). The quantity of extract depends on the strength of interaction between sorbent and analyte and the elution strength of the solvent.

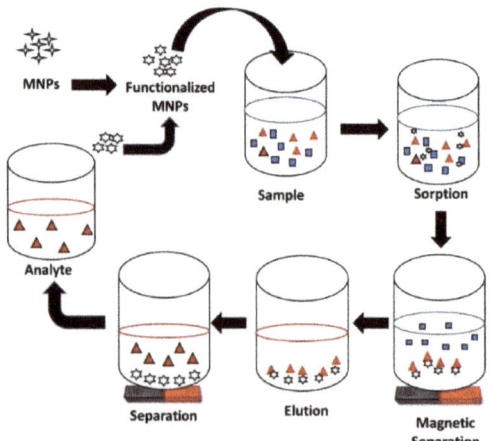

Figure 4. Schematic illustration of magnetic solid phase extraction.

In such applications, the magnetic core of the sorbent is mainly composed of nickel, cobalt, iron and their oxides. Pure iron oxide, for example, magnetite and maghemite are most commonly used but MNPs based on these oxides tend to be highly reactive and prone to aggregation. Therefore, surface modification with stabilizing groups is usually required. The major challenges associated with the use of MNPs are: the acquisition of high magnetic gradient to control transport properties of the MNPs present inside the matrix, poor dispersibility, strong aggregation tendency, inadequate stability in aqueous/acidic media and low selectivity for a specific target and so forth. Some of these challenges have been addressed by tuning the MNPs surface with appropriate functional groups in order to make them stable and selective for the analyte of interest, enabling them to be used as capture probes. As an example of application in the food sector, a magnetic nanocomposite composed of iron oxide NPs and polythionine was used as a sorbent in MSPE to capture and enrich the cobalt II ions [59]. The procedure enabled extraction and concentration of Co ions by 50 folds, with a limit of detection (LOD) of 0.3 ng L^{-1}. Similarly, a Schiff base/magnetite/silica nanocomposite was used as magnetic sorbent to pre-concentrate trace metals including Pb, Cu, Cd in biological and environmental samples [60]. Table 1 summarizes MNPs-based procedures for sample pretreatment.

Apart from being used as sorbent in MSPE, modified MNPs are also being used directly as capture probes. A nanoprobe based affinity mass spectrometry NBAMS technique was developed by Lin et al. to capture and analyze small molecule targets. MNPs served dual function, at first as capture probe to extract and enrich the analyte from a complex matrix and secondly as a solid laser desorption to detect the analyte from nanoprobe. The technique enabled separation and preconcentration of mefenamic acid, salicylamide, flufenamic acid, ketoprofen, prednisolone, mannose and sulindac. Chen et al. designed an immunoassay to capture proteins from a matrix using antibody conjugated iron oxide NPs. Analyte capturing and detection efficiency of the antibody-modified MNPs were compared with superparamagnetic microbeads, demonstrating higher performance of MNPs for such applications [61]. Alumina coated iron oxide NPs were also used to capture viruses. Iron oxide NPs modified with nitrilotriacetic acid (NTA), acting as a chelating agent for transition metals such as Zr(IV), Gd(III) and Ni(II) and so forth, formation of MNP-NTA-metal ion complexes were efficiently utilized to capture protein molecules [62].

Table 1. Application of silica modified magnetic nanoparticles (MNPs) as capture probe for pre-concentration of analytes.

Magnetic Nanomaterial	Analytes	Detection Technique	Amount of Sorbent (mg)	Sample Volume (mL)	LOD (ng L^{-1})	Enrichment Factor	Adsorption Capacity (mg g^{-1})	Precision (RSD, %)	Recovery (%)	Ref.
Fe$_3$O$_4$-SiO$_2$-γ- MPTMS	Cd Cu Hg Pb	ICP-MS	50	250	0.024 0.092 0.107 0.056	500	45.2 56.8 83.8 70.4	6.7 9.6 8.3 3.7	94	[63]
Fe$_3$O$_4$-SiO$_2$-SA	Cr(III) Cu(II) Ni(II) Cd(II)	FAAS	110	4	150 220 270 110	200	39.9 39.8 27.8 17.3	4.0 3.1 2.2 3.3	-	[64]
Fe$_3$O$_4$-SiO$_2$-γ- MPTMS	Te(IV)	ICP-MS	50	160	0.079	320	10.1	7.0	88–109	[65]
Fe$_3$O$_4$-SiO$_2$-L	Pb(II) Cd(II) Cu(II)	FAAS	130	350	140 190 120	-	-	1.4 1.6 1.8	97.8–102.9	[60]
Fe$_3$O$_4$-SiO$_2$-MIL-101	PAHs	HPLC-PDA	0.6+1.0	20	2.8–27.2	101–180	-	3.1–8.7	81.3–105	[66]
Fe$_3$O$_4$-SiO$_2$-diphenyl	PAHs	GC-MS	25	0.8	-	-	-	-	88–97	[67]
Fe$_3$O$_4$-SiO$_2$–AAPTS	As(V)	ICP-MS	50	150	0.21	3001	13.1	6.8	104.1	[68]
Fe$_3$O$_4$-SiO$_2$-IDA	Cd(II) Mn(II) Pb(II)	ICP-MS	40	100	0.16 0.26 0.26	200	45.1 30.5 73.1	4.8 4.6 7.4	95–106.6	[69]
Fe$_3$O$_4$-SiO$_2$- Bismuthiol-II	Cr Cu Pb	ICP-OES	100	100	43 58 85	96 95 87	8.6 5.3 9.4	3.5 4.6 3.7	90–104	[70]
Fe$_3$O$_4$-SiO$_2$-TiO$_2$	Cd(II) Cr(III) Mn(II) Cu(II)	ICP-MS	40	50	4.0 2.6 1.6 2.3	100	59.3 27.8 15.4 33.2	3.6 4.5 4.0 4.1	100–109	[71]
Aminated-CoFe$_2$O$_4$- SiO$_2$	Cd(II)	HG-AFS	20	50	3.15	50	5.0	4.9	98.0–100.4	[72]
Fe$_3$O$_4$-SiO$_2$-Zincon	Pb	GFAAS	20	100	10	200	21.5	7.8–9.2	84–104	[73]
Fe$_3$O$_4$-SiO$_2$-β-CD	BPA DES	HPLC	100	250	20.0 23.0	100–390	-	<7	80–105	[74]

Table 1. Cont.

Magnetic Nanomaterial	Analytes	Detection Technique	Amount of Sorbent (mg)	Sample Volume (mL)	LOD (ng L^{-1})	Enrichment Factor	Adsorption Capacity (mg g^{-1})	Precision (RSD, %)	Recovery (%)	Ref.
Fe$_3$O$_4$-SiO$_2$	Sudan dyes	UFLC	40	4	82–120	500	-	1.93–8.11	87.10–111.4	[75]
Fe$_3$O$_4$-SiO$_2$-DAPD	Cu(II) Zn(II)	FAAS	10	100	140 220	125	45 32	2.3 3.6	97–104	[76]
Fe$_3$O$_4$-SiO$_2$-DPC	Hg(II)	AAS	100	200	160	100	-	2.2	97.5	[77]
Fe$_3$O$_4$-HMS	DDT	GC-MS	10	35	-	-	-	-	-	[78]

DCP 1,5-diphenylcarbazide, HMS hexagonal mesoporous silica, HPLC-PAD High performanace liquid chromatography-photodiode array detection, ICP-OES Inductively coupled plasma optical emission spectroscopy, HG-AFS Hydride genreation atomic fluorescence spectroscopy.

Protein separation and purification is highly demanded in food, biosciences and biomedical applications. Precipitation, co-precipitation, chromatography, filtration, ultrafiltration, centrifugation and dialysis are the most commonly used methods for protein bioprocessing. However, these methods suffer limitations such as time consuming, the need for sample pre-treatment and skilled operators and so forth, which could be overcome through magnetic separation. MNPs-based magnetic separation is a powerful technique for such applications requiring protein isolation and purification. Figure 5 presents the different stages involved in the magnetic separation of proteins using MNPs modified with ligands having high affinity for targeted proteins. Ligand-functionalized MNPs are designed to specifically recognize and capture the target protein followed by magnetic separation. Separation using an indirect approach is also possible, in which ligands are first added into the crude sample, to form make complexes with corresponding proteins. Meanwhile, MNPs functionalized with suitable functional groups recognize the ligand-protein complex and will be separated by applying an external magnetic field. Subsequently, separated proteins are eluted from the surface of MNPs after several rounds of magnetic separation and washing.

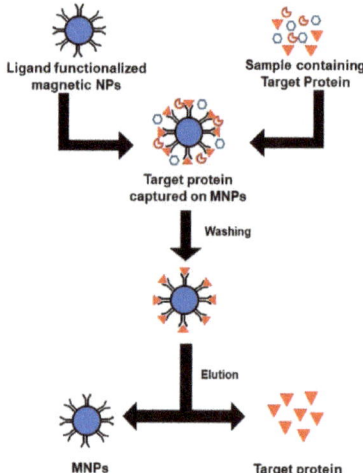

Figure 5. Schematic illustration of magnetic affinity separation of proteins.

The selection and design of the ligand and its binding to MNPs are the most important steps in order to obtain a high yield of purified protein. A good ligand must have high physical and chemical stability, low cost, high specificity for target and high bonding capacity. Several ligands are being used in magnetic affinity separation of proteins such as enzymes, antibodies, DNA and aptamers [79]. Such ligands offer high specificity but are expensive and some have low stability and bonding capacity. As an alternative, pseudo affinity ligands [80] and ion exchange groups [81] having well defined chemical structure have been designed to capture proteins. There are basically three classes of such ligands—amino acids, metal chelates and triazine dyes [82]. These ligands possess relatively low specificity but have higher physical and chemical stability, are easy to elute, have low cost and high bonding capacity. In general, pseudo affinity ligands are preferable over ion exchange groups due to their higher bonding capacity and greater specificity towards targeted proteins. Triazine dyes such as Cibacron Blue F3GA and some metal ions have been widely used as pseudo affinity ligands due to their high selectivity for large number of proteins [83].

Elution methods and buffer conditions used for the separation of proteins from ligand-immobilized MNPs are equally important to obtain high yields. The basic principle of elution is to change the pH or salt concentration of buffer that changes the surface charge of protein, which causes weakening of the interaction between the ligand and the protein. In this way, MNPs are regenerated and ready to be used for the next cycle of protein purification. Two buffers 0.05 mol/L glycine NaOH (pH 11) and 0.05 mol/L citrate (pH 3) have been reported to desorb IgG protein from modified MNPs with elution rates 35% and 64%, respectively [84]. The protein recoveries were satisfactory; however, extreme pH values significantly decreased the bioactivity of protein. Likewise, an increase in salt concentration reduces the electrostatic interaction between protein and ligands. Therefore, buffers containing higher salt concentration are good eluting reagents that can completely desorb proteins. Proteins that could not easily desorb from the surface of ligand-functionalized MNPs due to strong interaction between ligand and protein require specific elution such as affinity elution to displace the adsorbed proteins. A summary of different MNP-based protein purification procedures is provided in Table 2.

Table 2. Protein purification using functionalized MNPs.

Protein	Magnetic Carrier	Ligand	Elution Method	Binding Capacity (mg/g)	Reference
Lipase	Fe_3O_4-PAA	–COOH	Phosphate buffer (pH 9)	605	[85]
Antibody	Fe_3O_4-gum Arabic-Artificial Protein	Artificial Protein A/ artificial Protein L	Citrate buffer (pH 3) and Glycine NaOH buffer (pH 11)	133 65	[84]
Superoxide dismutase	Fe_3O_4-IDA-Cu^{+2}	IDA-Cu^{+2}	Potassium phosphate containing NH_4Cl	n/a	[86]
Bovine haemoglobin	Fe_3O_4-SiO_2-GPS–IDA-Zn^{+2}	IDA-Zn^{+2}	n/a	207.2	[87]
Lactoferrin	Fe_3O_4-PGMA-EA-heparin	Heparin	NaCl Solution	164	[88]
His-Tagged Protein	Fe_3O_4-PMIDA-Ni^{+2}	PMIDA-Ni^{+2}	Sodium phosphate, imidazole and NaCl	n/a	[80]
Bromelain	Fe_3O_4-PAA	–COOH	Phosphate buffer containing NaCl	476	[89]
Lysozyme	Magnetic PHEMA beads-Cibacron Blue-F3GA	Cibacron Blue F3GA	Tris/HCl buffer containing NaCl	342	[90]
	Fe_3O_4-PEG-CMCTs	–COOH	PBS + NaCl	256.6	[91]
	Fe_3O_4-PAA	–COOH	PBS + NaSCN	224	[92]
	Fe_3O_4-SiO_2-GPS-Tris	Tris		108.6	[81]

PAA polyacrylic acid, IDA iminodiacetic acid, PHEMA poly(2-hydroxyethyl methacrylate, PGMA polyglycidyl methacrylate, PMIDA N-phosphonomethyl iminodiacetic acid, CM-CTS carboxymethyl chitosan, PEG polyethylene glycol, GPS 3-glycidoxypropyltrimethoxysilane.

5. Food Analysis Using MNPs

Food analysis, and the need to develop analytical methods for the analysis of food samples, has gained significant attention during the past decades. The presence of chemical contaminants in food poses a major concern affecting the food safety and security for public health. The main application of MNPs in food analysis is for sample pre-concentration and analyte extraction, typically for inorganic and organic contaminants. Other uses have been reported in the development of emerging electroanalytical methods in which MNPs are used as electrode modifier. In most cases, MNPs are stabilized using silane chemistries, which can be further functionalized with specific ligands selected to capture their corresponding analyte. For enhancing specificity and detection capabilities of food contaminants, magnetic extraction methods are coupled with instrumental techniques such as spectrophotometry or chromatography, for example, High Performance Liquid Chromatography (HPLC), Polymerase chain reaction (PCR), immunoassays, Gas Chromatography (GC)/ Liquid Chromatography- mass spectrometry (LC-MS) and so forth, Enzyme immunoassays and aptamer-based assays are commonly used in food analysis to detect different immunogenic (antibody-antigen based) and biochemical reactions. MNPs have been integrated with these techniques to increase the efficiency. Contaminants such as mycotoxins, pesticide residue and food allergens and so forth, have been analyzed by using MNPs integrated immunoassays. Immunomagnetic separation (IMS) using antibody functionalized magnetic particles has been used successfully in a number of studies for affinity capture of targets and subsequent enzyme-linked immunosorbent assay (ELISA) or real-time polymerase chain reaction (PCR) detection. Speroni et al. reported a magnetic particle-based ELISA assay for detection and quantification of a peanut allergen. PAMAM-sodium, carboxylate modified magnetic micro-particles were used as a solid support to immobilize antibodies. Afterwards, these antibody coated magnetic microparticles were suspended in a sample solution to capture and detect the Ara h3/4 peanut allergen in food matrices. The limit of detection (LOD) obtained using this method was 0.2 mg/Kg with good precision and reliability [93]. PCR is generally used for the pathogens detection. The reliability of PCR depends on the purity and amount of target DNA in the sample. In the presence of various inhibitors in the food matrix, rapid enrichment of target DNA is mandatory to yield the full strength of PCR [94]. MNPs are the best pre-concentrator in this regard. Yang et al., used submicron sized superparamagnetic anion exchangers to pre-concentrate bacteria for multiplexed PCR-based detection. By integrating MNPs in PCR, the LOD was lowered from 10^5 CFU/mL to 10^2 CFU/mL using *Agrobacterium tumefaciens* and *Escherichia coli* as model bacteria [95]. Integration of superparamagnetic anion exchangers has also been studied in freshly produced samples and a slight change in LOD (i.e., 10^3 CFU/mL) was observed. Furthermore, integration of MNPs in chromatographic detection techniques such as HPLC, LC-MS and optical methods have been reported for detection and extraction of contaminants for example, mycotoxins and veterinary medicines and so forth. Fe_2O_3 NPs based magnetic molecularly imprinted polymers (MIPs) were used for the extraction of β-lactam antibiotics from milk. Subsequently, the antibiotic was detected by LC-MS with LOD and recovery valued of 1.6–2.8 ng/mL and 71.6–90.7%, respectively [96].

An area of continuous development is the biosensors field which holds promise for fast and easy detection of different compounds. MNPs have been integrated in biosensors to increase sensitivity. Varshney et al., reported a MNPs-antibody based impedimetric biosensor for the detection of *E. coli* demonstrating a 35% increase in sensitivity due to incorporation of MNPs. The developed biosensor was based on interdigitated array microelectrode (IDAM) coupled with magnetic nanoparticle–antibody conjugates (MNAC). MNACs were prepared by immobilizing biotin-labeled polyclonal goat anti-*E. coli* antibodies onto streptavidin-coated magnetic nanoparticles, which were used to separate and concentrate *E. coli* O157:H7. The sensor had a LOD of 7.4×10^4 CFU/mL in pure culture and 8.0×10^5 CFU/mL in ground beef samples, requiring a total assay time of 35 min [97]. The same biosensing design can be applied for the detection of other pathogens by changing the type of immobilized antibodies [98]. Another MNP based biosensor has been developed for the detection of an herbicide 2,4-dichlorophenoxyacetic acid (2,4-D). The biosensor is based on immobilized alkaline phosphatase (ALP)-MNPs and the reaction of ALP with ascorbic acid 2-phosphate (AA2P). Fe_3O_4 nanoparticles and ALP were incorporated into a sol gel/chitosan biosensor membrane which led to an enhancement of the biosensor response. Using the inhibition property of the ALP, the biosensor was applied to the determination of the 2,4-D. The use of MNPs gives a two fold increase in sensitivity (LOD 0.3–0.4 µg/L with 95–100% recoveries) but the method suffered from interferences from heavy metals such as Hg^+ Cu^+ Pb^+ and Ag^+ and so forth. [99]. Similarly, MNPs have been incorporated in glucose biosensors for the detection of glucose in food samples. Kaushik et al. developed a Fe_2O_3 NPs-chitosan composite based glucose biosensor. MNPs were dispersed in chitosan (CH) solution to fabricate a nanocomposite film on an indium–tin oxide (ITO) glass plate. Glucose oxidase (GOx) was immobilized onto this CH–MNPs nanocomposite film via physical adsorption. The incorporation of MNPs increased the stability of the oxidase enzyme and subsequently the shelf life of the biosensor to up to 8 weeks under refrigeration conditions. This biosensor demonstrated a good linear range between 0.1–4 mg/mL, a sensing time of 5 s and a LOD of 9.3×10^{-2} mA/(mg mL cm^2) [100].

5.1. Analysis of Inorganic Species in Food Using MNPs

Metals such as lead, cadmium, mercury, silver and gold and so forth, have been analyzed in food samples using bare and functionalized MNPs. Functionalization normally increases the efficiency and selectivity of MNPs for different analytes. Mirabi and coworkers used sodium dodecyl sulfate (SDS) to functionalize MNPs with diphenylcarbazone enabling extraction of Cd through MDSPE with a LOD of 1 ng L^{-1} [101]. Huang achieved a lower LOD by using γ-mercaptopropyl trimethoxysilane (MPTMS) functionalized MNPs where the -SH group interacted more efficiently with the metal ions [63]. Pirouz et al. functionalized calcium ferrite NPs with (3-Aminopropyl)triethoxysilane (APTES) and phthalic anhydride PA, reporting higher selectivity and stability for these modified particles [102]. To improve performance, ionic liquids (ILs) have been used as an MNPs modifier for enhancing selectivity for extraction of food contaminants such as metal ions (Cd, Pb, Cu), synthetic dyes and pesticides [103,104] and so forth. ILs can be used in two different ways to enhance extraction of metal ions: modification of MNPs with ILs and using the ILs as ferro-fluid carriers.

Mahdinia et al. [105] reported the use of tricaprylmethyl ammoniumchloride thiosalicylate (Aliquat®336, [A336] [TS]) modified Fe$_3$O$_4$ MNPs for the isolation of cadmium from fruits (apple, orange, banana) and water samples by DMSPE with a pre-concentration factor of 50. The thiol groups present in Aliquat®336 increase the selectivity of the functionalized MNPs for Cd. After optimization of all the important parameters of DMSPE, a quantification range of 2.5–260 ng mL^{-1} and a LOD of 0.5 ng mL^{-1} was achieved using atomic absorption spectroscopy as detection method. Soylak et al. developed a method based on the complexation of Cd^{2+} with pyrrolidine dithiocarbamate used as chelate, which was then extracted by adding fine droplets of an ionic liquid (1-butyl-3-methylimidazolium hexafluorophosphate) with subsequent acid elution of Cd^{2+}, quantified using flame atomic absorption spectroscopy, with a LOD of 0.32 ng mL^{-1} and a preconcentration factor of 80. The method was applied to determine the amount of Cd^{2+} in spinach leaves and other fruits and vegetables [106]. Comparing these two methods for Cd analysis, the one reported by Soylak and Yilmaz (2015) showed good sensitivity and reliability based on the LOD and enrichment factors reported by the authors. A similar methodology was adopted for Cu analysis, in which Cu was complexed with diethyldithiocarbamate, followed by extraction of the chelate with ILs mixed with MNPs. Cu ions were then eluted from the surface of MNPs by acid digestion. Several ILs were tested for the extraction of chelates and a maximum recovery (90%) was found with 1-hexyl-3-methylimidazolium tetrafluoroborate [Hmim][BF$_4$] [107]. Table 3 summarizes representative work for the analysis of metals in food using functionalized MNPs.

Table 3. MNPs-based analysis of metals in food samples.

Analyte	Samples	Magnetic Functionalized Material	Detection Technique	Eluent	LOD (ng mL^{-1})	Recovery %	Reference
Hg	Fish	Fe$_3$O$_4$-IIP	ICP-OES	EDTA	0.03	98.4–102.4	[108]
Pb	Water, milk, canned tuna fish, parsley and canned tomato paste	CaFe$_2$O$_4$-SiO$_2$-NH$_2$_PA	FAAS	HNO$_3$	0.78	91.3–100	[102]
Ag	Rice, tuna fish and tea leaves	Fe$_3$O$_4$-SiO$_2$-SH	ICP-OES CV-AAS	Thiourea	0.07	96.2	[109]
Cu					0.09	99.8	
Cd					0.06	98.4	
Pb					0.08	95.4	
Hg					0.01	97.1	
Cd	Green tea. Lettuce, ginseng, rice, spice and carrot	Fe$_3$O$_4$-SDS-carbazone	FAAS	HCL	3.71	NR	[101]
Cd	Milk powder	Fe$_3$O$_4$-SiO$_2$-SH	ICP-MS	HCL	2 × 10^{-5}	97	[63]
Cu					9 × 10^{-5}	96	
Hg					1.1 × 10^{-4}	104	
Pb					6 × 10^{-5}	97	
Pb	Tuna fish, rice and shrimp	Fe$_3$O$_4$-SiO$_2$-3-(4-methoxybenzylideneamino)-2-Thioxothiazolodin-4-0ne	FAAS	MeOH-HNO$_3$	0.14	97.8–102.9	[60]
Cd					0.19	98.7–101.4	
Cu					0.12	98.6–102.6	

5.2. Analysis of Organic Species in Food Using MNPs

MNPs have also been used as a solid support in the extraction and analysis of organic food contaminants, including drugs such as sulphonamides (sulfisoxazole, sulfadoxine, sulfamethizole, sulfamethoxazole and sulfamerazine) in milk and honey samples, β-agonists in meat, different hormones for example, estrogens (estrone, estradiol and diethylstilbestrol) and cytoquinine. Other applications include the extraction of various bioactive compounds such as chlorogenic acid, phenolic acid and gallic acid and so forth. Selective analysis of gallic acid was achieved by Hao et al. who designed a magnetic molecularly imprinted polymer (MIPs) consisting of magnetic carbon nanotubes (CNTs) acting as a carrier and branched polyethylineimine as a functional monomer [110]. Extraction and detection of chlorogenic acid by using MNPs -MIPs was also reported, with a LOD and a linear range of 0.01 µg mL^{-1} and 0.05–100 µg mL^{-1} respectively. For the preparation of the MIP polymer, PEI was used as a functional monomer and NH$_2$ functionalized MNPs as carriers while chlorogenic acid was used as template. Application of this methodology was demonstrated for the analysis of chlorogenic acid in apples, peaches and grape juice [111].

MNPs have also been used to extract synthetic food dyes such as sudan IV, allura red and safranin T. SiO$_2$-MNPs coupled with [Hmim][PF$_6$] as ionic liquid were used for the fluorimetric analysis of safranin T in tomatoes and tomato sauce. Later, the ionic liquid and safranin T were recovered from the surface of magnetic NPs using ultrasound and an organic solvent. The optimized method was characterized by a linear range between 5–300 ng mL^{-1} with a LOD of 0.48 ng mL^{-1} [112]. Piao and Chen reported the extraction of Sudan dyes from chili powder by using magnetic MIPs. These imprinted polymers were composed of silica modified Fe$_3$O$_4$ NPs, methacrylic acid as a functional monomer and ethylene glycol dimethacrylate as cross-linking agent. The LOD reported by using this method was 6.2 ng g^{-1} with a linear range between 25–5000 ng g^{-1} [113]. Moreover, polystyrene covered MNPs were also tested for the extraction and analysis of Sudan food dyes from wine and grape juice and vinegar. In other applications, phathalates and bisphenol-A which are present in packaging of food and beverages were analyzed using functionalized MNPs. CNT functionalized magnetite NPs were used to extract phthalic esters from juices, carbonated beverages and mineral water. The excellent adsorption capability of these magnetic CNTs towards hydrophobic compounds was utilized to capture the organic target. The LOD and linear range obtained by using these MNPs were 0.013 ng ML^{-1} and 0.2–50 ng mL^{-1} respectively [114].

6. Conclusions

Magnetic NPs have found a large number of applications in the development of analytical platforms for food analysis because of their unique physical, magnetic and chemical properties. MNPs are characterized by a large surface area, rich functionalities and magnetic properties enabling their easy separation upon the application of an external magnetic field. This review paper summarized recent efforts dedicated to the synthesis and surface functionalization of MNPs and their application as capture probes and target amplifiers in a variety of analytical assays for the detection of organic and inorganic species. It was shown that the surface of MNPs can be modulated with other materials and linkers to perform a variety of functions. The functionalization of their surface was shown to enhance and improve the analytical features of the MNPs. Moreover, controlled modification is of vital importance to retain the original features of the particles, while imparting other characteristics. This review also summarized applications of MNPs such as support for bimolecular immobilization, protein purification and capture probes. The integration of MNPs in an analytical platform for food safety is widely explored to improve the food technology and this area is expected to continue. However, the potential risk of MNPs to human health and their impact on the environment should also be considered in future research.

Author Contributions: R.K. worked on the Sections 3–5 of the review paper. A.R. worked on the Sections 1 and 2 of the review paper. A.H. wrote abstract and conclusion part of the review paper, along with contribution in the design of review paper and final correction. S.A. planned the theme and idea of the review paper and performed the final correction.

Funding: This work was carried under NSF grant # 1561491 to S.A. R.K. and A.R. are financially supported by the Higher Education Commission (HEC) of Pakistan and the US-Pakistan Knowledge Corridor Program.

Acknowledgments: This work was supported by NSF grant # 1561491 to S.A. R.K. and A.R. gratefully acknowledge the Higher Education Commission (HEC) of Pakistan and the US-Pakistan Knowledge Corridor Program for support of their PhD studies at Clarkson University.

Conflicts of Interest: The authors declare no conflict of interest

References

1. Beveridge, J.S.; Stephens, J.R.; Williams, M.E. The Use of Magnetic Nanoparticles in Analytical Chemistry. *Annu. Rev. Anal. Chem.* **2011**, *4*, 251–273. [CrossRef] [PubMed]
2. Muldoon, L.L.; Sàndor, M.; Pinkston, K.E.; Neuwelt, E.A. Imaging, distribution, and toxicity of superparamagnetic iron oxide magnetic resonance nanoparticles in the rat brain and intracerebral tumor. *Neurosurgery* **2005**, *57*, 785–796. [CrossRef] [PubMed]
3. Puntes, V.F.; Krishnan, K.M.; Alivisatos, A.P. Colloidal nanocrystal shape and size control: The case of cobalt. *Science* **2001**, *291*, 2115–2117. [CrossRef] [PubMed]
4. Akbarzadeh, A.; Samiei, M.; Davaran, S. Magnetic nanoparticles: Preparation, physical properties, and applications in biomedicine. *Nanoscale Res. Lett.* **2012**, *7*, 144. [CrossRef] [PubMed]
5. Denizot, B.; Tanguy, G.; Hindre, F.; Rump, E.; Lejeune, J.; Jallet, P. The preparation of magnetite nanoparicles for biomedical. *J. Colloid Interface Sci.* **1999**, *209*, 10.1006.
6. Wang, W.-W.; Zhu, Y.-J.; Ruan, M.-L. Microwave-assisted synthesis and magnetic property of magnetite and hematite nanoparticles. *J. Nanopart. Res.* **2007**, *9*, 419–426. [CrossRef]
7. Wierucka, M.; Biziuk, M. Application of magnetic nanoparticles for magnetic solid-phase extraction in preparing biological, environmental and food samples. *Trac-Trends Anal. Chem.* **2014**, *59*, 50–58. [CrossRef]
8. Latham, A.H.; Williams, M.E. Controlling transport and chemical functionality of magnetic nanoparticles. *Acc. Chem. Res.* **2008**, *41*, 411–420. [CrossRef]
9. Burda, C.; Chen, X.B.; Narayanan, R.; El-Sayed, M.A. Chemistry and properties of nanocrystals of different shapes. *Chem. Rev.* **2005**, *105*, 1025–1102. [CrossRef]
10. Qiao, R.R.; Yang, C.H.; Gao, M.Y. Superparamagnetic iron oxide nanoparticles: From preparations to in vivo MRI applications. *J. Mater. Chem.* **2009**, *19*, 6274–6293. [CrossRef]
11. Gupta, A.K.; Gupta, M. Synthesis and surface engineering of iron oxide nanoparticles for biomedical applications. *Biomaterials* **2005**, *26*, 3995–4021. [CrossRef] [PubMed]
12. Laurent, S.; Forge, D.; Port, M.; Roch, A.; Robic, C.; Elst, L.V.; Muller, R.N. Magnetic iron oxide nanoparticles: Synthesis, stabilization, vectorization, physicochemical characterizations, and biological applications. *Chem. Rev.* **2008**, *108*, 2064–2110. [CrossRef] [PubMed]
13. Gao, J.H.; Gu, H.W.; Xu, B. Multifunctional Magnetic Nanoparticles: Design, Synthesis, and Biomedical Applications. *Acc. Chem. Res.* **2009**, *42*, 1097–1107. [CrossRef] [PubMed]
14. Baumgartner, J.; Antonietta Carillo, M.; Eckes, K.M.; Werner, P.; Faivre, D. Biomimetic magnetite formation: From biocombinatorial approaches to mineralization effects. *Langmuir* **2014**, *30*, 2129–2136. [CrossRef] [PubMed]
15. Biehl, P.; von der Lühe, M.; Dutz, S.; Schacher, F. Synthesis, characterization, and applications of magnetic nanoparticles featuring polyzwitterionic coatings. *Polymers* **2018**, *10*, 91. [CrossRef]
16. Timko, M.; Molcan, M.; Hashim, A.; Skumiel, A.; Muller, M.; Gojzewski, H.; Jozefczak, A.; Kovac, J.; Rajnak, M.; Makowski, M. Hyperthermic effect in suspension of magnetosomes prepared by various methods. *IEEE Trans. Magn.* **2012**, *49*, 250–254. [CrossRef]
17. Claudio, L.; Mitchell, B. *Nanoparticles from Mechanical Attrition. Synthesis, Functionalization and Surface Treatment of Nanoparticles*, Chapter 1; American Scientific Publishers: Valencia, CA, USA, 2002.
18. LaMer, V.K.; Dinegar, R.H. Theory, production and mechanism of formation of monodispersed hydrosols. *J. Am. Chem. Soc.* **1950**, *72*, 4847–4854. [CrossRef]

19. Khan, K.; Rehman, S.; Rahman, H.U.; Khan, Q. *Synthesis and Application of Magnetic Nanoparticles*; One Central Press (OCP): Atlantic Business Centre: Altrincham, UK, 2014; pp. 135–169.
20. Kudr, J.; Haddad, Y.; Richtera, L.; Heger, Z.; Cernak, M.; Adam, V.; Zitka, O. Magnetic nanoparticles: From design and synthesis to real world applications. *Nanomaterials* **2017**, *7*, 243. [CrossRef]
21. Salazar-Alvarez, G.; Qin, J.; Sepelak, V.; Bergmann, I.; Vasilakaki, M.; Trohidou, K.; Ardisson, J.; Macedo, W.; Mikhaylova, M.; Muhammed, M. Cubic versus spherical magnetic nanoparticles: The role of surface anisotropy. *J. Am. Chem. Soc.* **2008**, *130*, 13234–13239. [CrossRef]
22. Jana, N.R.; Chen, Y.; Peng, X. Size-and shape-controlled magnetic (Cr, Mn, Fe, Co, Ni) oxide nanocrystals via a simple and general approach. *Chem. Mater.* **2004**, *16*, 3931–3935. [CrossRef]
23. Rockenberger, J.; Scher, E.C.; Alivisatos, A.P. A new nonhydrolytic single-precursor approach to surfactant-capped nanocrystals of transition metal oxides. *J. Am. Chem. Soc.* **1999**, *121*, 11595–11596. [CrossRef]
24. Zhang, H.; Ding, J.; Chow, G.; Ran, M.; Yi, J. Engineering magnetic properties of Ni nanoparticles by non-magnetic cores. *Chem. Mater.* **2009**, *21*, 5222–5228. [CrossRef]
25. Sun, S.; Zeng, H.; Robinson, D.B.; Raoux, S.; Rice, P.M.; Wang, S.X.; Li, G. Monodisperse MFe_2O_4 (M = Fe, Co, Mn) nanoparticles. *J. Am. Chem. Soc.* **2004**, *126*, 273–279. [CrossRef] [PubMed]
26. Adschiri, T.; Hakuta, Y.; Sue, K.; Arai, K. Hydrothermal synthesis of metal oxide nanoparticles at supercritical conditions. *J. Nanopart. Res.* **2001**, *3*, 227–235. [CrossRef]
27. Yu, J.; Yu, X. Hydrothermal synthesis and photocatalytic activity of zinc oxide hollow spheres. *Environ. Sci. Technol.* **2008**, *42*, 4902–4907. [CrossRef]
28. Yang, T.; Li, Y.; Zhu, M.; Li, Y.; Huang, J.; Jin, H.; Hu, Y. Room-temperature ferromagnetic Mn-doped ZnO nanocrystal synthesized by hydrothermal method under high magnetic field. *Mater. Sci. Eng. B* **2010**, *170*, 129–132. [CrossRef]
29. Sander, D.; Oka, H.; Corbetta, M.; Stepanyuk, V.; Kirschner, J. New insights into nano-magnetism by spin-polarized scanning tunneling microscopy. *J. Electron Spectrosc. Relat. Phenom.* **2013**, *189*, 206–215. [CrossRef]
30. Wu, W.; He, Q.; Chen, H.; Tang, J.; Nie, L. Sonochemical synthesis, structure and magnetic properties of air-stable Fe3O4/Au nanoparticles. *Nanotechnology* **2007**, *18*, 145609. [CrossRef]
31. Ban, Z.; Barnakov, Y.A.; Li, F.; Golub, V.O.; O'Connor, C.J. The synthesis of core–shell iron@ gold nanoparticles and their characterization. *J. Mater. Chem.* **2005**, *15*, 4660–4662. [CrossRef]
32. Hernández-Hernández, A.A.; Álvarez-Romero, G.A.; Contreras-López, E.; Aguilar-Arteaga, K.; Castañeda-Ovando, A. Food analysis by microextraction methods based on the use of magnetic nanoparticles as supports: Recent advances. *Food Anal. Methods* **2017**, *10*, 2974–2993. [CrossRef]
33. Lu, H.; Yi, G.; Zhao, S.; Chen, D.; Guo, L.-H.; Cheng, J. Synthesis and characterization of multi-functional nanoparticles possessing magnetic, up-conversion fluorescence and bio-affinity properties. *J. Mater. Chem.* **2004**, *14*, 1336–1341. [CrossRef]
34. Yang, H.H.; Zhang, S.Q.; Chen, X.L.; Zhuang, Z.X.; Xu, J.G.; Wang, X.R. Magnetite-containing spherical silica nanoparticles for biocatalysis and bioseparations. *Anal. Chem.* **2005**, *77*, 354. [CrossRef]
35. Nakagawa, T.; Hashimoto, R.; Maruyama, K.; Tanaka, T.; Takeyama, H.; Matsunaga, T. Capture and release of DNA using aminosilane-modified bacterial magnetic particles for automated detection system of single nucleotide polymorphisms. *Biotechnol. Bioeng.* **2006**, *94*, 862–868. [CrossRef] [PubMed]
36. Yoza, B.; Arakaki, A.; Maruyama, K.; Takeyama, H.; Matsunaga, T. Fully automated DNA extraction from blood using magnetic particles modified with a hyperbranched polyamidoamine dendrimer. *J. Biosci. Bioeng.* **2003**, *95*, 21–26. [CrossRef]
37. Nakagawa, T.; Tanaka, T.; Niwa, D.; Osaka, T.; Takeyama, H.; Matsunaga, T. Fabrication of amino silane-coated microchip for DNA extraction from whole blood. *J. Biotechnol.* **2005**, *116*, 105–111. [CrossRef] [PubMed]
38. Anker, J.N.; Kopelman, R. Magnetically modulated optical nanoprobes. *Appl. Phys. Lett.* **2003**, *82*, 1102–1104. [CrossRef]
39. Baker, I. Magnetic nanoparticle synthesis. In *Nanobiomaterials*; Elsevier: Amsterdam, The Netherlands, 2018; pp. 197–229.
40. Berry, C.C.; Curtis, A.S. Functionalisation of magnetic nanoparticles for applications in biomedicine. *J. Phys. D Appl. Phys.* **2003**, *36*, R198.

41. Mateo, C.; Palomo, J.M.; Fernandez-Lorente, G.; Guisan, J.M.; Fernandez-Lafuente, R. Improvement of enzyme activity, stability and selectivity via immobilization techniques. *Enzym. Microb. Technol.* **2007**, *40*, 1451–1463. [CrossRef]
42. Bolivar, J.M.; Wilson, L.; Ferrarotti, S.A.; Fernandez-Lafuente, R.; Guisan, J.M.; Mateo, C. Stabilization of a formate dehydrogenase by covalent immobilization on highly activated glyoxyl-agarose supports. *Biomacromolecules* **2006**, *7*, 669–673. [CrossRef]
43. Li, Y.; Xu, X.; Deng, C.; Yang, P.; Zhang, X. Immobilization of trypsin on superparamagnetic nanoparticles for rapid and effective proteolysis. *J. Proteome Res.* **2007**, *6*, 3849–3855. [CrossRef]
44. Oh, C.; Lee, J.-H.; Lee, Y.-G.; Lee, Y.-H.; Kim, J.-W.; Kang, H.-H.; Oh, S.-G. New approach to the immobilization of glucose oxidase on non-porous silica microspheres functionalized by (3-aminopropyl) trimethoxysilane (APTMS). *Colloids Surf. B Biointerfaces* **2006**, *53*, 225–232. [CrossRef] [PubMed]
45. Palomo, J.M.; Muñoz, G.; Fernández-Lorente, G.; Mateo, C.; Fuentes, M.; Guisan, J.M.; Fernández-Lafuente, R. Modulation of Mucor miehei lipase properties via directed immobilization on different hetero-functional epoxy resins: Hydrolytic resolution of (R, S)-2-butyroyl-2-phenylacetic acid. *J. Mol. Catal. B Enzym.* **2003**, *21*, 201–210. [CrossRef]
46. Kim, J.; Grate, J.W.; Wang, P. Nanostructures for enzyme stabilization. *Chem. Eng. Sci.* **2006**, *61*, 1017–1026. [CrossRef]
47. Liu, X.; Lei, L.; Li, Y.; Zhu, H.; Cui, Y.; Hu, H. Preparation of carriers based on magnetic nanoparticles grafted polymer and immobilization for lipase. *Biochem. Eng. J.* **2011**, *56*, 142–149. [CrossRef]
48. Xie, T.; Wang, A.; Huang, L.; Li, H.; Chen, Z.; Wang, Q.; Yin, X. Recent advance in the support and technology used in enzyme immobilization. *Afr. J. Biotechnol.* **2009**, *8*, 4724–4733.
49. Zhu, H.; Pan, J.; Hu, B.; Yu, H.-L.; Xu, J.-H. Immobilization of glycolate oxidase from Medicago falcata on magnetic nanoparticles for application in biosynthesis of glyoxylic acid. *J. Mol. Catal. B Enzym.* **2009**, *61*, 174–179. [CrossRef]
50. Xu, J.; Sun, J.; Wang, Y.; Sheng, J.; Wang, F.; Sun, M. Application of iron magnetic nanoparticles in protein immobilization. *Molecules* **2014**, *19*, 11465–11486. [CrossRef]
51. López-Gallego, F.; Betancor, L.; Mateo, C.; Hidalgo, A.; Alonso-Morales, N.; Dellamora-Ortiz, G.; Guisán, J.M.; Fernández-Lafuente, R. Enzyme stabilization by glutaraldehyde crosslinking of adsorbed proteins on aminated supports. *J. Biotechnol.* **2005**, *119*, 70–75. [CrossRef]
52. Mateo, C.; Palomo, J.M.; Fuentes, M.; Betancor, L.; Grazu, V.; López-Gallego, F.; Pessela, B.C.; Hidalgo, A.; Fernández-Lorente, G.; Fernández-Lafuente, R. Glyoxyl agarose: A fully inert and hydrophilic support for immobilization and high stabilization of proteins. *Enzym. Microb. Technol.* **2006**, *39*, 274–280. [CrossRef]
53. Chang, M.-Y.; Juang, R.-S. Use of chitosan–clay composite as immobilization support for improved activity and stability of β-glucosidase. *Biochem. Eng. J.* **2007**, *35*, 93–98. [CrossRef]
54. Pan, C.; Hu, B.; Li, W.; Sun, Y.; Ye, H.; Zeng, X. Novel and efficient method for immobilization and stabilization of β-d-galactosidase by covalent attachment onto magnetic Fe_3O_4–chitosan nanoparticles. *J. Mol. Catal. B Enzym.* **2009**, *61*, 208–215. [CrossRef]
55. Huang, S.H.; Liao, M.H.; Chen, D.H. Direct binding and characterization of lipase onto magnetic nanoparticles. *Biotechnol. Prog.* **2003**, *19*, 1095–1100. [CrossRef] [PubMed]
56. Liu, W.; Bai, S.; Sun, Y. Preparation of magnetic nanoparticles and its application to enzyme immobilization. *Chin. J. Process Eng.* **2004**, *4*, 362–366.
57. Lu, A.H.; Salabas, E.e.L.; Schüth, F. Magnetic nanoparticles: Synthesis, protection, functionalization, and application. *Angew. Chem. Int. Ed.* **2007**, *46*, 1222–1244. [CrossRef] [PubMed]
58. Hemmati, M.; Rajabi, M.; Asghari, A. Magnetic nanoparticle based solid-phase extraction of heavy metal ions: A review on recent advances. *Microchim. Acta* **2018**, *185*, 160. [CrossRef] [PubMed]
59. Shegefti, S.; Mehdinia, A.; Shemirani, F. Preconcentration of cobalt (II) using polythionine-coated Fe_3O_4 nanocomposite prior its determination by AAS. *Microchim. Acta* **2016**, *183*, 1963–1970. [CrossRef]
60. Bagheri, H.; Afkhami, A.; Saber-Tehrani, M.; Khoshsafar, H. Preparation and characterization of magnetic nanocomposite of Schiff base/silica/magnetite as a preconcentration phase for the trace determination of heavy metal ions in water, food and biological samples using atomic absorption spectrometry. *Talanta* **2012**, *97*, 87–95. [CrossRef]

61. Chou, P.-H.; Chen, S.-H.; Liao, H.-K.; Lin, P.-C.; Her, G.-R.; Lai, A.C.-Y.; Chen, J.-H.; Lin, C.-C.; Chen, Y.-J. Nanoprobe-based affinity mass spectrometry for selected protein profiling in human plasma. *Anal. Chem.* **2005**, *77*, 5990–5997. [CrossRef]
62. Li, Y.-C.; Lin, Y.-S.; Tsai, P.-J.; Chen, C.-T.; Chen, W.-Y.; Chen, Y.-C. Nitrilotriacetic acid-coated magnetic nanoparticles as affinity probes for enrichment of histidine-tagged proteins and phosphorylated peptides. *Anal. Chem.* **2007**, *79*, 7519–7525. [CrossRef]
63. Huang, C.; Hu, B. Silica-coated magnetic nanoparticles modified with γ-mercaptopropyltrimethoxysilane for fast and selective solid phase extraction of trace amounts of Cd, Cu, Hg, and Pb in environmental and biological samples prior to their determination by inductively coupled plasma mass spectrometry. *Spectrochim. Acta Part B At. Spectrosc.* **2008**, *63*, 437–444.
64. Shishehbore, M.R.; Afkhami, A.; Bagheri, H. Salicylic acid functionalized silica-coated magnetite nanoparticles for solid phase extraction and preconcentration of some heavy metal ions from various real samples. *Chem. Cent. J.* **2011**, *5*, 41. [CrossRef] [PubMed]
65. Huang, C.; Hu, B. Speciation of inorganic tellurium from seawater by ICP-MS following magnetic SPE separation and preconcentration. *J. Sep. Sci.* **2008**, *31*, 760–767. [CrossRef] [PubMed]
66. Huo, S.-H.; Yan, X.-P. Facile magnetization of metal–organic framework MIL-101 for magnetic solid-phase extraction of polycyclic aromatic hydrocarbons in environmental water samples. *Analyst* **2012**, *137*, 3445–3451. [CrossRef] [PubMed]
67. Bianchi, F.; Chiesi, V.; Casoli, F.; Luches, P.; Nasi, L.; Careri, M.; Mangia, A. Magnetic solid-phase extraction based on diphenyl functionalization of Fe3O4 magnetic nanoparticles for the determination of polycyclic aromatic hydrocarbons in urine samples. *J. Chromatogr. A* **2012**, *1231*, 8–15. [CrossRef] [PubMed]
68. Huang, C.; Xie, W.; Li, X.; Zhang, J. Speciation of inorganic arsenic in environmental waters using magnetic solid phase extraction and preconcentration followed by ICP-MS. *Microchim. Acta* **2011**, *173*, 165–172. [CrossRef]
69. Zhang, N.; Peng, H.; Wang, S.; Hu, B. Fast and selective magnetic solid phase extraction of trace Cd, Mn and Pb in environmental and biological samples and their determination by ICP-MS. *Microchim. Acta* **2011**, *175*, 121. [CrossRef]
70. Suleiman, J.S.; Hu, B.; Peng, H.; Huang, C. Separation/preconcentration of trace amounts of Cr, Cu and Pb in environmental samples by magnetic solid-phase extraction with Bismuthiol-II-immobilized magnetic nanoparticles and their determination by ICP-OES. *Talanta* **2009**, *77*, 1579–1583. [CrossRef]
71. Zhang, N.; Peng, H.; Hu, B. Light-induced pH change and its application to solid phase extraction of trace heavy metals by high-magnetization Fe$_3$O$_4$@ SiO$_2$@ TiO$_2$ nanoparticles followed by inductively coupled plasma mass spectrometry detection. *Talanta* **2012**, *94*, 278–283. [CrossRef]
72. Wang, Y.; Tian, T.; Wang, L.; Hu, X. Solid-phase preconcentration of cadmium (II) using amino-functionalized magnetic-core silica-shell nanoparticles, and its determination by hydride generation atomic fluorescence spectrometry. *Microchim. Acta* **2013**, *180*, 235–242. [CrossRef]
73. Ozmen, E.Y.; Sezgin, M.; Yilmaz, A.; Yilmaz, M. Synthesis of β-cyclodextrin and starch based polymers for sorption of azo dyes from aqueous solutions. *Bioresour. Technol.* **2008**, *99*, 526–531. [CrossRef]
74. Ji, Y.; Liu, X.; Guan, M.; Zhao, C.; Huang, H.; Zhang, H.; Wang, C. Preparation of functionalized magnetic nanoparticulate sorbents for rapid extraction of biphenolic pollutants from environmental samples. *J. Sep. Sci.* **2009**, *32*, 2139–2145. [CrossRef] [PubMed]
75. Wang, Y.; Sun, Y.; Wang, Y.; Jiang, C.; Yu, X.; Gao, Y.; Zhang, H.; Song, D. Determination of Sudan dyes in environmental water by magnetic mesoporous microsphere-based solid phase extraction ultra fast liquid chromatography. *Anal. Methods* **2013**, *5*, 1399–1406. [CrossRef]
76. Zhai, Y.; He, Q.; Han, Q. Solid-phase extraction of trace metal ions with magnetic nanoparticles modified with 2, 6-diaminopyridine. *Microchim. Acta* **2012**, *178*, 405–412. [CrossRef]
77. Zhai, Y.; He, Q.; Yang, X.; Han, Q. Solid phase extraction and preconcentration of trace mercury (II) from aqueous solution using magnetic nanoparticles doped with 1, 5-diphenylcarbazide. *Microchim. Acta* **2010**, *169*, 353–360. [CrossRef]
78. Tian, H.; Li, J.; Shen, Q.; Wang, H.; Hao, Z.; Zou, L.; Hu, Q. Using shell-tunable mesoporous Fe$_3$O$_4$@ HMS and magnetic separation to remove DDT from aqueous media. *J. Hazard. Mater.* **2009**, *171*, 459–464. [CrossRef] [PubMed]

79. Fang, X.; Zhang, W.-W. Affinity separation and enrichment methods in proteomic analysis. *J. Proteom.* **2008**, *71*, 284–303. [CrossRef] [PubMed]
80. Sahu, S.K.; Chakrabarty, A.; Bhattacharya, D.; Ghosh, S.K.; Pramanik, P. Single step surface modification of highly stable magnetic nanoparticles for purification of His-tag proteins. *J. Nanopart. Res.* **2011**, *13*, 2475–2484. [CrossRef]
81. Zhang, G.; Cao, Q.; Li, N.; Li, K.; Liu, F. Tris (hydroxymethyl) aminomethane-modified magnetic microspheres for rapid affinity purification of lysozyme. *Talanta* **2011**, *83*, 1515–1520. [CrossRef]
82. Vijayalakshmi, M. Pseudo-biospecific affinity ligand chromatography. In *Molecular Interactions in Bioseparations*; Springer: Berlin, Germany, 1993; pp. 257–275.
83. Hilbrig, F.; Freitag, R. Protein purification by affinity precipitation. *J. Chromatogr. B* **2003**, *790*, 79–90. [CrossRef]
84. Batalha, I.L.; Hussain, A.; Roque, A. Gum Arabic coated magnetic nanoparticles with affinity ligands specific for antibodies. *J. Mol. Recognit.* **2010**, *23*, 462–471. [CrossRef]
85. Huang, S.-H.; Liao, M.-H.; Chen, D.-H. Fast and efficient recovery of lipase by polyacrylic acid-coated magnetic nano-adsorbent with high activity retention. *Sep. Purif. Technol.* **2006**, *51*, 113–117. [CrossRef]
86. Meyer, A.; Hansen, D.B.; Gomes, C.S.; Hobley, T.J.; Thomas, O.R.; Franzreb, M. Demonstration of a strategy for product purification by high-gradient magnetic fishing: Recovery of superoxide dismutase from unconditioned whey. *Biotechnol. Prog.* **2005**, *21*, 244–254. [CrossRef] [PubMed]
87. Ma, Z.-Y.; Liu, X.-Q.; Guan, Y.-P.; Liu, H.-Z. Synthesis of magnetic silica nanospheres with metal ligands and application in affinity separation of proteins. *Colloids Surf. A Physicochem. Eng. Asp.* **2006**, *275*, 87–91. [CrossRef]
88. Chen, L.; Guo, C.; Guan, Y.; Liu, H. Isolation of lactoferrin from acid whey by magnetic affinity separation. *Sep. Purif. Technol.* **2007**, *56*, 168–174. [CrossRef]
89. Chen, D.-H.; Huang, S.-H. Fast separation of bromelain by polyacrylic acid-bound iron oxide magnetic nanoparticles. *Process Biochem.* **2004**, *39*, 2207–2211. [CrossRef]
90. Başar, N.; Uzun, L.; Güner, A.; Denizli, A. Lysozyme purification with dye-affinity beads under magnetic field. *Int. J. Biol. Macromol.* **2007**, *41*, 234–242. [CrossRef] [PubMed]
91. Sun, J.; Su, Y.; Rao, S.; Yang, Y. Separation of lysozyme using superparamagnetic carboxymethyl chitosan nanoparticles. *J. Chromatogr. B* **2011**, *879*, 2194–2200. [CrossRef]
92. Liao, M.-H.; Chen, D.-H. Fast and efficient adsorption/desorption of protein by a novel magnetic nano-adsorbent. *Biotechnol. Lett.* **2002**, *24*, 1913–1917. [CrossRef]
93. Speroni, F.; Elviri, L.; Careri, M.; Mangia, A. Magnetic particles functionalized with PAMAM-dendrimers and antibodies: A new system for an ELISA method able to detect Ara h3/4 peanut allergen in foods. *Anal. Bioanal. Chem.* **2010**, *397*, 3035–3042. [CrossRef]
94. Yang, H.; Qu, L.; Wimbrow, A.N.; Jiang, X.; Sun, Y. Rapid detection of Listeria monocytogenes by nanoparticle-based immunomagnetic separation and real-time PCR. *Int. J. Food Microbiol.* **2007**, *118*, 132–138. [CrossRef]
95. Yang, K.; Jenkins, D.M.; Su, W.W. Rapid concentration of bacteria using submicron magnetic anion exchangers for improving PCR-based multiplex pathogen detection. *J. Microbiol. Methods* **2011**, *86*, 69–77. [CrossRef] [PubMed]
96. Zhang, X.; Chen, L.; Xu, Y.; Wang, H.; Zeng, Q.; Zhao, Q.; Ren, N.; Ding, L. Determination of β-lactam antibiotics in milk based on magnetic molecularly imprinted polymer extraction coupled with liquid chromatography–tandem mass spectrometry. *J. Chromatogr. B* **2010**, *878*, 3421–3426. [CrossRef] [PubMed]
97. Varshney, M.; Li, Y. Interdigitated array microelectrode based impedance biosensor coupled with magnetic nanoparticle–antibody conjugates for detection of Escherichia coli O157: H7 in food samples. *Biosens. Bioelectron.* **2007**, *22*, 2408–2414. [CrossRef] [PubMed]
98. Varshney, M.; Li, Y. Interdigitated array microelectrodes based impedance biosensors for detection of bacterial cells. *Biosens. Bioelectron.* **2009**, *24*, 2951–2960. [CrossRef]
99. Loh, K.-S.; Lee, Y.; Musa, A.; Salmah, A.; Zamri, I. Use of Fe_3O_4 nanoparticles for enhancement of biosensor response to the herbicide 2, 4-dichlorophenoxyacetic acid. *Sensors* **2008**, *8*, 5775–5791. [CrossRef]
100. Kaushik, A.; Khan, R.; Solanki, P.R.; Pandey, P.; Alam, J.; Ahmad, S.; Malhotra, B. Iron oxide nanoparticles–chitosan composite based glucose biosensor. *Biosens. Bioelectron.* **2008**, *24*, 676–683. [CrossRef]

101. Mirabi, A.; Dalirandeh, Z.; Rad, A.S. Preparation of modified magnetic nanoparticles as a sorbent for the preconcentration and determination of cadmium ions in food and environmental water samples prior to flame atomic absorption spectrometry. *J. Magn. Magn. Mater.* **2015**, *381*, 138–144. [CrossRef]
102. Pirouz, M.J.; Beyki, M.H.; Shemirani, F. Anhydride functionalised calcium ferrite nanoparticles: A new selective magnetic material for enrichment of lead ions from water and food samples. *Food Chem.* **2015**, *170*, 131–137. [CrossRef]
103. Yang, M.; Wu, X.; Jia, Y.; Xi, X.; Yang, X.; Lu, R.; Zhang, S.; Gao, H.; Zhou, W. Use of magnetic effervescent tablet-assisted ionic liquid dispersive liquid–liquid microextraction to extract fungicides from environmental waters with the aid of experimental design methodology. *Anal. Chim. Acta* **2016**, *906*, 118–127. [CrossRef]
104. Chen, J.; Zhu, X. Ionic liquid coated magnetic core/shell Fe_3O_4@SiO_2 nanoparticles for the separation/analysis of linuron in food samples. *Spectrochim. Acta Part A Mol. Biomol. Spectrosc.* **2015**, *137*, 456–462. [CrossRef]
105. Mehdinia, A.; Shegefti, S.; Shemirani, F. A novel nanomagnetic task specific ionic liquid as a selective sorbent for the trace determination of cadmium in water and fruit samples. *Talanta* **2015**, *144*, 1266–1272. [CrossRef] [PubMed]
106. Soylak, M.; Yilmaz, E. Determination of cadmium in fruit and vegetables by ionic liquid magnetic microextraction and flame atomic absorption spectrometry. *Anal. Lett.* **2015**, *48*, 464–476. [CrossRef]
107. Farahani, M.D.; Shemirani, F.; Ramandi, N.F.; Gharehbaghi, M. Ionic liquid as a ferrofluid carrier for dispersive solid phase extraction of copper from food samples. *Food Anal. Methods* **2015**, *8*, 1979–1989. [CrossRef]
108. Najafi, E.; Aboufazeli, F.; Zhad, H.R.L.Z.; Sadeghi, O.; Amani, V. A novel magnetic ion imprinted nano-polymer for selective separation and determination of low levels of mercury (II) ions in fish samples. *Food Chem.* **2013**, *141*, 4040–4045. [CrossRef] [PubMed]
109. Mashhadizadeh, M.H.; Amoli-Diva, M.; Shapouri, M.R.; Afruzi, H. Solid phase extraction of trace amounts of silver, cadmium, copper, mercury, and lead in various food samples based on ethylene glycol bis-mercaptoacetate modified 3-(trimethoxysilyl)-1-propanethiol coated Fe_3O_4 nanoparticles. *Food Chem.* **2014**, *151*, 300–305. [CrossRef]
110. Hao, Y.; Gao, R.; Liu, D.; Tang, Y.; Guo, Z. Selective extraction of gallic acid in pomegranate rind using surface imprinting polymers over magnetic carbon nanotubes. *Anal. Bioanal. Chem.* **2015**, *407*, 7681–7690. [CrossRef] [PubMed]
111. Hao, Y.; Gao, R.; Liu, D.; He, G.; Tang, Y.; Guo, Z. Selective extraction and determination of chlorogenic acid in fruit juices using hydrophilic magnetic imprinted nanoparticles. *Food Chem.* **2016**, *200*, 215–222. [CrossRef]
112. Zhang, L.; Wu, H.; Liu, Z.; Gao, N.; Du, L.; Fu, Y. Ionic liquid-magnetic nanoparticle microextraction of safranin T in food samples. *Food Anal. Methods* **2015**, *8*, 541–548. [CrossRef]
113. Piao, C.; Chen, L. Separation of Sudan dyes from chilli powder by magnetic molecularly imprinted polymer. *J. Chromatogr. A* **2012**, *1268*, 185–190. [CrossRef]
114. Luo, Y.-B.; Yu, Q.-W.; Yuan, B.-F.; Feng, Y.-Q. Fast microextraction of phthalate acid esters from beverage, environmental water and perfume samples by magnetic multi-walled carbon nanotubes. *Talanta* **2012**, *90*, 123–131. [CrossRef]

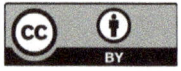

© 2019 by the authors. Licensee MDPI, Basel, Switzerland. This article is an open access article distributed under the terms and conditions of the Creative Commons Attribution (CC BY) license (http://creativecommons.org/licenses/by/4.0/).

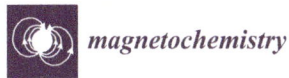

Review

Magnetic Beads in Marine Toxin Detection: A Review

Greta Gaiani [1], Ciara K. O'Sullivan [2,3] and Mònica Campàs [1,*]

[1] Institut de Recerca i Tecnologia Agroalimentàries, Ctra. Poble Nou km 5.5, 43540 Sant Carles de la Ràpita, Spain; greta.gaiani@irta.cat
[2] Deparment d'Enginyeria Química, Universitat Rovira i Virgili, Av. Països Catalans 26, 43007 Tarragona, Spain; ciara.osullivan@urv.cat
[3] Institut de Recerca i Estudis Avançats, Pg. Lluís Companys 23, 08010 Barcelona, Spain
* Correspondence: monica.campas@irta.cat

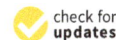

Received: 21 October 2019; Accepted: 9 November 2019; Published: 12 November 2019

Abstract: Due to the expanding occurrence of marine toxins, and their potential impact on human health, there is an increased need for tools for their rapid and efficient detection. We give an overview of the use of magnetic beads (MBs) for the detection of marine toxins in shellfish and fish samples, with an emphasis on their incorporation into electrochemical biosensors. The use of MBs as supports for the immobilization of toxins or antibodies, as signal amplifiers as well as for target pre-concentration, is reviewed. In addition, the exploitation of MBs in Systematic Evolution of Ligands by Exponential enrichment (SELEX) for the selection of aptamers is presented. These MB-based strategies have led to the development of sensitive, simple, reliable and robust analytical systems for the detection of toxins in natural samples, with applicability in seafood safety and human health protection.

Keywords: Magnetic bead; marine toxin; toxin capture; toxin detection; antibody; aptamer; immunoassay; immunosensor; electrochemical biosensor

1. Marine Toxins

Oceans and their resources have sustained nations for millennia, with seafood being a strong part of cultural identity and tradition. Marine toxins accumulate in shellfish, fish and other seafood, and, even if they do not all represent a threat for the hosting organism, they can be hazardous for human health, and have thus drawn attention from food safety agencies, the seafood industry and scientists worldwide [1]. The presence of marine toxins can have socio-economic impacts, including the closure of production and recreational areas, as well as enforcing changes in the diet of entire populations [2]. Diverse toxins cause different intoxications, which are grouped according to their effects: diarrheic shellfish poisoning (DSP), paralytic shellfish poisoning (PSP), amnesic shellfish poisoning (ASP), neurologic shellfish poisoning (NSP), ciguatera fish poisoning (CFP) and pufferfish poisoning [3]. The marine toxins responsible for these intoxications are produced by microalgae, except for pufferfish poisoning, in which the toxin producer is a bacterium [4].

In recent years, the use of traditional toxicity screening tests such as the mouse bioassay (MBA) is increasingly avoided due to their low sensitivity, low specificity and ethical problems. Chromatographic techniques coupled with several detection methods are powerful and accurate analysis tools, and are routinely used as reference methods for many marine toxins. However, the required instrumentation is expensive and requires trained personnel, and to address these shortcomings, the European Commission encourages the development and use of alternative or complementary methods [5], which are usually based on a functional or structural recognition of the toxin [6]. Cell-based assays (CBAs) are easy to perform, give an overall view of the toxicity of a sample and can detect the presence of unknown toxins. However, they show high variability, which hampers their harmonization, and may not be able to discriminate compounds that share the same mechanism of action. Some enzyme inhibition assays have been developed, and these assays are relatively easy to apply, but may suffer from enzyme instability as well as from matrix effects, which may interfere with the response. Receptor-based assays (RBAs) are based on the structural recognition of ligands, but the isolation of receptors from animals is not a trivial task, and, additionally, the affinity may not correlate with the toxicity. Immunoassays, based on the affinity between antibodies and target antigens, show high sensitivity. Whilst the structural recognition may not be necessarily related to the toxicity, antibodies are easier to obtain than receptors, and are also more robust, facilitating an easier implementation of immunoassays, as well as immunosensors, which have the added potential benefit of being miniaturisable and portable [7,8].

2. Magnetic Beads

Magnetic beads (MBs) are particles that consist of magnetite (Fe_3O_4) or maghemite (mostly in the face-centered cubic crystal modification γ-Fe_2O_3) and they have a superparamagnetic or a ferromagnetic behaviour, depending on their size and magnetic content [9]. Superparamagnetism is a particular kind of magnetism that occurs in sufficiently small ferromagnetic or ferrimagnetic particles, which exhibit magnetic properties only when placed in a magnetic field, with no residual magnetism once the magnetic field is removed or switched off. Because of the absence of a remnant magnetization, the previously magnetized superstructure decomposes into single particles. Ferromagnetic magnetism, instead, keeps a magnetic moment even when the magnetic field is removed, not allowing superstructures to decompose.

According to Laurent and co-workers [10], numerous chemical methods can be used to synthesize MBs, such as microemulsions, sonochemical reactions, sol-gel syntheses, hydrothermal reactions, hydrolysis and thermolysis of precursors, electrospray syntheses and flow injection syntheses. All these methods have been used to prepare particles with a regular composition and small size. Nevertheless, the most common method for the production of magnetite and maghemite MBs is still the chemical co-precipitation of iron salts.

MBs of different materials, sizes and functionalizations are now commercially available, enabling their conjugation to a broad range of biomolecules or compounds though different reaction chemistries or affinity interactions [11–13].

3. Magnetic Beads in Marine Toxin Detection

The use of MBs, mainly superparamagnetic, in the development of immunoassays and immunosensors for food analysis and clinical diagnosis is garnering increasing interest [14–16], due to the various advantages that the use of MBs can entail, including an increased surface-to-volume ratio, improved assay kinetics, a higher washing efficiency and lower matrix effects. Herein, we describe the exploitation of MBs in different approaches related with the detection of marine toxins, classifying them according to their use as supports, signal amplifiers, capture agents and, finally, for the production of biorecognition molecules. Table 1 gives an overview of the MB uses and functionalizations taken in consideration for this manuscript.

Table 1. Overview of the magnetic bead (MB) uses and functionalizations for their applicability in the detection of marine toxins.

MB Use	Target	MB Functionalization	Conjugation to	Strategy	LOD	Applicability	Ref.
Support	OA	Streptavidin	Biotinylated OA	Colorimetric immunoassay Electrochemical immunosensor	0.8-1.99 µg/L 0.38-0.99 µg/L	Spiked mussels	[17]
Support	OA	Streptavidin	Biotinylated OA	Electrochemical immunosensor	0.15 µg/L	Spiked mussels	[18]
Support	OA	Carboxylic acid groups	OA-BSA	Fluorescence immunosensor	0.05 µg/L	-	[19]
Support	OA	Streptavidin	Biotinylated OA	Colorimetric immunoassay Fluorescence immunosensor	0.5 µg/L 0.05 µg/L	Spiked mussels	[20]
Support	OA	Protein G	Anti-OA mAb	Colorimetric immunoassay Electrochemical immunosensor	1 µg/L 0.5 µg/L	Spiked mussels	[21]
Support	OA	Ni-iminodiacetic acid	Hys tail of PP2A	Colorimetric enzyme assay	30.1 µg/L	Spiked mussels, wedge clams, flat oysters and Pacific oysters	[22]
Support	AZA	Protein G	Anti-AZA pAb	Colorimetric immunoassay Electrochemical immunoassay Electrochemical immunosensor	1.1 µg/L 1.0 µg/L 3.7 µg/L	Naturally-contaminated mussels	[23]
Support	TTX	Maleimide	TTX	Electrochemical immunosensor	1.2 µg/L	Pufferfish	[4]
Support	TTX	Polyethylene glycol	BSA-TTX	Electrochemical immunoassay	5 µg/L	Pufferfish	[24]
Support	TTX	Thiodiglycolic acid	Anti-TTX aptamer	Fluorescence aptamer assay	0.06 µg/L	Spiked human body fluids	[25]
Support	BTX-2/DTX-1	Epoxy groups	anti-BTX-2 mAb anti-DTX-1 mAb	Electrochemical immunoassay	1.8 ng/L 2.2 ng/L	Spiked mussels, razor clams and cockles	[26]
Support	STX	Avidin	Secondary Ab	Electrochemical immunosensor	1.2 ng/L	Spiked seawater and mussels	[27]
Support	STX	Protein G	Anti-STX pAb	Colorimetric immunoassay	~3 µg/L	-	[28]
Support	STX	Protein-G	Anti-STX pAb	Colorimetric immunoassay	~6 ng/L	Naturally-contaminated mussels	[29]
Support	CTX3C	Epoxy groups	Anti-CTX3C mAbs	Electrochemical immunoassay	0.09 ng/L	Spiked and naturally-contaminated fish	[30]
Signal amplifier	OA	Protein G	Anti-OA mAb	SPR immunosensor	1.2 µg/L	Naturally-contaminated mussels	[31]
Capture agent	PSP toxins	Glutaraldehyde	Anti-PSP mAb	HPLC	-	*Alexandrium tamarense* culture	[32]
Capture agent	STX	Protein G	Anti-STX mAb	LC-MS/MS	0.526 µg/L	Spiked human urine	[33]
Capture agent	OA	Protein G	Anti-OA mAb	LC-MS/MS	0.3 µg/L	Naturally-contaminated oysters, mussels, clams and scallops	[34]

Table 1. *Cont.*

Capture agent				MALDI-TOF			
Production of biorecognition molecules	DA	C8 alkyl groups	-	Antibody phage display	-	Sea lion serum	[35]
Production of biorecognition molecules	CTX3C	Streptavidin	Biotinylated CTX3C fragment	-	-	-	[36]
Production of biorecognition molecules	STX	Epoxy groups	KLH-STX	Aptamer SELEX	-	-	[37]
Production of biorecognition molecules	GTX1/4	Amino groups	Carboxylated GTX1/4	Aptamer SELEX	-	-	[38]
Production of biorecognition molecules	PlTX	Carboxylic acid groups	PlTX	Aptamer SELEX; biolayer interferometry aptasensor	0.04 ng/L	Spiked shellfish and seawater	[39]
Production of biorecognition molecules	DA STX TTX	-	GO	Multiplex aptamer SELEX; fluorescence aptamer assay	0.45 µg/L 1.21 µg/L 0.39 µg/L	-	[40]
Production of biorecognition molecules	OA	Tosyl groups	Anti-OA F(ab')² fragment	Aptamer SELEX	0.33 µg/L	-	[41]

3.1. Magnetic Beads as Supports

The first report of the use MBs as a support for marine toxin detection was in the development of an immunosensor for okadaic acid (OA) [17] (Figure 1A). OA is a lipophilic marine toxin produced by microalgae of the genera *Dinophysis* and *Prorocentrum*. This toxin is accumulated in shellfish and, since its mode of action is related to the inhibition of protein phosphatases (PPs), it can cause DSP in humans. OA was conjugated to biotin and then captured on streptavidin-coated MBs. Once OA was immobilized on the MBs, a colorimetric indirect competitive enzyme-linked immunosorbent assay (ELISA) was performed, where OA in solution competed for interaction with an anti-OA monoclonal antibody (mAb). The authors tested two different sizes of MBs, achieving limits of detection (LODs) of 0.8 µg/L with 2.8 µm-diameter MBs and 1.99 µg/L with 1 µm-diameter MBs. The functionalized MBs were then exploited in an electrochemical immunosensor, where they were magnetically immobilized on screen-printed electrodes (SPEs), and, again, a competitive assay performed. Differential pulse voltammetry (DPV) was used to measure the oxidation of 1-naphthol resulting from the dephosphorylation of 1-naphthyl phosphate by the alkaline phosphatase (ALP) enzyme label, and slightly lower LODs were obtained, with the larger MBs again performing better (0.38 µg/L vs. 0.99 µg/L). It should be noted that whilst larger MBs imply a higher surface area, the amount of MBs used was 10-fold lower and the whole available surface area was lower when using the larger MBs. This immunosensor was then easily integrated into an automated flow-through system [18], one of the advantages of using MBs, achieving an improved LOD of 0.15 µg/L.

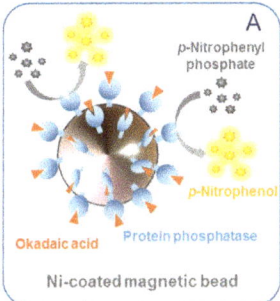
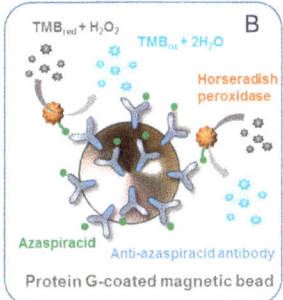
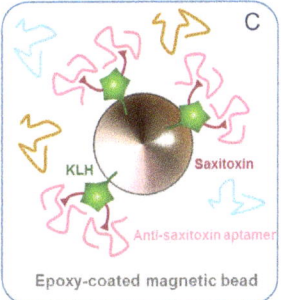

Figure 1. Examples of uses and functionalizations of MBs: (**A**) MBs as supports for enzymes, (**B**) MBs as supports for antibodies, and (**C**) MBs for the production of aptamers.

Moving towards the development of portable devices for field analysis, Pan and collaborators [19,20] described fluorescence immunosensors for the detection of OA. In the first work [19], carboxylic acid-modified MBs were used as a support for the immobilization of OA–bovine serum albumin (OA–BSA), which competed with OA in the sample to bind with an anti-OA mAb. The fluorescence of CdTe quantum dots (QDs) linked to the reporter antibody was detected using a portable flow cytometer (Moxi-Flow), facilitating on-site OA detection and quantification of OA, and achieving an LOD of 0.05 µg/L [19]. In the second work [20], the authors modified the system, using streptavidin-coated MBs with biotinylated OA and a secondary antibody labelled with R-phycoerythrin (R-PE) dye, again achieving an LOD of 0.05 µg/L.

Hayat and co-workers [21] also exploited MBs in a direct immunoassay/immunosensor format for the detection of OA. Instead of conjugating the toxin to the MBs, the anti-OA mAb was immobilized on protein G-coated MBs. OA labelled with horseradish peroxidase (HRP) was used as a tracer in the colorimetric assay, whilst, for the electrochemical immunosensor, no label was used. DPV measurements in a 1 mM $[Fe(CN)_6]^{3-/4-}$ solution showed that the interaction between the toxin and the antibody decreases the current peak of the ferri/ferrocyanide redox probe. Using this detection strategy, they obtained an LOD of 0.5 µg/L, lower than that obtained with the colorimetric immunoassay (1 µg/L).

An interesting and different approach for the detection of OA is presented in the work of Garibo et al. [22]. In this work, the PP inhibition was measured to detect and quantify the toxin. The authors used genetically engineered PPs with extra-His tails to conjugate the enzymes to Ni-modified MBs. The colorimetric assay attained an LOD of 30.1 µg/L. Although this LOD was more than an order of magnitude higher than that achieved with free enzymes, the immobilization of the PP on the MBs provided higher enzyme activity stability, a crucial parameter, especially when working with these enzymes.

Azaspiracids (AZAs) are lipophilic marine toxins produced by microalgae of the genera *Azadinium* and *Amphiodioma*. Those toxins accumulate in shellfish, and the ingestion of contaminated seafood can lead to azaspiracid shellfish poisoning (AZP), first reported in 1995 [42]. Leonardo and co-workers [23] developed an MBs-based direct immunoassay for AZA detection (Figure 1B). Protein G-coated MBs were functionalized with anti-AZA polyclonal antibody (pAb), and free AZA competed with HRP-labelled AZA (HRP–AZA) for binding to the immobilized antibody in suspension, achieving LODs of 1.1 and 1.0 µg/L, using 3,3′, 5,5′-tetramethylbezidine (TMB) as an enzyme mediator and optical and electrochemical detection, respectively. Additionally, the assay was completed in just 15 min, due to the faster kinetics provided by the use of MBs in suspension. When the biorecognition was performed, immobilizing the Ab-MBs magnetically on the electrode surface, the LOD increased to 3.7 µg/L, which could be attributable to mass transfer limitations. Furthermore, naturally-contaminated mussels were analyzed, and results were similar to the ones obtained with liquid chromatography coupled to tandem mass spectrometry (LC–MS/MS), demonstrating the applicability of the system for monitoring purposes.

Tetrodotoxin (TTX) is a potent natural neurotoxin produced by bacteria that live in endosymbiosis with some other organisms such as pufferfish. Consumption of this contaminated animal may cause intoxication and even death, and the rapid and reliable detection of TTX in pufferfish is thus of enormous importance. Recently, an electrochemical MB-based immunosensor has been developed for the detection of TTX [4]. Oriented and stable TTX immobilization was achieved through the formation of a cysteine monolayer on maleimide-activated MBs, for the subsequent covalent biding of TTX. A competitive assay was again pursued, with TTX in solution competing with the immobilized TTX for binding to an anti-TTX mAb and using an HRP-labelled secondary antibody as a reporter antibody. The immunocomplexes were magnetically captured on an 8-electrode array, and using amperometric detection, an LOD of 1.2 µg/L was achieved. The authors applied the biosensor to the detection of TTX in muscle, skin and the internal organs of two juvenile pufferfishes (*Lagocephalus sceleratus*) from Greece, achieving a good degree of correlation with LC–MS/MS. It had previously been observed that the liver tissue matrix had a marked effect on assay performance, and this effect was almost completely eliminated due to the use of MBs as a support. This work thus demonstrates the advantages that MBs provide in terms of reduction of matrix effects. An alternative electrochemical immunoassay for TTX was described by Zhang and co-workers [24], who synthesized MBs and coated them with polyethylene glycol for subsequent reaction with BSA–TTX. After competition between immobilized TTX and free TTX for a primary anti-TTX antibody, and incubation with an enzyme-labelled secondary antibody, the enzyme product was electrochemically measured. The modification of the working electrode with ionic liquids and carbon nanotubes significantly avoided electrode surface fouling by the enzyme product and improved the sensitivity as compared to bare electrodes, achieving an LOD of 5 µg/L.

Aptamers have also been used for the detection of TTX, as described by Jin and co-workers [25], who conjugated an NH_2-terminated anti-TTX aptamer to thiodiglycolic acid-stabilized Fe_3O_4 MBs. Carxboxylated carbon dots (CDs) were then added, forming Fe_3O_4/aptamer/CDs nanocomposites. When excited at 780 nM, those nanocomposites were observed to have a decreased up-conversion fluorescence emission at 475 nm, attributed to the photo-induced electron transfer (PET) from the CDs to the aptamer. The addition of TTX caused the unwinding of CDs from the aptamer and subsequent recovery of the up-conversion fluorescence. The system attained an LOD of 0.06 µg/L, and showed high selectivity when tested against other toxins (aflatoxin B_1 and B_2, botulin neurotoxin A and B and *Staphylococcus aureus* enterotoxin A and B), biomolecules (histidine, cysteine, uric acid, ascorbic acid, glucose, glutathione and thiohydracrylic acid) and anions (Cl^-, PO_4^{3-} and CO_3^{2-}) that could interfere in the analysis of human body fluids. The good recoveries obtained in the analysis of spiked gastric juice, serum and urine samples demonstrated the applicability of this aptamer-based optical assay.

Brevetoxin B (BTX-2) is a neurotoxin produced by microalgae such as *Ptychodiscus brevis* and *Gymnodinium breve*. This toxin accumulates in shellfish and, when ingested, can result in death. Additionally, aerosol exposure to BTX-2 during microalgae blooms can cause respiratory irritation [43]. This particular toxin together with dinophysistoxin-1 (DTX-1), an OA analog also responsible for DSP and produced by some *Prorocentrum* and *Dinophysis* species, were selected as targets for the development of a flow-through electrochemical immunoassay [26]. Anti-BTX-2 and anti-DTX-1 mAbs were co-immobilized on MBs. Tracers were synthesized by conjugation of the toxins with cadmium and copper nanoclusters. The incubation of the functionalized MBs with both toxins and their tracers, and the subsequent dissolution of the metal labels and injection into the detection cell, allowed the selective detection of the two toxins using square wave anodic stripping voltammetry, with no cross-reactivity observed. The system showed high cross reactivity with BTX-1, BTX-3, DTX-2 and DTX-3, as expected, and no false positive results from OA, pectenotoxin-6 (PTX-6) or yessotoxin (YTX). LODs of 1.8 ng/L and 2.2 ng/L were achieved for BTX-2 and DTX-1, respectively.

The PSP toxin group comprises saxitoxin (STX) and related compounds produced by marine dinoflagellates of *Alexandrium*, *Gymnodinium*, and *Pyrodinum* species. PSP toxins can accumulate in bivalves, crabs, lobsters and even carnivorous snails [44]. The ingestion of contaminated vectors causes neurotoxic illness that can result in paralysis and, at its acute expression, death. With this target in mind, Jin and co-workers [27] developed a magnetic electrochemical immunosensor for the detection of STX in seawater and seafood. The immunosensor used anti-STX antibody-functionalized MBs and palladium-doped graphitic carbon nitride nanoparticles (peroxidase mimetic) to generate the electrochemical signal. Unlike the other approaches described so far, the assay was non-competitive, because they took advantage of the electrostatic interaction between the electro-positive STX and the electro-negative palladium nanoparticles. The immunosensor successfully detected trace STX amounts in seawater and shellfish samples with an LOD of 1.2 ng/L. Moving towards compact analytical devices, Kim and Choi [28] proposed a lab-on-a-chip (LOC) system for the immunodetection of STX. The LOC system was composed of a sample chamber and a detection chamber connected via a channel. MBs functionalized with anti-STX antibodies were added to the sample chamber together with STX-HRP and the sample containing STX. After incubation, a magnet was used to transport the MBs from the sample chamber to the detection chamber, which had been previously filled with enzyme substrate. The LOD was around 3 µg/L, far below the regulatory level of PSP toxins (800 µg STX per kg shellfish). In 2017, Yu and Choi [29] improved the system by adding an extra washing chamber between the two existing ones, resulting in a decrease in the LOD to around 6 ng/L.

CFP is a human intoxication caused by the ingestion of contaminated fish and is a worldwide health problem. This disease is characterized by severe neurological, gastrointestinal and cardiovascular disorders. Causative toxins of CFP are produced by marine dinoflagellates of the genera *Gambierdiscus* and *Fukuyoa* and are known as ciguatoxins (CTXs). An electrochemical immunoassay for the detection of CTX3C was developed by Zhang et al. [30], where sample injection, incubation, capillary electrophoresis separation and electrochemical detection were all performed in a capillary system. An anti-CTX3C antibody was immobilized on MBs and injected into the capillary system, followed by the addition of CTX3C standard/contaminated samples. A rotating magnetic field was applied to increase mixing efficiency and molecular binding rates. An anti-CTX3C antibody linked to HRP-functionalized gold nanoparticles was then added and sandwich immunocomplexes were formed. Finally, the enzyme product was electrochemically detected, and the system achieved a very low LOD (0.09 ng/L), almost 17,000 times lower than that obtained with high performance liquid chromatography coupled to mass spectrometry (HPLC–MS). The authors claim that the enhanced sensitivity can be attributed to the use of gold nanoparticles as multi-enzyme carriers, resulting in a high HRP/Ab molar ratio.

3.2. Magnetic Beads as Signal Amplifiers

One of the functionalities of MBs is their ability to amplify signals, as exemplified in the work of Garibo et al. [31], who described the development of a competitive surface plasmon resonance (SPR) optical immunosensor for OA. Protein G-coated MBs were used to immobilize anti-OA antibodies, whilst OA was immobilized on the sensor chip surface. The antibodies were added to the sensor together with a free OA standard/sample, and any binding of molecules to the immobilized OA generated a response proportional to the bound mass. SPR analysis demonstrated that, with conjugates, it is possible to attain similar responses to free antibodies, but using an 8-fold lower antibody concentration. The Ab–MBs resulted in a 3-fold lower LOD, even in the presence of mussel matrix (from 4.7 µg/L to 1.2 µg/L), demonstrating the ability of MBs to be used as signal amplifiers.

3.3. Magnetic Beads as Capture Agents

Immunomagnetic capture (IMC) represents an innovative technique for toxin extraction and purification from complex environmental or biological matrices and is much simpler and more rapid than the use of chromatographic columns. The first example of IMC with marine toxins was reported by Devlin and co-workers [32], who covalently immobilized an antibody to MBs using glutaraldehyde crosslinking for the immunoaffinity extraction of PSP toxins from cultures of the dinoflagellate *Alexandrium tamarense*. After steel ball bearing beating for cell lysis, HPLC measurements showed that toxin recovery increased with increasing amounts of MBs (up to 96.2%), and that the process could be completed within an hour. Recently, Bragg and collaborators [33] coupled IMC with LC–MS/MS for the extraction and detection of STX from human urine. The method showed advantages over conventional protocols, such as an improved selectivity (reducing matrix interference), a 5-fold increase in sensitivity, and requirement of only one third of the sample volume.

IMC combined with LC–MS/MS has also been used by Chen and collaborators [34], in this case for the extraction of OA from shellfish samples. MBs were able to capture the toxin in just 10 min, due to their use of suspension. Additionally, shellfish matrix effects were minimized, and recovery values between 82.2% and 95.5% were obtained for the analysis of oysters, mussels and scallops.

MBs have also been used as capture agents in the work of Neely et al. [35]. In their study, the researchers reported the exposure of C8-coated MBs to blood serum samples from California sea lions to identify patterns of domoic acid (DA) toxicosis. DA can cause ASP and can affect not only humans but also common predators that live in and around marine habitats. Detection of DA was achieved using matrix-assisted laser desorption ionization time-of-flight (MALDI-TOF) mass spectrometry. Artificial neuronal networks (ANN) were trained using MALDI-TOF data from serum analysis, and the obtained models were good predictors of acute DAT. The strategy resulted in a highly sensitive (100% negative predictive value) and a highly specific (100% positive predictive value) diagnostic tool.

3.4. Magnetic Beads to Produce Biorecognition Molecules

Marine toxins are not always easy to find and isolate from field samples. The limited availability of marine toxins has hindered the development of biorecognition molecules and, consequently, of systems for their detection. To address this problem, specifically for CTXs, the use of synthetic toxin fragments has been exploited in the production of antibodies [36]. In this work, streptavidin-coated MBs were used for the panning of phages. In the experiment, a biotinylated synthetic ABC-ring fragment of CTX3C (ABC-PEG-biotin) was incubated with a phage library, and then captured on the streptavidin-coated MBs together with the positive phages expressing hapten-binding antibodies. To select antibodies to the left side of CTX3C, elution was performed with a synthetic CTX3C fragment, instead of the scarce

CTX3C. Following three rounds of selection and amplification, the authors observed an increased recovery of eluted phages, as well as the enrichment of phages bearing Fab fragments. The gene fragments from the sorted phage were sub-cloned for the production of three soluble recombinant Fabs, which had dissociation constants (K_d) of about 10^{-5} M.

MBs have also been used for the production of aptamers, oligonucleotides able to bind to specific target molecules with high affinity and specificity and used as biorecognition molecules in bioanalysis. The in vitro process to obtain aptamers is termed systematic evolution of ligands by exponential enrichment (SELEX), and MBs are frequently used as a support and for the effective partitioning of bound and unbound DNA because they improve the binding kinetics and the washing steps. The first example was described by Handy and co-workers [37], who conjugated STX to keyhole limpet hemocyanin (KLH) using 2,2′-(ethylenedioxy)bis(ethylamine) (Jeffamine) as a spacer compound, for its subsequent covalent binding to epoxy-coated MBs (Figure 1C). The modified MBs were incubated with a random ssDNA library. Bound and unbound DNA were magnetically separated, and the bound ssDNA was eluted from the MBs, PCR-amplified and finally used to enrich the ssDNA library for the following round of selection. After 10 rounds, the PCR product was cloned and sequenced. Preliminary results using SPR showed the affinity of the selected aptamer for STX. A sensor chip modified with DA was used to evaluate the specificity of the aptamer towards this marine toxin, which often co-occurs with STX. Binding was not observed, further supporting that the selected aptamer was specific to STX. Gao and co-workers [38] used a SELEX with MBs to produce aptamers for gonyautoxins 1/4 (GTX1/4). They immobilized the GTX1/4-carboxylated derivative on amine-modified MBs via the EDC/NHS chemistry. In round 2, negative MBs were introduced to remove the ssDNA that bound non-specifically to improve the screening efficiency. In round 3, free competitive counter-molecules were added in the positive incubation system to improve the specificity of screening. After eight rounds of selection, appropriate sequences were obtained. However, these sequences were not further investigated. The same research group developed an aptamer for the detection of palytoxin (PlTX), a toxin initially isolated from soft corals and later found in shellfish, sea urchins and crabs, usually associated with *Ostreopsis* blooms [39]. Counter SELEX was performed against potential interferents, including OA, microcystin-LR (MC-LR), STX, and brevetoxin-A/B, resulting in a highly selective aptamer. The selected aptamer was used to develop an optical biosensor based on biolayer interferometry, where PlTX was immobilized on the biosensor surface, and competed with free PlTX for binding to HRP-labelled aptamer. The addition of 3,3′-diaminobenzidine substrate solution resulted in the formation of a precipitated polymeric product directly on the biosensor surface. Changes in the optical thickness and mass density of biosensor layer were measured, resulting in an LOD of 0.04 ng/L.

Gu and collaborators [40] developed a magnetic separation-based multiple SELEX to simultaneously select aptamers against three different marine biotoxins: DA, STX and TTX. The first 12 rounds entailed mixed screening against the three toxins, and the subsequent four rounds of single screening were against each individual toxin. Additionally to the multiplexing strategy, the authors provided the novelty of combining the advantages of MBs and graphene oxide (GO) for efficient partitioning. A fluorescence assay was developed to determine the affinity of the aptamers, showing K_d values of of 62, 44 and 61 nM for DA, TTX and STX, respectively. Additionally, two multi-target aptamers, which can bind with either DA or TTX, were also obtained.

Finally, an aptamer specific to the antigen binding site of a mAb against OA has been produced using MB–SELEX [41]. The aptamer produced following this strategy mimics the OA structure. In this approach, F(ab′)$_2$ fragments (obtained by pepsin digestion of the anti-OA mAb) were conjugated to MBs and subsequently incubated with the ssDNA library. Negative selection with bare MBs and six additional mAbs (against STX, BTX-2, TTX, DA, nodularin (NOD) and MC-LR) was applied to remove non-specifically bound ssDNA. The produced aptamer was used in two different immunoassays. In the first one, biotinylated aptamer competed with free OA for binding to immobilized anti-OA mAb, followed by the addition of streptavidin-HRP, with the aptamer thus acting as a tracer. In the second assay, immobilized OA competed with the aptamer for binding to anti-OA mAb, which was subsequently detected using a secondary antibody.

4. Conclusions and Perspectives

Marine toxins play a crucial role in shellfish poisoning, and reliable, rapid and cost effective detection of very low concentrations of these toxins is critical. Currently, MBs have been used in the field of marine toxin detection as supports in assays and biosensors, capture agents for toxin pre-concentration and as tools to produce biorecognition molecules such as phages and aptamers. Because of their advantages in terms of increased surface-to-volume ratio, improved assay kinetics, increased washing efficiency and reduced matrix effects, efficient and highly sensitive analytical systems for the detection of marine toxins have been developed.

The use of MB-based strategies in marine environments can facilitate the confirmation of toxin presence in shellfish at the occurrence of harmful algal blooms (HABs), and speed up monitoring programs. However, to provide biotechnological tools for seafood safety and human health protection, it will be necessary to validate these MB-based approaches. Validation studies will include analyses of multiple samples, of different natures and from different geographic locations, some of them with multi-toxin profiles, and maybe with emerging toxins as challenging targets.

Author Contributions: M.C. conception; G.G. and M.C. literature search and collection; G.G., C.K.O. and M.C. design, writing and critical reviewing.

Funding: The authors acknowledge support from the Ministerio de Ciencia, Innovación y Universidades through the CIGUASENSING (BIO2017-87946-C2-2-R) project and from CERCA Programme/Generalitat de Catalunya. G. Gaiani acknowledges IRTA-Universitat Rovira i Virgili for her PhD grant (2018PMF-PIPF-19).

Conflicts of Interest: The authors declare no conflict of interest.

References

1. Zhao, L.; Huang, Y.; Dong, Y.; Han, X.; Wang, S.; Liang, X. Aptamers and Aptasensors for Highly Specific Recognition and Sensitive Detection of Marine Biotoxins: Recent Advances and Perspectives. *Toxins* **2018**, *10*, 427. [CrossRef] [PubMed]
2. Rongo, T.; van Woesik, R. Socioeconomic consequences of ciguatera poisoning in Rarotonga, southern Cook Islands. *Harmful Algae* **2012**, *20*, 92–100. [CrossRef]
3. Campàs, M.; Garibo, D.; Prieto-Simón, B. Novel nanobiotechnological concepts in electrochemical biosensors for the analysis of toxins. *Analyst* **2012**, *137*, 1055–1067. [CrossRef] [PubMed]
4. Leonardo, S.; Kiparissis, S.; Rambla-Alegre, M.; Almarza, S.; Roque, A.; Andree, K.B.; Christidis, A.; Flores, C.; Caixach, J.; Campbell, K. Detection of tetrodotoxins in juvenile pufferfish Lagocephalus sceleratus (Gmelin, 1789) from the North Aegean Sea (Greece) by an electrochemical magnetic bead-based immunosensing tool. *Food Chem.* **2019**, *290*, 255–262. [CrossRef] [PubMed]
5. European Comission. Regulation (EU) No 15/2011 of 10 January 2011 amending Regulation (EC) No 2074/2005 as regards recognised testing methods for detecting marine biotoxins in live bivalve molluscs. *Off. J. Eur. Union* **2011**, *6*, 3–6.
6. Reverté, L.; Soliño, L.; Carnicer, O.; Diogène, J.; Campàs, M. Alternative methods for the detection of emerging marine toxins: Biosensors, biochemical assays and cell-based assays. *Mar. Drugs* **2014**, *12*, 5719–5763. [CrossRef] [PubMed]
7. Reverté, L.; Prieto-Simón, B.; Campàs, M. New advances in electrochemical biosensors for the detection of toxins: Nanomaterials, magnetic beads and microfluidics systems. A review. *Anal. Chim. Acta* **2016**, *908*, 8–21. [CrossRef] [PubMed]
8. Leonardo, S.; Toldrà, A.; Campàs, M. Trends and prospects on electrochemical biosensors for the detection of marine toxins. In *Recent Advances in the Analysis of Marine Toxins, Comprehensive Analytical Chemistry*, 1st ed.; Diogène, J., Campàs, M., Eds.; Elsevier: Amsterdam, The Netherlands, 2017; Volume 78, pp. 303–341. [CrossRef]
9. Ruffert, C. Magnetic bead—Magic bullet. *Micromachines* **2016**, *7*, 21. [CrossRef] [PubMed]

10. Laurent, S.; Forge, D.; Port, M.; Roch, A.; Robic, C.; Vander Elst, L.; Muller, R.N. Magnetic iron oxide nanoparticles: Synthesis, stabilization, vectorization, physicochemical characterizations, and biological applications. *Chem. Rev.* **2008**, *108*, 2064–2110. [CrossRef] [PubMed]
11. Wu, W.; Wu, Z.; Yu, T.; Jiang, C.; Kim, W.-S. Recent progress on magnetic iron oxide nanoparticles: Synthesis, surface functional strategies and biomedical applications. *Sci. Technol. Adv. Mater.* **2015**, *16*, 023501. [CrossRef] [PubMed]
12. Chen, Z.; Wu, C.; Zhang, Z.; Wu, W.; Wang, X.; Yu, Z. Synthesis, functionalization, and nanomedical applications of functional magnetic nanoparticles. *Chin. Chem. Lett.* **2018**, *29*, 1601–1608. [CrossRef]
13. Duan, M.; Shapter, J.G.; Qi, W.; Yang, S.; Gao, G. Recent progress in magnetic nanoparticles: Synthesis, properties, and applications. *Nanotechnology* **2018**, *29*, 452001. [CrossRef] [PubMed]
14. Cardoso, V.F.; Francesko, A.; Ribeiro, C.; Bañobre-López, M.; Martins, P.; Lanceros-Mendez, S. Advances in magnetic nanoparticles for biomedical applications. *Adv. Healthc. Mater.* **2018**, *7*, 1700845. [CrossRef] [PubMed]
15. Xianyu, Y.; Wang, Q.; Chen, Y. Magnetic particles-enabled biosensors for point-of-care testing. *TrAC Trends Anal. Chem.* **2018**, *106*, 213–224. [CrossRef]
16. Pastucha, M.; Farka, Z.; Lacina, K.; Mikušová, Z.; Skládal, P. Magnetic nanoparticles for smart electrochemical immunoassays: A review on recent developments. *Microchim. Acta* **2019**, *186*, 312. [CrossRef] [PubMed]
17. Hayat, A.; Barthelmebs, L.; Marty, J.-L. Enzyme-linked immunosensor based on super paramagnetic nanobeads for easy and rapid detection of okadaic acid. *Anal. Chim. Acta* **2011**, *690*, 248–252. [CrossRef] [PubMed]
18. Dominguez, R.B.; Hayat, A.; Sassolas, A.; Alonso, G.A.; Munoz, R.; Marty, J.-L. Automated flow-through amperometric immunosensor for highly sensitive and on-line detection of okadaic acid in mussel sample. *Talanta* **2012**, *99*, 232–237. [CrossRef] [PubMed]
19. Pan, Y.; Zhou, J.; Su, K.; Hu, N.; Wang, P. A novel quantum dot fluorescence immunosensor based on magnetic beads and portable flow cytometry for detection of okadaic acid. *Procedia Technol.* **2017**, *27*, 214–216. [CrossRef]
20. Pan, Y.; Wei, X.; Liang, T.; Zhou, J.; Wan, H.; Hu, N.; Wang, P. A magnetic beads-based portable flow cytometry immunosensor for in-situ detection of marine biotoxin. *Biomed. Microdevices* **2018**, *20*, 60. [CrossRef] [PubMed]
21. Hayat, A.; Barthelmebs, L.; Sassolas, A.; Marty, J.-L. Development of a novel label-free amperometric immunosensor for the detection of okadaic acid. *Analytica Chim. Acta* **2012**, *724*, 92–97. [CrossRef] [PubMed]
22. Garibo, D.; Devic, E.; Marty, J.-L.; Diogène, J.; Unzueta, I.; Blázquez, M.; Campàs, M. Conjugation of genetically engineered protein phosphatases to magnetic particles for okadaic acid detection. *J. Biotechnol.* **2012**, *157*, 89–95. [CrossRef] [PubMed]
23. Leonardo, S.; Rambla-Alegre, M.; Samdal, I.A.; Miles, C.O.; Kilcoyne, J.; Diogène, J.; O'Sullivan, C.K.; Campàs, M. Immunorecognition magnetic supports for the development of an electrochemical immunoassay for azaspiracid detection in mussels. *Biosens. Bioelectron.* **2017**, *92*, 200–206. [CrossRef] [PubMed]
24. Zhang, Y.; Fan, Y.; Wu, J.; Wang, X.; Liu, Y. An Amperometric Immunosensor based on an ionic liquid and single-walled carbon nanotube composite electrode for detection of Tetrodotoxin in pufferfish. *J. Agric. Food Chem.* **2016**, *64*, 6888–6894. [CrossRef] [PubMed]
25. Jin, H.; Gui, R.; Sun, J.; Wang, Y. Facilely self-assembled magnetic nanoparticles/aptamer/carbon dots nanocomposites for highly sensitive up-conversion fluorescence turn-on detection of tetrodotoxin. *Talanta* **2018**, *176*, 277–283. [CrossRef] [PubMed]
26. Zhang, B.; Hou, L.; Tang, D.; Liu, B.; Li, J.; Chen, G. Simultaneous multiplexed stripping voltammetric monitoring of marine toxins in seafood based on distinguishable metal nanocluster-labeled molecular tags. *J. Agric. Food Chem.* **2012**, *60*, 8974–8982. [CrossRef] [PubMed]
27. Jin, X.; Chen, J.; Zeng, X.; Xu, L.; Wu, Y.; Fu, F. A signal-on magnetic electrochemical immunosensor for ultra-sensitive detection of saxitoxin using palladium-doped graphitic carbon nitride-based non-competitive strategy. *Biosens. Bioelectron.* **2019**, *128*, 45–51. [CrossRef] [PubMed]
28. Kim, M.-H.; Choi, S.-J. Immunoassay of paralytic shellfish toxins by moving magnetic particles in a stationary liquid-phase lab-on-a-chip. *Biosens. Bioelectron.* **2015**, *66*, 136–140. [CrossRef] [PubMed]
29. Yu, E.; Choi, S.-J. Development of an improved stationary liquid-phase lab-on-a-chip for the field monitoring of paralytic shellfish toxins. *BioChip J.* **2017**, *11*, 30–38. [CrossRef]

30. Zhang, Z.; Zhang, C.; Luan, W.; Li, X.; Liu, Y.; Luo, X. Ultrasensitive and accelerated detection of ciguatoxin by capillary electrophoresis via on-line sandwich immunoassay with rotating magnetic field and nanoparticles signal enhancement. *Anal. Chim. Acta* **2015**, *888*, 27–35. [CrossRef] [PubMed]
31. Garibo, D.; Campbell, K.; Casanova, A.; De La Iglesia, P.; Fernández-Tejedor, M.; Diogène, J.; Elliott, C.; Campàs, M. SPR immunosensor for the detection of okadaic acid in mussels using magnetic particles as antibody carriers. *Sensors and Actuators B Chem.* **2014**, *190*, 822–828. [CrossRef]
32. Devlin, R.; Campbell, K.; Kawatsu, K.; Elliott, C. Physical and immunoaffinity extraction of paralytic shellfish poisoning toxins from cultures of the dinoflagellate Alexandrium tamarense. *Harmful Algae* **2011**, *10*, 542–548. [CrossRef]
33. Bragg, W.A.; Garrett, A.; Hamelin, E.I.; Coleman, R.M.; Campbell, K.; Elliott, C.T.; Johnson, R.C. Quantitation of saxitoxin in human urine using immunocapture extraction and LC–MS. *Bioanalysis* **2018**, *10*, 229–239. [CrossRef] [PubMed]
34. Chen, J.; Tan, Z.; Wu, H.; Peng, J.; Zhai, Y.; Guo, M. Selective enrichment and quantification of okadaic acid in shellfish using an immunomagnetic-bead-based liquid chromatography with tandem mass spectrometry assay. *J. Sep. Sci.* **2019**, *42*, 1423–1431. [CrossRef] [PubMed]
35. Neely, B.A.; Soper, J.L.; Greig, D.J.; Carlin, K.P.; Favre, E.G.; Gulland, F.M.; Almeida, J.S.; Janech, M.G. Serum profiling by MALDI-TOF mass spectrometry as a diagnostic tool for domoic acid toxicosis in California sea lions. *Proteome Sci.* **2012**, *10*, 18. [CrossRef] [PubMed]
36. Nagumo, Y.; Oguri, H.; Tsumoto, K.; Shindo, Y.; Hirama, M.; Tsumuraya, T.; Fujii, I.; Tomioka, Y.; Mizugaki, M.; Kumagai, I. Phage-display selection of antibodies to the left end of CTX3C using synthetic fragments. *J. Immunol. Methods* **2004**, *289*, 137–146. [CrossRef] [PubMed]
37. Handy, S.M.; Yakes, B.J.; DeGrasse, J.A.; Campbell, K.; Elliott, C.T.; Kanyuck, K.M.; DeGrasse, S.L. First report of the use of a saxitoxin–protein conjugate to develop a DNA aptamer to a small molecule toxin. *Toxicon* **2013**, *61*, 30–37. [CrossRef] [PubMed]
38. Gao, S.; Hu, B.; Zheng, X.; Cao, Y.; Liu, D.; Sun, M.; Jiao, B.; Wang, L. Gonyautoxin 1/4 aptamers with high-affinity and high-specificity: From efficient selection to aptasensor application. *Biosens. Bioelectron.* **2016**, *79*, 938–944. [CrossRef] [PubMed]
39. Gao, S.; Zheng, X.; Hu, B.; Sun, M.; Wu, J.; Jiao, B.; Wang, L. Enzyme-linked, aptamer-based, competitive biolayer interferometry biosensor for palytoxin. *Biosens. Bioelectron.* **2017**, *89*, 952–958. [CrossRef] [PubMed]
40. Gu, H.; Duan, N.; Xia, Y.; Hun, X.; Wang, H.; Wang, Z. Magnetic Separation-Based Multiple SELEX for Effectively Selecting Aptamers against Saxitoxin, Domoic Acid, and Tetrodotoxin. *J. Agric. Food Chem.* **2018**, *66*, 9801–9809. [CrossRef] [PubMed]
41. Lin, C.; Liu, Z.-S.; Wang, D.-X.; Li, L.; Hu, P.; Gong, S.; Li, Y.-S.; Cui, C.; Wu, Z.-C.; Gao, Y. Generation of internal-image functional aptamers of okadaic acid via magnetic-bead SELEX. *Mar. Drugs* **2015**, *13*, 7433–7445. [CrossRef] [PubMed]
42. McMahon, T.; Silke, J. Winter toxicity of unknown aetiology in mussels. *Harmful Algae News* **1996**, *14*, 2.
43. Mello, D.F.; De Oliveira, E.S.; Vieira, R.C.; Simoes, E.; Trevisan, R.; Dafre, A.L.; Barracco, M.A. Cellular and transcriptional responses of Crassostrea gigas hemocytes exposed in vitro to brevetoxin (PbTx-2). *Mar. Drugs* **2012**, *10*, 583–597. [CrossRef] [PubMed]
44. Deeds, J.; Landsberg, J.; Etheridge, S.; Pitcher, G.; Longan, S. Non-traditional vectors for paralytic shellfish poisoning. *Mar. Drugs* **2008**, *6*, 308–348. [CrossRef] [PubMed]

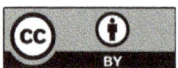

© 2019 by the authors. Licensee MDPI, Basel, Switzerland. This article is an open access article distributed under the terms and conditions of the Creative Commons Attribution (CC BY) license (http://creativecommons.org/licenses/by/4.0/).

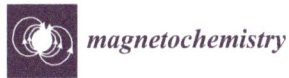

Review

Magnetic Janus Particles for Static and Dynamic (Bio)Sensing

Susana Campuzano, Maria Gamella, Verónica Serafín, María Pedrero, Paloma Yáñez-Sedeño and José Manuel Pingarrón *

Departamento de Química Analítica, Facultad de CC. Químicas, Universidad Complutense de Madrid, E-28040 Madrid, Spain
* Correspondence: pingarro@quim.ucm.es; Tel.: +34-913944315

Received: 29 July 2019; Accepted: 19 August 2019; Published: 22 August 2019

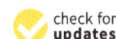

Abstract: Magnetic Janus particles bring together the ability of Janus particles to perform two different functions at the same time in a single particle with magnetic properties enabling their remote manipulation, which allows headed movement and orientation. This article reviews the preparation procedures and applications in the (bio)sensing field of static and self-propelled magnetic Janus particles. The main progress in the fabrication procedures and the applicability of these particles are critically discussed, also giving some clues on challenges to be dealt with and future prospects. The promising characteristics of magnetic Janus particles in the (bio)sensing field, providing increased kinetics and sensitivity and decreased times of analysis derived from the use of external magnetic fields in their manipulation, allows foreseeing their great and exciting potential in the medical and environmental remediation fields.

Keywords: magnetic Janus particles; (bio)sensing; static; self-propelled

1. Introduction

In 1989, Casagrande et al. [1] described the preparation of spherical particles from commercial glass spheres with diameters in the 50–90 μm range bearing half-hydrophilic half-hydrophobic surfaces. These particles were coined as "Janus beads" after the Roman God Janus depicted with twin faces, one looking to the future and the other to the past [2]. Unlike conventional particles, two-faced Janus particles provide asymmetry and directionality and can combine different or even incompatible properties within a single particle [3,4]. The surface anisotropy of these particles spatially decouples analytical functions (e.g., targeting and sensing) and allows spatial-selective bioconjugation that would otherwise be difficult to combine within the uniform composition or heterogeneous nanoparticles. Therefore, Janus nanoparticles have properties and functions, such as dual-targeting [5] and molecular sensing, which are incompatible when combined in a single structural unit or in heterogeneous "not Janus" nanoparticles, thus, opening opportunities for the construction of truly multifunctional entities [6,7]. Moreover, the asymmetry of the Janus particles surface (ratio of surface area devoted to different surface types on the two sides of the particle) can be varied at will depending on the particular applications without altering, interfering or losing the intrinsic properties of both faces, which makes them a unique category of materials in contrast to other particles. Since their development, these particles and their synthetic methods have evolved rapidly as they have been adapted to different applications and profited of the important advances in micro- and nano-manipulation systems and fabrication procedures. This evolution may include the introduction of a magnetic component (i.e., iron, nickel, Fe-Ti, CoNi) that allows driving them by means of a magnetic field towards different places in the human body where therapeutic drugs are released (i.e., drug delivery), to trap undesired entities (i.e., microorganisms), to be used for magnetic resonance imaging, separation of biological molecules or (bio)chemical sensing [8] or to perform many other applications as magnetically triggered devices in the biomedical area [9]. This displacement based on the magnetic field is useful for in vivo biomedical applications because these nano-systems can be precisely controlled by magnetic forces while their speed remains constant regardless of the medium through which they move. Moreover, these biocompatible, non-toxic particles are capable of travelling along the human body without harming cells and tissues. Therefore, a variety of magnetic micro- and nano-systems have already been reported in the literature for several biomedical applications with no adverse interactions with human tissues no matter the biological fluid conditions [10].

The great importance, applicability and future prospects that these devices promise have been already reviewed in articles focused on self-propelled affinity biosensors [11], biosensing with different magnetic particle labels, including Janus particles [12], Janus particles for biological imaging and sensing [7], or for biosensing [4], magnetically driven micro- and nano-robots [10], micro-/nano-robots for biomedicine [13], nano-/micro-systems for delivery and (bio)sensing at the cellular level [8], targeting and isolation of cancer cells [14], or the use of micromotors for biosensing applications [15]. Considering that the application of magnetic Janus particles in the (bio)sensing field is gaining importance rapidly, this review article is focused to the recent developments and applications of these particles both as static and dynamic (bio)sensing systems. Outstanding developments, current trends, challenges and prospects in this exciting field are highlighted and discussed.

2. Synthesis of Magnetic Janus Particles

The methods for the synthesis of magnetic Janus particles are diverse and difficult to classify [16]. A variety of synthetic strategies has been reported in the literature which, at least in part, can be classified as belonging to one of the following categories: (a) Masking or template; (b) direct deposition; (c) phase separation; and (d) self-assembly. An optional preparation method also includes bubble-templated assembly [17]. In the masking approach, the particles, trapped at the interface between two phases, are modified only on one side. Similarly, the template methods involve the use of sacrificial material to cover a part of the particle, while the other is modified [18]. In a direct deposition, the functionalizing material is driven only to the desired area of the particle. Fabrication methods based on phase separation require the use of two immiscible precursors and the existence of an interface. Microfluidics or emulsification with two immiscible fluids, where a liquid-liquid interface is formed, are alternatives explored for the preparation of anisotropic magnetic particles [19–22]. Regarding solid-liquid interfaces, the solid particle is usually employed as a nucleation site for the condensation of the liquid. Self-assembly methods are based on the spontaneous assembling of particles which act as building blocks for simple structures by entropy minimization [23]. Assembling may be directed by application of magnetic or electric fields and depends largely on the properties of the surrounding solution. In this section, some recent methods reported for the synthesis of magnetic Janus particles noted for their relevance and the practical utility of the resulting materials are reviewed.

Fe_3O_4 amphiphilic Janus nanoparticles (Fe_3O_4@AJNPs) bearing β-cyclodextrin (β-CD) and aminopyridine (APD) functionalized polymethyl methacrylate (PGMA) were prepared to construct pH-stimuli responsive co-assemblies through host-guest interactions between β-CD and APD [24]. As it is shown in Figure 1, hydrophilic superparamagnetic Fe_3O_4 nanoparticles (NPs) were used to obtain Fe_3O_4 wax microspheres employing Pickering emulsion by stirring in paraffin wax and dispersion in dimethylformamide (DMF). A further condensation reaction occurred between the particles and polyethylene glycol (PEG) to yield PEG-Fe_3O_4/wax composite microspheres which were washed with chloroform to dissolve the wax. PEG-Fe_3O_4-Br NPs were obtained by reaction with bromoacetic acid, and the ARGET ATRP technique (activators regenerated by the electron transfer for atom transfer radical polymerization) [25] was applied to graft polymethyl methacrylate-methacrylate (PMMA-MA) brushes onto the opposite hemisphere of PEG-Fe_3O_4-Br NPs, thus, obtaining the amphiphilic Janus PEG-Fe_3O_4-PMMA-MA. Finally, hydroxypropyl-β-CD reacted with PEG-Fe_3O_4-PMMA-MA through the condensation among the carboxyl groups in PMMA-MA and the hydroxyls in CD to obtain the functionalized amphiphilic Janus PEG-Fe$_3$O$_4$-PMMA-MA (CD), which were also named as Fe$_3$O$_4$@AJNPs.

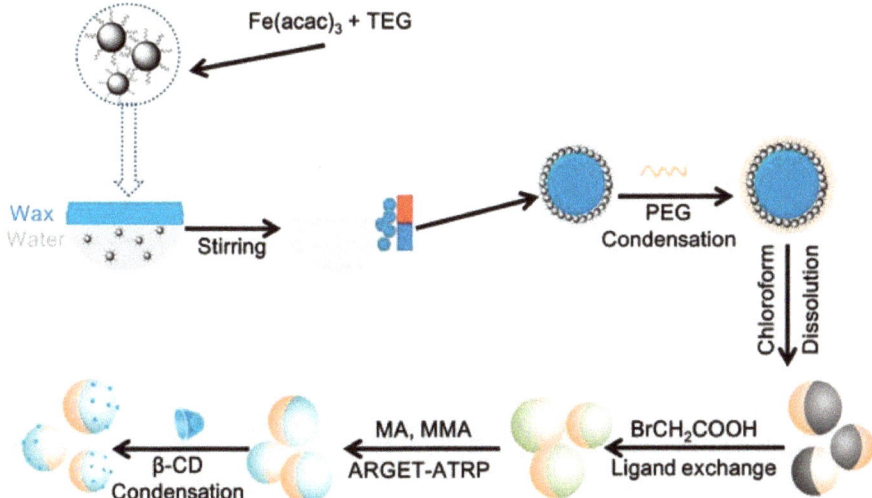

Figure 1. Schematic display of the method for the synthesis of Fe$_3$O$_4$@AJNPs. Reproduced from Reference [24] with permission.

Pickering emulsion was employed recently by Shaghaghi et al. [26] for the preparation of various types of Janus superparamagnetic iron oxide nanoparticles (SPIONs) decorated with folic acid (FA) and doxorubicin (DOX) with the aim of accumulating target cancerous cells through the FA ligands and deliver chemotherapy drugs. SPIONs were firstly masked and immobilized in paraffin wax particles for the subsequent synthesis of drug-conjugated Janus NPs (Figure 2). The waxed magnetic cores were half-coated by (3-mercaptopropyl) triethoxysilane (MPTES), and then dewaxed in solvents for a further anchoring of azide-3-aminopropyl-triethoxysilane (N$_3$-APTES) on the free side of the particle. Then, mono(acryloyl)-star-poly-(ethylene glycol) (Acl-sPEG) was conjugated to the core via thiolene click reaction in the presence of azobisisobutyronitrile (AIBN). Thereafter, N-hydroxysuccinimide (NHS)-ester of folic acid was grafted to sPEG to obtain SPION-sPEG-FA. The preparation of DOX-PCL-SPION (PCL = poly(ε-caprolactone)) involved grafting of DOX-PCL-yne to the particle via azid-yne click reaction in the presence of N,N,N′,N″,N″-pentamethyl diethylene-triamine (PMDETA).

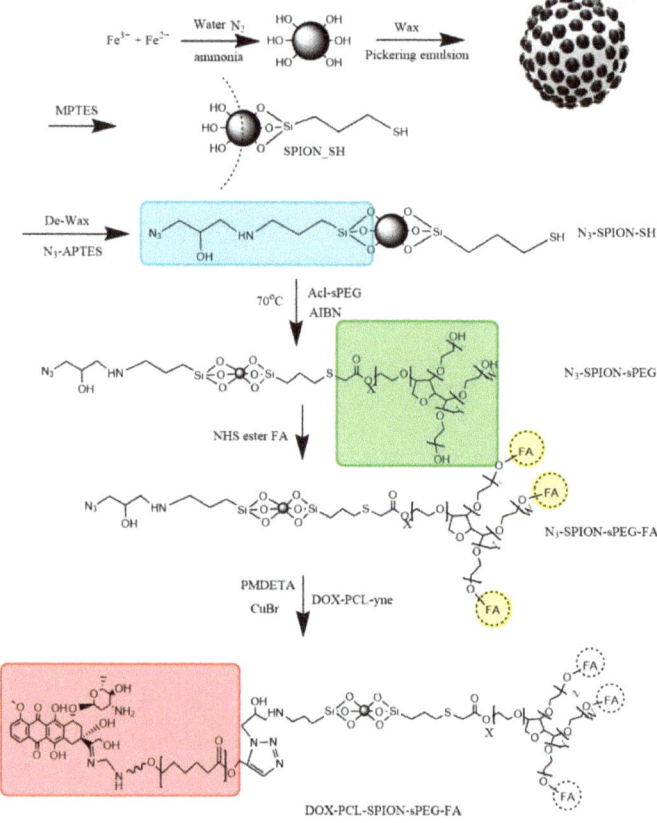

Figure 2. Scheme of the steps involved in the synthesis of drug-conjugated Janus nanoparticles (NPs). Reprinted from Reference [26] with permission.

Fe_3O_4-metal Janus nanoparticles have been used for a variety of interesting applications. An illustrative example is the recent synthesis of Fe_3O_4-Ag nanocomposites through a two-step solvothermal method. Once Fe_3O_4 particles were prepared, they were added to an $AgNO_3$ solution in acetic acid/acetate ethanolic mixture under ultrasonic dispersion followed by heating in an autoclave [27]. The prepared material exhibited not only magnetic properties, but also surface-enhanced Raman scattering (SERS) effect and was used as a substrate to detect adsorbed molecules on surfaces. Another interesting work implies the synthesis of Janus bifunctional composite Au-Fe_3O_4 NPs by means of a microwave heating. Two types of amphiphilic Janus Au-Fe_3O_4 NPs were prepared by coating with bi-compartment polymer brushes exhibiting opposite amphiphilic properties on Au and Fe_3O_4 surfaces by the ligand exchange method. Specifically, Au@PEGFe_3O_4@polystyrene (PS) Janus NPs, with PEG coating on the Au surface, and PS coating on the Fe_3O_4 surface were obtained by adding a mixture of thiolated polyethylene glycol (PEG-SH) and phosphonated polystyrene (PS-P) to the Au-Fe_3O_4 NPs. In addition, Au@PSFe_3O_4@PEG Janus NPs, with PS grafting on Au and PEG on Fe_3O_4, were prepared by adding a PEG-P and PS-SH mixture to Janus NPs. Double-layered plasmonic-magnetic vesicles were prepared from the synthesized NPs (Figure 3). Moreover, the amphiphilic distribution of the polymer grafts on the Janus Au-Fe_3O_4 surface, allows easily reversing the positions of the Au and Fe_3O_4 in the vesicular shell by changing the amphiphilic properties of the polymer brushes coated on their surface, with Au extended mostly to the outside and Fe_3O_4 localized inside the shell, or conversely. The resultant vesicles exhibited greatly enhanced optical and magnetic properties taking advantage from both the interparticle plasmonic coupling of the Au NPs and the magnetic interaction of the Fe_3O_4 localized in the doubled vesicular shell [28].

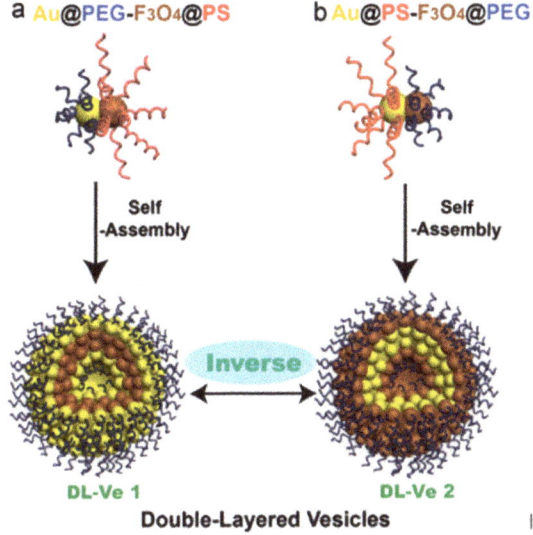

Figure 3. Schematic illustration of the Janus Au-Fe_3O_4 NPs grafted with hydrophilic polyethylene glycol (PEG) on Au and hydrophobic PS on Fe_3O_4 (a), and with PS on Au and PEG on Fe_3O_4 (b), and the hierarchical self-assembly of the resulting Janus amphiphilic nanoparticles into double-layered plasmonic-magnetic vesicles in aqueous media. Reprinted from Reference [28] with permission.

Taking advantage of the selective affinities of ferrite and metals to bind different ligands, an asymmetric functionalization method was reported by Jishkariani et al. [29] to prepare Janus heterodimers from Fe_3O_4-Pt and Fe_3O_4-Au nanoparticles. Dendritic phosphonic acid and disulfide groups were used to coat the iron oxide and Pt, respectively, or Au parts of the heterodimer to prepare amphiphilic structures (Figure 4). The synthesis involved 2,2-bis(hydroxymethyl)propionic acid (bis-MPA)-type disulfide dendrons 2, 4 and 6 with polar end-groups and a second-generation, stearate terminated, phosphonic acid bearing dendron 7 as the non-polar counterpart. Janus particles were prepared through sequential ligand exchange of the Fe_3O_4-Pt (or Fe_3O_4-Au) heterodimers.

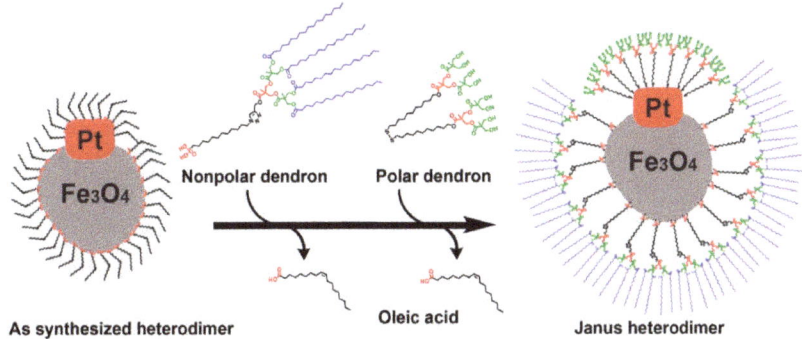

Figure 4. Schematic representation of the two-step ligand exchange process using dendritic ligands 7 and 6. Reprinted from Reference [29] with permission.

With the smart materials' development, self-propelled motors have drawn great attention in biomedical science or environmental remediation fields [30]. Among the different synthetic strategies, the introduction of magnetic materials results in an efficient method to make controllable motors to perform tasks in targeted areas [31]. With this objective, recent efforts have focused on metal-oxide based materials. Peng et al. [32] reported an easy method for the fabrication of hollow three-dimensional graphene oxide (GO)/MnFe$_2$O$_4$ motors by coupling shear force with capillarity. Figure 5 shows that the addition of aniline to aqueous suspensions of GO mixed with MnFe$_2$O$_4$ provoked a strong interaction which induced the effective aggregation of GO sheets giving rise to the subsequent turbulent flow structure under strong electric stirring. As a result, GO sheets spontaneously precipitated and gradually self-assembled into small 3D ball-shaped GO/MnFe$_2$O$_4$ hydrogels with embedded MnFe$_2$O$_4$ particles. The surface was coated with a thin GO layer by dipping it again into aqueous GO. Then, a capillary force arising from the evaporation process was used to pull the GO sheets together and reassembled the aerogel into a 3D bowl-shaped macrostructure (GO/MnFe$_2$O$_4$ motor) with a great ability to adsorb heavy metal ions, this favoured by the abundant oxygen-containing groups on the GO surface.

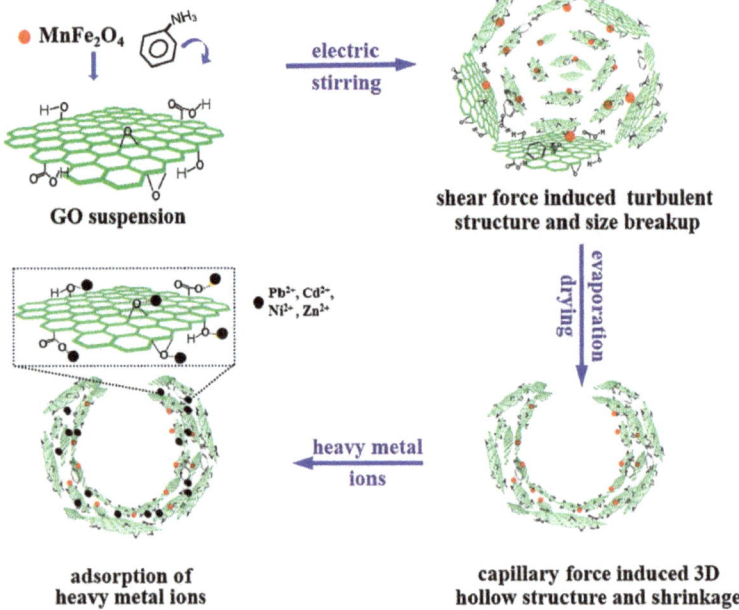

Figure 5. Scheme illustrating the self-assembly synthesis of a GO/MnFe$_2$O$_4$ motor for the removal of heavy metal ions by shearing force driven breakup combined with capillary force induced shrinkage. Reproduced from Reference [32] with permission.

Magnetically steerable self-propelled Janus micromotors with ability to selectively remove radioactive Cs from contaminated water were synthesized from mesoporous silica microspheres functionalized with copper ferrocyanide and coating half of the surface with ferromagnetic Ni and catalytic Pt layers (Figure 6). Mesoporous silica was firstly functionalized with ethylenediamine (S-EDA), followed by preparation of Cu(II) coordination complexes (S-EDA-Cu) and reaction with sodium ferrocyanide (FC) to obtain S-CuFC particles. Thereafter, a poly(vinylpyrrolidone) (PVP)-coated glass slide was placed in a humidity-controlled chamber, where the humidity was raised until PVP became adhesive, so that when the synthesized S-CuFC particles were dispersed across the PVP layer, half of them were fixed inside the film and only the top surfaces of the particles were coated sequentially with a Ni layer and a Pt layer. The prepared S-CuFC/Ni/Pt Janus micromotors were released from the

PVP-coated glass slide by sonication in ethanol [33]. It is important to note that the adsorption of Cs by the self-propelling micromotor adsorbents and their subsequent magnetic recovery provided the selective removing of more than 98% of the radioactive 137Cs ions from aqueous solutions.

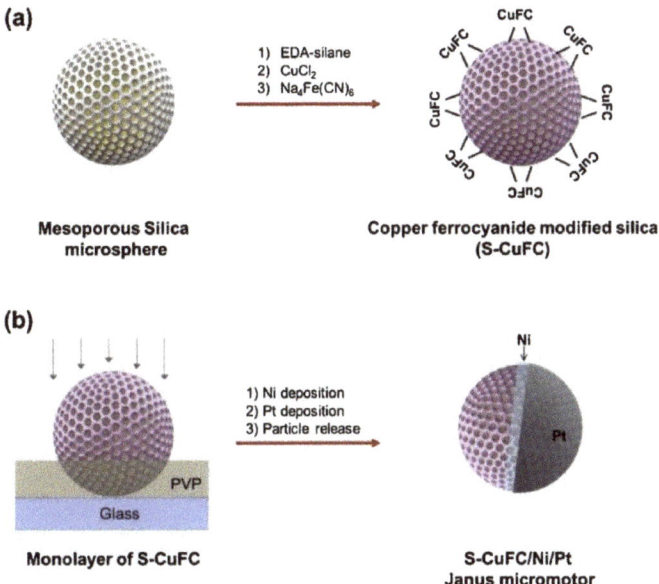

Figure 6. Scheme of the S-CuFC microspheres synthesis (**a**), and the sequential deposition of ferromagnetic Ni and catalytic Pt on half of the S-CuFC surface (**b**) for the fabrication of S-CuFC/Ni/Pt Janus micromotors. Reproduced from Reference [33] with permission.

3. Magnetic Janus Particles for (Bio)Sensing

Magnetic Janus particles combine anisotropy with magnetic properties, thus, delivering the ability to perform challenging tasks that would be impossible with isotropic particles. For example, a Janus particle may have the dual ability to stabilize an interface and to perform a catalytic reaction on some part of its surface [34]. This unique combination makes magnetic Janus particles interesting tools for a wide range of applications in different fields, such as catalysis [35], theranostic [36], drug delivery [37], biomedical imaging [7], biological probing, self-propelled carrier and remote manipulation of devices [7,38]. In addition, magnetic Janus particles can be used as surfactants, water-repellent coatings, or building blocks for supramolecular structures [38]. This section focuses on the implementation of Janus nanoparticles with a magnetic component for applications in static biosensing, but also including some examples of bioimaging, drug delivery and theranostic applications that involve a previous biosensing (target) step, as well as their use as biosensing self-propelled nanomachines. It is worth remarking here that even rare-earth-based Janus microparticles with magnetic and fluorescent functions have been reported and mostly used for drug delivery and bioapplications [39,40].

3.1. Static Janus Magnetic Particles for (Bio)Sensing

The anisotropy in shape, composition, and surface chemistry of Janus nanoparticles allows their users to perform complementary functions, achieving an outcome not possible with conventional nanoparticles in the field of biosensing. Lu et al. reported an article showing the advantages of a magnetic bifunctional particle for glucose sensing using Janus particles with peroxidase-like activity for colorimetric detection of glucose in one step. The particles were more stable over a wider range of pH than the enzyme horseradish peroxidase (HRP) and, because of their magnetic nature, they allow easy sample separation/concentration, and can be reused by simple isolation through magnetic separation [41]. Taking advantage of this methodology, magnetic tailored microparticles with Janus structure, generated by using a centrifugal microfluidic chip, were exploited in a multi-assay format for the simultaneous sensing of glucose and cholesterol [42]. A competitive binding assay using fluorescein isothiocyanate-dextran as a competing ligand was employed for sensing glucose, and microparticles embedded with γ-Fe_2O_3 nanoparticles were used as a catalyst for the oxidation of tetramethylbenzidine by H_2O_2, a product of the enzymatic hydrolysis of cholesterol. Both sensing assays were integrated into the same Janus type particle, thus, allowing simultaneous monitoring of glucose and cholesterol in human serum.

Janus magnetic nanoparticles have also been used for DNA [43,44] and protein detection [45,46]. Doyle's group brilliantly developed polymeric magnetic Janus particles with separate detection and barcoding compartments [44,47]. The barcoding region displayed arrays of dots, while the sensing compartment was functionalized with DNA probe molecules for multiplexed detection. The magnetic microparticles incorporated into the Janus disks allowed rotation by an external magnetic field, enabling solution exchange through immobilization, particle decoding through orientation control and reaction enhancement through active stirring [44]. Regarding protein detection, multifunctional dumbbell-shaped magnetic Janus particles were prepared and modified on one face with anti-CD14 antibody for cell attachment and coated with anti-TNFα antibody on the other face (Figure 7a). The system allowed specific cell targeting and in situ multi-detection of cytokines [46].

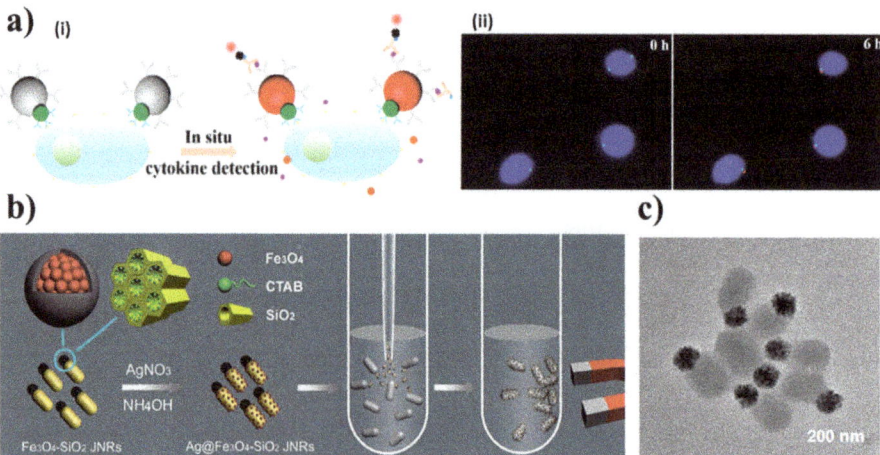

Figure 7. Scheme illustrating attachment of dumbbell particles to single cells and in situ sandwich Enzyme-Linked ImmunoSorbent Assay (ELISA) detection of cells released cytokine (i). Merged fluorescence images of the cell (blue) and dumbbell particles (green, small magnetic microspheres (sMS); red, big magnetic microspheres (bMS)) after ELISA detection. The images were taken at 6 h lipopolysaccharide (LPS) stimulation time. Cells were stained with CellTracker Blue CMAC (7-amino-4-chloromethylcoumarin) dye. Scale bar: 10 µm (ii) (a). Schematic illustration of a typical procedure for the in situ synthesis of AgNPs@Fe_3O_4-SiO_2 Janus nanorods (JNRs) and their sterilization and separation process (b). Magnetic Janus mesoporous silica nanoparticles Transmission Electron Microscope (TEM) images (bar = 200 nm) (c). Reprinted and adapted from Reference [46] (a), Reference [48] (b) and Reference [49] (c).

In several studies, magnetic JNPs have been used for the effective separation/concentration of biomaterials. Mirkin and coworkers developed triblock Au-Ni-Au nanorods for the detection and separation of protein mixtures [50,51]. The Au segments from the two-component triblock (Au-Ni-Au) nanorods were functionalized with nitrostreptavidin for capturing biotinylated proteins, and the Ni interior block was used as affinity template for simple and efficient separation of His-tagged proteins. In addition, the Ni portion of the nanorods is ferromagnetic, which enables easy isolation under a magnetic field. In this way, the authors demonstrated how the two-component triblock magnetic nanorods could be used to magnetically separate biotin-tagged proteins and His-tagged proteins from a mixed solution, thereby using a single material to separate and selectively remove multiple proteins and providing an alternative to the currently used affinity chromatography [51].

Multifunctional nanoplatforms based on the use of magnetic Janus mesoporous silica nanoparticles were designed to integrate bacterial capture, separation, and elimination into a single system [48,49,52]. In an interesting work, novel magnetic silica JNRs decorated with Ag nanoparticles (Figure 7b) showed superior magnetic sensitivity, strong binding to bacteria, and more effective and long-term antimicrobial activity than pure Ag nanoparticles. This was attributed to the properties of the formed nanocomposites with a variable AgNPs loading, which can significantly improve the dispersion and stability of the deposited AgNPs and enhance their bacteria binding capture efficiency [48]. Dong's group proposed the use of magnetic Janus mesoporous silica nanoparticles (MSNs) with hexadecyltrimethylammonium bromide (CTAB) loading, used both as a soft cationic template for mesoporous silica synthesis and anti-bacterial agent for bacterial elimination, and functionalized with amine groups, as nonselective ligands to bind both Gram-positive and Gram-negative bacteria via electrostatic attraction [53], as anti-bacterial drug [54]. In this way, the mesoporous silica body enhanced bacterial capture, due to its large surface, while the exposed Fe_3O_4 head maintained the strong paramagnetic property for bacterial separation [49]. To address specific bacteria targeting, fluorescent-magnetic Janus mesoporous silica nanoparticles were modified with a specific antibody. These JNPs acted as fluorescent identification and separation tools which enabled bacterial identification through Matrix-Assisted Laser Desorption Ionization Time-of-Flight Mass Spectrometry (MALDI-TOF-MS) directly from food matrixes [52].

Table 1 summarizes the main characteristics of the methodologies using magnetic Janus particles for static (bio)sensing applications.

Magnetic Janus Particles for Targeted Biomedical Applications

Nanoparticles have received great attention in the field of therapeutic and diagnostic. In particular, Janus particles, due to their two functional surfaces, can be used to selectively conjugate specific chemical moieties for drug delivery, non-invasive imaging, and/or targeted therapeutic intervention on a single-particle system [55]. Anisotropic nanoparticles have attracted great attention as multimodal imaging agents. In particular, magnetic nanoparticles can be used as contrast agents for magnetic resonance imaging (MRI) [7]. The incorporation of metallic nanoparticles provides plasmonic properties [56], and the subsequent modification with fluorescent dyes or quantum dots allows fluorescent imaging [57]. However, only a few systems have been reported involving specific target capacity into the magnetic Janus particles for imaging purposes. Dumbbell-shaped Au-Fe_3O_4 [58] and Ag-Fe_3O_4 [59] nanoparticles functionalized with specific antibodies against A431 human epithelial carcinoma cells and Raji and HeLa cells, respectively, were described. The high reflectance of the nanoparticles, due to the presence of the Au and Ag compartments, respectively, enabled optical visualization of cancer cells without fluorescence labeling, as well as MRI [58]. Recently, Sánchez et al. reported an elegant Janus nanoplatform by combining a Fe_3O_4NPs/mesoporous silica core@shell face together with an Au nanoparticle face [60]. Due to its anisotropy, the resulting hybrid nanocarriers successfully allowed the in vivo tumor-targeted (by its modification with a targeting peptide for cancer detection cRGD motif) multimodal MRI (Fe_3O_4 core), computed tomography (CT, AuNP face) and fluorescent tracking (fluorescent dye loading) in a fibrosarcoma-bearing mouse model (Figure 8). Moreover, in vitro experiments performed by 24 h incubation with HEK293, HepG2, RAW 264.7, adult fibroblasts (MAF), and fibrosarcoma (MF) mouse cells confirmed the biocompatibility of these Janus particles within the tested concentration range (35–350 µg mL^{-1}).

Table 1. Janus magnetic particles for static (bio)sensing.

Composition	Morphology	Preparation Method	Application	Target Analyte	Ref.
Magnetic Janus mesoporous silica nanoparticles	Rod	Sol-gel method	Capture, separation and elimination	*Escherichia coli* and *Staphylococcus aureus* on LB-agar plates	[49]
Magnetic Janus mesoporous silica nanoparticles	Rod	Sol-gel method	Capture and identification	Foodborne bacteria in milk samples	[52]
Au-Ni-Au	Rod	Porous template synthesis	Therapeutics and separations	Separation His-tagged proteins and Ab to poly-His	[50]
Encoded particles	-	Stop-flow lithography	Determination and identification	miRNAs	[44]
γ-Fe_2O_3- SiO_2/Glucose oxidase	Sphere	One-step flame-assisted spray-pyrolysis	Enzymatic biosensing	Glucose	[41]
NitroStrep-Au-Ni-Au-NitroStrep	Rod	Porous template synthesis	Magnetic protein separation	Separation of a mixture of Histag-Uniquitin, Biotin-BSA and protein A	[51]
Con A/dextran-γ-Fe_2O_3/esterase	Sphere	Centrifugal microfluidic chip	Enzymatic biosensing	Glucose and cholesterol in serum samples	[42]
EMG 507 ferrofluid/polymeric phase (PEGDA)	Sphere	Droplet micromagnetofluidic technique	Protein detection	BSA	[45]
Janus Hydrogel particles (Fe_3O_4/PEG/Darocur)	Acorn	Microfluidic synthesis	Bioimaging and imaging-guided therapies	DNA detection	[43]
AgNPs@Fe_3O_4-SiO_2	Rod	Sol-gel method	Antimicrobial	*Escherichia coli* and *Bacillus subtilis*	[48]
TCO-bMS and Tz-sMS	Dumbbell	Click Chemistry	Bioimaging, single-cell analysis and biomedical diagnostics	In situ TNFα detection released by cancer cells.	[46]

Ab, antibody; bMS, big magnetic microspheres; BSA, bovine serum albumin; LB, Luria-Bertani broth; PEG, polyethylene glycol; PEGDA, polyethylene glycol diacrylate; TCO, trans-cyclooctene; TzMS, tetrazine magnetic microspheres.

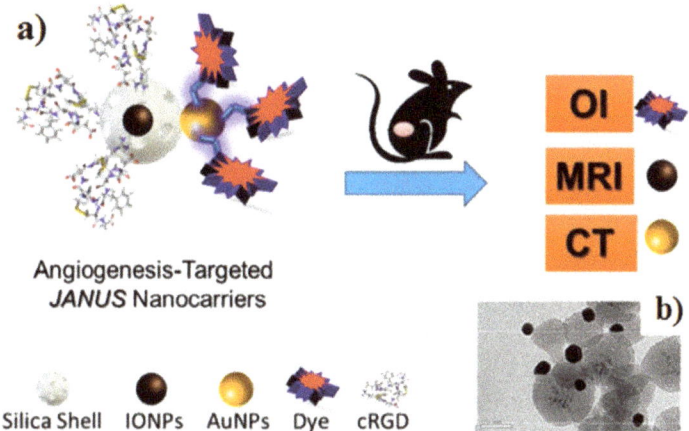

Figure 8. Strategy for multimodal molecular imaging assessment of targeted Janus nanoparticles in tumor-bearing mouse model (OI, optical imaging; MRI, magnetic resonance imaging; CT, computed tomography; IONPs, iron oxide nanoparticles; cRGD, peptide cyclo[Arg-Gly-Asp-D-Phe-Lys]). Reprinted and adapted from Reference [60].

The intrinsic heterogeneity of Janus particles makes them suitable for delivering drugs with different properties, unlike core-shell nanoparticles [61]. In drug delivery systems, specific targeting is crucial to avoid damage to healthy cells and to enhance the drug bioavailability [20]. Thus, some controlled release magnetic Janus particles have been conjugated with specific ligands for specific drug release targeting. In this context, dumbbell-like Au-Fe_3O_4 nanoparticles were prepared as target-specific nanocarriers to deliver cis-Pt complexes into epidermal growth factor receptor 2 (HER2)-positive breast cancer cells. In this structure, the Pt complex was anchored on the Au side and the HER2-specific monoclonal antibody Herceptin, chosen as a targeting agent, was linked to Fe_3O_4 side [62]. Following a similar strategy of active targeting and drug delivery, cell targeting and intracellular DNA magnetic-controlled release in cancer cells were also achieved by using magnetic Janus nanocapsules [63]. In addition, Wang et al. prepared super-paramagnetic Janus nanocomposites of polystyrene/Fe_3O_4@SiO_2 structure with dual functionalities for drug delivery applications. To achieve simultaneous cell targeting and stimulus-induced drug release, the polystyrene matrix was surface-decorated with carboxyl groups where the tumor cell targeting was attempted by the conjugation of folic acid, whereas the antitumor agent DOX was immobilized to the silica shell via a pH-sensitive hydrazone bond, thus, facilitating pH-induced drug release [64].

An exciting trend in drug delivery is incorporating therapeutic, targeting, and imaging all in one particle. Kilinc et al. synthesized Fe-Au nanorods for combined cell targeting, therapy and imaging able to specifically target breast cancer cells. In this design, the Au block was modified with heregulin, a ligand of HER family of receptors, whereas the magnetic response of the Fe block was used for mechanical perturbation and MRI [65]. A very nice work reported by Zhang et al. describes a method for the synthesis of uniform multifunctional Au/Fe_3O_4@C Janus nanoparticles. These nanoparticles were selectively functionalized with amino-poly(ethyleneglycol)thiol and folic acid on the exposed Au domains (Figure 9) to achieve high contrast for computed tomography imaging, excellent stability, good biocompatibility, as well as cancer cell-specific targeting. The mesoporous structure was used as a carrier for DOX, photothermal agent and MRI contrast agent [66]. New magnetic-luminescent multifunctional nanoparticles ($MnFe_2O_4$-$NaYF_4$) were modified with folic acid to target human esophagus carcinoma cells. The system exhibited multiple uses, including multimodal imaging, targeted drug delivery, and cancer imaging-guided therapies [67]. Following the same trend of theranostics approach, monodisperse Au-Fe_2C Janus nanoparticles were synthesized as multifunctional entities for cancer theranostics. The entities had triple-modal magnetic resonance/multispectral photoacoustic tomography/computed tomography imaging-guided for precise diagnosis and efficient tumor treatment through laser radiation. In vitro and in vivo targeting was achieved by modifying the Au-Fe$_2$C Janus particles with an affibody (ZHER2:342), showing a larger tumor accumulation and deeper tumor penetration than the non-targeted ones [68].

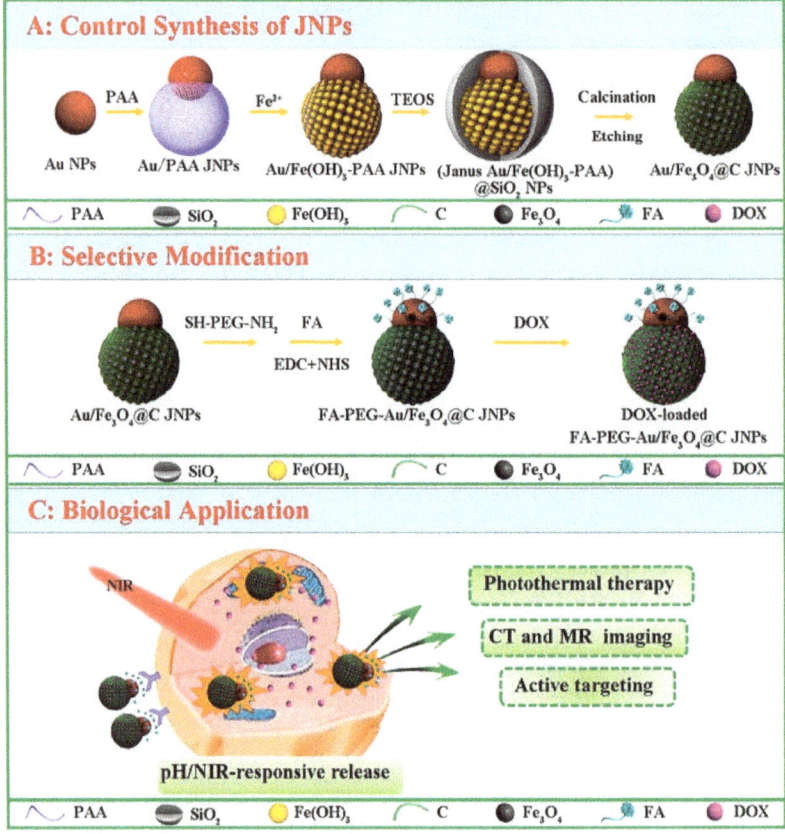

Figure 9. Scheme showing the controlled synthetic strategy for obtaining Au/Fe$_3$O$_4$@C JNPs (**A**). Selective modification of Au/Fe$_3$O$_4$@C JNPs (**B**). Biological application of FA-PEG-Au/Fe$_3$O$_4$@C JNPs for simultaneous dual-modal imaging and actively targeted chemo-photothermal synergistic therapy of cancer cells (**C**). Reprinted with permission from Reference [66].

The main aspects of targeted (bio)imaging and biomedical applications using magnetic Janus particles are outlined in Table 2.

Table 2. Janus magnetic particles for targeted (bio)imaging and biomedical applications.

Composition	Morphology	Preparation Method	Use	Application	Ref.
Au-Fe$_2$C/affibody	Snowman	Carburization process	Imaging-guided photothermal therapy	In vivo targeted tumor ablation and imaging	[68]
FITC-Fe$_3$O$_4$-PS$_{16}$-PAA10/DNA	Sphere	Phase separation	Target therapy	DNA release in cells	[63]
Fe-Au/PEG/Heregulin	Rod	Templated electrodeposition	Targeted diagnosis and therapy	Imaging and magnetic hyperthermia breast cancer cells	[65]
Au-IONP/Dye@MS	Snowman	Pickering emulsion interfacial synthesis	Fluorescence imaging, Magnetic resonance imaging, Computed tomography	In vitro and in vivo tumor-targeted imaging of Fibrosarcoma.	[60]
SiO$_2$ coated-Ag-Fe$_2$O$_3$/antibody	Snowman	Flame aerosol technology	Targeted bioimaging	Hela Cells	[59]
Folic acid/polystyrene/Fe$_3$O$_4$@SiO$_2$/DOX	Sphere	Combined process of miniemulsion and sol-gel reaction	Targeted drug release	Drug delivery in cancer cells	[64]
MnFe$_2$O$_4$-NaYF$_4$/folic acid	Dumbbell	Thermolysis	Targeted multimodal imaging and therapy.	Targeted photothermal therapy and imaging of human esophagus carcinoma cells	[67]
Au-Fe$_3$O$_4$/EGFR antibody	Dumbbell	Decomposing iron on the surfaces of Au nanoparticles	Bioimaging	Targeted bioimaging of human epithelial carcinoma cells	[57]
Pt complex/Au-Fe$_2$O$_3$/Herceptin	Dumbbell	Decomposition and oxidation	Target chemotherapy	Targeted Pt release to Her2-positive breast cancer cells	[62]
FA-PEG-Au/Fe$_3$O$_4$@C/DOX loaded	Snowman	-	Imaging, drug delivery and therapy	Targeted delivery of DOX, photothermal therapy, MRI and CT in Hela cells	[66]

CT, computed tomography; DOX, doxorubicin; EGFR, epidermal growth factor receptor; FA, folic acid; FITC, Fluorescein isothiocyanate; MRI, magnetic resonance imaging; MS, mesoporous silica; IONP, iron oxide nanoparticles; PEG, polyethylene glycol; PS16-PAA10, poly(styrene allyl alcohol).

3.2. Self-Propelled Janus Magnetic Particles for (Bio)Sensing

Under certain experimental conditions, Janus particles can be propelled autonomously (Janus motors). This self-propulsion can be achieved through certain electrochemical reactions or the incorporation of metals (Pt, Mg) capable of generating gaseous bubbles in the presence of certain fuels (H_2O_2, water). The inherent lack of a defined trajectory can be solved by including a magnetic component (usually nickel) in the Janus motor structure, which allows their guidance or isolation in the presence of an external magnetic field. Self-propelled Janus magnetic particles using metals, polymers or carbon materials have been reported so far.

Self-propelled Janus magnetic particles, unmodified or functionalized with appropriate bioreceptors, have demonstrated to possess unrivaled merits for optical and electrochemical on-site sensing and biosensing of a wide variety of analytes and biomolecules (nucleic acids, proteins, cancer and bacterial cells and other clinically relevant analytes, such as cortisol) in near real-time. Table 3 summarizes the main features of the biosensing strategies that were reported involving the use of self-propelled Janus magnetic particles. It is important to note that the autonomous movement of the Janus magnetic particles has been decisive in developing efficient and rapid biosensing strategies involving 'on-the-move' recognition and (bio)sensing events in complex samples without preparatory and washing steps [4,7,8,11,15,69–73]. This autonomous movement around the sample addresses the low binding efficiency associated with the slow analyte transport occurring in bioaffinity sensors working in quiescent sample droplets, thus, increasing the likelihood of target-receptor contacts and greatly enhancing the kinetic and sensitivity of the (bio)sensing event [11].

To date, the use of self-propelled Janus magnetic motors for biosensing involving trimetallic nanowires, tubular micromotors or spherical particles has been reported (Figure 10). In these biosensing applications, the signal transduction was achieved through: (1) Chemical sensing involving measurement of the speed and/or distance the motors travelled at fixed times in the presence of the target analytes [74,75]; (2) electrochemical sensing by electrochemical detection of electroactive compounds generated by degradation of non-electroactive compounds using Janus particles with artificial enzymatic activity [76] or by using particle-electrode impact voltammetry to quantify and qualify locomotion of self-propelled micromotors [77]; and (3) optical and fluorescent sensing by monitoring directly captured big target analytes (cells and bacteria) [78,79] or in connection with appropriate fluorescent labels [80,81] or quenching mechanisms [82,83].

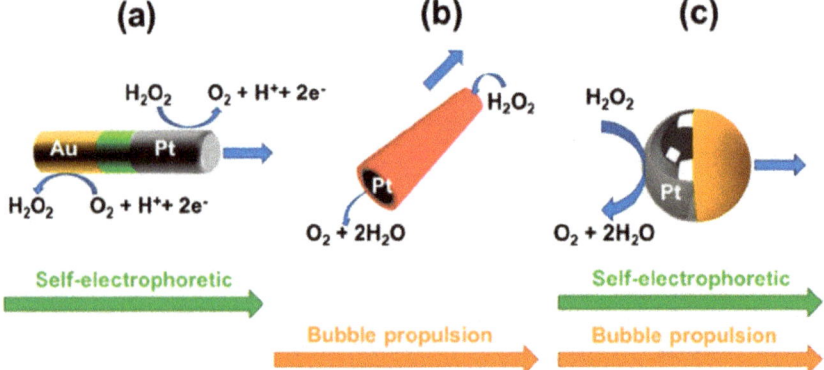

Figure 10. Magnetic Janus motors for biosensing applications and related propulsion mechanisms: Nanowires (**a**), tubular micromotors (**b**) and spherical particles (**c**). Reprinted from Reference [15] with permission.

Table 3. Self-propelled Janus magnetic particles for (bio)sensing.

Type of Self-Propelled Janus Magnetic Particles	Propulsion Mechanism (Fuel)	Fundamentals	Type of Detection	Target Analyte	Analytical Characteristics	Sample	Ref.
Au-Ni-Pt nanowires	Self-electrophoretic propulsion mechanism (H_2O_2)	Selective acceleration in the presence of silver ions (Ag^+) in connection with sandwich DNA hybridization approach onto a photolithography-prepared gold electrode	Optical (speed/distance travelled)	30-mer synthetic DNA or E. coli 16S mRNA	40 amol (synthetic DNA), 2000 cfus mL^{-1} of E. coli	untreated bacterial lysates	[75]
Photolithography prepared Pt/Au/Ni/Ti microtubes	Bubble propulsion (H_2O_2 + NaCh)	Sandwich DNA hybridization assay onto thiolated DNA capture probe modified microtubes	Indirect fluorescent (streptavidin fluorescent nanoparticles)	30-mer synthetic DNA or E. coli 16S mRNA	~25 nM synthetic target DNA	Spiked 100% human serum, 10% human urine and saliva and raw bacterial lysates	[80]
Photolithography prepared Pt/Au/Ni/Ti microtubes	Bubble propulsion (H_2O_2 + NaCh)	Sandwich aptameric assay onto thiolated aptameric capture probe modified microtubes	Indirect fluorescent (streptavidin fluorescent nanoparticles)	Human thrombin	~100 nM	Spiked untreated serum and plasma pretreated to precipitate fibrinogen	[81]
Photolithography prepared Pt/Au/Ni/Ti microtubes	Bubble propulsion (H_2O_2 + NaCh)	Selective recognition onto anti CEA-modified microtubes	Direct optical	CEA+ cancer cells	?	1:4 diluted human serum	[78]
Template electrodeposited Au/Ni/PANI/Pt microtubes	Bubble propulsion (H_2O_2 + NaCh)	Selective recognition onto ConA-modified microtubes	Direct optical	E. coli	?	Spiked drinking water, apple juice and seawater	[79]
Template electrodeposited Au/PEDOT/Ni/Pt microtubes	Bubble propulsion (H_2O_2 + NaCh)	Direct competitive immunoassay using cortisol-HRP onto anticortisol-modified microtubes	Indirect optical/naked-eye using H_2O_2/TMB	Cortisol	0.1 µg mL^{-1}	?	[84]
Au-Ni-Mg Janus particles	Bubble propulsion (water)	Produce OH^- ions to increase the medium pH and promote the paraoxon degradation	Amperometric (+0.9 V vs. Ag/AgCl)	Paraoxon	~4 mM	?	[76]
Magnetocatalytic hybrid Janus spherical particles (GQDs, PtNPs and Fe_3O_4NPs) modified with PABA	Magnetic and bubble propulsion (H_2O_2 + NaCh)	Interaction between PABA-modified GQDs and targeted bacterial LPS	Fluorescence quenching	E. coli	?	Unprocessed urine and serum samples	[82]
Magnetocatalytic hybrid Janus spherical particles (GQDs, PtNPs and Fe_3O_4NPs) modified with PABA	Magnetic and bubble propulsion (H_2O_2 + NaCh)	Interaction between PABA-modified GQDs and targeted bacterial LPS	Fluorescence quenching	Salmonella enterica	0.07 ng mL^{-1} of endotoxin	Spiked milk, mayo, egg yolk, and egg white	[83]

CEA, carcioembriogenic antigen; ConA, Concanavalin A; GQDs, graphene quantum dots; HRP, horseradish peroxidase; PABA, phenylboronic acid; LPS, lipopolysaccharides; PANI, polyaniline; PEDOT, poly(3,4-ethylenedioxythiophene); TMB, 3,3′,5,5′-tetramethylbenzidine.

Wang's group, from the University of California San Diego, pioneered the use of magnetic Janus motors for optical biosensing. In particular, Au-Ni-Pt nanowires were prepared for the determination of nucleic acids [75]. These catalytic nanowires are able to self-propel at speeds of ~10 µm s^{-1} in a solution containing 5–10% of H_2O_2. Platinum catalyzed the oxidation of H_2O_2, which generated electrons and free protons at that end of the nanomotor. Due to the structure of the nanowire, asymmetric distribution of charges and an electrical gradient was generated, which translated into the autonomous advancement of the nanomotor in the direction in which the platinum end pointed (Figure 11a). Taking advantage of the selective acceleration of these nanomotors in the presence of silver ions, attributed to the improved catalytic activity of platinum after underpotential deposition of silver on the nanowires [74], this group developed a strategy for nucleic acid biosensing using for the first time the distance traveled by the nanomotor as an analytical signal [75]. The biosensing strategy was used for the quantification of synthetic DNA and bacterial rRNA and involved a detector probe modified with Ag nanoparticles in a typical hybridization sandwich format. The assay implied co-self-assembly of a thiolated specific DNA capture probe and dithiotreitol (DTT) and post-treatment with mercaptohexanol (MCH) on a photolithography-prepared gold electrode followed by sequential incubation on this modified surface with the sample containing the target DNA and the Ag nanoparticles-modified detector probe. Upon placing a drop of an H_2O_2 solution on the electrode surface with the immobilized DNA sandwich, the Ag nanoparticles were rapidly dissolved and, after mixing the Ag$^+$ enriched solution with a nanomotors suspension, their speed was monitored for a fixed time (Figure 11a). The higher the concentration of target nucleic acid (30-mer synthetic DNA or *Escherichia coli* (*E. coli*) 16S mRNA), the larger the number of nanoparticles captured and, therefore, the higher the speed (or the distance travelled at a fixed time) of the nanomotors. This new biosensing principle was able to selectively detect 40 amol synthetic DNA and 2000 colony forming units (cfus) mL^{-1} of *E. coli* directly in untreated bacterial lysates. In addition, the principle facilitates the collection of multiple readings in a single experiment, reduces the likelihood of false positives or negatives, and can be easily extended to other biosensing strategies. Despite these interesting features, catalytic nanowires operation is restricted to low ionic strength environments, which limits their usefulness for biosensing purposes [11,69]. This is the reason why tubular micromotors and spherical particles, which efficiently propel in high ionic concentration environments and complex biological fluids, have been much more used for dynamic biosensing [15].

Microtubes with the internal catalytic surface of Pt are chemically propelled by O_2 bubbles generated by the decomposition of H_2O_2 in the presence of a suitable surfactant (Figure 11b) [69]. In addition, the incorporation of the ferromagnetic Ni intermediate layer makes it easy to be guided with a magnet. These microtubes were initially manufactured with standard photolithography techniques [80,81] and more recently by electrodeposition in commercial membranes [79,84], which is a much cheaper and simpler methodology that also allows the motor size to be modulated at will for each particular application. These micro-rockets can be modified with gold by electroplating, only on half of their external surface (Figure 11b,c) to facilitate their modification with different bioreceptors, and, therefore, they can be considered Janus motors.

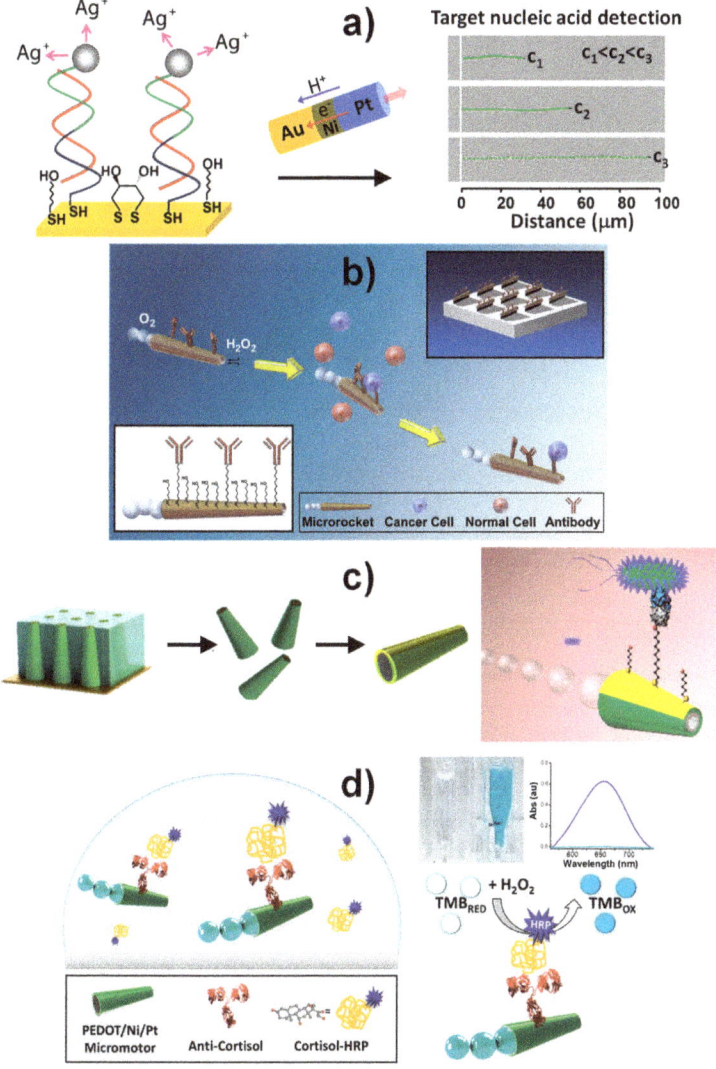

Figure 11. Optical biosensing using catalytic magnetic Janus motors (**a**) and tubular motors prepared by top-down photolithography (**b**) or template electrodeposition (**c**,**d**). Detection of: Nucleic acids with catalytic Au-Ni-Pt nanowires (**a**), cancer cells with Ti/Ni/Au/Pt microtubes modified with antibodies (**b**) bacteria with lectin-modified Au/Ni/PANI/Pt microtubular engines (**c**) and naked-eye detection of cortisol with antibodies-functionalized Au/PEDOT/Ni/Pt microtubes (**d**). Reprinted and adapted from Reference [75] (**a**), Reference [78] (**b**), Reference [79] (**c**) and Reference [84] (**d**) with permission.

Although these micro-rockets can travel at up to 2 mm s^{-1}, after the functionalization required conferring the necessary selectivity in biosensing applications they typically navigate at 100–200 μm s^{-1} (in biological samples supplemented with 1–5% (w/v) H_2O_2 and 0.25–2% (w/v) sodium cholate surfactant, NaCh). This is sufficient speed to ensure their prolonged navigation (>30 min) in complex and viscous biological media. The reported results show that the required H_2O_2 and NaCh concentrations affect neither the functionalization used to immobilize the bioreceptors nor the efficiency of the biological interactions required for biosensing. The speed of these microtransporters allows the rapid scanning of a sample, ensuring the probability of interaction of the target analyte with the surface-confined receptors. In addition, the convection currents and vortex effect associated with this movement and the generated bubbles create a very favorable hydrodynamic environment that accelerates the (generally slow) kinetics of the recognition reactions, allowing the development of efficient, simple biosensing strategies in near real-time [11,80].

Pt/Au/Ni/Ti microtubes were prepared by photolithography or by template electrodeposition of Pt and poly(3,4-ethylenedioxythiophene) (PEDOT) or polyaniline (PANI) on commercial membranes and modified with Au and Au+Ni (PANI/Pt or PEDOT/Pt) by electronic impact. After the functionalization of the sputtered gold external surface using the chemistry of thiol monolayers and the subsequent covalent immobilization of different receptors (antibodies, oligonucleotides and lectins), the resulting microtubes allowed direct optical biosensing of large target biomolecules, such as cancer cells [78] and bacteria [79], as well as indirect biosensing of smaller molecules (DNA [80], proteins [81] and hormones [84]) using different fluorescent labeling strategies.

Regarding direct detection, Janus tubular micromotors manufactured by photolithography and functionalized with a specific antibody were successfully used for the rapid and selective detection of pancreatic cancer cells that overexpressed the carcinoembryonic antigen (CEA) on their surface, in 1:4 diluted human serum (Figure 11b) [78].

Tubular micromotors of much smaller dimensions, manufactured by electroplating PANI/Pt using commercial membranes (Figure 11c) and successive electrodeposition of Ni and Au layers were applied to the biosensing of pathogenic bacteria. The manufacture of these micromotors is much simpler and cheaper than those prepared by photolithography and allows modulating their dimensions at demand depending on the size of the target biomolecule, enabling the visualization of the recognition process in real-time with no need for a later stage of additional labeling. For this purpose, these microtransporters were modified with the appropriate lectin for the efficient recognition of the target bacteria [79]. Using the affinity reaction of the lectin Concanavalin A by gram-negative bacteria, such as *E. coli*, it was possible to detect in real-time and at single-cell level this bacterium in drinking water, apple juice and seawater supplemented with the fuel required for the locomotion of the micromotors.

Regarding the indirect biosensing of small molecules, photolitographically prepared Pt/Au/Ni/Ti microtubes functionalized with a specific thiolated DNA probe were used for the determination of a 30-mer synthetic target DNA at the nanomolar level directly in biological matrices, such as serum, urine, saliva or longer target *E. coli* 16S rRNA in raw bacterial lysates without the need to apply previous pre-treatment or washing steps [80]. Pt/Au/Ni/Ti microtubes functionalized with aptamers were employed for sensitive and selective biosensing of circulating proteins (human thrombin) in biological fluids (serum and plasma) [81]. In both strategies, sandwich formats and fluorescent detection by labeling the biotinylated detector receptors (DNA or aptamer detector probes) with commercial fluorescent nanoparticles modified with streptavidin, were used.

More recently, Au-sputtered PEDOT/Ni/Pt microtubes were modified with a specific antibody and used, in connection with a direct competitive immunoassay using cortisol conjugated with horseradish peroxidase (HRP) and the 3,3′,5,5′-tetramethylbencidine (TMB)/H_2O_2 system, to develop and fast naked-eye biosensing strategy enabling "on the move" specific detection of cortisol down to 0.1 µg mL^{-1} in just 2 min and using microliter sample volumes (Figure 11d) [84].

Self-propelled spherical magnetic Janus particles also exhibit suitability for electrochemical and optical sensing and biosensing. In all cases, propulsion allows these particles to mix with liquids much better than the static ones, which significantly improves the biosensing efficiency. The applications include gold and magnesium micromotors, which operate thanks to corrosion reactions that generate bubbles on one side and propel the engine in the opposite direction. These Janus particles have demonstrated their ability to sense and degrade toxic pesticides or emerging contaminants in complex samples using simple and rapid protocols.

The remarkable capabilities offered by self-propelled spherical magnetic Janus particles in electrochemical sensing were shown by Wang's group [76]. Water-propelled Mg microparticles with a Ni-Au bilayer patch for magnetic guidance [85], exerted a dual function as "autonomous stirrers" significantly enhancing mass transport and as "natural enzyme mimics", inducing localized pH gradients for non-electroactive analytes degradation. These interesting features hold great promise for electrochemical measurements in microvolume samples at screen-printed electrodes [71,76]. In a pioneering approach, water-driven magnetic Au-Ni-Mg Janus particles were magnetically confined onto the surface of printable sensor strips through the intermediate Ni layer [76]. The particles served as artificial enzymes toward the alkaline and selective hydrolysis of the non-electrochemically detectable pesticide paraoxon into p-nitrophenol, an electroactive and non-hazardous compound (Figure 12a). The method exhibited 15-fold times higher sensitivity towards target analyte detection in the presence of the propelled particles, which was attributed to the enhanced mixing induced by the motion of self-propelled Janus magnetic particles.

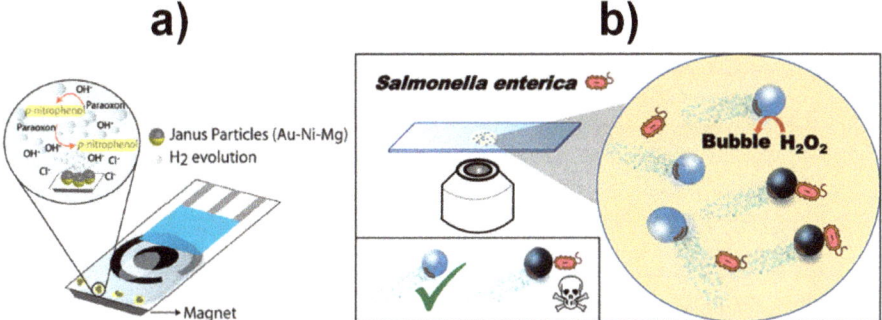

Figure 12. Electrochemical (**a**) and optical (**b**) biosensing using self-propelled spherical magnetic Janus particles. Electrochemical detection of organophosphorous nerve agents through their hydrolysis to non-hazardous, but electrochemically detectable by-product (p-nitrophenol) at screen-printed electrodes (**a**); optical biosensing of enterobacterial contamination by rapid quenching of the native fluorescence of the PABA-functionalized magnetocatalytic hybrid Janus spherical particles upon interaction with the target LPS from *Salmonella enterica* (**b**). Reprinted and adapted from (**a**) [76] and (**b**) [83] with permission.

Regarding optical sensing, Escarpa's group has used Janus magnetic motors for ultra-fast and sensitive biosensing of highly toxic species, such as deadly bacteria endotoxins [82,83]. The methods involve the use of highly efficient magnetocatalytic hybrid Janus spherical particles, synthesized using an oil-in-water emulsion containing graphene quantum dots (GQDs), PtNPs and Fe_3O_4NPs and modified with phenylboronic acid (PABA), to detect endotoxins released from *E. coli* [82] and *Salmonella enterica* [83] bacteria. The analytical readout relied on the fluorescence quenching upon the interaction of GQDs with the target bacterial lipopolysaccharides (Figure 12b). Due to their two active differentiated regions, these Janus particles can be propelled efficiently both in the presence of H_2O_2 and under a magnetic field. Authors reported that these particles can detect selectively the bacterial toxins at a 0.07 ng mL^{-1} endotoxin concentration, far below the 275 μg mL^{-1} level considered toxic to humans [83], in spiked clinical (urine and human serum) and food (milk, mayo, egg yolk and egg white) samples in just 15 min compared with the several hours required by the existing gold standard methods.

4. Conclusions, Main Challenges to Solve and Future Perspectives

The relevant progress in the design, fabrication and applications of magnetic Janus particles are reviewed in this article. Details on their synthesis procedures and on (bio)sensing applications of both static and self-propelled systems are highlighted and discussed.

A unique advantage of magnetic Janus particles is their easy manipulation, also together with their cargo (cells, bacteria, drugs and other biological material) through the application of external magnetic fields which, in turn, avoids the need of using chemical propellants with short lifetimes. In addition, this kind of Janus particles are also prone for functionalization and stand out for their high biocompatibility allowing their use as labels for biosensing, which also results in advantages connected with sensitivity and time of analysis. Moreover, they exhibit intrinsic peroxidase-like catalytic activity useful for such purpose. Furthermore, their anisotropy in shape, composition and surface chemistry allows for the combination of diverse, but complementary analytical functions in a single particle, which is difficult in non-Janus micro and nanoparticles. Moreover, their magnetic property may allow the plain use of magnetic-field based separation and recycling of these particles.

Static magnetic Janus nanoparticles have found application in the simultaneous determination of molecules of biological importance, such as glucose and cholesterol in serum, or multi-detection of DNA and proteins. In addition, they have been used for the effective separation and pre-concentration of biomaterials, thus, meaning an alternative to the usually employed affinity chromatography. Moreover, they have been applied in the integration of bacterial capture, separation and elimination in a single system and, what is more, they can also be used as imaging agents and in drug delivery allowing specific targeting with no damage to healthy cells. In this last field, a single system, including multimodal imaging, targeted drug delivery and cancer imaging-guided therapy has been proposed.

Self-propelled Janus magnetic particles have been used for optical and electrochemical biosensing of clinically relevant analytes, such as nucleic acids, proteins, cancer and bacterial cells, etc. Their autonomous movement has, in fact, allowed the development of efficient and quick biosensing systems able to recognize the target analytes in complex biological samples with no need for sample pretreatment or washing steps. What is more, these particles with free movement around the sample raise the probability of target-receptor contacts, which greatly increases the kinetics and sensitivity of the biosensing events.

Nevertheless, there are major challenges to be confronted before these particles can be introduced, for example, in routine medical care. On the one hand, it is necessary to find a way to easily fabricate at large scale environmentally friendly and low-cost biofunctionalized particle labels with high stability and adequate long-term storage. Quite a number of Janus particles synthetic methods have been reported to date. However, this is still a major challenge to be solved, indeed being one of the main facts hindering the wide applicability of these particles in many fields. Procedures to synthesize magnetic Janus particles are all but simple. Moreover, the synthesis of nano-sized Janus particles is even more complicated, requiring complex chemicals and resulting in the production of low amounts of particles, which is a burden for applications requiring high quantities of this material. For sure, an improvement in the control and yield of synthetic methods together with the preparation of modified JNPs with new capabilities should result in an increase of their potential applicability, thus, helping to introduce them in new practical applications and real-world systems. In fact, modern technologies, such as direct laser writing (DLW) and 3D printing in combination with experimental prototype simulations will allow manufacturing of improved complex architectures which is envisaged as a solution to solve problems associated with the synthesis of magnetic Janus particles.

Also, a more thorough study on the interactions between magnetic Janus particles and biological systems is necessary to allow the prediction of the biological response of multi-functional JNPs which would, in turn, result in more rational designs of these particles as (bio)sensing tools.

Another main challenge relies on the design of point-of-care (POC) devices using magnetic Janus particles, which would be of great interest mostly if they are fitted to the multiplexed analysis of several biomarkers for a single sample. Neither should be forgotten that collaboration among research laboratories and medical centers is highly needed to test the newly developed methodologies by full-scale clinical trials and to actually demonstrate the advantages they can provide as opposed to traditional sensing systems.

Author Contributions: Writing—review and editing, S.C., M.G., V.S., M.P., P.Y.-S. and J.M.P.; funding acquisition, S.C., P.Y.-S. and J.M.P.

Funding: This research was funded by Spanish Ministerio de Economía y Competitividad, research project CTQ2015-64402-C2-1-R; Ministerio de Ciencia, Innovación y Universidades, research project RTI2018-096135-B-I00; Comunidad de Madrid TRANSNANOAVANSENS-CM Program, Grant P2018/NMT-4349.

Acknowledgments: The financial support of the CTQ2015-64402-C2-1-R (Spanish Ministerio de Economía y Competitividad) and RTI2018-096135-B-I00 (Ministerio de Ciencia, Innovación y Universidades) Research Projects and the TRANSNANOAVANSENS-CM Program from the Comunidad de Madrid (Grant P2018/NMT-4349) are gratefully acknowledged.

Conflicts of Interest: The authors declare no conflict of interest. The funders had no role in the design of the study; in the collection, analyses, or interpretation of data; in the writing of the manuscript, or in the decision to publish the results.

References

1. Casagrande, C.; Fabre, P.; Raphaël, E.; Veyssie, M. "Janus Beads": Realization and Behaviour at Water/Oil Interfaces. *Europhys. Lett.* **1989**, *9*, 251–255. [CrossRef]
2. De Gennes, P.G. Soft matter. *Rev. Mod. Phys.* **1992**, *64*, 645–648. [CrossRef]
3. Shao, Z.; Cao, H.; Yang, Y.; Chen, X. Intelligent Janus nanoparticles for intracellular real-time monitoring of dual drug release. *Nanoscale* **2016**, *8*, 6754–6760.
4. Yáñez-Sedeño, P.; Campuzano, S.; Pingarrón, J.M. Janus particles for (bio)sensing. *Appl. Mat. Today* **2017**, *9*, 276–288. [CrossRef]
5. Jung, C.W.; Jalani, G.; Ko, J.; Choo, J.; Lim, D.W. Synthesis, characterization, and directional binding of anisotropic biohybrid microparticles for multiplexed biosensing. *Macromol. Rapid Commun.* **2014**, *35*, 56–65. [CrossRef] [PubMed]
6. Li, B.; Wang, M.; Chen, K.; Cheng, Z.; Chen, G.; Zhang, Z. Synthesis of Biofunctional Janus Particles. *Macromol. Rapid Commun.* **2015**, *36*, 1200–1204. [CrossRef] [PubMed]
7. Yi, Y.; Sanchez, L.; Gao, Y.; Yu, Y. Janus Particles for Biological Imaging and Sensing. *Analyst* **2016**, *141*, 3526–3539. [CrossRef] [PubMed]
8. Campuzano, S.; Esteban-Fernández de Ávila, B.; Yáñez-Sedeño, P.; Pingarrón, J.M.; Wang, J. Nano/microvehicles for efficient delivery and (bio)sensing at the cellular level. *Chem. Sci.* **2017**, *8*, 6750–6763. [CrossRef]
9. Cohn, D.; Sloutski, A.; Elyashiv, A.; Varma, V.B.; Ramanujan, R. In Situ Generated Medical Devices. *Adv. Health Mater.* **2019**, *8*, e1801066.
10. Chen, X.-Z.; Hoop, M.; Mushtaq, F.; Siringil, E.; Hu, C.; Nelson, B.J.; Pané, S. Recent developments in magnetically driven micro- and nanorobots. *Appl. Mater. Today* **2017**, *9*, 37–48. [CrossRef]
11. Wang, J. Self-propelled affinity biosensors: Moving the receptor around the sample. *Biosens. Bioelectron.* **2016**, *76*, 234–242. [CrossRef] [PubMed]
12. Schrittwieser, S.; Pelaz, B.; Parak, W.J.; Lentijo-Mozo, S.; Soulantica, K.; Dieckhoff, J.; Ludwig, F.; Guenther, A.; Tschöpe, A.; Schotter, J. Homogeneous Biosensing Based on Magnetic Particle Labels. *Sensors* **2016**, *16*, 828. [CrossRef] [PubMed]
13. Li, J.; De Ávila, B.E.-F.; Gao, W.; Zhang, L.; Wang, J. Micro/nanorobots for biomedicine: Delivery, surgery, sensing, and detoxification. *Sci. Robot.* **2017**, *2*, eaam6431. [CrossRef]
14. Gao, W.; de Ávila, B.E.; Zhang, J.; Wang, J. Targeting and isolation of cancer cells using micro/nanomotors. *Adv. Drug Deliv. Rev.* **2018**, *125*, 94–101. [CrossRef]
15. Jurado-Sánchez, B. Nanoscale Biosensors Based on Self-Propelled Objects. *Biosensors* **2018**, *8*, 59. [CrossRef]
16. Walther, A.; Müller, A.H.E. Janus Particles: Synthesis, Self-Assembly, Physical Properties, and Applications. *Chem. Rev.* **2013**, *113*, 5194–5261. [CrossRef]
17. Brugarolas, T.; Tu, F.; Lee, D. Directed assembly of particles using microfluidic droplets and bubbles. *Soft Matter* **2013**, *9*, 9046–9058. [CrossRef]
18. Zhang, L.; Zhang, F.; Dong, W.-F.; Song, J.-F.; Huo, Q.-S.; Sun, H.-B. Magnetic-mesoporous Janus nanoparticles. *Chem. Commun.* **2011**, *47*, 1225–1227. [CrossRef] [PubMed]
19. Ning, Y.; Wang, C.; Ngai, T.; Yang, Y.; Tong, Z. Hollow magnetic Janus microspheres templated from double Pickering emulsions. *RSC Adv.* **2012**, *2*, 5510–5512. [CrossRef]

20. Yang, S.; Guo, F.; Kiraly, B.; Mao, X.; Lu, M.; Leong, K.W.; Huang, T.J. Microfluidic synthesis of multifunctional Janus particles for biomedical applications. *Lab Chip* **2012**, *12*, 2097–2102. [CrossRef]
21. Kim, J.H.; Jeon, T.Y.; Choi, T.M.; Shim, T.S.; Kim, S.-H.; Yang, S.-M. Droplet microfluidics for producing functional microparticles. *Langmuir* **2014**, *30*, 1473–1488. [CrossRef]
22. Varma, V.B. Development of Magnetic Structures by Micro-Magnetofluidic Techniques. Ph.D. Thesis, Nanyang Technological University, Singapore, 2017.
23. Lattuada, M.; Hatton, T.A. Preparation and Controlled Self-Assembly of Janus Magnetic Nanoparticles. *J. Am. Chem. Soc.* **2007**, *129*, 12878–12889. [CrossRef]
24. Cai, S.; Luo, B.; Zhan, X.; Zhou, X.; Lan, F.; Yi, Q.; Wu, Y. pH-responsive superstructures prepared via the assembly of Fe_3O_4 amphipathic Janus nanoparticles. *Regen. Biomater.* **2018**, *5*, 251–259. [CrossRef] [PubMed]
25. Kwak, Y.; Matyjaszewski, K. ARGET ATRP of methyl methacrylate in the presence of nitrogen-based ligands as reducing agents. *Polym. Int.* **2009**, *58*, 242–247. [CrossRef]
26. Shaghaghi, B.; Khoee, S.; Bonakdar, S. Preparation of multifunctional Janus nanoparticles on the basis of SPIONs as targeted drug delivery system. *Int. J. Pharm.* **2019**, *559*, 1–12. [CrossRef]
27. Li, Y.; Yang, S.; Lu, X.; Duan, W.; Moriga, T. Synthesis and evaluation of the SERS effect of Fe_3O_4–Ag Janus composite materials for separable, highly sensitive substrates. *RSC Adv.* **2019**, *9*, 2877–2884. [CrossRef]
28. Song, J.; Wu, B.; Zhou, Z.; Zhu, G.; Liu, Y.; Yang, Z.; Lin, L.; Yu, G.; Zhang, F.; Zhang, G.; et al. Double-Layered Plasmonic-Magnetic Vesicles by Self-Assembly of Janus Amphiphilic Gold-Iron(II,III) Oxide Nanoparticles. *Angew. Chem.* **2017**, *129*, 8222–8226. [CrossRef]
29. Jishkariani, D.; Wu, Y.; Wang, D.; Liu, Y.; Van Blaaderen, A.; Murray, C.B. Preparation and Self-Assembly of Dendronized Janus Fe_3O_4–Pt and Fe_3O_4–Au Heterodimers. *ACS Nano* **2017**, *11*, 7958–7966. [CrossRef]
30. Parmar, J.; Vilela, D.; Villa, K.; Wang, J.; Sanchez, S. Micro- and Nanomotors as Active Environmental Microcleaners and Sensors. *J. Am. Chem. Soc.* **2018**, *140*, 9317–9331. [CrossRef] [PubMed]
31. Li, T.; Li, J.; Zhang, H.; Chang, X.; Song, W.; Hu, Y.; Shao, G.; Sandraz, E.; Zhang, G.; Li, L.; et al. Magnetically Propelled Fish-Like Nanoswimmers. *Small* **2016**, *12*, 6098–6105. [CrossRef]
32. Peng, X.; Gao, F.; Zhao, J.; Li, J.; Qu, J.; Fan, H.; Qu, J.Y. Self-assembly of a graphene oxide/$MnFe_2O_4$ motor by coupling shear force with capillarity for removal of toxic heavy metals. *J. Mater. Chem. A* **2018**, *6*, 20861–20868. [CrossRef]
33. Hwang, J.; Yang, H.-M.; Lee, K.-W.; Jung, Y.-I.; Lee, K.J.; Park, C.W. A remotely steerable Janus micromotor adsorbent for the active remediation of Cs-contaminated water. *J. Hazard. Mater.* **2019**, *369*, 416–422. [CrossRef] [PubMed]
34. Indalkar, Y.R.; Gaikwada, S.S.; Ubale, A.T. Janus particles recent and novel approach in drug delivery: An overview. *Curr. Pharma Res.* **2013**, *3*, 1031–1037.
35. Wu, Z.; Li, L.; Liao, T.; Chen, X.; Jiang, W.; Luo, W.; Yang, J.; Sun, Z. Janus nanoarchitectures: From structural design to catalytic applications. *Nano Today* **2018**, *22*, 62–82. [CrossRef]
36. Zhang, Y.; Huang, K.; Lin, J.; Huang, P.; Zhang, Y. Janus nanoparticles in cancer diagnosis, therapy and theranostics. *Biomater. Sci.* **2019**, *7*, 1262–1275. [CrossRef] [PubMed]
37. Tran, L.-T.-C.; Lesieur, S.; Faivre, V. Janus nanoparticles: Materials, preparation and recent advances in drug delivery. *Expert Opin. Drug Deliv.* **2014**, *11*, 1061–1074. [CrossRef] [PubMed]
38. Teo, B.M.; Young, D.J.; Loh, X.J. Magnetic anisotropic particles: Toward remotely actuated applications. *Part. Part. Syst. Charact.* **2016**, *33*, 709–728. [CrossRef]
39. Li, P.; Niu, X.; Fan, Y. Electrospraying magnetic-fluorescent bifunctional Janus PLGA microspheres with dual rare earth ions fluorescent-labeling drugs. *RSC Adv.* **2016**, *6*, 99034–99043. [CrossRef]
40. Li, K.; Li, P.; Jia, Z.; Qi, B.; Xu, J.; Kang, D.; Liu, M.; Fan, Y. Enhanced fluorescent intensity of magnetic-fluorescent bifunctional PLGA microspheres based on Janus electrospraying for bioapplication. *Sci. Rep.* **2018**, *8*, 17117. [CrossRef] [PubMed]
41. Lu, C.; Liu, X.; Li, Y.; Yu, F.; Tang, L.; Hu, Y.; Ying, Y. Multifunctional Janus Hematite–Silica Nanoparticles: Mimicking Peroxidase-Like Activity and Sensitive Colorimetric Detection of Glucose. *ACS Appl. Mater. Interfaces* **2015**, *7*, 15395–15402. [CrossRef] [PubMed]
42. Sun, X.-T.; Zhang, Y.; Zheng, D.-H.; Yue, S.; Yang, C.-G.; Xu, Z.-R. Multitarget sensing of glucose and cholesterol based on Janus hydrogel microparticles. *Biosens. Bioelectron.* **2017**, *92*, 81–86. [CrossRef] [PubMed]

43. Yuet, K.P.; Hwang, D.K.; Haghgooie, R.; Doyle, P.S. Multifunctional Superparamagnetic Janus Particles. *Langmuir* **2010**, *26*, 4281–4287. [CrossRef] [PubMed]
44. Lee, J.; Bisso, P.W.; Srinivas, R.L.; Kim, J.J.; Swiston, A.J.; Doyle, P.S. Universal process-inert encoding architecture for polymer microparticles. *Nat. Mater.* **2010**, *13*, 524–529. [CrossRef] [PubMed]
45. Varma, V.B.; Wu, R.G.; Wang, Z.P.; Ramanujan, R.V. Magnetic Janus particles synthesized by droplet micro-magnetofluidic techniques for protein detection. *Lab Chip* **2017**, *17*, 3514–3525. [CrossRef] [PubMed]
46. Zhao, P.; George, J.; Li, B.; Amini, N.; Paluh, J.; Wang, J. Clickable Multifunctional Dumbbell Particles for in Situ Multiplex Single-Cell Cytokine Detection. *ACS Appl. Mater. Interfaces* **2017**, *9*, 32482–32488. [CrossRef] [PubMed]
47. Appleyard, D.C.; Chapin, S.C.; Srinivas, R.L.; Doyle, P.S. Bar-coded hydrogel microparticles for protein detection: Synthesis, assay and scanning. *Nat. Protoc.* **2011**, *6*, 1761–1774. [CrossRef]
48. Zhang, L.; Luo, Q.; Zhang, F.; Zhang, D.-M.; Wang, Y.-S.; Sun, Y.-L.; Dong, W.-F.; Liu, J.-Q.; Huo, Q.-S.; Sun, H.-B. High-performance magnetic antimicrobial Janus nanorods decorated with Ag nanoparticles. *J. Mater. Chem.* **2012**, *22*, 23741–23744. [CrossRef]
49. Chang, Z.; Wang, Z.; Lu, M.; Li, M.; Li, L.; Zhang, Y.; Shao, D.; Dong, W. Magnetic Janus nanorods for efficient capture, separation and elimination of bacteria. *RSC Adv.* **2017**, *7*, 3550–3553. [CrossRef]
50. Lee, K.-B.; Park, S.; Mirkin, C.A. Multicomponent Magnetic Nanorods for Biomolecular Separations. *Angew. Chem.* **2004**, *116*, 3110–3112. [CrossRef]
51. Oh, B.-K.; Park, S.; Millstone, J.E.; Lee, S.W.; Lee, K.-B.; Mirkin, C.A. Separation of Tri-Component Protein Mixtures with Triblock Nanorods. *J. Am. Chem. Soc.* **2006**, *128*, 11825–11829. [CrossRef]
52. Chang, Z.-M.; Wang, Z.; Shao, D.; Yue, J.; Lü, M.-M.; Li, L.; Ge, M.; Yang, D.; Li, M.-Q.; Yan, H.; et al. Fluorescent-magnetic Janus nanorods for selective capture and rapid identification of foodborne bacteria. *Sens. Actuators B Chem.* **2018**, *260*, 1004–1011. [CrossRef]
53. Pu, L.; Xu, J.; Sun, Y.; Fang, Z.; Chan-Park, M.B.; Duan, H. Cationic polycarbonate-grafted superparamagnetic nanoparticles with synergistic dual-modality antimicrobial activity. *Biomater. Sci.* **2016**, *4*, 871–879. [CrossRef] [PubMed]
54. Hao, N.; Chen, X.; Jayawardana, K.W.; Wu, B.; Sundhoro, M.; Yan, M. Shape Control of Mesoporous Silica Nanomaterials Templated with Dual Cationic Surfactants and Their Antibacterial Activities. *Biomater. Sci.* **2016**, *4*, 87–91. [CrossRef]
55. Choi, J.-S.; Jun, Y.-W.; Yeon, S.-I.; Kim, H.C.; Shin, J.-S.; Cheon, J. Biocompatible Heterostructured Nanoparticles for Multimodal Biological Detection. *J. Am. Chem. Soc.* **2006**, *128*, 15982–15983. [CrossRef]
56. Zijlstra, P.; Orrit, M. Single metal nanoparticles: Optical detection, spectroscopy and applications. *Rep. Prog. Phys.* **2001**, *74*, 106401–106456. [CrossRef]
57. Selvan, S.T.; Patra, P.K.; Ang, C.Y.; Ying, J.Y. Synthesis of Silica-Coated Semiconductor and Magnetic Quantum Dots and Their Use in the Imaging of Live Cells. *Angew. Chem. Int. Ed.* **2007**, *46*, 2448–2452. [CrossRef]
58. Xu, C.; Ho, D.; Xie, J.; Wang, C.; Kohler, N.; Walsh, E.G.; Morgan, J.R.; Chin, Y.E.; Sun, S. Au-Fe_3O_4 Dumbbell Nanoparticles as Dual-Functional Probes. *Angew. Chem. Int. Ed.* **2008**, *47*, 173–176. [CrossRef]
59. Sotiriou, G.A.; Hirt, A.M.; Lozach, P.-Y.; Teleki, A.; Krumeich, F.; Pratsinis, S.E. Hybrid, silica-coated, Janus-like plasmonic-magnetic nanoparticles. *Chem. Mater.* **2011**, *23*, 1985–1992. [CrossRef]
60. Sánchez, A.; Paredes, K.O.; Ruiz-Cabello, J.; Martinez-Ruiz, P.; Pingarron, J.M.; Villalonga, R.; Filice, M. Hybrid Decorated Core@Shell Janus Nanoparticles as Flexible Platform for Targeted Multimodal Molecular Bioimaging of Cancer. *ACS Appl. Mater. Interfaces* **2018**, *10*, 31032–31043. [CrossRef] [PubMed]
61. Tao, G.; Bai, Z.; Chen, Y.; Yao, H.; Wu, M.; Huang, P.; Yu, L.; Zhang, J.; Dai, C.; Zhang, L. Generic synthesis and versatile applications of molecularly organic–inorganic hybrid mesoporous organosilica nanoparticles with asymmetric Janus topologies and structures. *Nano Res.* **2017**, *10*, 3790–3810. [CrossRef]
62. Xu, C.; Wang, B.; Sun, S. Dumbbell-Like Au-Fe_3O_4 Nanoparticles for Target-Specific Platin Delivery. *J. Am. Chem. Soc.* **2009**, *131*, 4216–4217. [CrossRef] [PubMed]
63. Hu, S.-H.; Chen, S.-Y.; Gao, X. Multifunctional Nanocapsules for Simultaneous Encapsulation of Hydrophilic and Hydrophobic Compounds and On-Demand Release. *ACS Nano* **2012**, *6*, 2558–2565. [CrossRef] [PubMed]
64. Wang, F.; Pauletti, G.M.; Wang, J.; Zhang, J.; Ewing, R.C.; Wang, Y.; Shi, D. Dual Surface-Functionalized Janus Nanocomposites of Polystyrene/Fe_3O_4 @SiO_2 for Simultaneous Tumor Cell Targeting and Stimulus-Induced Drug Release. *Adv. Mater.* **2013**, *25*, 3485–3489. [CrossRef]

65. Kilinc, D.; Lesniak, A.; Rashdan, S.A.; Gandhi, D.; Blasiak, A.; Fannin, P.C.; Von Kriegsheim, A.; Kolch, W.; Lee, G.U. Mechanochemical Stimulation of MCF7 Cells with Rod-Shaped Fe-Au Janus Particles Induces Cell Death Through Paradoxical Hyperactivation of ERK. *Adv. Health Mater.* **2014**, *4*, 395–404. [CrossRef] [PubMed]
66. Zhang, Q.; Zhang, L.; Li, S.; Chen, X.; Zhang, M.; Wang, T.; Li, L.; Wang, C. Designed Synthesis of Au/Fe$_3$O$_4$ @C Janus Nanoparticles for Dual-Modal Imaging and Actively Targeted Chemo-Photothermal Synergistic Therapy of Cancer Cells. *Chem. Eur. J.* **2017**, *23*, 17242–17248. [CrossRef] [PubMed]
67. Wu, Q.; Lin, Y.; Wo, F.; Yuan, Y.; Ouyang, Q.; Song, J.; Qu, J.; Yong, K.-T. Novel Magnetic-Luminescent Janus Nanoparticles for Cell Labeling and Tumor Photothermal Therapy. *Small* **2017**, *13*, 1701129. [CrossRef] [PubMed]
68. Ju, Y.; Zhang, H.; Yu, J.; Tong, S.; Tian, N.; Wang, Z.; Wang, X.; Su, X.; Chu, X.; Lin, J.; et al. An attractive multifunctional material for triple-modal imaging-guided tumor photothermal therapy. *ACS Nano* **2017**, *11*, 9239–9248. [CrossRef]
69. Ruiz, S.C.; Kagan, D.; Orozco, J.; Wang, J. Motion-driven sensing and biosensing using electrochemically propelled nanomotors. *Analyst* **2011**, *136*, 4621–4630.
70. Jurado-Sanchez, B.; Escarpa, A. Milli, micro and nanomotors: Novel analytical tools for real-world applications. *TrAC Trends Anal. Chem.* **2016**, *84*, 48–59. [CrossRef]
71. Jurado-Sánchez, B.; Escarpa, A. Janus micromotors for electrochemical sensing and biosensing applications: A review. *Electroanalysis* **2017**, *29*, 14–23. [CrossRef]
72. Jurado-Sánchez, B.; Pacheco, M.; Maria-Hormigos, R.; Escarpa, A. Perspectives on Janus micromotors: Materials and applications. *Appl. Mater. Today* **2017**, *9*, 407–418. [CrossRef]
73. Kong, L.; Guan, J.; Pumera, M. Micro- and nanorobots based sensing and biosensing. *Curr. Opin. Electrochem.* **2018**, *10*, 174–182. [CrossRef]
74. Kagan, D.; Calvo-Marzal, P.; Balasubramanian, S.; Sattayasamitsathit, S.; Manesh, K.M.; Flechsig, G.-U.; Wang, J. Chemical sensing based on catalytic nanomotors: Motion-based detection of trace silver. *J. Am. Chem. Soc.* **2009**, *131*, 12082–12083. [CrossRef] [PubMed]
75. Wu, J.; Balasubramanian, S.; Kagan, D.; Manesh, K.M.; Campuzano, S.; Wang, J. Motion-based DNA detection using catalytic nanomotors. *Nat. Commun.* **2010**, *1*, 36. [CrossRef] [PubMed]
76. Valdés-Ramírez, G.; Cinti, S.; Gao, W.; Li, J.; Palleschi, G.; Wang, J. Microengine-assisted electrochemical measurements at printable sensor strips. *Chem. Commun.* **2015**, *51*, 8668–8671.
77. Moo, J.G.S.; Pumera, M. Self-Propelled Micromotors Monitored by Particle-Electrode Impact Voltammetry. *ACS Sens.* **2016**, *1*, 949–957. [CrossRef]
78. Balasubramanian, S.; Kagan, D.; Hu, C.-M.J.; Campuzano, S.; Lobo-Castañon, M.J.; Lim, N.; Kang, D.Y.; Zimmerman, M.; Zhang, L.; Wang, J. Micromachine-Enabled Capture and Isolation of Cancer Cells in Complex Media. *Angew. Chem.* **2011**, *123*, 4247–4250. [CrossRef]
79. Campuzano, S.; Orozco, J.; Kagan, D.; Guix, M.; Gao, W.; Sattayasamitsathit, S.; Claussen, J.C.; Merkoçi, A.; Wang, J. Bacterial isolation by lectin-modified microengines. *Nano Lett.* **2012**, *12*, 396–401. [CrossRef] [PubMed]
80. Kagan, D.; Campuzano, S.; Balasubramanian, S.; Kuralay, F.; Flechsig, G.-U.; Wang, J.; Ruiz, S.C. Functionalized Micromachines for Selective and Rapid Isolation of Nucleic Acid Targets from Complex Samples. *Nano Lett.* **2011**, *11*, 2083–2087. [CrossRef]
81. Orozco, J.; Campuzano, S.; Kagan, D.; Zhou, M.; Gao, W.; Wang, J.; Ruiz, S.C. Dynamic Isolation and Unloading of Target Proteins by Aptamer-Modified Microtransporters. *Anal. Chem.* **2011**, *83*, 7962–7969. [CrossRef]
82. Jurado-Sánchez, B.; Pacheco, M.; Rojo, J.; Escarpa, A.; Jurado-Sánchez, B.; Jurado-Sánchez, B. Magnetocatalytic Graphene Quantum Dots Janus Micromotors for Bacterial Endotoxin Detection. *Angew. Chem. Int. Ed.* **2017**, *56*, 6957–6961. [CrossRef]
83. Pacheco, M.; Escarpa, A.; Sánchez, B.J. Sensitive Monitoring of Enterobacterial Contamination of Food Using Self-Propelled Janus Microsensors. *Anal. Chem.* **2018**, *90*, 2912–2917. [CrossRef] [PubMed]

84. Esteban-Fernández de Ávila, B.; Zhao, M.; Campuzano, S.; Ricci, F.; Pingarrón, J.M.; Mascini, M.; Wang, J. Rapid micromotor-based naked-eye immunoassay. *Talanta* **2017**, *167*, 651–657. [CrossRef] [PubMed]
85. Gao, W.; Feng, X.; Pei, A.; Gu, Y.; Li, J.; Wang, J. Seawater-driven magnesium based Janus micromotors for environmental remediation. *Nanoscale* **2013**, *5*, 4696–4700. [CrossRef] [PubMed]

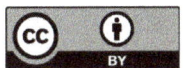 © 2019 by the authors. Licensee MDPI, Basel, Switzerland. This article is an open access article distributed under the terms and conditions of the Creative Commons Attribution (CC BY) license (http://creativecommons.org/licenses/by/4.0/).

MDPI
St. Alban-Anlage 66
4052 Basel
Switzerland
Tel. +41 61 683 77 34
Fax +41 61 302 89 18
www.mdpi.com

Magnetochemistry Editorial Office
E-mail: magnetochemistry@mdpi.com
www.mdpi.com/journal/magnetochemistry

www.ingramcontent.com/pod-product-compliance
Lightning Source LLC
LaVergne TN
LVHW071936080526
838202LV00064B/6615